FOURTH EDITION

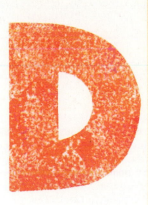

Drugs and Society

Glen Hanson
Department of Pharmacology and Toxicology
University of Utah
Salt Lake City, Utah

Peter J. Venturelli
Department of Sociology
Valparaiso University
Valparaiso, Indiana

Jones and Bartlett Publishers
Boston London

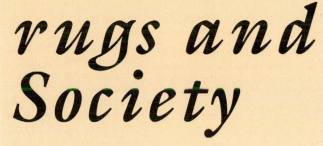

Editorial, Sales, and Customer Service Offices
Jones and Bartlett Publishers
One Exeter Plaza
Boston, MA 02116
617-859-3900
800-832-0034

Jones and Bartlett Publishers International
7 Melrose Terrace
London W6 7RL
England

Library of Congress Cataloging-in-Publication Data

Hanson, Glen, (Glen R.)
Drugs and society / Glen Hanson, Peter Venturelli.—4th ed.
p. cm.
Includes bibliographical references and index.
ISBN 0-86720-830-9
1. Drugs 2. Drugs—Toxicology. 3. Drug abuse.
I. Venturelli, Peter J., 1949- II. Title.
RM301.W58 1995
615'.1—dc20 94-46298
CIP

Acquisitions Editor: Joseph E. Burns
Developmental Editor: B. Czar Productions, Inc.
Assistant Production Manager/Coordination: Judy Songdahl
Manufacturing Buyer: Dana L. Cerrito
Photo Researcher: Kristi Dailey
Design: Melinda Grosser for *silk*
Editorial Production Service: The Book Company
Typesetting and Color Separation: Pre-Press Company, Inc.
Cover Design: Marshall Henrichs
Cover Printing: John P. Pow Company
Printing and Binding: Rand McNally

Cover photograph: © James Blank/Stock, Boston

Printed in the United States of America
99 98 97 96 95 10 9 8 7 6 5 4 3 2 1

Photo Credits

p 2: © Eric Nelson/Custom Medical Stock Photo; p. 19: © Rob Nelson/Stock, Boston; p 32: James C. Smalley/The Picture Cube; p 62: Reuters/Bettmann; p 69: Leonard McCombe/Life Magazine © Time Inc.; p 100: Barry Bomzer/Tony Stone Images; p 111: © Science Photo Library/Custom Medical Stock Photo; p 113: John Griffin/The Image Works, Inc.; p 128: UPI/Bettmann Newsphotos; p 148: UPI/Bettmann; p 152: Bruce Ayres/Tony Stone Images; p 157: Rodger Kingston/The Picture Cube; p 169: Michael Siluk/The Image Works, Inc.; p 174: D&I MacDonald/The Picture Cube; p 187: left, © M. Huberland/Photo Researchers; right, © Martin M. Rotker, Science Source/Photo Researchers; p 189: Courtesy of Kenneth Lyons Jones, MD; p 192: John Coletti/The Picture Cube; p 209: © Will and Deni McIntyre/Photo Researchers; p 232: Gary Wagner/Stock, Boston; p 235: Rick Strange/The Picture Cube; p 243: Jonathan L. Barkan/The Picture Cube; p 246: Reuters/Bettmann; p 248: NIDA Notes, Volume 7, Number 4. Courtesy of National Institute on Drug Abuse; p 258: Ebsin-Anderson/The Image Works, Inc.; p 271: Photo by Jeremy Bigwood. Courtesy of the Fitz Hugh Ludlow Memorial Library, San Francisco; p 272: Courtesy of the Drug Enforcement Administration, Washington, DC; p 273: Bettmann; p 274: © 1991 Time Inc. Reprinted by permission; p 277: Courtesy of the Drug Enforcement Administration, Washington, DC; p 279: Reuters/Bettmann; p 288: Carlos Goldin/D. Donne Bryant Stock; p 298: Beringer, Dratch/The Picture Cube; p 310: Michael Edrington/The Image Works, Inc.; p 312: George Goodwin/The Picture Cube; p 321, Courtesy Ciby-Greigy Corp.; p 330: Arnold J. Kaplan, APSA-AFIAP/The Picture Cube; p 334: Bettmann; p 342: Courtesy of the Drug Enforcement Administration, Washington, DC; p 343: Courtesy of Dr. Glen Hanson; p 346: Courtesy of the Drug Enforcement Administration, Washington, DC; p 348: Courtesy of the Drug Enforcement Administration, Washington, DC; p 358: Courtesy of W.R. Spence, MD, Editor: Giles Bateman, © 1991 HEALTH EDCO ®, a division of WRS Group, Inc., Waco TX, 76702-1207; p 364: Cindy Loo/The Picture Cube; p 368: Photos courtesy of the Drug Enforcement Administration, Washington, DC; p 379: Mark M. Walker/The Picture Cube; p 401: © L. Steinmark/Custom Medical Stock Photo; p 408: Kindra Clineff/The Picture Cube; p 409: © Custom Medical Stock Photo p 418: Science Photo Library/Custom Medical Stock Photo; p 426: John Coletti/The Picture Cube; p 429: Jeff Greenberg/dMRp/The Picture Cube; p 434: Reuters/Bettmann; p 438: UPI/Bettmann; p 447: Reuters/Bettmann; p 450: Reuters/Bettmann; p 455: Reuters/Bettmann; p 464: © Blair Seitz, Science Source/Photo Researchers; p 472: © Richard Hutchings/Photo Researchers; p 490: Marty Heitner/The Picture Cube; p 497: © Keith/Custom Medical Stock Photo

BRIEF CONTENTS

CONTENTS

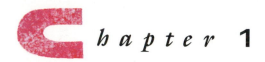

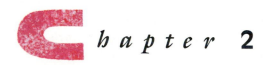

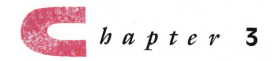

Chapter 4

Chapter 5

Chapter 6

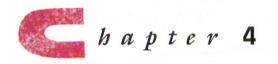

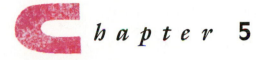

Chapter 7

Chapter 8

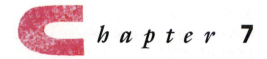

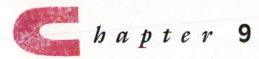

Chapter 12

Hallucinogens 330

Chapter 13

Marijuana 364

Chapter 14

Drugs and Therapy 390

Chapter 15

Drug Abuse Among Special Populations 426

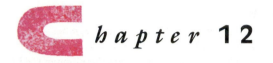

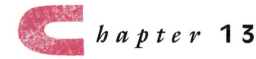

PREFACE

The fourth edition of *Drugs and Society* is a much improved text intended to help university students from a wide range of disciplines gain a fundamental understanding of drug-related problems in our society. We have included the most current views on drug abuse in an objective and easily understood fashion. The intent of the authors is to help students learn to apply basic understanding gained from the study of this text to their personal and professional lives in order to make informed and responsible choices with regard to drugs and drug-abuse problems. This new edition has been critically reviewed by those who teach drug-abuse courses, such as sociologists, social workers, health educators and by many experts in the drug-abuse field. The text has been revised according to their insightful chapter-by-chapter recommendations.

Features and Benefits

The fourth edition includes the most up-to-date information on the pharmacological, sociological, and psychological perspectives of commonly abused drugs. In response to reviewers' recommendations several features have been added and organized in an interesting and provocative manner to help students assimilate the material. The new features include:

- **Case in Point** Examples of relevant clinical issues relating to each major group of drugs discussed.
- **Here and Now** Current events that illustrate the personal and social consequences of drug abuse issues.
- **Cross Currents** Controversial topics presented in a debate format to encourage critical thinking by the student on important drug abuse concerns of the day.
- **Healthy People 2000** These national health objectives are integrated into each chapter to help students understand the role of national governmental policy in dealing with drug abuse problems.

Each chapter also includes improved learning aids for students. These aids help students understand new terminology and concepts as well as encourage students to think about the application of the information in practical settings. Throughout the book the readers will find many real-life examples of drug effects or drug principles to help them appreciate the relevance of the concepts presented. The learning aids found in each chapter are:

- **Highlighted definitions** New terminology is defined throughout the chapters as well as in a complete glossary at the end of the book.
- **"Learning Objectives"** These lists are included in each chapter and identify major concepts to be taught.
- **Summary statements** These concise summaries are found at the end of each chapter and correlate with the learning objectives mentioned above.
- **"Did You Know" sections** Interesting facts are presented at the beginning of each chapter and discussed in the text.
- **Chapter questions** Provocative questions are listed in each of the chapters to encourage students to discuss, ponder, and critically analyze their own feelings and biases about the information presented in the book.
- **Concise and well-organized tables and figures** These updated features are found throughout the book in order to present the latest information to students in an easily understood format.
- **New color photographs and drawings** These additions help to graphically illustrate important concepts and facilitate comprehension as well as retention of information.

Because of these new and updated features, we believe that this edition of *Drugs and Society* is much more "user friendly" than previous editions and will substantially enhance student learning and interest.

New and Improved Topical Coverage

The new topical coverage includes:

- **Extensive, updated material and references** Approximately 50% of the citations in this edition are 1992 or later references. These sources of the most current drug information available are listed after each chapter to assist students who want to pursue topics introduced in the text.
- **A new chapter and a thoroughly revised chapter on alcohol** Chapters 7 and 8 are devoted to the most current and important issues and topics related to alcohol use and abuse.
- **A new chapter on special populations** The new Chapter 15 delves into the special drug-abuse problems of adolescents, females, athletes, and victims of AIDS.
- **A new chapter on drugs and therapy** Chapter 14 includes a revised section on nonprescription medication as well as a new section on the most commonly used prescription drugs. The objective of this important chapter is to help students appreciate how all types of drugs should be used properly.
- **DSM IV** The recent publication of the fourth edition of the *Diagnostic and Statistical Manual (1994) of Mental Disorders* (DSM IV) includes major sections on the problems of substance abuse in general and each of the major drugs of abuse in particular. This widely acclaimed manual published by the American Psychiatric Association is considered by most health professionals to be the most authoritative work on the diagnosis of drug dependence, intoxication, and drug-induced psychiatric disorders. Our text integrates DSM IV criteria and insights throughout its chapters to help readers better understand the causes and consequences of substance abuse, making it an authoritative text for instructing students about drug abuse issues.

These extensive topical revisions have made the fourth edition of *Drugs and Society* an exceptional text on drug abuse and an excellent reference for a wide spectrum of college and university classes dealing with drug abuse problems and issues. Thus, students in nursing, physical education and other health sciences, psychology, social work, and sociology will find that our text provides useful current information and perspectives to help them understand the following aspects of drug abuse: (1) why and how drug abuse occurs; (2) the results of drug abuse; (3) how to prevent drug abuse; and (4) how drugs can be effectively used.

Topical Sequence

The material in the text encompasses both biomedical and social-psychological views. *Drugs and Society* begins in chapter 1 by distinguishing between drug use and abuse and examining how and why people use and abuse drugs. In this chapter, basic drug-related terminology is introduced and the overall historical and current patterns of drug abuse in the U.S. are presented. Chapter 2 presents and evaluates the major theories that explain why people misuse drugs: these include sociological, psychological and biological explanations and the significance of the association between mental disorders and drug abuse. Chapter 3 reviews the historical evolution of drug use and regulation so that students can appreciate how and why drugs are classified and controlled today. Such knowledge helps students to understand the differences between drug use, misuse and abuse and their consequences. Chapter 4 instructs students about the factors that determine how drugs affect the body. This chapter details the physiological and psychological variables that determine how and why people respond to drugs used for therapeutic and recreational purposes. Because the addicting properties of most, if not all, substances of abuse are due to the effects of drugs on the reward centers of the brain, chapter 5 helps the student understand the basic biochemical operations of the nervous and endocrine systems and explains how psychoactive drugs and anabolic steroids alter such functions.

Chapters 6 through 13 deal with specific drug groups that are commonly abused in this country. Those drugs which depress brain activity are discussed in chapters 6 (sedative/hypnotic agents), 7 and 8 (alcohol), and 9 (narcotics). The drugs which stimulate brain activity are covered in chapters 10 (amphetamines, cocaine, and caffeine) and 11 (tobacco and nicotine). The last main category of substances of abuse is the hallucinogens. Such drugs alter the senses and create dreamlike and/or distorted experiences. These substances are discussed in chapters 12 (hallucinogens such as LSD, mescaline, and PCP) and 13 (marijuana). Although most drugs that are abused cause more than one effect (for example, cocaine can be a stimulant and a hallucinogen), the classification we have chosen for this text is frequently used by experts and pharmacologists in the drug abuse field and is based on the drug effect that is most likely to predominate following abuse. All of the chapters in this section are similarly organized. They discuss the historical origins and evolution of the agents so students can better understand society's attitudes toward, and regulation of, these drugs. Previous and current clinical uses of these drugs are discussed to help students appreciate distinctions between therapeutic use and abuse. Next, the patterns of abuse of these substances and special features which contribute to their abuse potential are discussed. Finally, nonmedicinal and medicinal therapies for drug-related dependence, withdrawal, and abstinence are presented.

Chapter 14 explores the topic of drugs and therapy. As with illicit drugs of abuse, nonprescription and prescription drugs can be misused if not understood. This chapter helps the student to appreciate the uses and benefits of proper drug use as well as appreciate that legal drugs can also be problematic.

Chapter 15 helps the student to recognize that substance abuse and its consequences are dependent on the psychosocial identity and biological makeup of those who become addicted to these substances. This new chapter examines adolescents, women, athletes, and AIDS victims—groups that present special drug abuse problems in terms of identification, prevention and treatment.

Chapter 16 of *Drugs and Society* acquaints students with the treatment, rehabilitation, and prevention of the major drugs of abuse. This final chapter describes the principal sociological, psychological and pharmacological strategies used to treat and prevent substance abuse and details their advantages and disadvantages. The discussion in this chapter helps students to better understand why drug abuse occurs, how society currently deals with this problem on an individual and group basis, and the likelihood of rehabilitation of persons dependent on these substances.

Authors' Perspective

Due to the pervasive nature of drug abuse in our society, this text integrates material from the authors who represent distinct but essential perspectives of this problem. Dr. Hanson and Professor Venturelli are respected experts in their fields. They have taught thousands of students in drug-related classes at their universities, are actively involved in drug-abuse research, and represent the disciplines of sociology, psychology and pharmacology. The authors have served on editorial boards of pharmacological textbooks and journals, published many articles on drug-abuse topics in national and international journals, have been members of national and local committees that deal with drug-abuse problems, and have served as consultants to law enforcement agencies for abuse-related issues.

Instructor's Aids

For instructors adopting this fourth edition for classroom use, a revised instructor's manual containing over 1,000 test questions is available. In addition, a computerized test bank, written and supervised exclusively by Venturelli and Hanson, and 30 overhead acetate transparency masters are also available to the instructors. A video library is available to qualified institutions. Please call the marketing department at Jones and Bartlett for further details.

Acknowledgements

The numerous improvements that have made this edition could not have occurred without the hard work and dedication of numerous people.

First, we gratefully acknowledge the efforts of Joseph Burns, vice-president at Jones and Bartlett Publishers, for his professional direction throughout the revision process. His ability to identify the best developmental specialists in textbook publishing was essential. Also at Jones and Bartlett, the production specialists, Judy Songdahl and Paula

Carroll, are to be congratulated for their invaluable assistance and expertise. Likewise, we thank Amina Sharma at Jones and Bartlett for her ability to maintain communication between the authors and the many experts critiquing the latest edition.

Other individuals include Maxine Effenson Chuck, an editor who provided invaluable suggestions and encouragement with an endless flow of queries and rewrites.

We are indebted to the many reviewers who evaluated the manuscript at different stages of development. Large sections of the manuscript were reviewed and greatly improved by the comments of:

Charles Arokiasamy, Louisiana State University
Eileen Clifford, North Hennepin Community College
Lynne Durrant, University of Utah/Salt Lake City
Kathy Elliott, University of Southwestern Louisiana
Georgia Lynn Keeney, University of Minnesota/Duluth
William London, Kent State University
Beverly Mahoney, Pennsylvania State University
Linda Marshall, Mankato State University
Kerry Redican, Virginia Polytechnic and State University
Thomas Rowe, University of Wisconsin/Stevens Point

We are also deeply grateful to the following individuals who provided thoughtful criticism that improved the topical coverage and pedagogy for this new edition: Marvin Feit, The University of Akron; Melissa Fleming, Northern Essex Community College; Mark Freeman, Rollins College; Karl Herrmann, Lock Haven University; Barry Hunt, Northwestern State University of Louisiana; Nancy Li, Tyler Junior College; Jim Matney, Wichita State University; Mark Minelli, Central Michigan University; Richard Morales, Rochester Institute of Technology; James Pahz, Central Michigan University; Margarete Parrish, Rutgers University; George Poole, Pepperdine University; Sallye Raymond, University of New Orleans; J. C. Rodriguez, University of North Florida; Adam Rok, Northeast Wisconsin Technical College; Alex Rubins, Cuyahoga Community College; Jeffrey Schaler, American University; Martin Turnauer, Radford University; S. Marie Walter, College of St. Catherine; Noah Young, Pepperdine University; and Paul Young, Houghton College.

The authors would like to acknowledge the comments and suggestions of those users of previous editions of *Drugs and Society* who responded to our book evaluation surveys.

Other scholars with expertise in social work are gratefully acknowledged for their careful reviews and criticisms of our manuscript: Keith Kilty at Ohio State University (Chapter 16); Bryan Y. Byers, a friend and colleague at Valparaiso University (Chapter 2); and sociologists David J. Pittman at Washington University and David R. Rudy at Morehead State University (Chapter 8).

At our respective institutions the authors wish to thank a multitude of people too numerous to list individually but who have given us invaluable assistance for meeting publication deadlines.

At Valparaiso University, Professor Venturelli's secretary, Lynn Shimala, and students Leah Piepkorn and Nicole Doctor (Chapter 16) top the list. We also thank Leah's conscientious efforts as a permissions editor. At the University of Utah, we thank the secretarial staff for their support and flawless transcriptions.

Last, and most of all, Dr. Hanson especially thanks his wife, Margaret, for her patience and encouragement. Professor Venturelli appreciates the patience of his students while he tried to meet publication deadlines throughout the revision process.

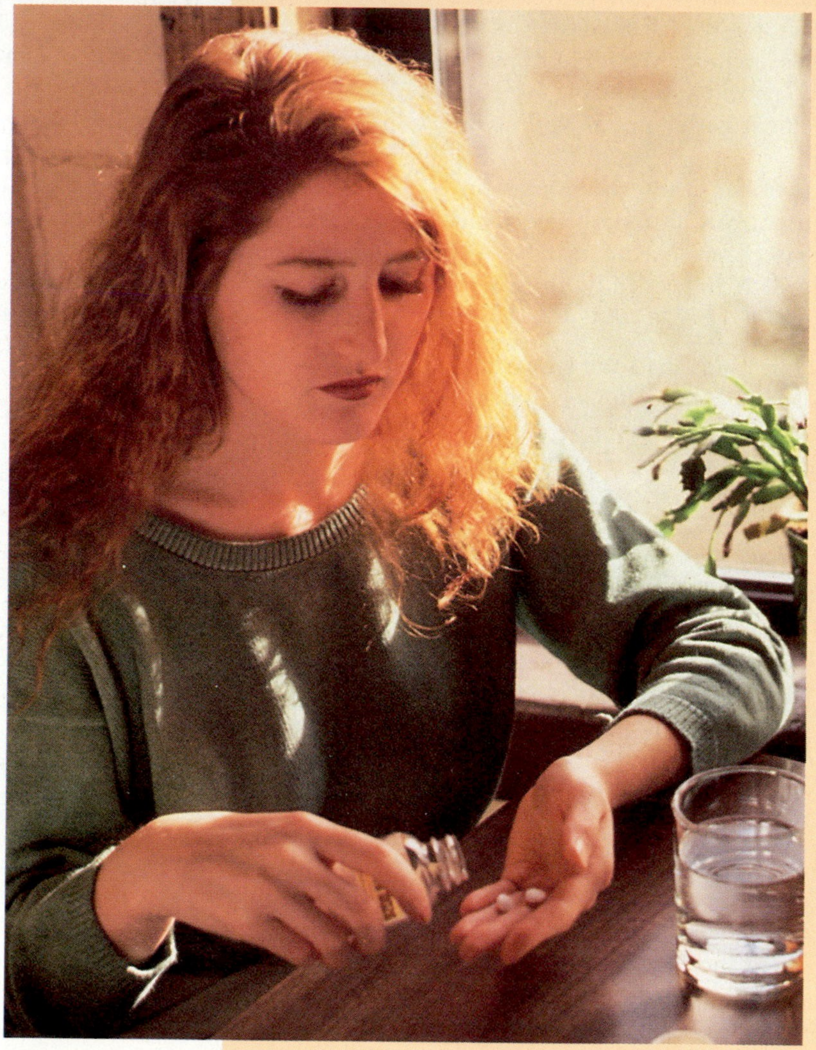

Chapter 1

DID YOU KNOW THAT . . .

- Drug abuse has the ability to destroy our society.
- Designer drugs are created for profit and were created as a method for circumventing the laws that make certain substances illegal.
- People in the 18- to 25-year-old age group are by far the heaviest users of, and experimenters with, both licit and illicit drugs.
- Approximately 1.5 billion prescriptions for psychoactive drugs are written each year.
- The majority of young drug abusers come from homes in which drugs are used extensively.
- The alcohol industry alone spends more than $1 billion on yearly advertising.
- The majority of illicit drug users are employed.
- In comparison to nonusers, drug users are nearly twice as likely to have quit their jobs or to have been fired.
- Drug addiction is an "equal opportunity" affliction, found in all races, religions, social classes, and age groups.
- Despite the media influences, illicit drug use has been steadily declining since 1981.
- For college students, illicit drug use has been declining steadily since 1980.

An Introduction to Drug Use

LEARNING OBJECTIVES

On completing this chapter, you will be able to

1. Give two reasons why it is important to understand drug use and abuse in today's world.
2. Explain how drug use is affected by pharmacological, cultural, social, and contextual factors.
3. Explain when drugs were first used and under what circumstances.
4. Describe the role mass media play in promoting drug use.
5. Indicate how widespread drug use is and who the potential drug abusers are.
6. Explain when drug use leads to drug abuse.
7. Name the three types of drug users, and explain how they differ.
8. Name the four different uses of drugs.
9. Explain what gender differences exist in the use of drugs.

continued

Healthy People 2000

Eliminate or severely restrict all forms of tobacco product advertising and promotion to which youth younger than age 18 are likely to be exposed.

Extend adoption of alcohol and drug policies for the work environment to at least 60% of worksites with 50 or more employees.

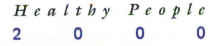

LEARNING OBJECTIVES

10 Rank in descending order from highest to lowest the most commonly used drugs.
11 Characterize the employment status of most illicit drug users.
12 Explain how positive wellness and holistic health relate to current drug use problems.
13 Define the following terms: *drug(s)*, *"gateway drugs," medicine, prescription medicines, over-the-counter drugs (OTCs), drug misuse, drug abuse,* and *drug addiction.*

This fourth edition of *Drugs and Society* is particularly strengthened by the varied expertise of its authors, who specialize in pharmacology and toxicology, social psychology, and sociology, with social work and health perspectives. The book is enhanced by the information and approaches of these varied fields of expertise, and by the study of drug use from multi- and cross-disciplinary perspectives.

This chapter introduces the following four major subject areas of the general topic, drugs and society. The first section looks at the dimensions of drug use and drug abuse, and emphasizes the most commonly abused illicit drugs. The second section gives an overview of drugs in society—extent and frequency of use, statistics and trends, and how the mass media influence our use of drugs. The third section focuses on the topic of how people are attracted to drug use. This section explores when use leads to abuse, who becomes a user, and how widespread drug abuse is. The fourth section discusses the new holistic approach to drug use and emphasizes the underlying theme of this book, that promoting drug use knowledge strengthens out own awareness of drug use and increases our ability to help others who may have problems with drugs.

Although drug use dates back thousands of years, the use and abuse of drugs are today more prevalent and widespread throughout the world than ever before. Understanding how drugs are used and often abused is important for two reasons. First, drug abuse is both a national and an international crisis. Second, there is a danger that the conditions surrounding abuse can harm many customary and traditional values and attitudes responsible for holding society together. When drug use becomes widespread in neighborhoods and communities, the stability of the social order becomes undermined by unpredictability, mistrust, suspicion, doubt, and confusion.

The Dimensions of Drug Abuse

Generally speaking, any substance that modifies the nervous system and states of consciousness is a **drug**. Such modification can enhance, inhibit, or distort the functioning of the body, thus also affecting patterns of behavior and social functioning. Individual drug use produces a complex ripple of effects that this book describes in terms of pharmacological, behavioral, cultural, and social factors. We examine pharmacological factors in terms of how the ingredients of a particular drug affect the functions of the body and how the nervous system reacts to the drugs by affecting social behavior. Behavioral changes in response to drug use occur in social and cultural contexts that involve a society's views about drug use, its historical conventions and traditions. Social factors that affect drug use develop through the values and attitudes of drug-using communities, subcultures, peers, and families, as well as through the extent and quality of users' experiences with personal and social use of drugs. Examining these aspects of drug use leads us

Self-Check

Drug Quiz

A test of what people knew about illicit drugs and their effects would have been a brief exercise a decade ago. Now the list of questions is uncomfortably long, the answers more disturbing than ever. How much do you know?

1. Name the major drug problem among teenagers today.
2. How fast can a child become an alcoholic?
3. Why are grade-school children drawn to wine coolers?
4. Are some drugs gateways that may lead to further substance abuse?
5. How does today's marijuana compare with the marijuana of a generation ago?
6. Does the use of marijuana cause damage to the brain?
7. Do marijuana and cigarettes inflict about the same lung damage?
8. How did "crack" get its name?
9. How long does alcohol stay in the bloodstream after a round of heavy drinking?
10. How long do traces of marijuana remain in the body after it has been smoked?
11. What does "crack" look like?
12. What is "crank"?
13. How long does a "crack" high last?
14. How does marijuana affect mood?
15. How many children ages 12 to 17 say they have tried hallucinogens like LSD, PCP, peyote, or mescaline at least once?
16. Can geneticists figure out which people are most likely to become addicts?
17. What is the price of a single dose of "crack"?
18. Blotter paper is associated with which drug?
19. Which drug temporarily gives its user abnormal physical strength?
20. What is "Ecstasy"?

Answers on next page.

Source: V. Sussman, "How to Beat Drugs." *U.S. News and World Report* (11 September 1989): 69–72.

to explore the sociology and psychology of drug use. Finally, we will be considering the particular circumstances under which drugs are used for diminishing physical pain, curing illness, providing relaxation, relieving stress or anxiety, heightening awareness, providing visual, auditory or sensory distortion, or bolstering confidence. Contexts that define personal dispositions toward drug use as well as the social and physical surroundings in which drugs are used: whether drugs are taken out of doors, in private homes, or at rock concert settings.

Although the common term for substances that affect both mind and body functioning is popularly called a *drug*, researchers use the term **psychoactive drugs** or *psychoactive substances* because these are more precise in explaining how drugs affect the body. The term *psychoactive drugs* refers to the effect these substances have on the central nervous system and how these drugs alter consciousness or perceptions. Because of their effects on the brain, these drugs can be used to treat physical or mental illness. However, because the body can tolerate increasingly large doses, many psychoactive drugs may be used in

DRUG any substance that modifies the nervous system and states of consciousness

PSYCHOACTIVE DRUGS or **PSYCHOACTIVE SUBSTANCES** substances that affect the central nervous system and alter consciousness or perceptions

Self-Check

Drug Quiz Answers

1. Alcohol
2. As quickly as six months. An early start on drinking and an immature brain and body make youngsters vulnerable.
3. Because they look and taste much like soda. (Girls especially like them because they don't look or taste like beer.) But wine coolers average 6% alcohol content, compared with 4% for beer and 10% to 14% for wine. Wine typically is served in smaller amounts, so a 12-ounce cooler delivers more alcohol than a glass of wine.
4. Yes. Researchers say it is rare to find abusers of cocaine, heroin, or virtually any addictive drug who did not start with some combination of alcohol, tobacco, and marijuana.
5. It is much more potent. The National Institute on Drug Abuse reports that the amount of THC, the active ingredient in marijuana, averaged 1% by weight in 1970. Today's dope averages 3% to 3.5%. Sinsemilla, an increasingly popular type of marijuana, averages 6.5% THC and may contain as much as 10% to 15%.
6. Animal studies demonstrate that ingesting the daily equivalent of a joint or two for several years destroys brain cells.
7. Researchers say one to three joints daily produces lung damage and cancer risks comparable with smoking five times as many cigarettes.
8. From the crackling made by the crystals of cocaine when smoked.
9. Alcohol leaves the body in 24 hours or less.
10. Traces of THC show up in the urine 10 to 35 days after marijuana is smoked.
11. Soaplike shavings or broken chalk.
12. It is the street term for *methamphetamine*, a class of stimulants also called "speed."
13. Six to eight minutes.
14. Whatever a person's conscious or unconscious emotional state, marijuana magnifies it. After the initial effect, however, it acts as a depressant.
15. According to a federally sponsored 1988 National Household Survey on Drug Abuse, 704,000 youngsters have tried hallucinogens at least once.
16. No method can reliably predict who will become chemically dependent.
17. Generally $2 to $5 in major urban centers but $25 and up in smaller cities, depending on supply and demand.
18. "Acid," or LSD.
19. Known as "angel dust," PCP has pain-killing properties that make users extraordinarily difficult to restrain physically.
20. Also known as XTC or "Adam" (from its chemical acronym MDMA), "Ecstasy" is a hallucinogen currently popular with college students. It appears to cause brain damage.

Source: V. Sussman, "How to Beat Drugs." *U.S. News and World Report* (11 September 1989): 69–72.

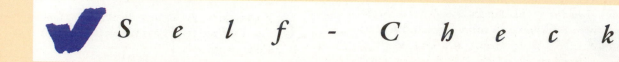

progressively greater and more uncontrollable amounts. For many substances, a user is at risk of moving from occasional to more regular use, and from moderate use to heavy and chronic use. A chronic user may then risk addiction and withdrawal symptoms whenever the drug is not supplied to the body.

Psychoactive drugs are classified as either **licit** (legal) or **illicit** (illegal). Coffee, tea, cocoa, alcohol, tobacco, and over-the-counter (OTC) drugs are licit, or legal substances, and, when used in moderation, are usually socially acceptable. Marijuana, cocaine, and LSD are examples of illicit drugs.

Researchers have made some interesting findings regarding legal and illegal drug use:

1. The use of such legal substances as alcoholic beverages and tobacco is considerably more common than is the use of illegal drugs such as marijuana, heroin, and LSD. Other legal drugs such as depressants and stimulants, though less popular than alcohol and tobacco, are still more widely used than the illegal heroin and LSD.
2. The popular use of legal drugs, particularly alcohol and tobacco, has caused far more deaths, sickness, violent crimes, economic loss, and other social problems than the use of illegal drugs.
3. Societal reaction to various drugs changes with time and place. Opium is today an illegal drug and widely condemned as a *panopathogen* (a cause of all ills), but in the last two centuries it was a legal drug and popularly praised as a *panacea* (a cure of all ills). Alcohol use was widespread in the United States in the early 1800s, became illegal by the 1920s, and then was relegalized and has been widely used again since the 1930s. In contrast, cigarette smoking is legal in all countries today, but in the seventeenth century it was illegal in most countries and the smoker was harshly punished in some. For example, the penalty for cigarette smoking was having the nose cut off in Russia, lips sliced off in Hindustan (India), and head chopped off in China (Thio 1983, 332–333).

Today, new emphasis in the United States on public health hazards from cigarettes are again leading some people to consider new measures to restrict or even outlaw tobacco smoking.

Most Commonly Abused Illicit Drugs

This book examines the drugs most subject to abuse—those that are taken for pleasure or relief from boredom or stress:

1. *Narcotics*—opium, morphine, codeine, and heroin
2. *Depressants, such as sedatives and hypnotics*—barbiturates, benzodiazepines (such as Valium), methaqualone (Quaalude), and alcohol
3. *Stimulants*—cocaine (and crack), amphetamines, and caffeine as well as coffee, tea, and tobacco
4. *Hallucinogens*— LSD (lysergic acid diethylamide), mescaline, and peyote
5. *Cannabis*—marijuana and hashish
6. *Organic solvents*—inhalants such as gasoline, airplane glue, and paint thinner, as well as certain foods, herbs, and vitamins

Appendix 1-1 (at the end of this chapter) lists the most commonly abused drugs in society, outlining their medical uses, trade names, slang terms, physical or psychological dependence, tolerance, duration, usual methods of administration, possible effects, effects of overdose, and withdrawal syndromes. The Here and Now box on page 10 shows some current "street terms" for the substances and processes involved in illicit use of these drugs.

Designer Drugs In addition to these traditional categories for abused illicit drugs, innovations in technology have produced new categories known as **"designer" drugs.** These are relatively recent types that are created as **structural analogs**

LICIT DRUGS legal drugs, such as coffee, alcohol, and tobacco

ILLICIT DRUGS illegal drugs, such as marijuana, cocaine, and LSD. Other commonly used terminology for drug use is highlighted in the Here and Now box.

DESIGNER DRUGS new categories of hybrid drugs

STRUCTURAL ANALOGS drugs that result from altered chemical structures of already illicit drugs. These drugs are produced for profit and mimic current effects of controlled substances

Here and Now

Commonly Used Terms

Here are some of the most important definitions used for understanding drug use and/or abuse.

Gateway drugs	The word **gateway** suggests a path leading to something else. Alcohol, tobacco, and marijuana are the most commonly used drugs. Almost all abusers of more powerfully addictive drugs have first experimented with these three substances.
Medicines	Medicines are used to prevent or treat the symptoms of an illness. Medicines are drugs prescribed by a physician.
Prescription medicines	These are drugs prescribed by a physician. Common examples include drugs prescribed to eliminate drowsiness, stimulation, or relaxation.
Over-the-counter (OTC) drugs	These are drugs sold without a prescription. Recently OTC drugs accounted for "$12 billion a year in retail sales" (Goode 1993, 36). OTC drugs can be purchased at will, without first seeking medical advice. Often these drugs are misused or abused.
Drug misuse	The unintentional or inappropriate use of prescribed or OTC drugs. Misuse includes, but is not limited to (1) taking more drugs than prescribed, (2) using OTC or psychoactive drugs in excess without medical supervision, (3) mixing drugs with alcohol, (4) using old medicines for self-treating new symptoms of an illness or ailment, (5) discontinuing certain prescribed drugs at will and/or against a physician's recommendation, and (6) administering prescription drugs to family members without medical consultation and supervision.
Drug abuse	Also known as *chemical* or *substance abuse*. The willful misuse of either licit or illicit drugs for recreation, perceived necessity, or convenience. Drug abuse differs from drug use in that drug *use* is taking or using drugs, while *abuse* is a more intense misuse of drugs, often to the point of addiction.
Drug addiction	Drug addiction involves noncasual or nonrecreational drug use. A frequent symptom includes intense psychological preoccupation with obtaining and consuming drugs. Both physiological and psychological symptoms of withdrawal are often manifested when the craving for the drug is not satisfied. Recently more emphasis has been placed on defining the psychological craving for drug use than on the more biologically based determinants of addiction. (See Chapter 16 for more precise information regarding addiction and the addiction process.)

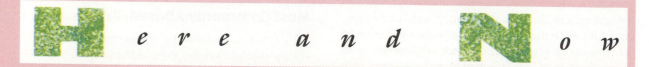

of substances already scheduled (forbidden) under the Controlled Substances Act (CSA). The term *structural analogs* refers to drugs that result from altered chemical structures of already existing illicit drugs (see Chapter 3, "Drugs, Regulations, and the Law"). Generally, these drugs are prepared by underground chemists, whose goal for profit is to mimic the psychoactive effects of controlled substances. The number of designer drugs that are created and sold illegally is very large. Anyone with knowledge of college-level chemistry can alter the chemical ingredients and produce new designer-type drugs although it may be nearly impossible to predict their properties or effects except by trial and error. Currently, there are three major types of synthetic analog drugs available through the illicit drug market: analogs of phencyclidine (PCP), analogs of fentanyl and meperidine (both synthetic narcotic analgesics), such as Demerol, MPPP, (called MPTP), PEPAP, and analogs of amphetamine and methamphetamine (which have stimulant and hallucinogenic properties) such as **MDMA**, known as "Ecstasy" or "Adam," which is widely used on college campuses as a euphoriant and, to some extent, by clinicians as an adjunct to psychotherapy (National Institute on Drug Abuse [NIDA] 1986). The arrival of these high-technology psychoactive substances is a sign of the new high levels of risk and unpredictable outcome faced by drug users in the 1990s and beyond. As the pace of such risks in substance use increases, the need for a broader, more well-informed view of drug use becomes even more important than in the past.

An Overview of Drugs in Society

Many people think that problems with drugs are unique to this era. However, drug use and abuse has always been part of human society. For example, the Grecian oracles of Delphi used drugs, Homer's Cup of Helen induced sleep and provided freedom from care, and the mandrake root mentioned in Genesis supplied hallucinogenic belladonna compound. In Genesis 30:14–16, the mandrake is mentioned in association with love making:

> In the time of wheat harvest Reuben went out and found some mandrakes in the open country and brought them to his mother Leah. Then Rachel asked Leah for some of her son's mandrakes, but Leah said, "Is it so small a thing to have taken away my husband, that you should take my son's mandrakes as well?" But Rachel said, "Very well, let him sleep with you tonight in exchange for your son's mandrakes." So when Jacob came in from the country in the evening, Leah went out to meet him and said, "You are to sleep with me tonight; I have hired you with my son's mandrakes." That night he slept with her.

Ancient literature is filled with references to the use of mushrooms, datura, hemp, marijuana, opium poppies, and so on. Under the influence of some of these drugs, many people experienced extreme ecstasy or sheer terror. Some old pictures of demons and devils look very much like those described by modern drug users during so-called bummers, or bad trips. The belief that witches could fly may also have been drug induced because many natural preparations used in so-called witches' brews induced the sensation of dissociation from the body, as in flying or floating.

There are some indications that, as far back as 2240 B.C., attempts to regulate drug use were made. For instance, in that year, problem drinking was addressed in the Code of Hammurabi and is described as "a problem of men with too much leisure time and lazy dispositions." Nearly every culture has, as part of its historical record, laws controlling the use of a wide range of drugs.

GATEWAY DRUGS drugs that often lead to the use of more serious drugs. Alcohol, tobacco, and marijuana are the most commonly used gateway drugs.

MDMA a type of illicit drug known as "Ecstasy" or "Adam" having stimulant and hallucinogenic properties

Here and Now

Street Terms: Cocaine, Heroin, Marijuana

What do 1990s users call various forms of drug administration?

Inhaling cocaine

Blow
Blow coke
Do a line
Geeze
Hitch up the reindeers
Pop
Sniff
Snort
Toot

Smoking cocaine (crack)

Chase
Freebasing
Ghost busting

Smoking marijuana

Blast
Blast a joint
Blast a roach
Blast a stick
Blow
Burn one
Do a joint
Dope smoke
Fire it up
Get a gage up
Hit
Hit the hay
Mow the grass
Poke
Puff the dragon
Tea party
Toke
Toke up
Up against the stem = addicted to smoking marijuana

Injecting an opiate

Blackjack
Backup = prepare vein for injection
Bang
Bingo
Flow a fix/blow a shot = injection misses the vein and the opiate is wasted in the skin
Boot
Channel swimmer = one who injects heroin
Chipping = using only occasionally
Cooker
Cranking up
Cushion = the vein the drug is injected into; also channel, gutter, pipe, sewer
Emergency gun = instrument used to inject other than syringe
Fix
Flag = appearance of blood in the vein
Fuete = hypodermic needle; also
gaffus
glass
glass gun
hype stick
Geezer
Get off
Hit the main line
Hot load/hot shot = lethal injection of an opiate
Jolt
Joy pop
Main line
Shoot/shoot up
Skin popping
Slam
Spike

Source: Bureau of Justice Statistics (BJS). *A National Report: Drugs, Crime and the Justice System.* U.S. Department of Justice, Office of Justice Programs. Washington, DC: U.S. Government Printing Office, December 1992: 24.

Extent and Frequency of Drug Use in Society

Erich Goode, a much-respected sociologist, lists four different uses of drugs:

1. *Legal instrumental use or medical use*—prescription drugs and OTC drugs used to relieve or treat mental or physical symptoms
2. *Legal recreational use*—the consumption of such illicit drugs as tobacco, alcohol, and caffeine to achieve pleasure or satisfaction
3. *Illegal instrumental use*—taking a drug without medical supervision or prescription to

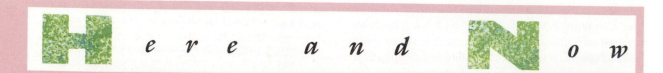

accomplish a task or goal, such as taking nonprescribed amphetamines to drive through the night
4. *Illegal recreational use*— taking illicit drugs for fun or pleasure to experience euphoria

(Goode 1993)

Why has there been such an increase in drug use? There are several possible answers, none of which by itself offers a satisfactory solution. One interesting perspective is that practically all of us are drug *users,* and what constitutes drug *abuse* is just a matter of degree. Another explanation is that more varieties of both licit and illicit drugs are available today. Evidence for this is found in numerous citations. One source estimates that 70% of all currently marketed drugs were either unknown or unavailable 15 years ago (Lipton and Lee 1988, 136). Another source, *Drug Use Around the World* (Kusinitz 1988, p. 149) asserts that "in the modern age, increased sophistication has brought with it techniques of drug production and distribution that have resulted in worldwide epidemic of abuse." Finally, other reliable estimates report that as much as one-third of the American population over age 12 has tried an illegal substance (Goode 1990, 97). For example, in 1991 approximately 37% of the American population over age 12 had tried at least one illegal substance during their lifetimes (Goode 1993, 95). This percentage translates into approximately 75 million Americans! The extent of drug use has also permeated the workplace affecting our nation's employees. The adjacent Here and Now boxes show (1) the latest findings on drugs in the workplace, and (2) how employed adults are affected by certain drugs.

Drug Use: Statistics and Trends An incredible amount of money is spent each year for legal chemicals that alter consciousness, awareness, or mood. There are four classes of these legal chemicals:

1. *Social drugs*—$58.9 billion for alcohol; $25.2 billion for cigarettes (add another $1.4 billion for cigars, chewing, pipe, and roll-your-own tobacco, and snuff tobacco); $5.7 billion for coffee, tea, and cocoa
2. *Prescription or ethical drugs*—$30 billion (Goode 1993, 35)
3. *Over-the-counter (OTC) or patent drugs*—12 billion, including cough and cold items, external and internal analgesics, antacids, laxatives, antidiarrheals, and sleep aids and sedatives
4. *Miscellaneous drugs* (such as aerosols, nutmeg, morning glory seeds, and others)—amount unknown

Studies from the Social Research Group of George Washington University; the Institute for Research in Social Behavior in Berkeley, California; and others provide detailed, in-depth data showing that drug use is universal. A major purpose of these studies was to determine the level of psychoactive drug use in the population aged 18 through 74, excluding those people hospitalized or in the armed forces. Data were collected to identify people using specific categories of drugs: caffeine, sleeping pills, nicotine, alcohol, and other psychoactive drugs. Other studies show that people in the 18- to 25-year-old age groups are by far the heaviest users and experimenters (see also Table 1.2, page 21).

Over 80% of respondents in the studies report that they drank coffee during the previous year, and over 50% said that they drank tea. Another finding from these data shows that nearly one-third of the population drinks more than five cups of caffeine-containing beverages each day. In 1989, 295 billion doses of caffeine were consumed in the United States. These figures exclude caffeine sources such as chocolate, cocoa, cola drinks, No Doz, and other OTC products with caffeine, such as Excedrin, Anacin, and others.

The number of cigarettes smoked in the United States in 1987 was approximately 550 billion (Forster, Jacobs, and Siegel 1989). Almost 22 gallons of beer were consumed by each man, woman, and child, as were more than 2 gallons of wine and more than 2.8 gallons of distilled spirits. Studies show that many people have used marijuana at least once in their lives: about 13% of youth (3.4 million), 51% of young adults (13.5 million), and 24% of adults (34 million) (NIDA 1993).

The average household owns about 35 drugs, of which one out of five is a prescription drug and the other 4 are over-the-counter drugs (NIDA 1993). Of the many prescriptions written by physicians, approximately one-fourth modify moods and behaviors in one way or another. Surveys report that over 50% of adults in the United States have, at some time in their lives, taken a psychoactive drug (one that affects mood or conscious-

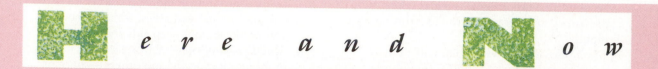

Here and Now

Research on Drugs in the Workplace

Given that a large majority of the adult population of the United States is employed, worksite programs have unique potential for success in reducing drug use and its adverse consequences in a large proportion of the drug-using population. The social and fiscal contingencies related to employment provide the basis for potentially powerful techniques for modifying behavior. Research data are beginning to emerge on the prevalence and impact of workplace-related drug use and on industry programs to reduce them.

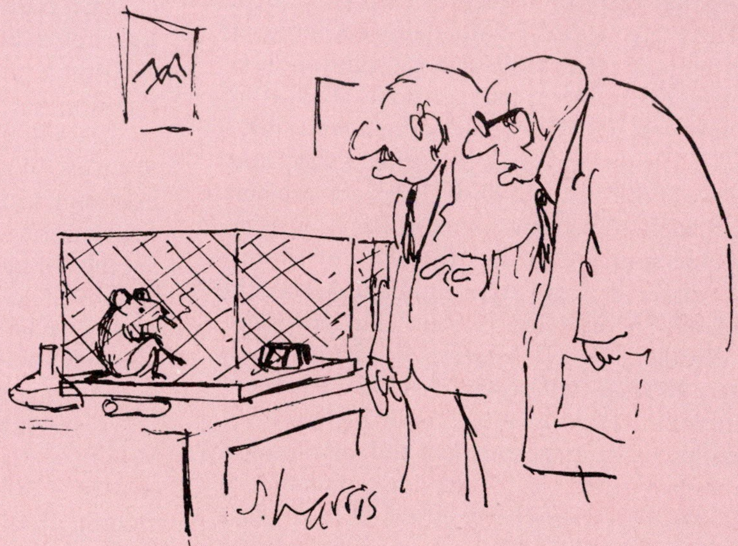

"HE'S THE TYPICAL AMERICAN MOUSE— LIKES A DRINK BEFORE DINNER, SMOKES A LITTLE, WATCHES TV..."

Source: ® Sidney Harris, *American Scientist* magazine. Used with permission.

Prevalence of Drug Use in the Workforce

The majority of illicit drug users are *employed*. Data from the 1988 NIDA National Household Survey show that 70% of those reporting current illicit drug use (defined as having used at least once in the previous month) were employed (55% full time; 15% part time). This suggests that over 10 million employed people are current users of illicit drugs.

Among full-time employees, 8.2% overall report current use of illicit drugs, but there are significantly higher rates of use in certain demographic groups. For example, 24% of males aged 18–25 years, and 15% of males aged 26–34 years are current users. Marijuana and cocaine are the most commonly used illicit drugs.

This significant drug use by members of the U.S. workforce carries with it the risk of drug dependence as well as a host of problems related to decreased job performance and productivity. Other findings regarding

Current Drug Use Among Full-time Employed

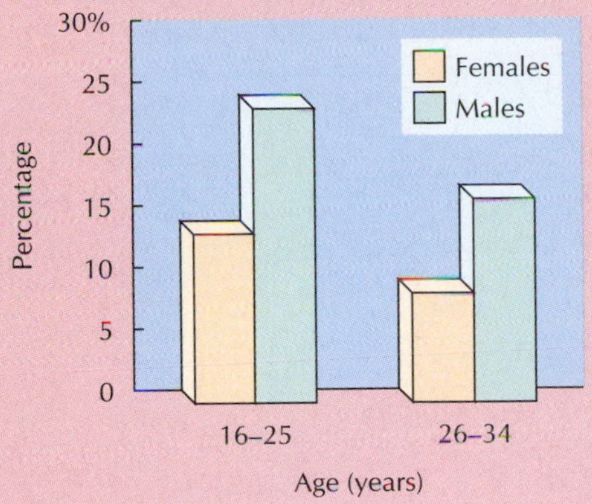

Current Users of Illicit Drugs

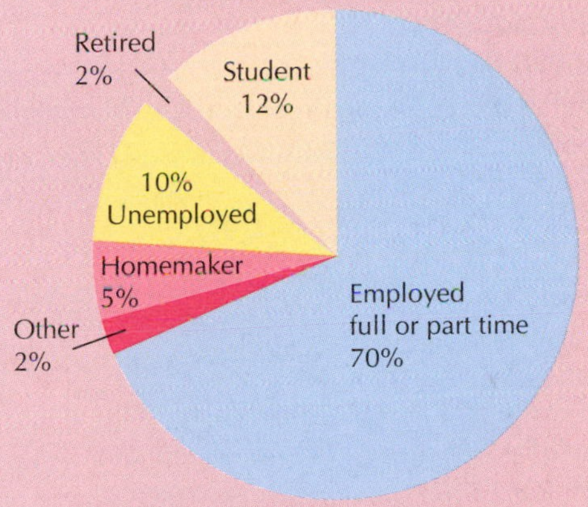

Source: National Institute on Drug Abuse. "Research on Drugs and the Workplace." *Capsules CAP 24.* Rockville, MD: U.S. Department of Health and Human Services.1990b. Revised June 1993.

the topic of drugs and the workplace include additional statistics that negatively impact on job performance: Drug users are:

1.6 times as likely than nonusers to have quit their jobs or have been fired
1.5 times as likely to have had an accident, and twice as likely to have been injured
1.5 times as likely to have been disciplined by a supervisor
1.8 times as likely to be absent

In addition,

6% of full- and part-time employees reported current marijuana use.
1% of full-time employers reported current cocaine use. In summary, 7 million workers report marijuana and cocaine use.

What do you think are the primary reasons why apparently employed workers use drugs?

Source: Parts excerpted from U.S. Department of Justice. *Drugs, Crime, and the Justice System: A National Report from the Bureau of Justice Statistics.* Washington, DC: U.S. Government Printing Office, 1992.

Here and Now

Current Marijuana and Cocaine Use Among Employed Adults by Type of Employment

The following list summarizes findings of a survey conducted by George Washington University and the National Institute on Drug Abuse of 3,000 adults, of whom 1,716 were employed in jobs outside the home and the remainder were students, homemakers, or retirees.

1. Most youths do not cease drug use when they begin working.
2. Of the total sample, 18% reported past-year marijuana use, and 6% reported past-year cocaine use.
3. Significant differences were found among occupational categories in marijuana use: no differences found in current cocaine use.
4. Age was the most significant predictor of marijuana and cocaine use. Younger employees (18–24 years old) were more likely to report drug use than older employees (25 years plus).
5. Marijuana and cocaine use were significantly higher among male than female employees.

Job Category	Marijuana Use Current	Cocaine Use Current
Professional or Managerial ($n = 546$	7%	1%
Business or Farm owner ($n = 77$)	13%	2%
Sales or Manufacturers' representative ($n = 99$)	15%	3%
Clerical ($n = 212$)	7%	1%
Skilled trade ($n = 251$)	16%	3%
Semiskilled trade ($n = 19$)	12%	1%
Laborer ($n = 36$)	10%	5%
Service worker ($n = 170$)	12%	4%
Other ($n = 68$)	24%	2%
	Chi sq = 19.5 $\rho < .05$	Chi sq = 6.6 NS

With regard to marijuana and cocaine use among younger employees 18 to 34 years old:

6. Employees with less than a high school education had higher rates of marijuana and cocaine use than employees with higher levels of education. Current marijuana use ranged from 35% for employees who had not finished high school to 16% for employees who had attended or graduated from college.
7. Within the 18- to 34-year-old subgroup, there were no significant differences in marijuana and cocaine use rates across five educational categories (18–24; 25–34; 35–44; 45–54; 55+).

Source: R. F. Cook and ISA Associates. "Drug Use Among Working Adults: Prevalence Rates and Estimation Methods," in *Drugs in the Workplace: Research and Evaluation Data*, edited by S. W. Gust and J. M. Walsh, 17–23. NIDA Research Monograph 91. Rockville, MD: National Institute on Drug Abuse, 1989.

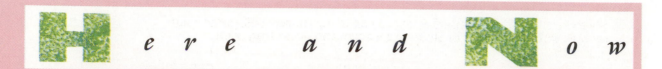

TABLE 1.1 National Household Survey on Drug Abuse, 1993: percentage and estimated number of alcohol, tobacco, and illicit drug users

	Lifetime [a]		Past Month	
	Percentage	Number of Users (Thousands)	Percentage	Number of Users (Thousands)
Alcohol	85%	171,710	51%	103,232
Cigarettes	73	147,557	27	54,825
Marijuana and Hashish	33	67,379	5	9,721
Smokeless Tobacco	14	28,555	3	6,885
Nonmedical Use of Any Psychotherapeutic [b]	13	25,422	2	3,275
Cocaine	12	23,396	c	c
Hallucinogens	8	16,381	c	c
Stimulants	7	14,249	0.3	667
Analgesics	6	12,330	0.7	1,457
Inhalants	5	10,953	0.6	1,218
Tranquilizers	6	11,289	0.5	1,043
Sedatives	4	8,684	0.4	785
PCP	4	7,307	1	c
Crack	2	3,898	0.2	479
Any Illicit Drug	37	75,071	6.3	12,813

Source: National Institute on Drug Abuse. *National Household Survey on Drug Abuse, Highlights 1993.* Rockville, MD: NIDA, February 1993: 71.

Note: Total population 202.8 million.

[a] Lifetime refers to ever used.

[b] Nonmedical use of any prescription stimulant, sedative, tranquilizer, or analgesic; does not include over-the-counter drugs.

[c] Low precision; no estimate reported.

ness). Over one-third of adults have used or are using depressants or sedatives.

In summarizing the *National Household Survey on Drug Abuse, 1993* (NIDA 1993) (Table 1.1), the following patterns appear:

1. Alcohol was by far the most widely used drug, with 85% lifetime use and 51% in the past month before the survey was taken—171.7 million had ever used alcohol during their lifetimes.
2. Next highest was cigarettes, 73% and 27%—147.6 million lifetime users.
3. A total of 75.1 million had ever used illicit-drugs.
4. The most commonly used illicit drug was marijuana—33% and 5% were current users.
5. The next most commonly used types of illicit drugs in 1993 were prescription psychotherapeutic drugs and cocaine. The lifetime use was 13% for psychotherapeutic drugs and 12% for cocaine.
6. Other illicit drugs, hallucinogens, inhalants, or heroin (not listed in table) were used by fewer than 9% in their lifetimes.
7. Finally, 2% reported using crack in their lifetimes and 1% in the last month.

An NIDA study indicates drug use trends

based on gender. Men are most likely to use stimulants in their thirties, depressants in their forties and fifties, and sedatives from age 60 on. Women however, are most likely to use stimulants from age 21 through age 39 and depressants more frequently in their thirties. Women's use of sedatives is similar to the pattern of use by men, with the frequency of use increasing with age. Women tend to use pills to cope with problems, whereas men tend to use alcohol. In addition, people over 35 are more likely to take pills, whereas younger people prefer alcohol. Among those using pills, younger people and men are more likely to use stimulants than older people and women, who take sedatives (Chambers and Griffey 1975).

The actual figures for use of all psychoactive drugs are probably 35% higher than reported. This discrepancy exists partly because a large number of people get psychoactive drugs on the "black market" and from friends and relatives who have legitimate prescriptions. An estimated 70% of all psychoactive prescription drugs used by people under 30 are obtained without the user having a prescription. Pharmacists' records show that about $60.7 billion are spent on psychoactive drug prescriptions (U.S. Bureau of the Census 1993, 108) with the rate of increase estimated at about 9% per year. Such figures show that it may be more difficult to find people who do not use psychoactive drugs than people who do.

Mass Media Influences on Drug Use in Everyday Life

Studies have shown that the majority of young users come from homes in which drugs are used extensively (Goode 1993; Coombs 1988). Thus children frequently witness drug use at home. For instance, in the morning, parents may consume large quantities of coffee to wake up and other forms of medication throughout the day: tablets for an upset stomach, vitamins for stress, or aspirin for a headache. Finally, before retiring, the grown-ups may take a "little night cap" or a sleeping pill to relax. Pills alone are taken in almost unbelievable volume. Such everyday consumption of legal drugs—caffeine, prescription or over-the-counter drugs and alcohol—is based on demand fueled by the pace of modern lifestyles and greatly accelerated by the influence of today's increasingly sophisticated mass media.

If you look around your classroom building, the dormitories at your college, or the surroundings of your own homes, evidence of mass media and electronic equipment can be found everywhere. Cultural knowledge and information is transmitted via media and electronic gadgets we simply "can't live without" to the point where these surroundings help us define *and* shape our everyday reality.

Although over 70% of the adult population are regular newspaper readers, television remains the most influential medium. Almost 93 million American homes have television sets; 59% have more than one set, and 96% have color sets. In the United States, the number of hours spent watching television is staggering. Statistics indicate that the average household spends 49 hours and 49 minutes per week watching television (Nielsen 1986). This is over 7 hours per day!

Advertisers invest huge amounts of money in television commercials because of the popularity of the medium. For example, $65 billion per year is generated by the alcohol industry. They spend more than $1 billion on yearly advertising (Kilbourne 1989). "The advertising budget for one beer—Budweiser—is more than the entire budget for research on alcoholism and alcohol abusers" (Kilbourne 1989, 13). If there are any doubts that advertising is not effective in promoting drinking, why would a multinational corporation such as Budweiser allocate over $1 billion yearly for advertising?

Radio, newspapers, and magazines are also saturated with advertisements for OTC drugs, constantly offering relief from whatever illness you may have. There are pills for inducing sleep and staying awake, as well as for treating indigestion, headache, backache, tension, constipation, and the like. Mood, level of consciousness, and physical discomfort can be significantly altered by using these medicinal compounds.

Furthermore, experts warn that drug advertising will increase geometrically. A few years ago, the FDA lifted a two-year ban on consumer advertising of prescription drugs (Wang 1985).

In their attempts to sell drugs, product advertisers use the authority of a physician or health expert or the seemingly sincere testimony of a mesmerized product user. Adults are strongly affected by testimonial advertising because these drug commercials can appear authentic and convincing to large numbers of viewers, listeners, or readers. More recently R. J. Reynolds Nabisco in the late 1980s strategized using "Joe Camel" to promote Camel cigarettes. This cartoon figure has strengthened Camel's market share, despite the large number of antismoking protest groups claiming that Joe Camel is really designed to appeal to children and teens (see Chapter 11, "Tobacco," for discussion on tobacco companies venturing to foreign markets as U.S. cigarette sales continue to decline).

The constant barrage of commercials, including many for OTC drugs, relay the message that, if you are experiencing restlessness or uncomfortable symptoms, drug taking is acceptable. As a result, adults and eventually children are led to believe that drugs are necessary to maintain well-being.

The Attraction of Drug Use and Some Patterns of Drug Abuse

Why are people so attracted to drugs? Like the ancient Assyrians, who sucked on opium lozenges, and the Romans, who ate hashish sweets some 2,000 years ago, many users claim to be bored, in pain, frustrated, unable to enjoy life, or alienated. They turn to drugs in the hope of finding oblivion, peace, "togetherness," or euphoria. The fact that few drugs cause all the effects for which they are taken doesn't seem to be a deterrent. People continue to take drugs for a number of reasons:

1. They may be searching for pleasure, and drugs may make them feel good.
2. Drugs may relieve stress or tension or provide a temporary escape for people with anxiety.
3. Peer pressure is strong, especially for young people. The use of drugs has become a rite of passage in some levels of society.
4. In some cases, drugs may enhance religious or mystical experiences. A few cultures teach children how to use specific drugs for this purpose.
5. Drugs can relieve pain and symptoms of illness.

Since historically, many people have been unsuccessful in eliminating the fascination with drugs, it is important that we come to understand it. To reach such an understanding, we will address why people are attracted to drugs, how different types of drugs affect the body and the mind, and what forms of treatment are available for eliminating abuse. These questions are addressed at a general level in Chapter 2, and at the level of specific substances in each chapter from 6 through 13.

When Does Use Lead to Abuse?

Views on the use of drugs depend on one's perspective. For example, from a pharmacological perspective, if a patient is suffering severe pain because of car collision injuries, high doses of a narcotic such as morphine or Demerol should be given to control discomfort. While someone is in pain, there is no reason not to take the drug. From a medical standpoint, once healing has occurred and pain has been relieved, drug use should cease. If the patient continues using the narcotic because it provides a sense of well-being or has become a habit, the pattern of drug intake would then be considered abuse. Thus, the amount of drug taken or the frequency of dosing does not necessarily determine abuse (although those that abuse drugs do usually consume frequent high doses). Rather, the *motive* for taking the drug is the principal factor in determining abuse.

Initial drug abuse symptoms are excessive use, constant preoccupation over the availability and supply of the drug, refusing to admit excessive use, early symptoms of withdrawal whenever the user attempts to stop taking the drug, and neglect of important goals and/or ambitions in favor of using the drug. Even the legitimate use of a drug can be controversial. Often physicians cannot decide even among themselves what constitutes legitimate use of a drug. For example, MDMA ("Ecstasy") is a drug currently prohibited for therapeutic use, but in 1985, when the Drug Enforcement Administration (DEA) was deciding MDMA's status, some 35 to 200 physicians (mostly psychiatrists) were using it in their practice. These clinicians claimed that MDMA relaxed inhibitions and enhanced communications and was useful as a psychotherapeutic adjunct to assist in dealing with psychiatric patients (Shecter 1989). From the perspective of these

CROSSCURRENTS

Are Drugs Good or Bad?

Without culture and society, drugs are neither good nor bad. Drugs are simply compounds that cause or produce certain effects in individuals. Whether drug use is good or bad becomes a matter of opinion when it is viewed culturally, socially, economically, politically, and religiously. The particular cultural context becomes complicated when individual versus collective rights are considered.

The issue of placing limits on drug use is similar to such "hot button" issues as abortion and euthanasia. For example, the question of drug use becomes value laden when viewed and applied in specific cultural, social, political, religious, and biological contexts. In a sense, these perspectives complicate and confuse the simple, neutral act of taking drugs. Consider these propositions: (1) Whose business is it if a group of mature adults privately enjoys the occasional use of drugs mainly for recreational purposes? (2) What if a group of ninth-graders finds the same pleasures in the use of drugs on weekends?

Without any other additional assumptions, the first example may not raise much consternation for many people. However, the second example can easily lead to many emotional and intellectual arguments.

Current plausible solutions to our drug use problems are contained in the legalization, decriminalization (see Chapter 3) and harm reduction (see Chapter 16, pp. 470–471) proposals for "dealing" with drug use and/or abuse. Initially, the issue of limiting drug use appears simple, but on closer inspection it is a complicated problem.

Three possible positions outlined here are

Position 1: Legalize all drugs; let people do what they want with drug use.

Position 2: Keep the current practice, legalize a few drugs such as alcohol and nicotine, and continue to legally prohibit other drugs.

Position 3: Prohibit the use of all drugs (except caffeine) that are not for medical purposes prescribed by health care providers.

Each of these three positions have positive and negative tradeoffs. For example, if drugs were legalized, would all users maintain rational control over drug use? What about minors—should they be legally allowed to use drugs? What about pregnant women, should they be allowed to use drugs at their discretion? Does society have a responsibility to protect self-harm?

If the second position is selected, we find ourselves as we are currently. Many drugs are prohibited, while drugs such as alcohol and tobacco are legalized. Does this work? Is drug use and/or abuse under control? Do minors escape drug enforcement laws? Are the legalized drugs safer than prohibited ones? Are there safe drunk drivers? What is the rationale for legalizing certain drugs proven to be more damaging and costly to our nation's citizens while others are illegal?

The third position also has some problems. Do you think that if all drugs—with the exceptions of tea, coffee, or cocoa—were prohibited, this would stop inappropriate use and misuse of drugs? Is it possible to legally prohibit drug use given that individuals have inalienable rights under our U.S. Constitution?

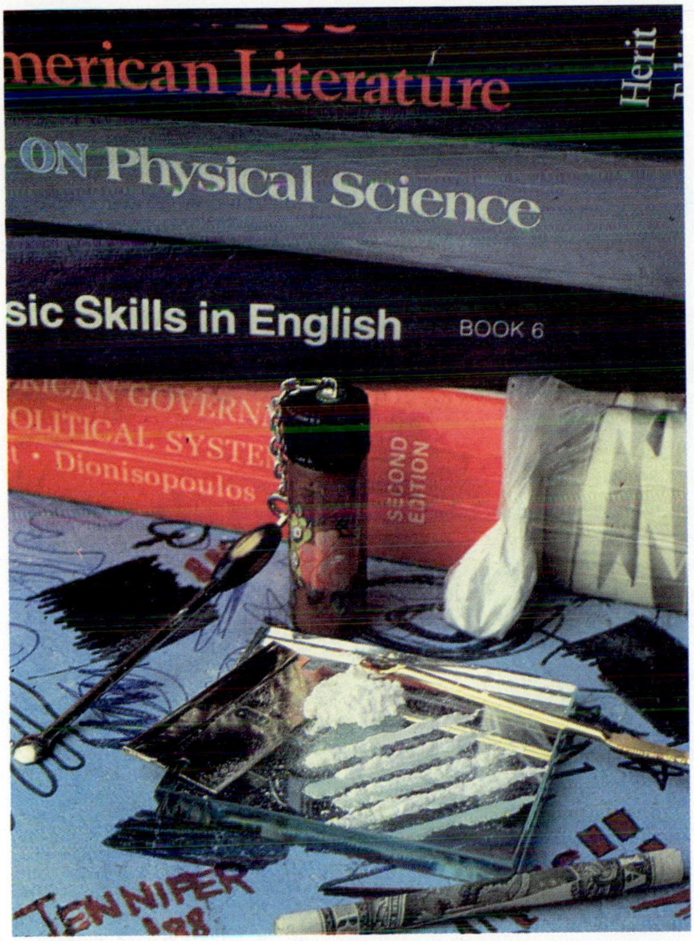

Over the past 10 to 15 years, cocaine abuse has become one of the greatest drug concerns in U.S. society.

physicians, Ecstasy was a useful medicinal tool. However, the DEA did not agree and made Ecstasy a Schedule I drug (see Chapter 3). This classification excludes any legitimate use of a drug in therapeutics; consequently, according to this ruling, anyone taking Ecstasy is guilty of drug abuse.

Other special-interest groups take a more liberal view. They consider drug abuse a statutory problem and describe it as "the use of drugs in an illegal manner." According to such a limited definition, excessive use of alcohol by anyone over 21 years of age would not be considered a form of drug abuse, in spite of the consequences. Obviously, such a narrow view of drug abuse is not very useful in trying to deal with the consequences of extreme inappropriate drug use, such as alcoholism.

If the problem of drug abuse is to be understood and solutions are to be found, identifying what causes the abuse is most important. When a drug is being abused, it is not legitimately therapeutic; that is, it does not improve the user's physical or mental health. If such drug use is not for therapeutic purposes, what is the motive for using it?

There are many possible answers to this question. Most drug abusers perceive some psychological advantage when using these compounds (at least initially). For many, the psychological lift is significant enough that they are willing to risk social exclusion, arrest, incarceration, and fines to have their drug. The psychological effects that these drugs cause may entail an array of diverse feelings. Different types of drugs have different psychological impacts. The type of drug an individual selects to abuse may ultimately reflect his or her own mental state.

That is, for people who experience chronic depression, feel intense job pressures, an inability to focus on accomplishing goals, or develop a sense of inferiority, a stimulant such as cocaine or

Case in Point

"You Wasn't In Unless You Were Getting High"

The following excerpt describes the impact of peer pressure on a youth who uses heroin to be "hip."

> Cats on the block had been using it for years and they had been trying to get me to use it but backed off. A couple of my partners went down and they pulled a stick-up and they had plenty of money, so they came back after buying dope for everybody. We seen the availability of it and they seemed to know what they were talking about. It was a thing where heroin was always talked about. We all went off in a vacant building, must have been about a dozen of us. We just lined up, rolled up our sleeves and started pushing the dope, you know, everybody got a shot.
>
> We was sitting around with friends of ours. We all grew up together and they were into it before we were. We wanted to know what kind of feeling that was, the way we watched them high. And they looked like they felt so good. So I stayed awhile and tried it.
>
> When we used to play hooky, we used to have hooky parties, and the older crowd of dudes used to try to come to the party to mess with the women. Then they'd sneak off in the bathroom and start shooting heroin. And they'd come out and say, "Hey, take [snort] a couple of blows, I think you'll like it." And we'd do, just being naive and wanting to hang out, we did it. At first I didn't like it. I don't know what it was that continued me with it because it made me more sick than pleasing.
>
> Using heroin in those days was a fad. You wasn't cool unless you had it and, you know, you want to be like everybody else, you want to be like your big brother, gang fightin'. You want to be hip, and you wasn't in the crowd unless you were getting high.

Source: Reprinted with the permission of Lexington Books, an imprint of Macmillan, Inc., from *Life with Heroin: Voices from the Inner City* by Bill Hanson, George Beschner, James M. Walters, and Elliot Bovelle. Copyright © 1985 by Lexington Books.

amphetamines may appear to provide a solution to such dilemmas; these drugs cause a spurt of energy, euphoria, a sense of superiority, and imagined confidence. In contrast, people who experience nervousness and anxiety and want instant relief from the pressures of life may choose a depressant such as alcohol or barbiturates; these agents sedate, relax, and provide relief, and even have some amnesiac properties, allowing users to suspend and/or forget their problems. People who perceive themselves as creative and/or who have artistic talents may select hallucinogenic-types of drugs to "expand" their mind, heighten their senses, and distort the confining nature of reality. As individuals come to rely more on drugs to inhibit, deny, accelerate, or distort their realities, they run the risk of becoming psychologically dependent on drugs—a process described in detail in Chapter 4.

Types of Drug Users

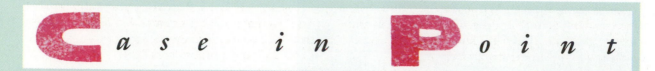

Some are occasional or moderate users of drugs, while others cannot let a day pass without use. Such variability in the frequency and extent of usage has been characterized by researchers in three basic patterns. Beschner (1986) distinguishes between **experimenters, compulsive users,** and **floaters** (these last are drug users who drift between experimenters and compulsive users). *Experimenters* begin using drugs largely because of peer pressure and curiosity, and do it within a generally fun atmosphere. Marijuana and alcohol are the usual limits of their drug-taking behavior, and they are more likely to know the difference between light, moderate, and chronic use. *Compulsive users*, in contrast, "... devote considerable time and energy to getting high, talk incessantly (sometimes exclusively about drugs), and become connoisseurs of street drugs" (Beschner 1986, 7). Other antecedents of compulsive use are serious needs to escape from perplexing problems and to avoid stress and anxiety. Often such users have difficulty with assuming personal responsibilities, suffer from low self-esteem, and are children of dysfunctional families. More serious psychological problems often underlie their compulsive drug-taking behavior.

Finally, *floaters* vacillate from the need for pleasure seeking and the desire to relieve moderately serious problems. As a result, floaters drift between experimental drug-taking peers to chronic drug-using peers. In a sense, floaters are marginal individuals, and they do not strongly identify with experimenters or compulsive users. An example of how various types of drug users are often adversely affected by peers is shown in the Case in Point box. (The significance of peers and how they affect the allure of drug usage is more elaborately discussed in Chapter 2.)

How Widespread Is Drug Abuse?

As mentioned earlier, drug abuse today is more acute and widespread than in any pervious age. The evidence for this is that drug busts are an everyday occurrence in the United States. On any given day, you can scan most major national and international newspapers and undoubtedly run across stories about illegal drug manufacturing, distribution, or use.

Substance abuse is not confined to any specific social or socioeconomic group. Many of us, for example, are a little dismayed when we discover that certain individuals we admire—such as celebrities, politicians, athletes, clergy, and academics—admit to or are apprehended for abusing illicit drugs. We are also taken aback when we hear that cigarettes, alcohol, and marijuana abuse are commonplace in some junior high and even grade schools. Further, most of us know of at least one close friend or family member who abuses drugs.

Drug use is an **"equal-opportunity affliction"** in that no one is immune and research shows that drug consumption cuts across income, social class, and age groups (see Table 1.2 page 22). Drugs are as seductive to the poor as they are to the wealthy, to the highly educated and the school dropout, to the young and the old.

Holistic Approach to Drug Use

Besides discussing the pharmacological, psychological, and social ramifications of most commonly used licit and illicit drugs, this book has a larger focus. This larger focus involves showing how drug use information can be used personally for improving yourself, others you care about, and your society. Learning that drug use never occurs in isolation—that drug use is affected by genetic inheritance, psychological conditioning, peer group pressure, tension or anxiety, unhealthy role modeling, dysfunctional families, serious personality problems, and ethnic and racial conflicts—is a good first step toward understanding why and how drug use occurs.

The chapters in this book discuss most of the major drugs of abuse and emphasize an under-

EXPERIMENTERS, COMPULSIVE USERS, and **FLOATERS** types of drug users: experimenters are novel users, compulsive users are often addicted users, and floaters are users who vacillate from the need to seek pleasure to the need to relieve serious psychological problems

EQUAL-OPPORTUNITY AFFLICTION drug use, in that it cuts across all members of society regardless of income, social class, and age category

TABLE 1.2 Trend data from the National Institute of Drug Abuse's National Household Survey on Drug Abuse, prevalence of illicit drug use, 1982–1992

		1982	1985	1988	1991[a]	1992[b]
Use in Past Month	All ages 12+	12.2%	12.1%	7.3%	6.3%	5.5%
	12–17	12.7	14.9	9.2	6.8	6.1
	18–25	30.4	25.7	17.8	15.4	13.0
	26–34	19.2	21.1	13.0	9.0	10.1
	35+	3.4	3.9	2.1	3.1	2.2
Use in Past Year	All ages 12+	18.7	19.6	14.1	12.7	11.1
	12–17	22.0	23.7	16.8	14.8	11.7
	18–25	43.4	42.6	32.0	29.1	26.4
	26–34	29.5	32.0	22.6	18.4	18.3
	35+	5.6	6.6	5.8	6.4	5.1
Use in Lifetime (ever used)	All ages 12+	32.3	36.9	36.6	37.0	36.2
	12–17	27.6	29.5	24.7	20.1	16.5
	18–25	65.3	64.3	58.9	54.7	51.7
	26–34	57.7	62.2	64.2	61.8	60.8
	35+	13.2	20.4	23.0	27.3	28.0

Note that this table shows a gradual yearly decline in drug use across all age groups through 1992.

Note: These figures include use of marijuana, cocaine, hallucinogens, inhalants (except in 1982), heroin, and nonmedical use of sedatives, tranquilizers, stimulants, and analgesics. Data on inhalant use were not collected in 1982, which may lower overall prevalence figures for that year, especially for 12- to 17-year-olds.

[a]Source for all figures in this column: National Institute on Drug Abuse, *National Household Survey on Drug Abuse* (Rockville, MD: NIDA, 1992).

[b]All figures in this column: National Institute on Drug Abuse, *National Household Survey on Drug Abuse* (Rockville, MD: NIDA, 1993).

Source: National Institute of Drug Abuse. *NIDA Notes* 5, no. 1 (Winter 1989–1990): 4.

standing of how drugs work and how they affect both the mind and the body.

How can such information be used constructively? First, it is important to keep in mind that since the mid-1970s drug use has been steadily declining. Figures 1.1 and 1.2 show steady declines in drug use for twelfth-graders and college students. Both these figures show that overall drug use in the younger generations continues to diminish (Johnston et al. 1993).

The recent declines in drug use reflect our current emphasis on viewing health as interrelated with positive wellness. The interrelatedness involves a compromise among physical, psychological, emotional, social, spiritual, and environmental factors. No longer are these domains of existence viewed as separate entities. Thus, "no part of the mind, body, or environment is truly separate and independent" (Edlin and Golanty 1992, 5).

The **positive wellness** approach says that health and wellness are ways of life (Edlin and Golanty 1992, 6). Gaining knowledge of how and why drugs work—the subject matter in these chap-

POSITIVE WELLNESS an approach advocating the maintenance of health and wellness as a way of life

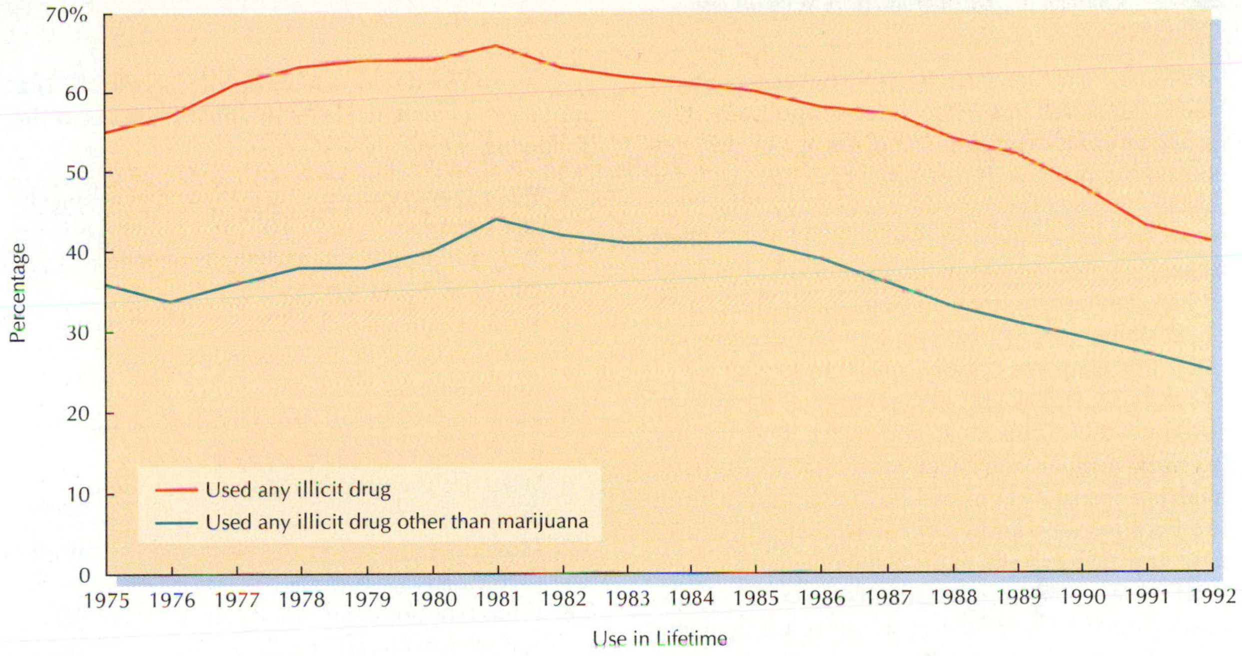

FIGURE 1.1 Trends in Lifetime Prevalence of an Illicit Drug Use Index for Twelfth-Graders *Source:* Lloyd P. Johnston, Patrick M. O'Malley, and Jerald G. Bachman. *National Survey Results from the Monitoring the Future Study, 1975–1992*. Vol. 1. Rockville, MD: National Institute on Drug Abuse, 1993: 79.

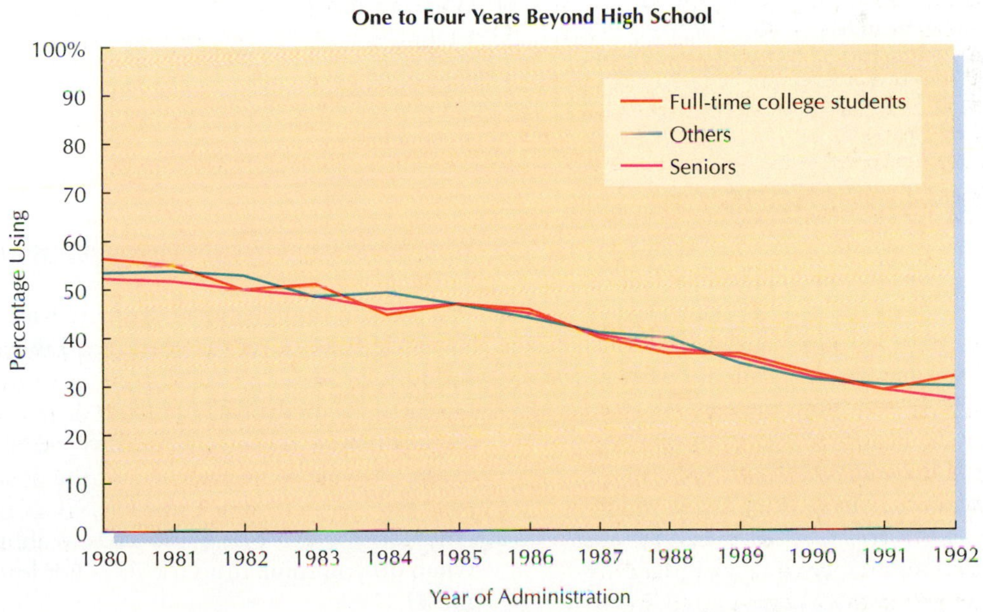

Note: "Others" refers to high school graduates one to four years beyond high school not currently enrolled full time in college.

FIGURE 1.2 Any Illicit Drug Trends in Annual Prevalence Among College Students Versus Others *Source:* Lloyd P. Johnston, Patrick M. O'Malley, and Jerald G. Bachman. *National Survey Results from the Monitoring the Future Study, 1975–1992*. Vol. 1. Rockville, MD: National Institute on Drug Abuse, 1993: 172.

ters—supports the current holistic approach to health and wellness. The knowledge gained in understanding drug use is important not only for comprehending your own health, but also for understanding (1) why others use drugs; (2) what to do (remedies and solutions) when loved ones, friends, and family members abuse drugs; (3) how to help and advise drug abusers about the pitfalls of substance use; (4) the best educational, preventive, and treatment options available for victims of drug abuse; and (5) the danger signals in yourself and/or others you care about when drug use exceeds normal and necessary use. A **holistic health** approach requires knowledge about drug use because such knowledge increases self-awareness and if necessary, your ability to help others with whom you are emotionally involved. Thus, putting such knowledge to use can result in aiding yourself as well as your society.

Holistic health requires self-awareness about the use and possible abuse of drugs. In essence, drug information prevents embracing simple "quick fix" solutions to drug use problems. Such information not only promotes your own self-maintenance by promoting self-healing, but also increases your ability to help others by promoting prevention, education, and treatment of deviant drug use.

As suggested by the title of this book, our inquiry into drug use and/or abuse delves into the following questions:

1. What types of drugs exist? (See Appendix 1-1 and Chapters 7, 8, 9, 10, 11, 12, and 13.)
2. Why are drugs used and/or abused? (See Chapters 2 and 4.)
3. Who uses drugs? (See Chapter 15.)
4. When does drug use become misuse or abuse? (See Chapters 3 and 4.)
5. How and when are drugs used? (See Chapter 4.)
6. What are the proper and improper use of drugs? (See Chapter 14.)
7. How do drugs affect the body and the mind? (See Chapter 5.)
8. What types of drugs are legally permissible, and what types are legally prohibited? (See Chapter 3.)
9. What are the legal ramifications of drug use? (See Chapter 3.)
10. What other social problems correlate with drug use or abuse? (See boxes in Chapters 15 and 16.)
11. What are the most effective methods for controlling and stopping drug use? (See Chapter 16.)

Review Questions

1. Are the authors overstating the view that extensive drug use can unravel the very fabric of our society?
2. Speculate on how you think slang street terms develop and become the vernacular of particular drug use (Here and Now, page 8).
3. Briefly review the historical uses of drugs. Do you think drug use is innate in our society?
4. Given our affluence, why is drug use so widespread?
5. Why would employees risk using drugs while working?
6. Why do you think national drug use has been slowly declining over the years (see Table 1.2)?
7. Do the mass media really *promote* drug use, or do they merely *reflect* our extensive use of drugs? Provide some evidence for the position you take.
8. When do you think drug use leads to abuse? When do you think drug use does not lead to abuse?
9. Analyze the cartoon in Here and Now on page 12–13. What do you think is the deeper meaning of the caption?
10. Since many experimental drug users do not gravitate to excessive drug use, should experimenters be left alone, perhaps just given legal warnings?

HOLISTIC HEALTH health perspective advocating knowledge about drug use to increase self-awareness and help others

11. From all you have read thus far, can you predict the type of family life from which future drug abusers come? How about future nonusers of illicit drugs?

12. Why do Americans use so many legal drugs ranging from alcohol, tobacco, to OTC drugs? What in our society causes the extensive use of drugs?

Key Terms

drug
psychoactive drugs or psychoactive substances
licit drugs
illicit drugs
gateway drugs
designer drugs
structural analogs
MDMA
experimenters, compulsive users, and floaters
equal-opportunity affliction
positive wellness
holistic health

Summary

1. Two reasons for the importance of understanding drug use are (1) drug abuse is a national and international problem, and (2) drug use can destroy social cohesion, which is a prerequisite for a fully functioning society.
2. The pharmacological factors in drug use involve how the ingredients of a particular drug affect the functioning of the body. Cultural factors include society's views of drug use, as determined by custom and tradition. Social factors involve the values and attitudes of drug-using subcultures within communities. The contextual view of drug use involves the particular reason(s) for drug use, and the social and physical surroundings when drugs are used.
3. Mentions of drug use date back to the Bible, including ancient literature dated 2240 B.C. Under the influence of drugs, many people experienced extreme ecstasy to sheer terror. At times drugs were used to induce sleep and provide freedom from care.
4. The mass media tend to promote drug use through advertising. The constant barrage of OTC drug commercials relays the message that if you are experiencing some symptom, drug taking is acceptable.
5. Drug users are found in all occupations and professions, income and social class levels, and across all age groups. No one is immune to drug use. Drug use is an "equal opportunity" affliction.
6. From a pharmacological perspective, drug use becomes excessive when psychoactive drugs are taken without medical reasons. *Initial drug* abuse symptoms are excessive use, overpreoccupation with the availability and supply of drugs, denial of excessive use, symptoms of withdrawal whenever the user attempts to stop taking the drug, and neglect of personal goals in favor of using the drug.
7. There are three types of drug users: experimenters, compulsive users, and floaters. *Experimenters* try out drugs because of curiosity and peer pressure. *Compulsive users* use drugs on a full-time basis and seriously desire to escape from or alter reality. *Floaters* vacillate between experimental drug use to chronic drug use.
8. Four different types of drug users exist according to sociologist Erich Goode: (a) legal instrumental use or medical use, (b) legal recreational use, (c) illegal instrumental use, and (d) illegal recreational use.
9. The gender differences that exist in the use of drugs are the following: men are more likely to use stimulants in their thirties, depressants in their forties and fifties, and sedatives from age 60 on. Women are more likely to use stimulants from age 21 through age 30 and depressants more frequently in their thirties. Women tend to use pills to cope with problems, whereas men are more likely to use alcohol.
10. The most commonly used and abused drugs from highest to lowest are alcohol, cigarettes,

marijuana, smokeless tobacco, nonmedical use of stimulants, sedatives, tranquilizers, or analgesics not sold over the counter; stimulants and OTC analgesics.

11. Contrary to popular opinion, most drug users are employed. Approximately 70% are either full- or part-time employees.
12. Positive wellness advocates say that health and wellness is a fundamental style of life, and holistic advocates believe that knowledge about drug use heightens self-awareness and increases our ability to help others who may have a drug problem.
13. Definitions of the following key terms for understanding drug use are *drug(s)*, any substance that modified biological, psychological, and/or social behavior. *Gateway drugs* are drugs that lead to the progressive use of other drugs. *Medicines* and *prescription medicines* are prescribed by a physician. *Over-the-counter drugs* are sold without a prescription. Drug misuse refers to unintentional or inappropriate use of prescribed or OTC drugs. *Drug abuse* refers to the willful misuse of either licit or illicit drugs for recreation, necessity, or convenience. *Drug addiction* involves an intense psychological preoccupation with obtaining and consuming drugs.

References

Beschner, George. "Understanding Teenage Drug Use." In *Teen Drug Use*, edited by George Beschner and Alfred Friedman. Lexington, MA: Heath 1986: 1–18.

Bureau of Justice Statistics (BJS). *A National Report: Drugs, Crime and the Justice System*. U.S. Department of Justice, Office of Justice Programs. Washington, DC: U.S. Government Printing Office, December 1992: 24.

Chambers, C. C., and M. S. Griffey. "Use of Legal Substances Within the General Population: The Sex and Age Variables." *Addictive Diseases 2* (1975): 7–19.

Coombs, R. H., ed. *The Family Context of Adolescent Drug Use*. New York: Harworth, 1988.

Edlin, Gordon, and Eric Golanty. *Health and Wellness: A Holistic Approach*, 4th ed. Boston, MA: Jones and Bartlett, 1992.

Forster, C. D., N. R. Jacobs, and M. A. Siegel, eds. *Drugs and Alcohol—America's Anguish*. Wylie, TX: Information Plus, 1989.

Goode, Erich. *Deviant Behavior*, 3d ed. Englewood Cliffs, NJ: Prentice Hall, 1990.

Goode, Erich. *Drugs in American Society*, 4th ed. New York: McGraw-Hill, 1993.

Hanson, B., G. Beschner, J. M. Walters, and E. Bovelle. *Life with Heroin: Voices from the Inner City*. Lexington, MA: Lexington Books, 1985.

Johnston, L. D., P. M. O'Malley, and J. G. Bachman. *Use of Licit and Illicit Drugs by America's High School Students: 1973–1984*. Rockville, MD: National Institute on Drug Abuse, 1985.

Johnston, L. D., P. M. O'Malley, and J. G. Bachman. *National Survey Results from the Monitoring the Future Study, 1975–1992. 2 vols.* Rockville, MD: National Institute on Drug Abuse, 1993.

Kilbourne, Jean. "Advertising Addiction: The Alcohol Industry's Hard Sell." *Multinational Monitor* (June 1989): 13–16.

Kumpfer, Karol L., and Charles W. Turner. "The Social Ecology Model of Adolescent Substance Abuse: Implications for Prevention." *International Journal of the Addictions*, no. 25 (1990–1991): 435–63.

Kusinitz, M. "Drug Use Around the World." In *Encyclopedia of Psychoactive Drugs*, edited by S. Snyder. Series 2. New York: Chelsea House, 1988.

"Let's All Work to Fight Drug Abuse." Dallas, TX: L.A.W. Publications, 1991.

Lipton, M. A., and H. J. Lee. *Psychopharmacology: A Generation of Progress*. New York: Raven Press, 1988.

National Institute on Drug Abuse (NIDA). "Designer Drugs."*Capsules (CAPS)*. Rockville, MD: June 1986.

National Institute on Drug Abuse (NIDA). *The 1988 Household Survey on Drug Abuse: What the Results Tell Us*. Rockville, MD: NIDA, 1988.

National Institute on Drug Abuse (NIDA). *NIDA Notes* 5, no. 1 (Winter 1989–1990): 4.

National Institute on Drug Abuse (NIDA). *Capsules (CAPS)*. "Research on Drugs and the Workplace." Rockville, MD: NIDA, 1990a.

National Institute on Drug Abuse (NIDA). "Study Finds Higher Drug Use Among Adolescents Whose Parents Divorce." *NIDA Notes* 5, no. 3 (Summer 1990b): 10.

National Institute on Drug Abuse (NIDA). *National Household Survey on Drug Abuse*. Rockville, MD: NIDA, 1992.

National Institute on Drug Abuse (NIDA). *National Household Survey on Drug Abuse: Highlights 1993.* Rockville, MD: NIDA, 1993: 7.

Nielsen Company. *Television: 1986 Nielsen Report.* Northbrook, IL: Nielsen, 1986.

Schecter. M. "Serotonergic-Dopaminergic Mediation of 3, 4-Methytenedioxy-Methamphetamine (MDMA, Ecstasy)." *Pharmacology, Biochemistry and Behavior* 31 (1989): 817–24.

Sussman, V. "How to Beat Drugs." *U.S. News and World Report* (11 September 1989): 69–72.

Thio, A. *Deviant Behavior,* 2d ed. Boston: Houghton Mifflin, 1983.

U.S. Bureau of The Census. *Statistical Abstract of the United States, 1993.* 113th ed. Washington, DC: U.S. Government Printing Office, 1993: 108.

U.S. Department of Justice. *Drugs, Crime, and the Justice System: A National Report from the Bureau of Justice Statistics.* Washington, DC: U.S. Government Printing Office, 1992.

Wang, P. "A New Way to Drugs." *Time* (30 December 1985): 33–34.

Appendix

Appendix 1-1: Drugs of Use and Abuse

The table that follows on pages 24–27 provides detailed information about the drugs listed. Note that the heading *CSA Schedules* refers to categorization under the Controlled Substances Act (CSA). The roman numeral(s) to the right of each drug name specifies each as a Schedule I, II, III, IV, or V drug. See Chapter 3, Appendix 3-1, for more information on scheduling.

Source: Adapted from Drug Enforcement Administration, U.S. Dept. of Justice, *Drugs of Abuse*. 1989 Edition. Washington, DC: Government Printing office, 1989: and "Let's All Work to Fight Drug Abuse." Dallas, TX: L.A.W. Publications, 1991.

APPENDIX 1-1 Drugs of use and abuse

Drugs/CSA Schedules		Medical Uses	Trade or Other Names	Slang Names
Narcotics				
Opium	II III V	Analgesic, antidiarrheal	Dover's Powder, Paregoric, Parepectolin	Opium
Morphine	II III	Analgesic, antitussive	Morphine, MS-Contin, Roxanol, Roxanol-SR	M, Morpho, Morph, Tab, White, Stuff, Miss, Emma, Monkey
Codeine	II III V	Analgesic, antitussive	Tylenol w/Codeine, Empirin w/Codeine, Robitussin A-C, Fiorinal w/Codeine	School Boy
Heroin	I	None	Diacetylmorphine	Horse, Smack, H, Stuff, Junk
Hydromorphone	II	Analgesic	Dilaudid	Little D, Lords
Meperidine (Pethidine)	II	Analgesic	Demerol, Mepergan	Isonipecaine, Dolantol
Methadone	II	Analgesic	Dolophine, Methadone, Methadose	Dollies, Dolls, Amidone
Other Narcotics	I II III IV V	Analgisic, antidiarrheal, antitussive	Numorphan, Percodan, Percocet, Tylox, Tussionex, Fentanyl, Darvon, Lomotil, Talwin[a]	T. and Blue's, Designer Drugs (Fentanyl Derivatives), China White
Depressants				
Chloral Hydrate	IV	Hypnotic	Noctec	—
Barbiturates	II III IV	Anesthetic, anticonvulsant, sedative, hypnotic, veterinary euthanasia agent	Amytal, Butisol, Fiorinal, Lotusate, Nembutal, Seconal, Tuinal, Phenobarbitol	Yellows, Yellow Jackets, Barbs, Reds, Redbirds, Tooies, Phennies
Benzodiazepines	IV	Antianxiety, anticonvulsant, sedative, hypnotic	Ativan, Dalmane, Diazepam, Librium, Xanax, Serax, Valium, Tranxene, Verstran, Versed, Halcion, Paxipam, Restoril	Downers, Goof Balls, Sleeping Pills, Candy
Methaqualone	I	Sedative, hypnotic	Quaalude	Lude, Quay, Guad, Mandrex
Glutethimide	III	Sedative, hypnotic	Doriden	—
Other Depressants	III IV	Anitanxiety, sedative, hypnotic	Equanil, Miltown, Noludar, Placidyl, Valmid	Tranquilizers, Muscle Relaxants, Sleeping Pills

Dependence Physical/ Psychological	Tolerance	Duration (hours)	Administration Methods	Possible Effects	Effects of Overdose	Withdrawal Syndrome
High/High	Yes	3–6	Oral, smoked	Euphoria, drowsiness, respiratory depression, constricted pupils, nausea	Slow and shallow breathing, clammy skin, convulsions, coma, possible death	Watery eyes, runny nose, yawning, loss of appetite, irritability, tremors, panic, cramps, nausea, chills and sweating
High/High	Yes	3–6	Oral, smoked, injected			
Mod./Mod.	Yes	3–6	Oral, injected			
High/High	Yes	3–6	Injected, sniffed, smoked			
High/High	Yes	3–6	Oral, injected			
High/High	Yes	3–6	Oral, injected			
High/ High–Low	Yes	12–24	Oral, injected			
High–Low/ High–Low	Yes	Variable	Oral, injected			
Mod./Mod.	Yes	5–8	Oral	Slurred speech, disorientation, drunken behavior without odor of alcohol	Shallow respiration, clammy skin, dilated pupils, weak and rapid pulse, coma, possible death	Anxiety, insomnia, tremors, delirium, convulsions, possible death
High–Mod./ High/Mod.	Yes	1–16	Oral			
Low/Low	Yes	4–8	Oral			
High/High	Yes	4–8	Oral			
High/Mod.	Yes	4–8	Oral			
Mod./Mod.	Yes	4–8	Oral			

[a] Not designated as a narcotic under C.S.A. (Controlled Substances Act).

APPENDIX 1-1 Drugs of use and abuse, continued

Drugs/CSA Schedules		Medical Uses	Trade or Other Names	Slang Names
Stimulants				
Cocaine[b]	II	Local anesthetic		Bump, Toot, C, Coke, Flake, Snow, Candy, Crack
Amphetamines	II	Attention deficit disorders, narcolepsy, weight control	Biphetamine, Desoxyn, Dexedrine	Pep Pills, Bennies, Uppers, Truck Drivers, Dexies, Black Beauties, Speed
Phenmetrazine	II	Weight control	Preludin	Uppers, Peaches, Hearts
Methylphenidate	II	Attention deficit disorders, narcolepsy	Ritalin	Speed, Meth, Crystal, Crank, Go Fast
Other Stimulants	III IV	Weight control	Adipex, Cylert, Didrex, Ionamin, Melfiat, Plegine, Sanorex, Tenuate, Tepanil, Prelu-2	—
Hallucinogens				
LSD	I	None		Acid, Microdot, Cubes
Mescaline and Peyote	I	None		Mesc Buttons, Cactus
Amphetamine Variants	I	None	2, 5-DMA, PMA, STP, MDA, MDMA, TMA, DOM, DOB	Ecstasy, Designer Drugs
Phencyclidine	II	None	PCP	PCP, Angle Dust, Hog, Peace Pill
Phencyclidine Analogues	I	None	PCE, PCPY, TCP	—
Other Hallucinogens	I	None	Bufotenine, Ibogaine, DMT, DET, Psilocybin, Psilocyn	Sacred Mushrooms, Magic Mushrooms, Mushrooms
Cannabis				
Marijuana	I	None		Pot, Grass, Reefer, Roach, Maui Wowie, Joint, Weed, Loco Weed, Mary Jane
Tetrahydrocannabinol	I II	Cancer chemotherapy antinauseant	THC, Marinol	THC
Hashish	I	None		Hash
Hashish Oil	I	None		Hash Oil
Inhalants		None	Gasoline, Airplane Glue, Veg. Spray, Hairspray, Deodorants, Spray Paint, Liquid Paper, Paint Thinner, Rubber Cement	Sniffing, Glue Sniffing Snorting

[b] Designated as a narcotic under C.S.A.

Dependence Physical/ Psychological	Tolerance	Duration (hours)	Administration Methods	Possible Effects	Effects of Overdose	Withdrawal Syndrome
Possible/High	Yes	1–2	Sniffed, smoked, injected	Increased alertness, excitation, euphoria, increased pulse rate and blood pressure, insomnia, loss of appetite	Agitation, increase in body temperature, hallucinations, convulsions, possible death	Apathy, long periods of sleep, irritability, depression, disorientation
Possible/High	Yes	2–4	Oral, injected			
Possible/High	Yes	2–4	Oral, injected			
Possible/Mod.	Yes	2–4	Oral, injected			
Possible/High	Yes	2–4	Oral, injected			
None/Unknown	Yes	8–12	Oral	Illusions and hallucinations, poor perception of time and distance	Longer, more intense "trip" episodes, psychosis, possible death	Withdrawal syndrome not reported
None/Unknown	Yes	8–12	Oral			
Unknown/ Unknown	Yes	Variable	Oral, injected			
Unknown/High	Yes	Days	Smoked, oral, injected			
Unknown/High	Yes	Days	Smoked, oral, injected			
None/Unknown	Possible	Variable	Smoked, oral, injected, sniffed			
Unknown/Mod.	Yes	2–4	Smoked, oral	Euphoria, relaxed inhibitions, increased appetite, disoriented behavior	Fatigue, paranoia, possible psychosis	Insomnia, hyperactivity and decreased appetite occasionally reported
Unknown/Mod.	Yes	2–4	Smoked, oral			
Unknown/Mod.	Yes	2–4	Smoked, oral			
Unknown/Mod.	Yes	2–4	Smoked, oral			
None/Unknown	Yes	30 min.	Sniffed	Euphoria, headaches, nausea, fainting, stupor, rapid heartbeat	Damage to lungs, liver, kidneys, bone marrow, suffocation, choking, anemia, possible stroke, sudden death	Insomnia, increased appetite, depression, irritability, headache

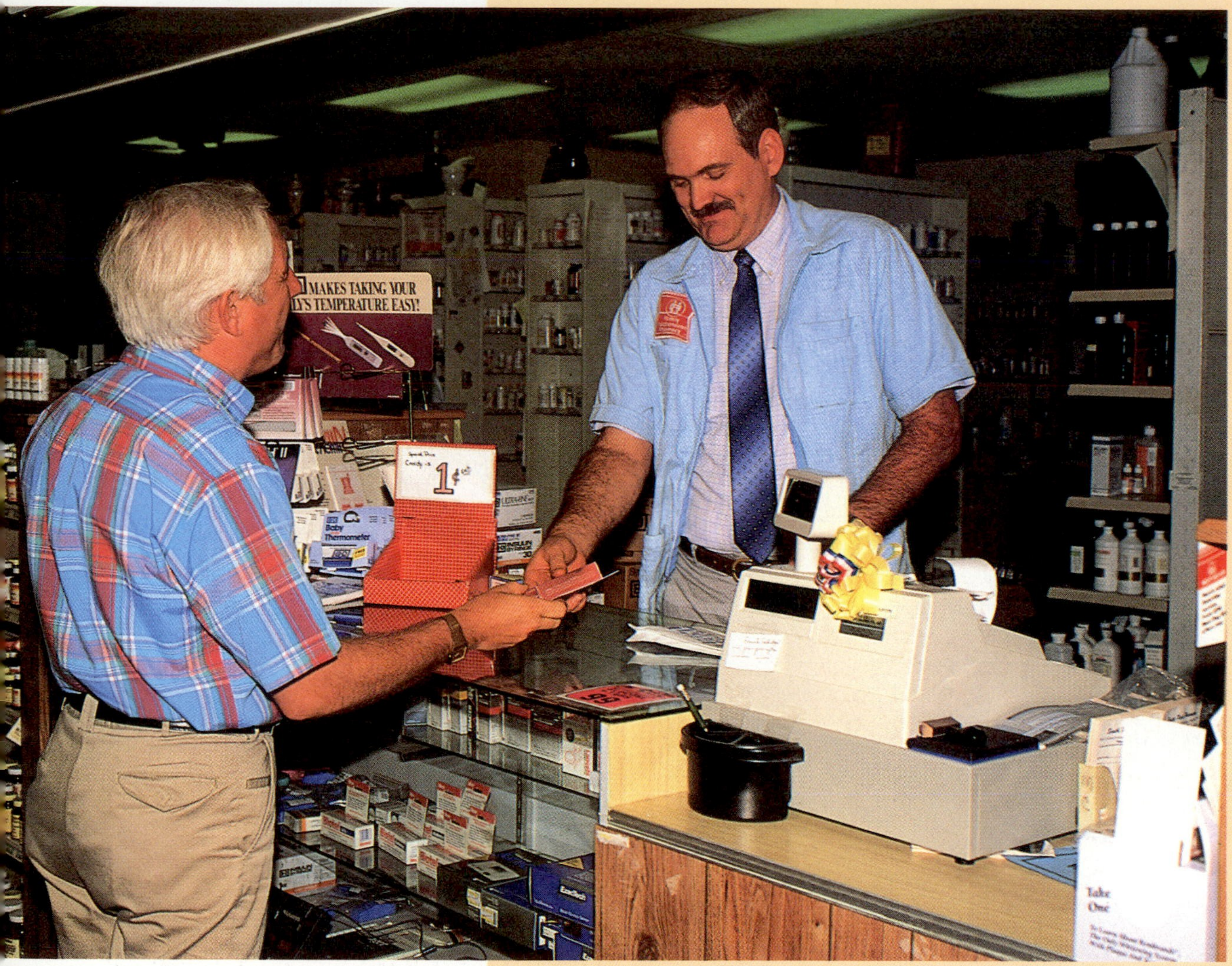

Chapter 2

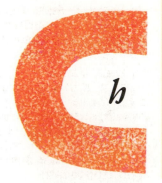

Did You Know That . . .

- Drug use and drug dealing are major factors in the growth of crime and violence among the young.
- Biological explanations of drugs trace the desire for drug use to innate physical beginnings and suggest that the tendency to abuse drugs may be an inherited predisposition.
- A strong relation exists between severe drug addiction and mental illness.
- Sigmund Freud believed that the addiction to drugs was an outgrowth of habitual (compulsive) masturbatory activity.
- Such personality traits as extreme forms of introversion and extraversion may explain why many people abuse drugs.
- Drug use is mostly learned from others.
- Whenever drug use becomes consistent and habitual, it usually occurs in the peer group setting, with people we like.
- Drugs are sometimes used to compensate for a lack of self-confidence.
- No single theory can explain why most people use drugs.
- Some theories advocate that an individual's alliance with drug-using peers largely results from an inability to cope with rapid societal change.
- People who perceive themselves as drug users are more likely to develop serious drug abuse problems.

Explaining Drug Use and Abuse

Learning Objectives

On completing this chapter, you will be able to

1. List six reasons why drug use or abuse is a more serious problem today than it was in the past.
2. List and briefly describe the following biological theories as they relate to drug use and abuse: genetic pursuit of pleasure, self-medication, and genetic influence.
3. Explain the relationships between some mental disorders and possible effects of certain drugs.
4. Explain the relationship between introverted or extraverted personality patterns and possible effects of stimulants or depressants.
5. Briefly define and explain reinforcement or learning theory and some of its applications to drug use and abuse.
6. List and briefly describe the following sociological theories as they relate to drug use and

continued

Healthy People 2000

Increase to at least 45% the proportion of people with major depressive disorders who obtain treatment.

Increase to at least 75% the proportion of people aged 10 and older who have discussed issues related to . . . tobacco, alcohol, other drugs, or safety with family members on at least one occasion during the preceding month.

L E A R N I N G   O B J E C T I V E S

abuse: (1) social influence theories, namely social learning, social influence (the role of significant others in the socialization process), labeling, and subculture theories; and (2) structural influence theories, namely social disorganization and social strain and control theories.

7 Describe symptoms and indicators of possible drug use or abuse in childhood behavior patterns.

8 List and describe three factors in the learning process that Howard Becker believes first-time users go through before they become attached to using illicit psychoactive drugs.

9 Define the following concepts: primary and secondary deviance, master status, and retrospective interpretation.

10 Explain why both internal and external controls against drug use are not sufficient to block the allure of drugs (Reckless's containment theory).

A Changing World

Historical records document drug use as far back as 2240 B.C., when Hammurabi, the Babylonian king and lawgiver, addressed the problems associated with drinking alcohol. Further, as noted in Chapter 1, virtually every culture has had problems with drug use and abuse. Based on this information, we can conclude that drug use and abuse is a very old problem. Some may wonder why we need to study and seek explanations for this age-old problem.

To suggest why the quest for explanations and information is more important than ever, we offer six reasons why drug use and abuse is an even more serious issue than it was in the past and thus worthy of study:

1. From 1960 to the present, drug use has become a widespread phenomenon. Before the 1960s, drug use was a serious problem only within certain isolated populations. Today, however, it affects nearly every social group.
2. Today, drugs are much more potent than they were years ago. For example, in 1960, the average THC content of marijuana was 1 to 2%. (THC is the ingredient responsible for making a person "high.") Today, the amount of THC in marijuana varies between 4 and 6%. Marijuana from Colombia ranges between 4 and 6%. Other more refined varieties usually grown without seeds, such as ***sinsemilla***, range between 6 and 8%. To a large extent, the increase of THC content is due to improved cultivation techniques (Mijuriya and Aldrich 1988). Crack and other manufactured drugs offer potent effects at low cost, vastly multiplying the damage potential of drug abuse.
3. Whether they are legal or not, drugs have become commonplace, and their sale is a multibillion-dollar-a-year business, with major influence on many national economies.
4. Drug use endangers the future of a society by physically harming its youth and potentially destroying the lives of many young men and women. When "gateway" drugs such as alcohol and tobacco are used at an early age, there is a strong possibility that the use will progress to other drugs, such as marijuana, cocaine, and amphetamines. Early drug use will likely lead to a lifelong habit, which has serious implications for the future.
5. Drug use and drug dealing is becoming a major factor in the growth of crime, especially among the young. Violent delinquent gangs are increasing at an alarming rate (Hutchinson and Kyle 1993; Moore 1993). Violent gun shootings, drive-by killings, car jacking, and "wilding" (Cummings 1993, 49) are common in cities (and increasing in small towns), such that the public has reacted with dismay, outrage, and fear (Moore 1993; Kunen 1989; and Will 1990, 64).

6. The possibility of serious accidents caused by drug users is greater as people become more dependent on technology. For instance, the operation of sophisticated machines and electronic equipment requires that workers and professionals be free of the effect of mind-altering drugs. Just imagine if several computer programmers responsible for supervising air traffic control were occasional cocaine users, or if technicians at a major x-ray diagnostic and cancer treatment center smoked marijuana during their lunch breaks.

Why does a nation such as ours have such a severe drug problem? With remarkable and unsurpassed excellence in scientific, technological, and electronic accomplishments, one might think that in the United States drug use and/or abuse could be controlled and would begin to diminish. One might also think that the allure of drugs could further diminish when we look at the statistically high proportions of accidents, crimes, marital strife and divorce, addiction, and death rates from the use and abuse of licit and illicit drugs. Yet such social, economic, and medical costs have not served as a deterrent to drug use.

Considering these costs, what explains the continuing use and abuse of drugs? What could possibly sustain and feed the allure of drugs? Why are drugs used when the consequences are so well documented?

In answering these questions, we need to recall from Chapter 1 some basic reasons why people take drugs:

1. People may be searching for pleasure, and drugs may make them feel good.
2. Drugs may relieve stress or tension or provide a temporary escape for people with anxiety.
3. Peer pressure is strong, especially for young people. The use of drugs has become a rite of passage in some levels of society.
4. In some cases, drugs may enhance religious or mystical experiences. A few cultures teach children how to use specific drugs for this purpose.
5. Drugs can relieve pain and symptoms of illness.

Although these reasons may suggest some underlying causes for excessive or abusive drug use, they also suggest that the variety and complexity of explanations and motivations are almost infinite. For any one individual, it is seldom clear when nondestructive use becomes abuse. When we consider the wide use of such licit drugs as alcohol, nicotine, and caffeine, we find that over 88% (U.S. Bureau of the Census 1990, 122) of the U.S. population are daily drug users in some form. Further, as we will see in the remaining chapters of this text, almost any of the hundreds of moods humans are capable of can be mimicked by some drug.

We can therefore begin to understand why the explanation for drug use and abuse is complicated and cannot be forced into one or two theories. In attempting to answer the question of why people use drugs, researchers have tackled the question from three major theoretical positions, namely, biological, psychological, and sociological perspectives. The remainder of this chapter discusses these three major explanations.

Biological Explanations

As noted in Chapter 1, biological explanations have tended to use genetic theories or to use the disease model for explaining drug addiction. The view that alcoholism is a sickness dates back approximately 200 years (Conrad and Schneider 1980). The specific disease perspective is based on E. M. Jellinek's (1960) view that alcoholism largely involves a loss of control over drinking and that the drinker experiences clearly distinguishable phases in his or her drinking patterns. Thus, the disease model views drug abuse as an illness in need of treatment or therapy. For example, concerning alcoholism, the illness affects the abuser to the point of loss of control.

According to biological theories, drug abuse has an innate physical beginning stemming from constitutional physical characteristics that cause certain individuals either to experiment or to crave

SINSEMILLA a more potent type of marijuana meaning "without seeds"

the drugs to the point of abusive use. **Genetic** and **biophysiological theories** explain addiction in terms of genetics, brain dysfunction, and biochemical patterns.

Biological explanations emphasize that the **central nervous system (CNS)** reward sensors are more sensitive to drugs that are abused, making the drug experience more pleasant and more alluring for these individuals (Jarvik 1990). (The CNS is defined as one of the major divisions of the nervous system, composed of the brain and spinal cord.) In contrast, others find the effects of drugs of abuse very unpleasant; such people are not likely to be attracted to these drugs (Farrar and Kearns 1989).

Most experts acknowledge that biological factors play an essential role in drug abuse. These factors likely determine how the brain responds to these drugs and why such substances are addictive. It is thought that by identifying the nature of the biological systems that contribute to drug abuse problems that improved therapy can be developed (Halloway 1991).

All the major biological explanations related to drug abuse assume that these substances exert their **psychoactive effects** (effects on the brain's mental functions) by altering brain chemistry. Specifically, the drugs of abuse interfere with the functioning of **neurotransmitters,** chemical messengers used for communication between brain regions (see Chapter 5 for details). The following are three principal biological theories that help explain why some drugs are abused and why certain people are more likely to become addicted when using these substances.

Drugs of Abuse Are Positive Reinforcers

Biological research has shown that stimulating some brain regions with an electrode causes very pleasurable sensations. In fact, laboratory animals would rather self-administer stimulation to these brain areas than eat or engage in sex. It has been demonstrated that drugs of abuse also activate these same pleasure centers of the brain, and because of this positive reinforcing property these drugs are repeatedly self-administered by animals and drug addicts (Koob 1992).

It is generally believed that most drugs with abuse potential enhance the pleasure centers by causing the release of a specific brain neurotransmitter called **dopamine** (Izenwasser and Kornetsky 1992): release of dopamine by the functional cells of the brain (neurons) leads to the drug-seeking behavior that is common to all drug addictions (Stolerman 1992). In addition, it has been proposed that overstimulation of these brain regions by continual drug use "exhausts" these dopamine systems and leads to depression and an inability to experience normal pleasure. It has been proposed that such a mechanism accounts for the craving and some of the other unpleasant effects experienced during withdrawal from these drugs (Imperato et al. 1992).

Drugs of Abuse and Psychiatric Disorders

Biological explanations are thought to be responsible for the substantial overlap that exists between drug addiction and mental illness. Because of the similarities, severe drug dependence itself is classified as a form of psychiatric disorder by the American Psychiatric Association (see the discussion of *DSM-IV* classifications later in this chapter). For example, abuse of drugs can themselves cause mental conditions that mimic major psychiatric illness such as schizophrenia, severe anxiety disorders, and suicidal depression (Halloway 1991;

GENETIC AND BIOPHYSIOLOGICAL THEORIES explanations of addiction in terms of genetic brain dysfunction and biochemical patterns

CNS (CENTRAL NERVOUS SYSTEM) one of the major divisions of the nervous system, composed of the brain and the spinal cord

PSYCHOACTIVE EFFECTS how drug substances alter and affect the brain's mental functions

NEUROTRANSMITTERS chemical messengers released by neurons (nerve cells) for communication with other cells

DOPAMINE the brain transmitter believed to mediate the rewarding aspects of most drugs of abuse

American Psychiatric Association 1994). It is believed that these similarities are due to the fact that common chemical factors (changes in neurotransmitter systems in the brain) are altered both by drugs of abuse and during episodes of psychiatric illness (Halloway 1991). Several important potential consequences of this relationship may help us understand the nature of drug abuse problems.

1. *Psychiatric disorders are potential risk factors for drug addiction, and* vice versa. This conclusion is supported by the fact that the incidence of mental illness is higher in the drug-abusing population than among those who do not abuse drugs. Thus, psychiatric illness is present in 37% of those with a severe alcoholic disorder and present in 53% of those with a severe nonalcohol drug disorder (Brady and Lydiard 1992). The issue of co-occurrence between drug abuse and mental illness is very important and research to study its prevalence is being encouraged by federal mental health and drug abuse programs ("Epidemiological and Services Research" 1994). Because of the common mechanisms, drug abuse is likely to expose or worsen psychiatric disorders (Halloway 1991). For example, in some urban hospitals as many as 38% of the patients admitted for acute psychiatric episodes have been using cocaine (Galanter et al. 1992).
2. *Therapies that are successful in treating psychiatric disorders may be useful in treating mental problems caused by the drugs of abuse.* In fact, the principal medications used to relieve psychosis, agitation, and suicidal behavior caused by intense use of drugs of abuse are the same therapeutic agents prescribed for the treatment of psychiatric disorders such as schizophrenia, anxiety disorders, and severe endogenous depression (Halloway 1991). It is likely that many of the therapeutic lessons we learn about dealing with psychiatric illnesses can be useful in drug abuse treatment, and *vice versa.*
3. *Abuse of drugs by some people may be an attempt to relieve underlying psychiatric disorders.* Such people commonly use CNS depressants such as alcohol to relieve anxiety, while CNS stimulants such as cocaine are frequently used by patients with depression disorders (Grinspoon 1993). In such cases, if the underlying psychiatric problem is relieved, the likelihood of successfully treating the drug abuse disorder improves substantially.

Genetic Explanations

One biological theory receiving close scrutiny is that inherited traits can predispose some individuals to drug addiction. Such theories have been supported by the observation that increased frequency of alcoholism and drug abuse exists among children of alcoholics and drug abusers (Uhl et al. 1993). Further support comes from reports from studies where separated and adopted identical twins (originated from the same genes) are more likely to have similar alcoholism and drug abuse problems than similarly treated fraternal twins (originated from two separate sets of genes). Such studies estimate that drug vulnerability due to genetic influences is approximately 38%, while environmental and social factors account for the balance (Uhl et al. 1993).

Other studies attempting to identify the specific genes that may predispose the carrier to drug abuse problems have suggested that a brain target site (called a *receptor*—see Chapter 5 for details) for dopamine is altered in a manner that increases the drug abuse vulnerability (Uhl et al. 1992). Although several genetic studies have confirmed these findings, others have not (Uhl et al. 1992). Studies that test for genetic factors in complex behaviors such as drug abuse are very difficult to conduct and interpret. It is sometimes impossible to design experiments that distinguish among genetic, social, environmental, and psychological influences in human populations. For example, it is well established that inherited traits are major contributors to psychiatric disorders, such as schizophrenia and depression (Gershon and Rieder 1992). It is also established that substance abuse disorders occur in approximately half of those with severe mental illness (Bartels et al. 1993). Thus, patients who abuse stimulants, such as cocaine, have a high incidence of depression (Grinspoon 1993). Because of this co-occurrence, a high incidence of an abnormal gene in a cocaine-abusing population may not be directly linked to drug abuse behavior, but may be associated with depression, which has a high representation in cocaine abusers (Uhl et al. 1992).

Theoretically genetic factors can directly or

CROSSCURRENTS

TOPIC: Drug abuse, or the tendency for drug abuse can be caused by biological forces that are beyond individual control or social forces that often involve self-selected or group influences.

1. Make a case, quoting at least three theories in this chapter that support ways in which drug abuse may develop biologically.
2. In opposition to the arguments supported by the three theories selected for part 1, cite at least three theories that support the argument that self-selected or group handicaps are largely responsible for the development of drug dependency.

(This assignment can easily be prepared as a class project where one group prepares and debates position 1, a second group prepares and debates position 2, and a third group summarizes and critiques the positions of groups 1 and 2.)

In conclusion, we find that although the evidence is convincing that biological factors are major contributors to drug abuse problems, clearly much more needs to be learned before we can fully understand their implications. However, as these factors are elucidated, we can hope they will generate greater appreciation of the nature of substance addiction and suggest better strategies to prevent or resolve drug abuse problems.

indirectly contribute to drug abuse vulnerability in several ways; for example,

1. Psychiatric disorders that are genetically determined may be relieved by drugs of abuse, thus encouraging their use.
2. In some people, reward centers of the brain may be genetically determined to be especially sensitive to addicting drugs; thus, use of drugs of abuse by these people would be particularly pleasurable and would lead to a high rate of addiction.
3. Character traits, such as insecurity and vulnerability, which often lead to drug abuse behavior, may be genetically determined, causing a high rate of addiction in these people.
4. Factors that determine how difficult it will be to break a drug addiction may be genetically determined, causing severe craving or very unpleasant withdrawal effects; such people are less likely to abandon their drug of abuse.

The appeal of the genetic theories for drug abuse is that once discovered they may help us to understand the reasons that drug addiction occurs in some individuals but not in others. In addition, if genetic factors play a major role in drug abuse, it might be possible to do genetic screening to identify people who are especially vulnerable to drug abuse problems and help such people avoid exposure to these substances. (See Crosscurrents box for an exercise that can promote your understanding of how biological determinants can affect drug abuse.)

Psychological Explanations

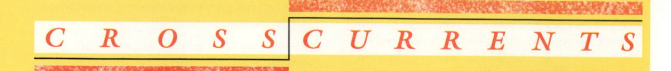

Psychological theories mostly deal with internal mental states, often associated with or exacerbated by social and environmental factors. Early psychological theories began with Freud, who linked "primal addictions" with masturbation, and postulated that all later addictions, including alcohol and other drugs, were caused by ego impairments. Freud felt that drugs fulfilled insecurities that stem from parental inadequacies, causing difficulty in adequately forming bonds of friendships. He said alcoholism (see Chapter 8) is an expression of the death instinct, as are self-destruction, narcissism, and oral fixations. Although Freud's views present interesting insights often not depicted in other theories, his theoretical concerns are difficult to operationalize, test, and provide data for verification.

Distinguishing Between Substance Abuse and Mental Disorders

Widely accepted categories of diagnosis for behavioral disorders, including substance abuse, have been established by the American Psychiatric Association. As standardized diagnostic categories, the characteristics of mental disorders have been analyzed by professional committees over many years and today are summarized in their fourth generation of development in a widely accepted book called the *DSM-IV,* or *Diagnostic and Statistical Manual,* 4th edition (American Psychiatric Association 1994). In addition to categories for severe psychotic disorders and more common neurotic disorders, experts in the field of psychiatry have established specific diagnostic criteria for various forms of substance abuse. All patterns of drug abuse that are described in the chapters of *Drugs and Society,* 4th edition, have a counterpart description in the *DSM-IV* manual for medical professionals. For example, the *DSM-IV* discusses the mental disorders resulting from the use or abuse of sedatives, hypnotics, or antianxiety drugs; alcohol; narcotics; amphetamine-like drugs; cocaine; caffeine; nicotine (tobacco); hallucinogens; phencyclidine (PCP); inhalants; and cannabis (marijuana). This manual of psychiatric diagnoses discusses in detail the mental disorders related to the taking of drugs of abuse, the side effects of medications and the consequence of toxic exposure to these substances (American Psychiatric Association 1994).

Because of the similarities between, and coexistence of, substance-related mental disorders and naturally occurring (referred to as *primary*) psychiatric disorders, it is sometimes difficult to distinguish between the two problems; however, in order for proper treatment to be rendered, the cause of the psychological symptoms needs to be determined. According to *DSM-IV* criteria, substance use (or abuse) disorders can be identified by the presence of the following features and their associated criteria:

1. *Substance dependence* that is distinguished by the presence of
   - Tolerance and a need for markedly increased amounts of drug
   - Withdrawal and continual use of the substance to prevent its occurrence
   - Unsuccessful efforts to reduce substance use despite knowledge of its harmful effects
   - A need to maintain a substantial supply of the substance
   - A change in lifestyle to accommodate use of the substance
2. *Substance abuse* that is distinguished by the presence of
   - Recurrent substance use causing an inability to fulfill major role obligations at work, school, or home
   - Recurrent substance use making some situations physically dangerous
   - Recurrent substance use leading to legal problems
   - Recurrent substance use leading to social and personal problems
3. *Substance intoxications* that are distinguished by
   - Development of reversible substance-related symptoms due to recent use of a drug
   - Expression of problematic behavioral or psychological changes due to the effects of substance on the brain
4. *Substance withdrawal* that is distinguished by
   - Development of a set of symptoms specifically related to the cessation of, or reduction in, substance use that has been heavy and prolonged
   - Associated symptoms that cause emotional and physical stress and interfere with social and occupational functioning

The occurrence and consequence of dependence, abuse, intoxication, and withdrawal are important distinguishing features of substance abuse disorders and are discussed in greater detail in Chapter 4 and in conjunction with each drug group.

According to the *DSM-IV,* other information that can also help distinguish between substance-induced and primary mental disorders are (1) personal and family medical, psychiatric, and drug histories; (2) physical examinations; and (3) laboratory tests to assess physiological functions and determine the presence or absence of drugs. However, the possibility of primary mental disorder should not be excluded just because the patient is using drugs—remember, many drug users are self-medicating primary psychiatric problems with substances of abuse. The coexistence of underlying psychiatric problems in a drug user is suggested by the following circumstances: (1) the psychiatric problems do not match the usual drug effects (for example, use of marijuana usually does not cause severe psychotic behavior); (2) the psychiatric disorder was present before the patient started abusing substances; and (3) the mental disorder persists for more than four weeks after substance use is stopped. The *DSM-IV* makes it clear that the relationship between mental disorders and substances of abuse is important for proper diagnosis, treatment, and understanding.

Personality and Drug Use

Since medieval times, personality theories of increasing sophistication have been used to classify long-term behavioral tendencies or traits that appear in individuals, and these traits have long been considered as influenced by biological or chemical factors. Although such classification systems have varied widely, nearly all have shared two commonly observed dimensions of personality: introversion and extraversion. Individuals who show a predominant tendency to turn their thoughts and feelings inward rather than to direct attention outward have been considered to show the trait of *introversion*. At the opposite extreme, a tendency to seek outward activity and sharing feelings with others has been called *extraversion*. Of course, every individual shows a mix of such traits in varying degrees and circumstances.

In some research studies, introversion and extraversion patterns have been associated with levels of neural arousal in brain stem circuits (Carlson 1990; J. A. Gray 1987), and these forms of arousal are similar and closely associated with effects caused by drug stimulants or depressants. Such research hypothesizes that people whose systems produce high levels of sensitivity to neural arousal may find high-intensity external stimuli to be painful, and may react by turning inward. With these extremely high levels of sensitivity, such people may experience neurotic levels of anxiety or panic disorders. On the other extreme, those whose systems provide them with very low levels of sensitivity to neural arousal may find that moderate stimuli are inadequate to produce responses. To reach moderate levels of arousal, they may turn outward to seek high-intensity external sources of stimulation (Eysenck and Eysenck 1985; Gray 1987).

Since high- and low-arousal symptoms are easy to create by using stimulants, depressants, or hallucinogens, it is possible that these personality patterns of introversion or extraversion may have some association with how a person reacts to substances. For people whose experience is predominantly introverted or extraverted, extremes of high or low sensitivity may be leading them to seek counteracting substances that become important methods of bringing experience to a level that seems bearable.

Theories Based on Learning

How are abuse patterns learned? Research on learning or conditioning explains how humans acquire new patterns of behavior by the close association or pairing of one significant reinforcing stimulus with another less significant or neutral stimulus. In learning by this method, people get used to certain behavior patterns. This process, known as *conditioning*, explains why pleasurable activities may become intimately connected with other activities that are also pleasurable, neutral, or even unpleasant. In addition, people can turn any new behavior into a recurrent and permanent one by the process of **habituation**—*repeating certain patterns of behavior until they become established or habitual.*

The basic process by which learning mechanisms can lead a person into drug use is described in Bejerot's **"addiction to pleasure" theory** (Bejerot 1965, 1972, 1975). The theory assumes that it is biologically normal to continue a pleasure stimulus when once begun. The pleasure derived from stimulation may become habitual when new and shorter nerve courses come into function and higher centers are disconnected. For example, the pleasure associated with getting high may become a learned conditioned response if opiate users discover that the drug and sexual stimulation are mutually reinforcing. Such mutual reinforcement makes opiate use become addictive when the two stimuli have become mutually reinforcing. At this point, drug use and sexual stimulation have become mutually reinforcing through paired associative learning.

Another example is when drug use is associated with receiving affection or approval in a social setting, such as within a peer group relationship. Initially, the use of particular drugs may not, in themselves, be very important or pleasurable to the individual. However, the affection experienced during intimate interaction when drugs are used becomes paired with the drug. The pleasure derived from peer approval, the intimacy often associated with such interaction coupled with drug use can become paired and associated. In this example, drug use and intimacy may become perceived as very worthwhile.

By the conditioning process, a pleasurable experience such as drug taking may become associated with a comforting or soothing environment. When this happens, two different outcomes may result. *One,* the user may feel uncomfortable taking the drug in any other environment (as marijuana or even a psychedelic drug, taken in another environment, may actually produce tension, insecurity, panic reactions), or—in the case of LSD, for example—a bad trip. *Two,* the user may become very accustomed or habituated to the familiar environment as part of the drug experience. The likely result is that through the process of developing drug tolerance (see Chapter 4), such a familiar environment may occur when the body begins to react less severely to the drug. Likewise, taking the drug in a different setting may cause a more severe or "fresh" reaction because the unfamiliar environment is not associated with the original habituated experience.

Finally, through this process of conditioning and habituation, a drug user can become accustomed to unpleasant effects of drug use such as withdrawal symptoms. Such unpleasant effects and experiences may become habituated—neutralized or less severe in their impact, so that the user continues taking drugs without feeling or experiencing the negative effects of the drug.

HABITUATION repeating certain patterns of behavior until they become established or habitual

"ADDICTION TO PLEASURE" THEORY theory that assumes that it is biologically normal to continue a pleasure stimulus when once begun

DIFFERENTIAL REINFORCEMENT the ratio between reinforcers favorable and disfavorable for sustaining drug use behavior

Sociological Social Psychology Learning Theories

Other extensions of reinforcement or learning theory focus on how positive social influences by drug-using peers reinforce the allure of drugs. Social interaction, peer *camaraderie* and approval, and drug use work together as positive reinforcers sustaining drug use (Akers 1992). Thus, if the effects of drug use become personally rewarding, "or become reinforcing through conditioning, the chances of continuing to use are greater than for stopping" (Akers 1992, 86). It is through learned expectations, association with others who reinforce drug use, that individuals *learn* the pleasures of drug taking (Becker 1963, 1967). Similarly, if the experiences are interpreted as *dis*favorable, as with a frightening LSD trip, then the experience will be negatively perceived and the distinctive appeal of the drug will diminish rapidly.

Note that positive reinforcers, such as peers, other friends and acquaintances, family members, and drug advertisements, do not act alone in inciting and sustaining drug use. Learning theory as defined here also relies on some variable amounts of imitation and trial-and-error learning methods.

Finally, **differential reinforcement**—defined as the ratio between reinforcers favorable and disfavorable for sustaining drug use behavior—must be considered. The use and eventual abuse of drugs can vary with certain favorable or unfavorable reinforcing experiences. The primary determining conditions are (1) the amount of exposure to drug-using peers versus non-drug-using peers, (2) the general preference for drug use in a particular neighborhood or community, (3) age of initial use (younger adolescents are more greatly affected than older adolescents), and (4) frequency of drug use among peer members.

Sociological Explanations

Sociological explanations for drug use share important commonalties with psychological explanations under social learning theories. The main distinguishing features determining psychological and sociological explanations are that psychological explanations focus more on how the *internal states* of the drug user are affected by social relationships within families, peers, and other more distant relationships. Sociological explanations, in contrast, focus on how factors *outside the individual may affect drug users.* Such outside forces could be the types of families, lifestyles of peer groups, or types of neighborhoods and communities. Sociology views the motivation for drug use as largely determined by the types and quality of bonds the drug user or potential drug user has with significant others or with physical surroundings. The degree of influence with which outside factors are believed to affect the drug user distinguishes psychological from sociological analyses.

As previously stated, no one biological and psychological theory can adequately explain why most people use drugs. People differ from one another in terms of such traits as introversion or extraversion, and differ extensively in the outlooks and problems they face, and as a result, take drugs for very different reasons. Theories may differ from each other partly because of these variations, and partly because the explanations are derived from different perspectives of biology, psychology, and sociology. Explanations may also differ because they simultaneously try to account for individual personality characteristics, unique social influences and situations, and specific circumstances regarding why drugs are used.

Two major sociological explanations in this section are *social influence theories* and *structural influence theories.* Micro- and macroscopic theoretical explanations divide the sociological theories for explaining drug use. This section begins with **microscopic explanations** based on social influence theories and concludes with **macroscopic** structural influence theories. Although both sets of theories focus on understanding why people use drugs, social influence theories direct their attention to the role of significant others and the impact this has on the individual. Structural influence theories, in contrast, are based on the belief that the particular organization of society has a major influence on drug use and abuse.

Social Influence Theories

The theories presented in this section are known as (1) social learning, (2) the role of significant others in socialization, (3) labeling, and (4) subculture theories. The bases of these theories are that an individual's motivation to seek drugs is caused by social influence or coercion.

Social Learning Theory **Social learning theory** explains drug use as a form of learned behavior. Conventional learning occurs through imitation, trial and error, improvisation, rewarding appropriate behavior, and cognitive mental processes. Social learning theory focuses directly on how drug use and abuse is acquired through interaction with others who use and abuse drugs.

The theory emphasizes the pervasive influence of *primary groups,* which are groups that share a high amount of intimacy and spontaneity and whose members are bonded emotionally. Families and residents of a close-knit urban neighborhood are examples of primary groups. In contrast, *secondary groups* are groups that share segmented relationships where interaction is based on prescribed role patterns. An example of a secondary group would be the relationship between you and a sales clerk in a grocery store or among a group of employees scattered throughout a corporation.

Social learning theory addresses a type of interaction that is *highly specific.* This type of interaction involves learning specific motives, techniques, and appropriate meanings that are commonly attached to a particular type of drug. (See

MICROSCOPIC EXPLANATIONS closeup, detailed, mostly day-to-day explanations for why people use drugs

MACROSCOPIC EXPLANATIONS comprehensive, overall structural or general explanations for why people use drugs

SOCIAL LEARNING THEORY explanations of drug use behavior as a form of learned behavior

Case in Point

This excerpt, from the author's files, illustrates social learning theory.

> I first started using drugs, mostly alcohol and pot, because my best friend in high school was using drugs. My best friend Tim (a pseudonym) learned from his older sister [to use drugs]. Before I actually tried pot, Tim kept telling me how great it was to be high on dope, he said it was much better than beer. I was really nervous the first time I tried pot with Tim and another friend even though I heard so much detail about it from Tim before that first time I tried it. The first time I tried it, it was a complete letdown. The second time (the next day, I think it was), I remember I was talking about a teacher we had and in the middle of the conversation, I remember how everything appeared different. I started feeling happy and while listening to Tim as he poked jokes at the teacher, I started to hear the background music more clearly than ever before. By the time the music ended, and a new CD started, I knew I was high. He gave me a smile I will never forget. Especially, I remember his eyes staring at me when he blurted out, "Welcome to the club, Peter."

Source: Interview with a 22-year-old male student at a private liberal arts college in the Midwest, conducted by Peter Venturelli on 9 October 1993.

Case in Point box as an example of social learning theory.)

As the sociologist Howard Becker points out in his well-known article "Becoming a Marijuana User," the novice who is perceived as a first-time user has to learn the technique:

> I was smoking like I did an ordinary cigarette. He said, "No, don't do it like that." He said, "Suck it, you know, draw in and hold it in your lungs till you . . . for a period of time."
>
> I said, "Is there any limit of time to hold it?"
>
> He said, "No, just till you feel that you want to let it out, let it out." So I did that three or four times. (Becker 1966, 47)

Learning to perceive the effects of the drug is the second major outcome in the process of becoming a regular user. Here, the ability to feel the authentic effects of the drug is being learned. The more experienced drug users in the group impart their knowledge to naive first-time users. The coaching information they provide describes how to recognize the euphoric effects of the drug, as illustrated in another excerpt:

> I just sat there waiting for something to happen, but I really didn't know what to expect. After the fifth "hit" [a hit consists of deeply inhaling a marijuana cigarette as it is being passed around and shared in a group], I was just about ready to give up ever getting "high."
>
> Then suddenly, my best buddy looked deeply into my eyes and said, "Aren't you 'high' yet?" Instead of just answering the question, I immediately repeated the same words the exact way he asked me. In a flash, we both simultaneously burst out laughing. This uncontrollable laughter went on for what appeared to be over five minutes. Then he said, "You silly ass, it's not like an alcohol 'high,' it's a 'high high.' Don't you feel it? It's a totally different kind of 'high.'"
>
> At that very moment, I knew I was definitely 'high' on the stuff. If this friend would not have said this to me, I probably would have continued thinking that getting 'high' on the hash was impossible for me.

Source: This three-paragraph excerpt is from an interview with a 17-year-old male attending a small, private liberal arts college in the Southeast, conducted by Peter Venturelli on 15 May 1984.

After learning the technique and how to perceive the effects of the drug, Becker informs us that members in groups teach first-time users how to enjoy the experience:

> Because they [first-time users] think they're going to keep going up, up, up till they lose their minds or begin doing weird things or something. You have to like reassure them, explain to them that they're not really flipping or anything, that they're gonna be all right. You have to just talk them out of being afraid. Keep talking to them, reassuring, telling them it's all right. And come on with your own story, you know: "The same thing happened to me. You'll get to like that after awhile." Keep coming on like that; pretty soon you talk them out of being scared . . . that gives them more confidence. (Becker 1966, 55)

Once drug use has begun, continuing the behavior involves the following learned sequence: (1) where and from whom the drug can be purchased, (2) how to maintain the secrecy of use from authority figures and casual acquaintances, and (3) justification(s) for continual use.

Role of Significant Others Once a pattern of drug use has been established, what part of the learning process sustains drug-taking behavior? Edwin Sutherland (1947, 5–9), a pioneering criminologist in sociology, believes that the mastery of criminal behavior depends on the frequency, duration, priority, and intensity of contact with others who are involved in similar behavior. This theory can also be applied to drug-taking behavior.

In applying Sutherland's principles of social learning to drug use, which he calls *differential association theory,* the focus is on how other members of social groups reward criminal behavior and under what conditions this deviance is perceived as important and pleasurable.

Becker and Sutherland's theories explain why adolescents use psychoactive drugs. Essentially, both theories say that the use of drugs is learned during intimate interaction with others who serve as a primary group. See Here and Now box for information on how the role of significant others can determine a child's disposition to illicit drug use.

Learning theory also explains how adults and the elderly acquire a favorable attitude toward drug-taking behavior. This occurs through such influences as drug advertising, with its emphases on testimonials by avid users, medical advice, or assurances from actors and actresses portraying physicians or nurses. Listeners, viewers, or readers who experience such commercials promoting particular brand-name over-the-counter drugs, are bombarded with the necessary motives, techniques, and appropriate attitudes for consuming drugs. When drug advertisements and medical experts recommend a particular drug for specific ailments, they in effect are authoritatively persuading viewers, listeners, or readers that taking a drug will soothe or cure the medical problem presented.

AMOTIVATIONAL SYNDROME intensive state of lethargy coinciding with heavy marijuana use

Are Drug Users Socialized Differently?

Social scientists, primarily sociologists and social psychologists, believe that most social development patterns are closely linked to drug use. Based on the age when an adolescent starts to consume alcohol, predictions can be made about his or her sexual behavior, academic performance, and other behaviors, such as lying, cheating, fighting, and marijuana use. The same predictions can be made when the adolescent begins using marijuana. Early intense use of alcohol or marijuana represents a move toward less conventional behavior, greater susceptibility to peer influence, increased delinquency, and lower achievement in school. In general, drug abusers have 14 characteristics in common:

1. Their drug use usually follows clear-cut developmental steps and sequences. Use of legal drugs, such as alcohol and cigarettes, almost always precedes use of illegal drugs.
2. Use of certain drugs, particularly marijuana, is linked to the **amotivational syndrome,** which causes a general change in personality. This change is characterized by apathy, a lack of interest in pursuing and accomplishing goals, and a noticeable lack of ambition.[1]

[1]Some argue that perhaps a general lack of ambition (also known as *lethargy*) may *precede* rather than *result from* marijuana use, or that aspects of the amotivational syndrome are already present in heavy marijuana users even before the drug is used and that the use of marijuana merely heightens the syndrome. In any case, the steady use of marijuana and the amotivational syndrome often occur together.

Here and Now

Symptoms of Drug and Alcohol Abuse

Profile of the Child Least Likely to Use Drugs

1. Child comes from a strong family.
2. Family has a clearly stated policy toward drug use.
3. Child has strong religious convictions.
4. Child is an independent thinker, not easily swayed by peer pressure.
5. Parents know the child's friends and the friends' parents.
6. Child often invites friends into the house and their behavior is open, not secretive.
7. Child is busy, productive, and pursues many interests.
8. Child has a good secure feeling of self.
9. Parents are comfortable with their own use of alcohol, drugs, and pills and set a good example in using these substances and are comfortable in discussing their use.
10. Parents set a good example in handling crisis situations.

Symptoms of Possible Drug Use

EDITOR'S NOTE: A child should display more than merely one of the symptoms below when experimenting with drugs. Please remember that any number of the symptoms could also be the result of a physical impairment or disorder.

1. Abrupt change in behavior. Example from very active to passive, loss of interest in previously pursued activities such as sports or hobbies.
2. Diminished drive and ambition.
3. Moodiness.
4. Shortened attention span.
5. Impaired communication such as slurred speech, jumbled thinking.
6. Significant change in quality of school work.
7. Deteriorating judgment and loss of short-term memory.
8. Distinct lessening of family closeness and warmth.
9. Sudden carelessness of appearance.
10. Inappropriate overreaction to even mild criticism.
11. Secretiveness about whereabouts and personal possessions.
12. Friends who avoid introduction or appearance in the child's home.
13. Use of words that have odd, underworld connotations.
14. Secretiveness and/or desperation for money.
15. Rapid weight loss or appetite loss.
16. "Drifting off" beyond normal daydreaming.
17. Extreme behavioral changes such as hallucination, violence, unconsciousness, etc., could indicate a dangerous situation is close at hand needing fast medical attention.
18. Unprescribed or unidentifiable pills.
19. Strange "contraptions" or hidden articles.
20. Articles missing from the house. Child could be stealing to receive money to pay for drugs.

Source: L.A.W. Publications, *Let's All Work to Fight Drug Abuse*, new ed. (Addison, TX: C & L Printing Company, 1985) 38. Used with permission of the publisher.

3. Immaturity, maladjustment, or insecurity usually precede the use of marijuana and other illicit drugs.
4. Those more likely to try illicit drugs especially before age 12 usually have a history of poor school performance and classroom disobedience.
5. Delinquent or repetitive deviant activities usually precede involvement with illicit drugs.
6. A set of values and attitudes that facilitates the development of deviant behavior exists before the person tries illicit drugs.
7. A social setting where drug use is common, such as communities and neighborhoods where peers use drugs indiscriminately and where "crack" houses and drug-using gangs dominate, are likely to reinforce and increase the predisposition to drug use.
8. Drug-induced behaviors and drug-related attitudes of peers are usually among the strongest predictors of subsequent drug involvement.
9. Children who feel their parents are distant from their emotional needs are more likely to become drug addicted.
10. The older people are when they start using drugs, the greater the probability of stopping drug use. The period of greatest risk of initiation into illicit drug use is usually over by the early twenties.
11. The family structure has changed. More than half the women in the United States work outside the home. How this affects the quality of child care and nurturing is difficult to assess. Also, a higher percentage of children are being raised in single-parent households, due to separation and divorce.
12. Mobility obstructs a sense of permanency, and it contributes to a lack of self-esteem. Often children are moved from one location to another, and their community can easily become nothing more than a group of strangers. There may be little pride in home or community and no commitment to society.
13. Among minority members, a major factor involved in drug dependence is a feeling of powerlessness due to discrimination based on race, gender, social standing, or other attributes. Groups subject to discrimination have a disproportionately high rate of unemployment and below-average income. The Carnegie Council on Children estimated that 19 million children grow up in poverty every year and feel powerless in their situation. The adults they have as role models are unemployed and powerless. There are higher rates of delinquency and drug addiction in such settings.
14. Abusers that become highly involved in selling drugs begin by witnessing that drug trafficking is a lucrative business, especially in rundown neighborhoods. In some communities, selling drugs is the only available alternative to real economic success (Blum and Richards 1979; Williams 1989; Wilson 1988).

Labeling Theory Although the controversy continues whether this is a theory or perspective (Akers 1968, 1992; Plummer 1979), the position we take is that labeling is a theory, for it explains something very important with respect to drug use. Labeling theory does not explain why initial drug use occurs; it does, however, detail the processes by which many people come to view themselves as socially deviant from others. Note that the terms *deviant* (in cases of individuals) or *deviance* (in cases of behavior), are sociologically defined as involving difference(s) from expected patterns of social behavior. The terms are not used in a judgmental manner, nor are the individuals or the behavior *judged* to be deviant; instead, the terms refer to norm violators or norm violations.

Labeling theory says that other people whose impressions of us we value have a determining influence over our self-image (Best 1994, 237; Goode 1994, 99). (For an example of how labeling theory applies to real-life situations, see Case in Point box.) Implied in this theory is that we have a small amount of control over the image we portray. Instead, members of society, especially those we consider to be significant others, have much power in defining or redefining our image. The image we have of ourselves is vested in the people

LABELING THEORY a theory stressing that other peoples' impressions have a direct influence over one's self-image

Here and Now

Study Finds Higher Drug Use Among Adolescents Whose Parents Divorce

Children who are adolescents when their parents divorce have more extensive drug use and more drug-related health, legal, and other problems than their peers, according to a recent study by NIDA grantee Dr. Richard Needle. The study has linked the extent of teens' drug use to their age at the time of their parents' divorce.

Dr. Needle, who performed the research at the University of Minnesota, found that teenagers whose parents divorce use more drugs and experience more drug-related problems than two other groups of adolescents: those who were 10 or younger when their parents divorced, and those whose parents remained married.

The research "contributes to our understanding of the crucial and changing roles the family plays in explaining adolescents' drug-using behavior," says Dr. Needle, who is serving a 2-year appointment as a senior staff fellow in NIDA's Community Research Branch.

The study also has important implications for drug abuse prevention efforts, says Dr. Meyer Glantz, of NIDA's Prevention Research Branch. "This study says that not everybody is at the same risk for drug use," says Dr. Glantz. "People at greater risk can be identified, and programs should be developed to meet their special needs."

Dr. Needle's 5-year study, which began in 1982, followed 508 randomly selected families with children ages 11, 12, or 13, who were participants in a large health maintenance organization. Over the course of the study, 67 families experienced disruption, including separation, divorce, and remarriage.

The study found that drug use among all adolescents increased over time. However, drug use was higher among adolescents whose parents had divorced, either when their children were preteens or teenagers. Drug use was highest for those teens whose parents divorced during their children's adolescent years. The latter group also reported more adverse consequences related to drug use, such as physical problems, family disputes, and arrests.

Dr. Needle found distinct gender differences in the way divorce affected adolescent drug use, whether the divorce occurred during the offspring's childhood or adolescent years. Males whose parents divorced reported more drug use and drug-related problems than females. Females whose care-taking parent remarried reported increased drug use after the remarriage. By contrast, males whose care-taking parent remarried reported a decrease in drug-related problems following the remarriage.

Dr. Needle cautions that the findings may be of limited applicability, since most of the families were White and had middle to high income levels. He also urges that the findings not be interpreted simplistically. "These data should not be interpreted as an argument for the nuclear family," Dr. Needle says.

The findings, says Dr. Glantz, indicate the complex ways in which factors such as divorce and remarriage can influence drug-using behavior, particularly when the disruptions occur during adolescence.

Since the latest statistics indicate that one out of every two marriages will end in divorce, does this accurately predict that most children from divorced families will use and abuse drugs? In cases of the children from divorced families, are there any other factors that can predict potential drug use?

Reference

Needle, Richard H.; Su, Susan S.; and Doherty, William J. Divorce, remarriage, and adolescent substance use: A prospective longitudinal study. *Journal of Marriage and the Family* 52:157–169, 1990.

Source: National Institute on Drug Abuse, "Study Finds Higher Use Among Adolescents Whose Parents Divorce." *NIDA Notes* 5, no. 3 (Summer 1990): 10.

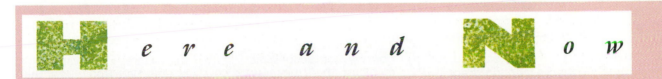

Case in Point

This excerpt, from the author's files, illustrates labeling theory.

> After my mom found out, she never brought it up again. I thought the incident was over—dead, gone, and buried. Well, . . . it wasn't over at all. My mom and dad must have agreed that I couldn't be trusted anymore. I'm sure she was regularly going through my stuff in my room to see if I was still smoking dope. Even my grandparents acted strangely whenever the news on television would report about the latest drug bust in Chicago. Several times that I can't ever forget was when we were together and I could hear the news broadcast on TV from my room about some drug bust. There they all were whispering about me. My grandma asking if I "quitta the dope." One night, I overheard my mother reassure my dad and grandmother that I no longer was using dope. You can't believe how embarrassed I was that my own family was still thinking that I was a dope fiend. They thought I was addicted to pot like a junkie is addicted to heroin! I can tell you that I would never lay such a guilt trip on my kids if I ever have kids. I remember that for two years after the time I was honest enough to tell my mom that I had tried pot, they would always whisper about me, give me the third degree whenever I returned late from a date, and go through my room looking for dope. They acted as if I was hooked on drugs. I remember that for a while back then I would always think that if they think of me as a drug addict, I might as well get high whenever my friends "toke up." They should have taken me at my word instead of sneaking around my personal belongings. I should have left syringes laying around my room!

Source: Interview with a 20-year-old male college student at a private university in the Midwest, conducted by Peter Venturelli on 19 November 1993.

we admire and look to for guidance and advice. If key people we admire or fear come to define our actions as deviant, then their definition becomes "facts" of our reality.

After having read about some of the main contributors to labeling theory, we can summarize by saying that the labels we use to describe people have a way of influencing their self-perceptions. In returning to our example, even if Jack does not initially believe he is an addict but instead an occasional user, the idea that his friends perceive him as a drug abuser will cause Jack to be uneasy whenever he is in their company. These uneasy feelings will interfere with Jack's ability to convey a non-drug-using image. At first Jack may deny the charge. Then he may poke fun at what others think of him. But eventually, Jack will begin to perceive himself more in line with the consistent perceptions of his accusers. This final perception occurs gradually. If he is unsuccessful in eradicating the addict image, Jack will reluctantly concur with the label that has been pinned on him *or* leave the group so that he can once again become acceptable in the eyes of other people.

Substance has been added to labeling theory by Edwin Lemert (1951, 133–141), who distinguishes between two types of deviance: primary and secondary deviance. **Primary deviance** is inconsequential deviance, which occurs without having a lasting impression on the perpetrator. Generally, most first-time violations of law, for example, are primary deviations. Whether the suspected or accused individual has committed the deviant act does not matter. What matters is whether the individual *identifies* with the deviant behavior.

Secondary deviance develops when the individual begins to identify and perceive himself or herself as deviant. The moment this occurs, deviance shifts from being primary to secondary. Many adolescents casually experiment with drugs. If, however, they begin to perceive themselves as drug users, then this behavior is virtually impossible to eradicate. The same holds true with OTC drug abuse. The moment an individual believes that he or she feels better after using a particular drug, the greater the likelihood that he or she will use the drug consistently.

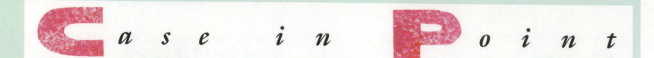

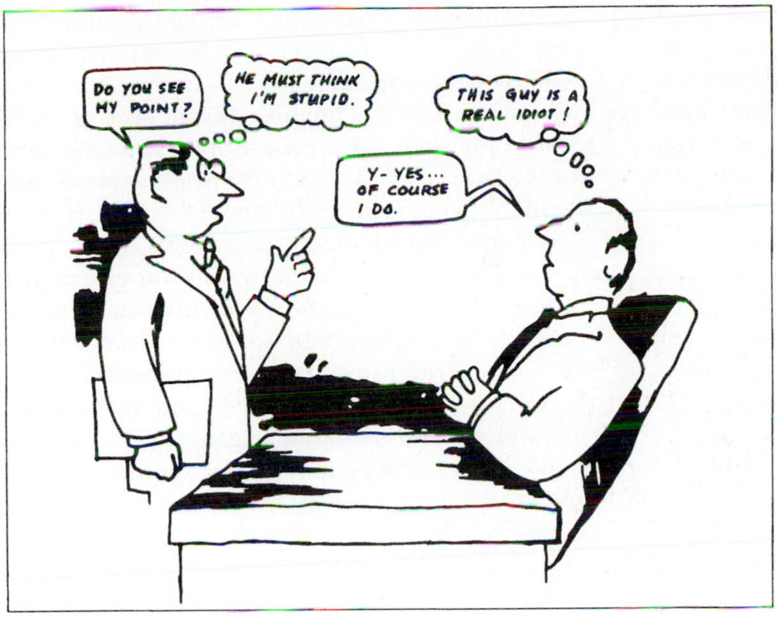

This is an illustration of the reflective process that often occurs in daily conversations when we think that our unspoken thoughts are undetectable and hidden. In reality, however, these innermost thoughts are clearly conveyed through body language and nonverbal gestures. *Source:* Reproduced with permission of Alex Silvestri.

Howard Becker (1963) believes that certain negative status positions (such as alcoholic, mental patient, criminal, drug addict, and so on) are so powerful that they dominate others. For example, if people who are important to Jack call him a "druggie," this becomes a powerful label that will take precedence over any other status positions Jack may occupy. This label becomes Jack's **master status**—that of an addicted drug user. Even if Jack is also an above-average biology major, an excellent drummer, and a very likeable individual, those factors become secondary. Furthermore, once a powerful label is attached, it becomes much easier for the individual to uphold the image dictated by members of society. Master status labels distort an individual's public image in that other people expect consistency in role performance.

Once a negative master status has been attached to an individual's public image, labeling theorist Edwin Schur asserts that retrospective interpretation occurs. **Retrospective interpretation** is a form of "reconstitution of individual character or identity" (1971, 52). This largely involves redefining a person's image within a particular social group.

Finally, William I. Thomas's (1923, 203–22) contribution to labeling theory can be summarized in the theorem that "If men define situations as real, they are real in their consequences." Thus, according to this dictum, when someone is perceived as a drug user, the perception functions as a label of that person's character and shapes his or her self-perception.

Subculture Theories **Subculture theory** largely explains drug use as caused by peer pressure. Sub-

PRIMARY DEVIANCE inconsequential deviant behavior in which the perpetrator does not identify with the deviance

SECONDARY DEVIANCE advanced type of deviant behavior that develops when the perpetrator identifies with the deviant behavior

MASTER STATUS the overriding status position in the eyes of others that clearly identifies an individual; for example, doctor, lawyer, alcoholic, HIV positive

RETROSPECTIVE INTERPRETATION the social psychological process of redefining a person's reputation as a member of a particular group

SUBCULTURE THEORIES explain drug use as caused by peer pressure culture theory asks, How does drug use result from peer group influence(s)? Social psychologically, in all groups, there are certain members who are very charismatic and, as a result, exert more social influence than other peer members. Often such appealing members are group leaders, task leaders, or emotional leaders, who maintain a strong ability to influence others. Drug use that results from peer pressure demonstrates the extent to which these more popular, charismatic leaders can influence and socially pressure others to initially use or abuse drugs. This excerpt from an interview illustrates subculture theory.

> I first started messing around with alcohol in high school. In order to be part of the crowd, we would sneak out during lunchtime at school and get "high." About six months after we started drinking, we moved on to other drugs. . . . Everyone in high school belongs to a clique, and my clique was heavy into drugs. We had a lot of fun being "high" throughout the day. We would party constantly. Basically, in college, it's the same thing.
>
> *Source:* Interview with a 19-year-old male student at a small, religiously affiliated private liberal arts school in the Southeast, conducted by Peter Venturelli on 9 February 1985.

In sociology, charismatic leaders are viewed as possessing status and prestige, defined as distinction in the eyes of others. In reality, as explained by the eminent sociologist Max Weber, such leaders have power over inexperienced drug users. Members of peer groups are often persuaded to experiment with drug use if leaders say, "Come on, try some, it's great" or "Trust me, you'll love it once you try it." In groups where drugs are consumed, the extent of peer influence with regard to drug use is affected by the more charismatic leaders. Such leaders find that the art of persuasion and camaraderie that drug use entails are very gratifying.

A further extension of subculture theory is the social and cultural support perspective. This perspective explains drug use and/or abuse in peer groups as resulting from an attempt by peers to solve problems collectively. In the neoclassic book, *Delinquent Boys: The Culture of the Gang* (1955), Cohen pioneered a study that showed for the first time that delinquent behavior is a collective attempt to gain social status and prestige within the peer group. Members of certain peer groups are unable to achieve respect within the larger society. Such status-conscious youths find that being able to commit delinquent acts without apprehension by the law is admirable in the eyes of their peers. In effect, Cohen believes, delinquent behavior is a subcultural solution for overcoming status frustration and feelings of low self-esteem largely determined by lower-class frustrations.

Although Cohen's emphasis is on explaining juvenile delinquency, his notion that delinquent behavior is a subcultural solution can easily be applied to drug use and abuse in primarily members of lower-class peer groups. Underlying drug use and abuse in delinquent gangs, for example, results from sharing common feelings of alienation and escape from a society that appears noncaring, distant, and hostile.

Consider the current upsurge in violent gang memberships (see also Chapter 15, "Drug Abuse Among Special Populations," for more detail on adolescents and gangs). In such groups, not only is drug dealing a profitable venture, but also drug use serves as a collective response to alienation and estrangement from conventional middle-class society. In cases of minority violent gang members, the alienation results from racism, increasing poverty, the effects of migration and acculturation, and the result of minority status in a white-male-dominated society such as the United States (Glick and Moore 1990; Moore 1978).

Structural Influence Theories

The focus of these theories is on how the organization of a society, group, or subculture is largely responsible for drug abuse by its members. The belief is that it is not the society, group, or subculture that is causing the behavior—in this case, drug use—but that the organization itself or the lack of an organization determines the resulting behavior.

Social disorganization and social strain theories identify the different kinds of social change that are disruptive and how, in a general sense, people are affected by such change. Social disorganization theory asks, what in the social order causes people to deviate? Social strain theory asks, can the way in which a society is organized cause social deviance? This theory believes that frustration results from being unable to achieve desired goals. This perceived shortcoming compels an individual to deviate in order to achieve desired needs.

Overall, social disorganization theory describes a situation where, because of rapid social change, previously affiliated individuals no longer find themselves integrated into a community's social, commercial, religious, and economic institutions. When this occurs, community members that were once affiliated become disaffiliated and lack effective attachment to the social order. As a result, these disaffiliated people begin to gravitate toward deviant behavior.

In order to develop trusting relationships, stability and continuity are essential for proper socialization. As will be discussed later in this chapter, if identity transformation occurs during the teen years, when drugs are first introduced, a stable environment is very important. Yet in a technological society, destabilizing and disorienting forces often result because technology causes rapid social change.

Although most people have little or no difficulty when confronted with rapid social change, others perceive this change as beyond their control. For example, consider an immigrant who experienced a nervous breakdown because he was unable to cope with the new society. The following interview shows how such confusion and lack of control lead to drug use, which is viewed as an attractive alternative to coping with confusion and stress:

> ***Interviewee***: The world is all messed up.
> ***Interviewer***: Why? In what way?
> ***Interviewee***: Nobody gives a damn anymore about anyone else.
> ***Interviewer***: Why do you think this is so?
> ***Interviewee***: It seems like life just seems to go on and on...I know that when I am under the influence, life is more mellow. I feel great! When I am "high," I feel relaxed and can take things in better. Before I came to Chalmers College [a pseudonym], I felt home life was one great big mess; now that I am here, this college is also a big pile of crap. I guess this is why I like smoking dope. When I am "high," I can forget my problems. My surroundings are friendlier; I am even more pleasant! Do you know what I mean?
>
> *Source:* Interview with a 19-year-old male marijuana user attending a small, private, liberal arts college in the Southeast, conducted by Peter Venturelli on 12 February 1984.

Current Social Change in Most Societies

Does social change per se cause people to use and abuse drugs? In response to this question, *social change*—defined as "any measurable change caused by technological advancement that disrupts cultural values and attitudes"—does not by itself cause widespread drug use. In most cases, social change materialistically advances a culture by profoundly affecting how things are accomplished. At the same time, however, rapid social change disrupts day-to-day behavior preserved by tradition, which has a tendency to fragment such conventional social groups as families, communities, and neighborhoods. By **conventional behavior,** we mean behavior that is largely dictated by custom and tradition and thus evaporates under rapid social change.

Examples are the number of youth subcultures that proliferated during the 1960s (Yinger 1982) and other more recent lifestyles and subcultures such as rappers, right to life, prochoice, Mothers Against Drunk Driving (MADD), gay liberation, punk rockers, and the recent new wave subcultures that are in existence. Furthermore, two other subcultures, teenagers and the elderly, both of which have become increasingly independent and in some subgroups alienated from other age groups in society, are discussed separately in Chapter 16.

Simply stated, today's social institutions no longer influence people as much as they did in the past. As a consequence, people are free to explore different means of expression and types of recreation. For most, this is a liberating experience leading to new and exciting outcomes; for others, the freedom to explore involves drug use and abuse.

The following two excerpts, gathered from various interviews, illustrate social disorganization and strain theory.

STRUCTURAL INFLUENCE THEORIES theories that view the organization of a society, group, or subculture as responsible for drug use and abuse by its members

CONVENTIONAL BEHAVIOR behavior largely dictated by custom and tradition and that is often jeopardized by rapid social change

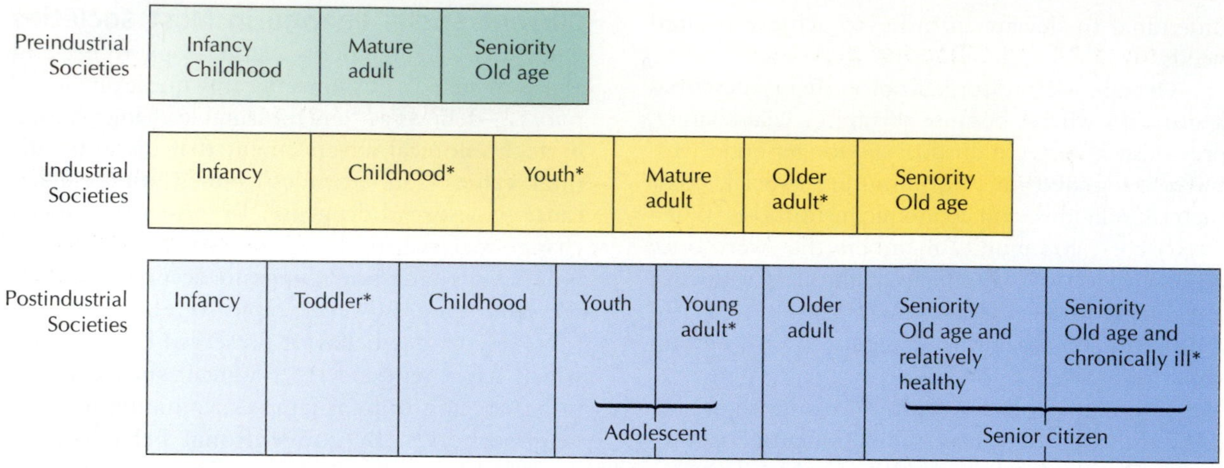

*Represents a newly developed and separate stage of identification and expression from the prior era.

FIGURE 2.1 Levels of technological development and corresponding subcultures

These days, everything is rush, rush, rush. There are just not enough hours in the day. I set aside weekends in order to relax. Alcohol and marijuana allow me to relax from the rest of the week.

I am into my own life because everyone is doing this. I see nearly everyone doing well around here. It's only those who are too stupid to succeed who are poor. I have had a rough time making it lately. Cocaine and speed help, but I know it's not the answer to all my problems. For now, drugs help me to put up with all the shit going on in my life.

Sources: First paragraph, interview with a 22-year-old, female, part-time college student at a public liberal arts college in the Southeast, conducted by Peter Venturelli, 10 April 1986; Second paragraph, interview with a 25-year-old male residing in the Southeast and receiving various forms of welfare, conducted by Peter Venturelli, 10 March 1985.

Is there any link between social change and drug use? Although no direct link exists, there is plenty of proof that certain dramatic changes occur in the organization of society and many eventually lead certain groups to use and abuse drugs. Figure 2.1 illustrates how the number of life cycle stages increases, depending on a society's level of technological development. Overall, this implies that, as societies advance from preindustrial to industrial to post-industrial, there is a greater likelihood that new subcultures will develop (see Fischer 1976, for similar thinking). In contrast to industrial and postindustrial societies, preindustrial societies do not have as many separate and distinct periods and cycles of social development. What is implied here is that the greater the number of distinct life cycles, the greater the fragmentation between the members of different stages of development. "Generation gaps" occur across age groups that are increasingly unable to share differing values and attitudes.

Control Theories This last structural influence theory we are reviewing places most of its primary emphasis on influences outside the self as the primary cause for deviating to drug use and/or abuse. Control theories place importance on positive socialization. **Socialization** is defined as "the process by which individuals learn to internalize the attitudes, values, and behaviors needed to become participating members of conventional society." Generally, control theorists believe that human beings can easily become deviant if left without social controls. Thus, theorists who specialize in control theory emphasize the necessity of maintaining bonds to family, school, peers, and other social, political, and religious organizations.

TABLE 2.1 Likelihood of drug use

	External Social Control	
Individual Internal Control	**Strong**	**Weak or Nonexistent**
Strong	Least likely (almost never)	Less likely (probably never)
Weak	More likely (probably will)	Most likely (almost certain)

In the 1950s and 1960s, criminologist Walter C. Reckless (1961) developed containment theory. According to this theory, the socialization process results in the creation of strong or weak internal and external control systems.

Internal control is determined by the degree of self-control, high or low frustration tolerance, positive or negative self-perception, successful or unsuccessful goal achievement, and either resistance or adherence to deviant behavior. Environmental pressures, such as social conditions, may limit the accomplishment of goal-striving behavior; such conditions include poverty, minority group status, inferior education, and lack of employment.

The external, or outer, control system consists of effective or ineffective supervision and discipline, consistent or inconsistent moral training, positive or negative acceptance, identity, and self-worth. Examples are latchkey children who become delinquent and alcoholic parents who are inconsistent with discipline. This is another example of breakdown in social control.

In applying this theory to the use or abuse of drugs, we could say that, if an individual has a weak external control system, the internal control system must take over to handle external pressure. Similarly, if an individual's external control system is strong from positive socialization based on discipline, moral training, and development of positive feelings of self-worth, then this individual's internal control system will not be seriously challenged. If, however, either the internal or external control system is mismatched—in that one happens to be weak and the other strong—the possibility of drug abuse increases.

If an individual's external and internal controls are both weak, he or she is most likely to use and abuse drugs. Table 2.1 shows the likelihood of drug use resulting from either strong or weak internal and external control systems. It indicates that, if both internal and external controls are strong, the use and abuse of drugs is not likely to occur. However, if the internal and external systems are both weak, drug use is most likely to occur (providing, of course, that drugs are available and presented by trusted friends).

Travis Hirschi (1971, 85, 159), a much respected sociologist and social control theorist, believes that delinquent behavior tends to occur whenever people lack (1) attachment to others, (2) commitment to goals, (3) involvement in conventional activity, and (4) belief in the common value system. If a child or adolescent is unable to become circumscribed within the family setting, school, and the nondelinquent peers, then the drift to delinquent behavior is inevitable.

We can apply Hirschi's theories to drug use as follows:

1. Drug users are less likely than nonusers to be closely tied to their parents.
2. Good students are less likely to use drugs.

CONTROL THEORIES believe that if left to their own nature, individuals have a tendency to deviate from expected cultural values, norms, and attitudes

SOCIALIZATION the learning process responsible for becoming human

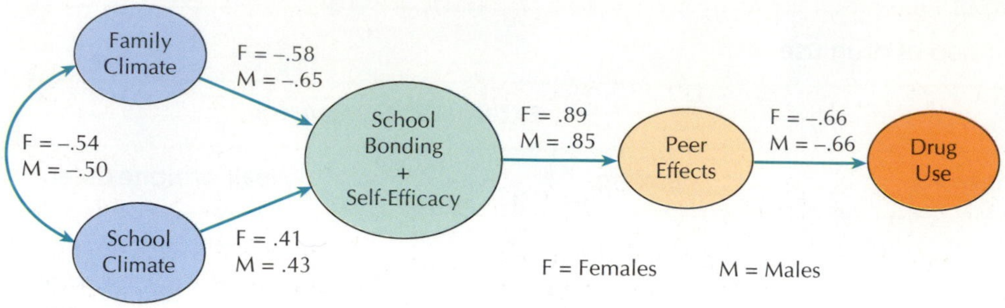

Note: The use of both licit and illicit drugs are included in this model.

FIGURE 2.2 Primary At-Risk Factors Responsible for Drug-Use: Final Social Ecology Model *Source:* Karol L. Kumpfer and Charles W. Turner. "The Social Ecology Model of Adolescent Substance Abuse: Implications for Prevention." *International Journal of the Addictions* 25, no. 4A (1991): 433–63.

3. Drug users are less likely to participate in social clubs and organizations and engage in team sport activities.
4. Drug users are very likely to have friends whose activities are congruent with their own attitudes.

The following excerpt illustrates control theory:

> I guess you could call me more of a loner type. I belong to groups, but I am never really involved much in them. I have just a few really close friends and these friends are also like me—mostly nonjoiners.
>
> Here I am in my early thirties, and I still enjoy getting "high." When I was in my early twenties, I thought that once my friends would eventually leave and get married or move away, I would quit using drugs. Now that most of these friends are no longer here, I still get "high," mostly on my own.
>
> *Source:* Interview with a 32-year-old male employed as a middle manager, residing in the Midwest, conducted by Peter Venturelli, 9 December 1986.

In conclusion, control theory depicts how conformity to conventional groups prevents deviance by demonstrating the relationship between the extent of group conformity and deviant drug use. The theories are similar in that both suggest that control is either internally or externally enforced by family, school, and peer group expectations. In addition, individuals who are either (1) not equipped with an internal system of self-control reflecting the values and beliefs of conventional society or (2) personally alienated from major social institutions such as family, school, and church may deviate without feeling guilty for their actions, often because of peer pressure resulting in a suspension or modification of internal beliefs.

Predicting the Risk Factors Responsible for Drug Use

To this point, the statistics and trends of drug use have been staggering, pointing to a nation nearly saturated with licit and illicit drug use. Kumpfer and Turner (1990–1991, 450) present a social ecology model predicting causes and effects responsible for drug use and/or abuse (see Figure 2.2 and see Here and Now box for how this model applied to a sample population of high school students).

Danger Signals of Drug Abuse

How does one know when the use of drugs moves beyond normal use? Many people are prescribed drugs that affect their moods. Using these drugs wisely can be important for physical and emotional health. But sometimes it is difficult to decide when using drugs to handle stress becomes inappropriate.

Here and Now

Applying the Kumpfer and Turner Social Ecology Model

Here are summary findings for males and females in a high school sample of 1,373 from a mixed urban–rural high school district in Utah (Kumpfer and Turner 1991):

1. There is a very strong relationship between illegal alcohol and drug use in high school students and close alliance with antisocial peers and involvement in socially deviant acts of behavior.
2. Positive self-esteem and positive school bonding affects the selection of positive peers. Similarly negative self-esteem and negative school bonding affects selection of negative or antisocial peers.
3. Family climate and to a lesser extent, school climate strongly influences the extent of school bonding and self-efficacy.
4. Students with poor sense of self or students who were unable to adequately bond to their school were more likely to come from poor family or school environments.
5. In essence, the quality of family and school climate predicts increased vulnerability to negative peers. (Kumpfer and Turner 1991, 455)

Do you think these summarized findings would *equally* explain recreational, moderate, and chronic drug users? In other words, do different types of users all come from inadequate nurturing homes and from deficient (socially deviant) school environments? Why or why not? If not, differentiate between the types of users and what affects them most or least.

It is important that your use of drugs does not result in catastrophe. Here are some danger signals that can help you evaluate your own way of using drugs.

1. Do those close to you often ask about your drug use? Have they noticed any changes in your moods or behavior?
2. Are you defensive if a friend or relative mentions your drug or alcohol use?
3. Are you sometimes embarrassed or frightened by your behavior under the influence of drugs or alcohol?
4. Have you ever gone to see a new doctor because your regular physician would not prescribe the drug you wanted?
5. When you are under pressure or feel anxious, do you automatically take a depressant or drink or both?
6. Do you take drugs more often or for purposes other than those recommended by your doctor?
7. Do you mix drugs and alcohol?
8. Do you drink or take drugs regularly to help you sleep?
9. Do you have to take a pill to get going in the morning?
10. Do you think you have a drug problem?

If you have answered yes to a number of these questions, you may be abusing drugs or alcohol. There are places to go for help at the local level. One such place might be a drug abuse program in your community, listed in the Yellow Pages under "Drug Abuse." Other resources include community crisis centers, telephone hotlines, and the Mental Health Association.

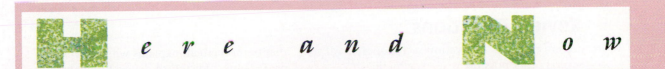

Review Questions

1. In addition to better cultivation techniques, cite several other possible reasons why the potency (THC content) of the average marijuana joint has increased since 1960.
2. Given that over 88% of the U.S. population members are daily drug users of some form, do you think we need to re-examine our strict drug laws, which may be punishing a sizable number of drug users in our society who simply want to use illicit drugs?
3. Is there any way to combine biological with sociological explanations for why people use drugs so that the two perspectives do not conflict? (Sketch out a synthesis between these two sets of theoretical explanations.)
4. What is the relationship between mental illness and drug abuse? For what reasons is this relationship important?
5. Do you accept the "rats in a maze" conception that psychology offers for explaining why people come to abuse drugs? (This is primarily the view that humans are like automatons and that reinforcement explains why certain people become addicted to drugs?) Explain your answer.
6. In reviewing the psychological and sociological drug use theories, which theories best explain drug use? Defend your answer.
7. Does differential association theory take into account non-drug-using individuals whose socialization environment was drug infested?
8. Do you believe drug users are socialized differently and that these alleged differences account for drug use? Defend your answer.
9. Can divorce be blamed for adolescent drug use? Why or why not, and if so, to what extent?
10. Can it be said that the current and alarming drug abuse statistics reflect the failure of social change in our society? Do you agree or disagree with this statement? Why or why not?
11. Critique the final social ecology model, Figure 2.2. What are its strengths and what are its weaknesses for predicting drug use?

Key Terms

sinsemilla
genetic and biophysiological theories
CNS (central nervous system)
psychoactive effects
neurotransmitter
dopamine
habituation
"addiction to pleasure" theory
differential reinforcement
microscopic explanations
macroscopic explanations
social learning theory
amotivational syndrome
labeling theory
primary deviance
secondary deviance
master status
retrospective interpretation
subculture theories
structural influence theories
conventional theories
control theories
socialization

Summary

1. Drug use is more serious today than in the past because (a) since 1960 to the present, drug use, and/or abuse has increased dramatically; (b) today, illicit drugs are more potent than in the past; (c) use of drugs is presented by the media as rewarding; (d) drug use physically harms members of society; and (e) drug use and drug dealing by violent gangs are steadily increasing at an alarming rate.
2. Genetic theory believes that the predisposition to drug use can be found in the gene structure. "Addiction to pleasure" theories believe that it is biologically normal to continue a pleasure stimulation when drugs are proven to be a pleasurable experience.
3. The American Psychiatric Association classifies severe drug dependence as a form of psychiatric disorder. Drugs that are abused can cause

mental conditions that mimic major psychiatric illnesses such as schizophrenia, severe anxiety disorders, and suicidal depression (Halloway 1991).

4. Introversion and extraversion patterns have been associated with levels of neural arousal in brain stem circuits (Carlson 1990; Gray 1987), and these forms of arousal are similar and closely associated with effects caused by drug stimulants or depressants.
5. Reinforcement or learning theory explains that the motivation to use and/or abuse drugs stems from how the "high" from alcohol and other drugs reduce anxiety, tension, and stress. This theory believes that drugs become rewarding as they chemically calm down and stimulate and/or depress the control centers of the brain. Positive social influences by drug-using peers also promote drug use.
6. Social influence theories include social learning, the role of significant others, and labeling and subculture theories. Social learning theory explains drug use as a form of learned behavior. Social influence and the role of significant others detail the learning process involved in drug use and/or abuse. Labeling theory says that other people we consider important can influence whether drug use becomes an option for us. If key people we admire or fear come to define our actions as deviant, then the definition becomes the "facts" of our reality. Subculture theories trace original drug experimentation, use, and/or abuse to peer pressure.
7. The following consistencies in socialization patterns are found among drug abusers: (a) immaturity, maladjustment, and/or insecurity; (b) poor school performance and classroom disobedience; (c) delinquency or repetitive deviant activities; (d) residence in drug-infested neighborhoods; (e) intensive pro-drug peer involvement; (f) parental relationships viewed as distant, uncaring, and aloof; (g) more than usual residential mobility (seven or more times); (h) personally felt discrimination, prejudice, and sexism and/or racism; and (i) exposure and belief that selling drugs is a very lucrative business venture.
8. Sociologist Howard Becker believes that first-time drug users become attached to drugs because of the following three factors; (1) they learn the techniques of drug use; (2) they learn to perceive the pleasurable effects of drugs; and (3) they learn to enjoy the drug experience.
9. *Primary deviance* is deviant behavior that the perpetrator does not identify with; hence, it is inconsequential deviant behavior. *Example:* "I just tried cocaine once. I'll never do it again; it's not for me." *Secondary deviance* is deviance that one readily identifies with. *Example:* "Maybe I am good at stealing, like my friends tell me." *Master status* refers to a primary status that upholds numerous other statuses, such as male or female, corporate executive, and full-time student. *Example:* "Did you know that my neighbor is a heroin addict?" *Retrospective interpretation* refers to redefining a person's image within a particular group. *Example:* "My roommate is an alcoholic; I never would have thought that of him. Now I know why he always wants to go to parties and stay late into the night."

   The concepts *primary* and *secondary deviance, master status,* and *retrospective interpretation* all relate to labeling theory. They help explain how a person can perceive himself or herself as being deviant and how others make this judgment, as well. During the onset of primary deviance, the accused perpetrator of deviant behavior is not perceived as truly deviant. Circumstantial causes are often attributed to his or her behavior. In a more advanced phase of deviant identity, secondary deviance results when the accused begins to identify with the deviant behavior. Master status is when an individual's deviant reputation predominates in the eyes of others. Retrospective interpretation involves redefining past behavior in light of the deviant image.
10. Both internal and external social control should prevail concerning drug use. Internal control deals with internal psychic and internalized social attitudes while external control is exemplified by living in a neighborhood and community where drug use and/or abuse is severely criticized or not tolerated as a means to seek pleasure or avoid stress and anxiety.

References

Akers, Ronald L. "Problems in the Sociology of Deviance: Social Definition and Behavior." *Social Forces* 6 (June 1968): 455–65.

Akers, Ronald L. *Drugs, Alcohol, and Society: Social Structure, Process, and Policy.* Belmont, CA: Wadsworth, 1992.

American Psychiatric Association. "Substance-Related Disorders." *Diagnostic and Statistical Manual of Mental Disorders,* 4th edition. Allen Frances, Chairperson. Washington, DC: American Psychiatric Association, 1994: 175–272.

Bartels, S., G. Teague, R. Drake, R. Clark, P. Bush, and D. Noordsy. "Substance Abuse in Schizophrenia: Service Utilization and Costs." *Journal of Nervous and Mental Disease* 181 (1993): 227–32.

Becker, H. S. *Outsiders: Studies in the Sociology of Deviance.* New York: Free Press, 1963.

Becker, Howard S. "History, Culture, and Subjective Experience: An Exploration of the Social Basis of Drug-Induced Experiences." *Journal of Health and Social Behavior* 8 (1967): 163–76.

Bejerot, N. "Current Problems of Drug Addicted." *Lakartidingen* (Sweden) 62, no. 50 (1965): 4231–38.

Bejerot, N. *Addiction: An Artificially Induced Drive.* Springfield, IL: Thomas, 1972.

Bejerot, N. "The Biological and Social Character of Drug Dependence." *Psychiatrie der Gegenwart, Forschung und Praxis.* Edited by K. P. Kisker, J. E. Meyer, C. Muller, and E. Stromogrew, Vol. 3. 2d ed., 488–518. Berlin: Springer-Verlag, 1975.

Beschner, G., and A. Friedman. *Teen Drug Use.* Lexington, MA: Heath, 1986.

Best, Joel, and David F. Luckenbill. *Organizing Deviance.* 2d ed. Englewood Cliffs, NJ: Prentice Hall, 1994.

Blum, R. H., and L. Richards. "Youthful Drug Use." In *Handbook on Drug Abuse,* edited by R. L. Dupont, A. Goldstein, and J. O. Darnell, 257–69. Washington, DC: National Institute on Drug Abuse, 1979.

Borton, T. "Pressure to Try Drugs and Alcohol Starts in Early Grades." *Weekly Reader,* 25 April 1983: 47–53.

Brady, K., and R. Lydiard, "Bipolar Affective Disorder and Substance Abuse." *Journal of Clinical Psychopharmacology* 12 (1992): 178–228.

Carlson, N. *Psychology: The Science of Behavior.* 3d ed. Boston: Allyn and Bacon, 1990.

Cershon, E., and R. Rieder, "Major Disorders of Mind and Brain." *Scientific American* 267 (September 1992): 127–33.

Cohen, A. K. *Delinquent Boys: The Culture of the Gang.* Glencoe, IL: Free Press, 1955.

Conrad, Peter, and Joseph W. Schneider. *Deviance and Medicalization.* St. Louis, MO: Mosby, 1980.

Cotton, N. A. "The Familial Incidence of Alcoholism." *Journal of Studies on Alcohol* 40 (1979): 89–116.

Cummings, Scott. "Anatomy of a Wilding Gang." In *Gangs: The Origins and Impact of Contemporary Youth Gangs in the United States,* edited by Scott Cummings and Daniel J. Monti, 49–73. Albany: State University of New York Press, 1993.

"Epidemiological and Services Research on Mental Disorders that Co-occur with Drug and/or Alcohol Disorders." *Prevention Pipeline* 7 (January–February 1994): 71.

Eysenck, H. J. and Eysenck, M. W. *Personality and Individual Differences: A Natural Science Approach.* New York: Plenum Press, 1985.

Farrar, H., and G. Kearns. "Cocaine: Clinical Pharmacology and Toxicology." *Journal of Pediatrics* 115 (1989): 665–75.

Fischer, C. S. *The Urban Experience.* New York: Harcourt Brace Jovanovich, 1976.

Galanter, M., S. Egelko, G. De Leon, C. Rohrs, and H. Franco. "Crack/Cocaine Abusers in the General Hospital: Assessment and Initiation of Care." *American Journal of Psychiatrity* 149 (1992): 810–15.

Glick, Ronald, and Joan Moore, eds. *Drugs in Hispanic Communities.* New Brunswick: Rutgers University Press, 1990.

Goode, Erich. *Deviant Behavior.* 4th ed. Englewood Cliffs, NJ: Prentice Hall, 1994.

Gray, J. A. *The Psychology of Fear and Stress.* 2d ed. Cambridge, England: Cambridge University Press, 1987.

Grinspoon, L. "Update on Cocaine." *Harvard Mental Health Letter* 10 (September 1993): 1–4.

Halloway, M. "Rx for Addiction." *Scientific American* (March 1991): 94–103.

Hirschi, T. *Causes of Delinquency.* 2d ed. Los Angeles: University of California Press, 1971.

Hutchinson, Ray, and Charles Kyle. "Hispanic Street Gangs in Chicago's Public Schools." In *Gangs: The Origins and Impact of Contemporary Youth Gangs in the United States,* edited by Scott Cummings and Daniel J. Monti, 113–36, Albany: State University of New York Press, 1993.

Imperato A., A. Mele, M. Serocco, and S. Puglisi-Allegra. "Chronic Cocaine Alters Limbic Extracellular Dopamine Neurochemical Basis for Addiction." *European Journal of Pharmacology* 212 (1992): 299–300.

Izenwasser, S., and C. Kornetsky. "Brain-stimulation Reward: A Method for Assessing the Neurochemical

Basis of Drug-Induced Euphoria." In *Drugs of Abuse and Neurobiology,* edited by R. Watson. Boca Raton, FL: CRC Press, 1992: 1–21.

Jarvik, M. "The Drug Dilemma: Manipulating the Demand." *Science* 250 (1990): 387–92.

Jellinek, E. M. *The Disease Concept of Alcoholism.* New Haven, CT: Hillhouse Press, 1960.

Koob, G. "Drugs of Abuse: Anatomy, Pharmacology and Function of Reward Pathways." *Trends in Pharmacological Sciences* 13 (May 1992): 177–84.

Kumpfer, Karol L., and Charles W. Turner, "The Social Ecology Model of Adolescent Substance Abuse: Implications for Prevention," *International Journal of the Addictions* 25, no. 4A (1991): 433–63.

Kunen, James S. "Madness in the Heart of the City." *People* (22 May 1989): 107–11.

Lemert, E. M. *Social Psychology: A Systematic Approach to the Theory of Sociopathic Behavior.* New York: McGraw-Hill, 1951.

Mijuriya, T. H., and M. R. Aldrich. "Cannabis 1988: Old Drug, New Dangers—The Potency Question." *Journal of Psychoactive Drugs* 20 (1988): 47–55.

Moore, Joan. "Gangs, Drugs, and Violence. In *Gangs: The Origins and Impact of Contemporoary Youth Gangs in the United States,* edited by Scott Cummings and Daniel J. Monti, 27–46. Albany: State University of New York Press, 1993.

Moore, Joan. *Homeboys: Gangs, Drugs and Prison in the Barrios of Los Angeles.* Philadelphia: Temple University Press, 1978.

Plummer, Kenneth. "Misunderstanding Labelling Perspectives." *Deviant Interpretations,* edited by David Downes and Paul Rock, 85–121. London: Robertson, 1979.

Reckless, W. C. "A New Theory of Delinquency." *Federal Probation* 25 (1961): 42–46.

Schur, E. M. *Labeling Deviant Behavior.* New York: Harper & Row, 1971.

Stolerman, I. "Drugs of Abuse: Behavioral Principles, Methods and Terms." *Trends in Pharmacological Sciences Reviews* 13 (May 1992): 170–76.

Sutherland, E. *Principles of Criminology.* 4th ed. Philadelphia: Lippincott, 1947.

Thomas, W. I., with D. S. Thomas. *The Child in America.* New York: Knopf, 1923.

Uhl, G., A Persico, and S. Smith. "Current Excitement with D-2 Dopamine Receptor Gene Alleles in Substance Abuse." *Archives of General Psychiatry* 49 (February 1992): 157–60.

Uhl, G., K. Blum, E. Noble, and S. Smith. "Substance Abuse Vulnerability and D-2 Receptor Genes." *Trends in Neurological Sciences* 16 (1993): 83–88.

U.S. Bureau of the Census, U.S. Department of Commerce. *Statistical Abstract of the United States, 1990, The National Data Book,* 110th edition. Washington, DC: U.S. Bureau of the Census, U.S. Department of Commerce, January 1990: 122.

Will, George. "America's Slide into the Sewers." *Newsweek* (30 July 1990): 64.

Williams, Terry. *The Cocaine Kids.* New York: Addison-Wesley, 1989.

Wilson, William J. *The Truly Disadvantaged.* Chicago: University of Chicago Press, 1990.

Wilson, M., and S. Wilson. *Drugs in American Life.* New York: Wilson, 1975.

Yinger, M. J. *Countercultures: The Promise and the Peril of a World Turned Upside Down.* New York: Free Press, 1982.

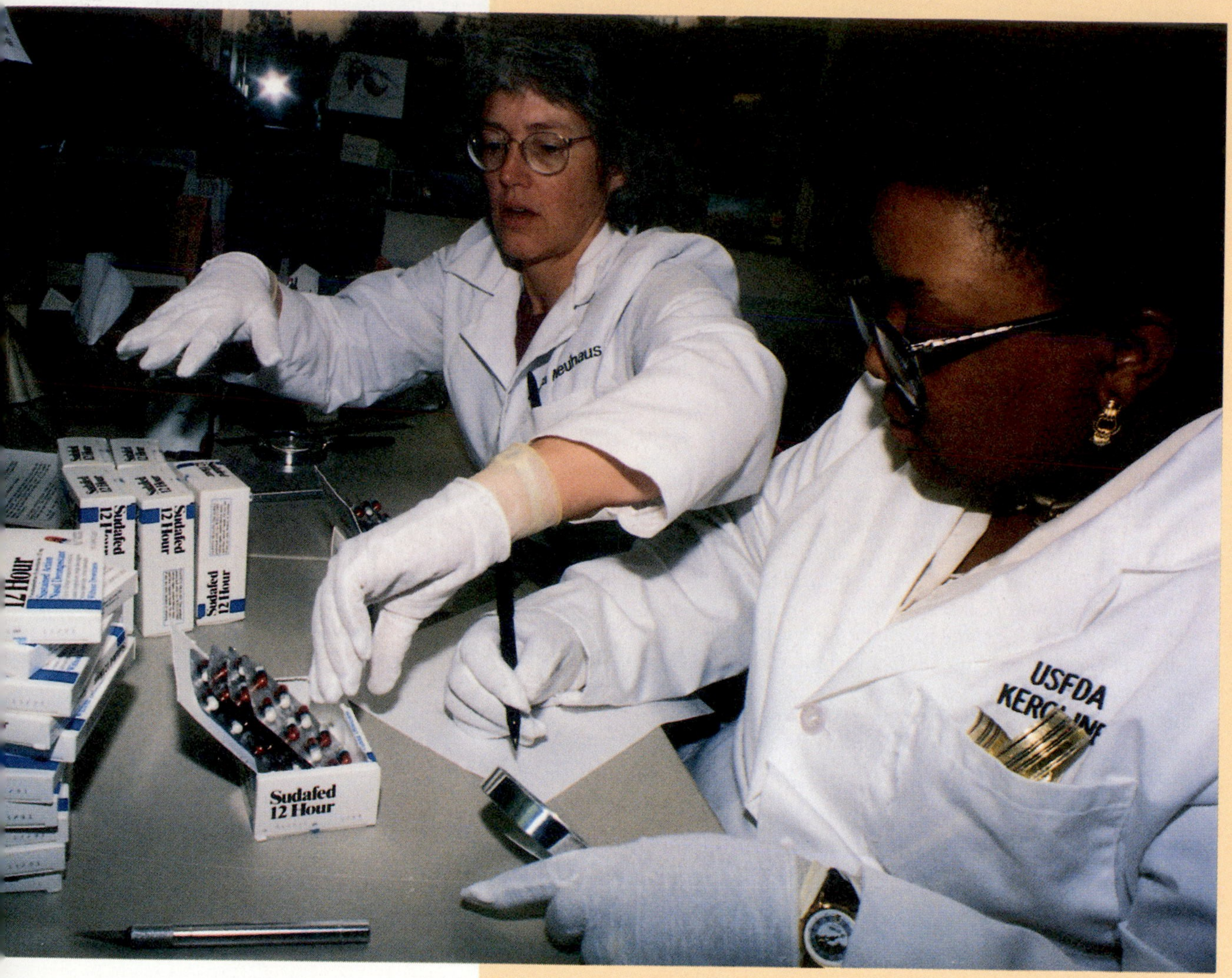

Chapter 3

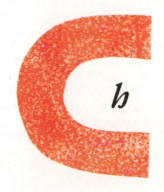

Drugs, Regulations, and the Law

DID YOU KNOW THAT . . .

- At the turn of the century, drug laws in the United States were more concerned with protecting the secret formulas of patent medicines than with protecting the public from the dangers of these products.
- Some patent medicines sold at the turn of the century contained opium and cocaine and were highly addictive.
- Before World War II, all drugs, except those classified as narcotics, were available without prescription.
- Not until the Kefauver-Harris Amendments of 1962 were drug companies required to demonstrate the effectiveness and safety of medications before they could be marketed.
- Today it can cost a drug company $500 million and require 10 years of testing before a new drug is approved for marketing.
- The FDA is in the process of switching many effective and safe prescription drugs to nonprescription status.
- The money spent by drug companies to promote their products is more than six times the combined educational budget of all the medical schools in the United States.
- Many medical experts consider drug abuse a mental disorder.
- Nearly one-fourth of prison inmates are incarcerated because of illegal drug activities.

LEARNING OBJECTIVES

On completing this chapter, you will be able to

1. Identify the major criteria that determine how society regulates drugs.
2. Describe how patent medicines influenced the early development of drug regulation in the United States.
3. Describe the similarities between opium and cocaine, and the roles each has played in the formation of drug legislation.
4. Explain the significance of the Pure Food and Drug Act of 1906 and why it was important in regulating drugs of abuse.
5. Identify the changes in drug regulation that occurred because of the 1938 Federal Food, Drug, and Cosmetic Act.
6. Explain the significance of the Durham-Humphrey Amendment of 1951.

continued

Healthy People 2000

Extend to 50 states administrative driver's license suspension and revocation laws or programs of equal effectiveness for people determined to have been driving under the influence of intoxicants.

Increase to 50 the number of states that have enacted and enforced policies, beyond those in existence in 1989, to reduce access to alcoholic beverages by minors.

LEARNING OBJECTIVES

7 Describe the changes in drug regulation that occurred because of the Kefauver-Harris Amendments of 1962.
8 Identify and explain the stages of testing for an investigational new drug (IND).
9 Discuss the special provisions (exceptions) made by the Food and Drug Administration (FDA) for drug marketing.
10 Outline the procedures used by the FDA to regulate nonprescription drugs.
11 Explain the FDA's *switching policy* and its significance to the over-the-counter (OTC) market.
12 List the principal factors that influence the formation of laws regulating drug abuse.
13 Identify and explain the Harrison Act of 1912.
14 Outline the major approaches used to reduce substance abuse.
15 Identify the major costs to society of drug abuse.
16 Describe advantages and disadvantages of legalizing drugs of abuse.

There is a tendency to assume that social sanctions and laws regarding drugs have always had aims similar to those we observe today in the United States. In fact, drug regulations and laws, as we know them in the United States and other industrialized countries, have developed only recently, often seemingly by a process of trial and error. Yet by contrasting conditions in industrialized and less developed countries, we see that not every society follows U.S. ways of regulating or outlawing drugs. Some seem more repressive, some seem more permissive, and some have raised and imported drugs that other countries have forbidden. As we look at developing societies now in the stage of industrialization that our grandparents experienced in the United States years ago, we can gain insight into how attitudes on drug regulation developed here. We may also appreciate some of the dilemmas that seem so puzzling to us today.

In this chapter, we examine the development of drug regulation in the United States as it applies both to manufacturing drugs and controlling their use and abuse. Although it might seem that the regulation of drug manufacturing and of drug abuse would be at opposite ends of the spectrum, in fact the two have evolved from the same process.

Cultural Attitudes Toward Drug Abuse

The current attitudes of U.S. culture toward the use of mind-altering substances is a blend of beliefs in individuals' rights to live their lives as they desire and society's obligation to protect its members from burdens due to uncontrolled behavior. The history of drug regulation consists of regulatory swings due to attempts by government to balance these two factors while responding to public pressures and perceived public needs. For example, a hundred years ago, most people expected the government to protect citizens' rights to produce and market new foods and substances; they did not expect or desire the government to regulate product quality or claims. Instead, the public relied on private morals and common sense to obtain quality and protection in an era of simple technology. Unfortunately, U.S. society had to learn by tragic experience that its trust was not well placed; many unscrupulous entrepreneurs were willing to risk the safety and welfare of the public in order to maximize profits and acquire wealth. In fact, most medicines of these earlier times were not only ineffective but often dangerous.

Because of high technology and the rapid

advancements society has made, we now rely on highly trained experts and government "watchdog" agencies for consumer information and protection. Out of this changing environment have evolved two major guidelines for controlling drug development and marketing:

1. *Society has the right to protect itself from the damaging impact of drug use.* This concept is closely aligned with the emotional and highly visible issues of drug abuse, but also includes protection from other drug side effects, as well. Thus, while we expect the government to protect society from drugs that can cause addiction, we also expect it to protect us from drugs that cause cancer, cardiovascular disease, or other threatening medical conditions.
2. *Society has the right to demand effective drugs.* This expectation is based on the philosophy "You get what you pay for." If drug manufacturers promise that their products relieve pain, these drugs should be analgesics; if they promise that their products relieve depression, those drugs should be antidepressants; if they promise that their products relieve stuffy noses, those drugs should be decongestants.

The public, through regulatory agencies and statutory enactments, has attempted to require that drug manufacturers produce *safe* and *effective* pharmaceutical products. Closely linked is the fact that society uses similar strategies to protect itself from the problems associated with the specific drug side effect of dependence or addiction, which is associated with drug abuse.

The Evolution of Drug Regulation

Governments have only recently required that drug manufacturers demonstrate the effectiveness and safety of their medicinal products. Although controversy continues as to how restrictive laws that regulate drug use and marketing should be, few would argue that we should return to the "good old days" of unregulated laissez-faire policies, when patients took all the risks and drug companies were without liability. Those were the days of patent medicines, nostrums, elixirs, restoratives, rejuvenators, and panacea medicines, which were sold freely and without question to a naive public.

The Great American Fraud: Patent Medicines

In the late 1800s and early 1900s, the sales of uncontrolled medicines flourished and became widespread. Many of these products were called **patent medicines**, which signified that the ingredients were secret, not that they were patented. The law of the day seemed to be more concerned with someone's recipe being stolen than with preventing harm to the naive consumer. Toxic ingredients in these medicines included acetanilid in Bromo-Seltzer and Orangeine and prussic (hydrocyanic) acid in Shiloh's Consumption Cure.

Most of the patent medicines appear to have been composed largely of either colored water or alcohol, with an occasional added ingredient such as opium or cocaine. Hostetter's Stomach Bitters, with 44% alcohol, could easily have been classified as liquor. Sale of Peruna (28% alcohol) was prohibited to Native Americans because of its high alcoholic content! Birney's Catarrh Cure contained 4% cocaine. Wistar's Balsam of Wild Cherry (see Figure 3.1), Dr. King's Discovery for Consumption, Mrs. Winslow's Soothing Syrup, and several others contained opiates as well as alcohol.

The medical profession of the mid- and late-nineteenth century was ill prepared to do battle with the ever-present manufacturers or distributors of patent medicines. Qualified physicians during this time were rare. Much more common were medical practitioners with poor training and little understanding. In fact, many of these early physicians practiced a brand of medicine that was generally useless and frequently more life threatening than the patent medicines themselves.

PATENT MEDICINES unregulated proprietary medicines often associated with fraudulent therapy

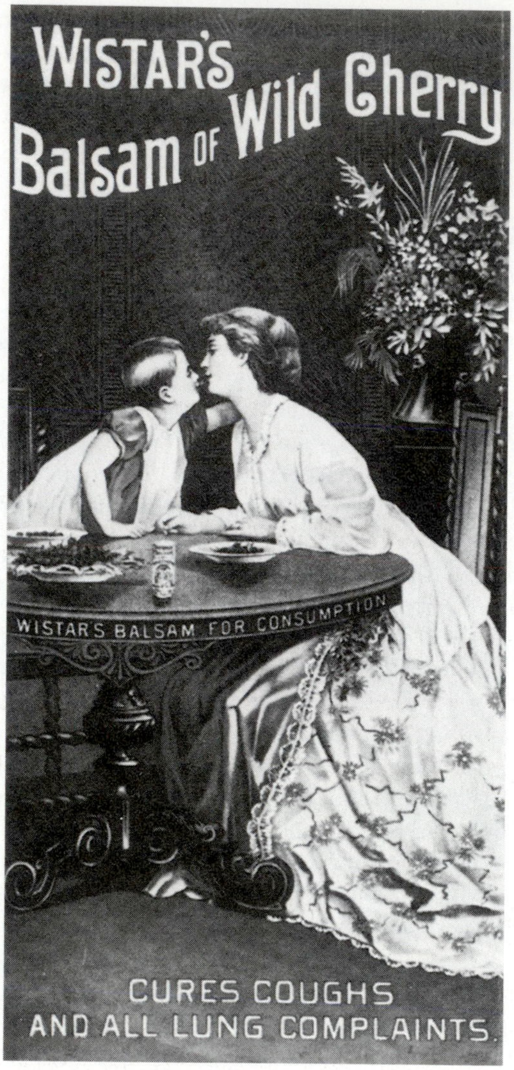

Figure 3.1 A poster of one of the patent medicines that contained liberal doses of opium and a high concentration of alcohol. Wistar's medicine was widely used around the turn of the century to treat tuberculosis ("consumption"), which was responsible for over 25% of all adult deaths in the United States. The federal government finally forced the remedy off the market by 1920.

In 1905, *Collier's Magazine* ran a series of articles called the "Great American Fraud," which warned of the abuse of patent medicines. This brought the problem to the attention of the public (Adams 1905). *Collier's* coined the phrase "dope fiend" from *dope,* an African word meaning "intoxicating substance." The American Medical Association (AMA) joined in and widely distributed reprints of the *Collier's* story to inform the public about the dangers of these medicines, even though the AMA itself accepted advertisements for patent medicines that physicians knew were addicting. The publicity caused mounting pressure on Congress and on President Roosevelt to do something about these fraudulent products. In 1905, the president proposed that a law be enacted to regulate interstate commerce of misbranded and adulterated foods, drinks, and drugs. This received further impetus when Upton Sinclair's book *The Jungle* was published in 1906—a nauseatingly realistic exposé describing in detail the filth, disease, and putrefaction in the Chicago stockyards.

Not all patent medicines were ineffective, watered-down concoctions without pharmacological activity. In fact, some of these so-called curatives were all too active and contained potent, dangerous, and addicting drugs. Two of these substances helped shape attitudes that would form the basis of regulatory policies for years to come: the opium derivatives (narcotic drugs, such as heroin and morphine) and cocaine (see Case in Point).

Stages in Recognizing a Health Hazard: The Case of Opium

People today do not realize how recently it was common to eat or smoke opium in the United States and throughout Europe. The opium "eaters" were typically middle-class Caucasians who often became hooked on opiates while using patent medicines to relieve pain. In addition, physicians at the time believed an opiate dependency was better than alcoholism and even encouraged substitution of one drug for the other. For example, the famous English physician Thomas Sydenhaum enthusiastically advocated the replacement of alcohol with laudanum, a concoction of opium dissolved in sherry-flavored cinnamon, cloves, and saffron. The most common uses of laudanum and other opium products were to treat pain and diarrhea and to promote a sense of relaxation and well-being. Many famous people of the nineteenth century, including writers such as Samuel Taylor Coleridge, became addicted to laudanum (Scott 1969).

Although such concoctions were used freely, physicians were aware of opium's dangerous properties; however, they maintained that the benefits of use far outweighed the dangers. One such clini-

Case in Point

"Wonder Drugs" That Fooled Even the Great Doctors

Some of the world's most famous doctors were fooled for a time by the untested but apparently beneficial effects of drugs that are now, a century later, notorious for their dangers to health and society.

Opium and morphine, which helped numb the pain for so many wounded in the American Civil War, were both candidates for the "wonder drug" that might help stressed and nervous people become calm and focused, according to George Wood, a prestigious University of Pennsylvania professor. In the years after the Civil War, Wood minimized the known addictive dangers of opium and wrote the most glowing medical endorsements for it. He said that opium produced "a universal feeling of delicious ease and comfort," as well as "an exaltation of our better mental qualities, a warmer glow of benevolence, a disposition to do great things, ... a higher devotional spirit." He announced that opium raised "the intellectual and imaginative faculties to the highest point." The prestige of such a famous doctor's endorsement went a long way in blinding Americans to the dangers of opium, which were becoming increasingly obvious over the years.

The next "wonder drug," cocaine, received a similar rave review from an even more famous physician, psychiatrist Sigmund Freud. He saw this stimulant as a cure for depression and as a relatively harmless substitute for opium addiction. In 1884, Freud described his medicinal use of cocaine: "I have been working with a miracle drug. I have had dazzling success in the treatment of a case of gastric catarrh. . . . I take very small doses of it regularly against depression and against indigestion, and with the most brilliant success." Freud wrote a treatise on cocaine entitled *"Uber Coca"* ("about coca"), which he described as "a song of praise for this magical substance."

Freud's enthusiasm for the substance diminished somewhat when he began to appreciate the dangers of this drug. He used cocaine as a substitute to help wean his friend, Fleischl, from morphine addiction (Aldrich and Barker 1976). Following administration of large doses of the powerful stimulant, Freud spent a frightful night nursing Fleischl through an episode of cocaine-induced psychosis. In the end, Fleischl's opium addiction was relieved, but an addiction to cocaine took its place. After this experience, Freud turned against the use of all drugs (Holmstedt 1967).

Are there any lessons in these experiences that have relevance to society's current problems with drugs of abuse?

cian was George Wood, a professor of medicine at the University of Pennsylvania. In 1868, he wrote that opium addiction could result in "total loss of self-respect, and indifference to the opinions of the community." In addition, he stated that for the truly addicted, "everything is sacrificed to the insatiable demands of the vice." In spite of these condemnations, like his fellow physicians, Wood believed that opium addiction was only marginally dangerous and less of a threat than alcohol addiction.

In the late 1850s and early 1860s, techniques for subcutaneous injection of morphia (an opium derivative related to morphine) became widely available. Prior to this time, opium was only taken by mouth, which was less effective and less addicting. With the advent of injected morphia, the addiction problems became much more severe and generalized (Morgan 1981). A large number of soldiers became addicted to morphine as a result of the use of this drug during the Civil War to treat dysentery, pain, and fatigue and took the habit home when the war was over. At this time, dependence on opium or morphine was considered undesirable and not respectable, but because the drugs were legal (and uncontrolled) and their moderate use did not appear to disrupt the life of the user, addiction caused no serious social concern. At the time, the only restriction on importation was a tax, passed in 1842, on all opiates brought into the United States.

Although public concern would probably have developed sooner or later because of the increasing occurrence of opiate addiction among the white middle class, the first restrictions were directed at opium smoking among Chinese immigrants. Tens of thousands of Chinese laborers were brought to the United States in the 1850s and 1860s to work on the railroad construction throughout the West. They brought with them their custom of smoking opium for relaxation. Labor contractors actually offered an allowance of half a pound of smoking opium a month as a bonus to recruit Chinese immigrant laborers. This policy continued until an economic depression affected areas with large concentrations of Chinese immigrants. Unemployed U.S. workers (there were no unemployment checks or welfare benefits then) unfairly blamed the Chinese laborers as the cause of their economic problems. The Chinese-run *opium dens* became a convenient scapegoat for unvented frustrations and often the focus of fabricated stories. White women and girls supposedly were induced to visit the opium dens, whereupon they were forced into addiction and became depraved "dope fiends."

It was possible in many states to buy smoking-grade opium in pharmacies and even in general stores. The state of Nevada, in 1877, was the first to prohibit retail sales of smoking opium. Twenty states—mostly in the West, with a substantial immigrant Chinese population—passed statutes to prohibit operation of opium dens or the smoking and possession of opium. The actual importation and selling of opium remained legal until 1887, when importation of opium by Chinese (but not by Americans!) was forbidden. The effect of this restriction was to encourage smuggling by organized groups. The tariff was increased further in 1890 and then halved in 1897 to discourage the smuggling and illegal manufacture by Chinese. In 1909, the Smoking Opium Exclusion Act banned the importation of smoking-grade opium, again as a response to inflammatory anti-Chinese publicity about U.S. girls and boys who were lured into addiction and "doomed, hopelessly doomed, beyond the shadow of redemption" (Austin 1978). This emotional attack on smoking opium is difficult to reconcile with the frequent use of laudanum and injected morphine by middle-class Americans at that time. In 1914, the tax was increased to $400 per pound on opium prepared in the United States, and the Harrison Act, also passed in 1914, increased penalties for illegal use of opiates even further.

With increased concern about the growing problem of opium addiction, attempts were made to treat and cure severe dependence. One of the most notable efforts for treatment was proposed by German physician Eduard Levinstein in 1878. He recommended that the addicted patient be isolated for one to two weeks in a room devoid of any means of committing suicide. The patient would be constantly attended, and withdrawal symptoms would be treated with hot baths, bicarbonate of soda, chloral hydrate (a CNS depressant; see Chapter 6), and unlimited quantities of brandy and champagne (apparently a rich person's cure). Levinstein believed that, once a cure had been achieved, there would be no relapse. He also felt that, if governments would rigidly regulate morphia and only permit physicians access to the drug, addiction would become a rare occurrence. Unfortunately, while Levinstein's approach was well intended (and actually incorporated some concepts that are still used today to treat drug dependence), it was relatively ineffective; there was only minimal success.

Changing Attitudes: The Dangers of Cocaine

The idea of weaning addicts from drug dependence by substituting another drug became popular as the incidence of opium addiction became more alarming. One drug commonly used to relieve opium users of their narcotic habit was the potent stimulant cocaine (Morgan 1981). Cocaine was first refined from the Peruvian coca plant in 1860 by Albert Niemann. Although the powers of the coca plant had been known in Europe as early as the sixteenth century, the properties of its active ingredient, cocaine, had not been studied. Once purified, many individuals became intrigued with its powerful effects on the nervous system. The famous psychiatrist Sigmund Freud was particularly interested in this potent stimulant as an antidepressant. He hoped it would be a harmless replacement for opium addiction, but he soon became disillusioned by the harmful effects of cocaine.

The American experience with cocaine in some ways mirrored that of Freud. Because of its numbing effects, cocaine was first used in America as a nerve tonic. Like Freud, the American people at first embraced this new miracle drug with great enthusiasm. It was included in tonics—the best known of which was called Coca-Cola—as well as in wines and an array of patent medicines promoted as cures for coughing to hemorrhoids (see Chapter 10 for more details) (Wallace et al. 1981). Exaggerated claims were the rule of the day (Morgan 1981). One advocate declared that cocaine "would supply the place of food, and make the coward brave and the silent eloquent." Actually, the continual use of this drug made the unsuspecting addicted, a lesson that the American people painfully learned and are learning again.

It was against this backdrop of ineffectual patent medicines and growing awareness of the dangers of addiction to opium and cocaine that legislation was first passed to provide safer and more effective pharmaceutical products to the public while restricting access to addicting substances.

The Road to Regulation and the FDA

The decline of patent medicines started with the 1906 Pure Food and Drug Act, which required manufacturers to indicate the amounts of alcohol, morphine, opium, cocaine, heroin, and marijuana extract on the label of each container. It became obvious at this time that many of the medicinal products on the market labeled as nonaddictive were in fact potent drugs "in sheep's labeling" and could cause severe dependence. However, most government interest centered on regulation of the food industry, not drugs. Even though federal drug regulation was based on the free-market philosophy that consumers could select for themselves, it was decided that the public should have information on possible dependence-producing drugs to ensure that they understood the risks associated with using these products. The Pure Food and Drug Act made misrepresentation illegal, so that a potentially addicting patent drug could not be advertised as nonhabit forming. This marked the beginning of new involvement by governmental agencies in drug manufacturing. (See Table 3.1 for a summary of federal regulation of drug marketing.)

The Pure Food and Drug Act was modified, although not in a consumer-protective manner, by the Sherley Amendment in 1912. The distributor of a cancer "remedy" was indicted for falsely claiming on the label that the contents were effective. The case was decided in the U.S. Supreme Court in 1911. Justice Holmes, writing for the majority opinion, said that, based on the 1906 act, the company had not violated any law because legally all it was required to do was accurately state the contents, their strength and quality. The accuracy of the therapeutic claims made by drug manufacturers was not controlled. Congress took the hint and passed the Sherley Amendment to add to the existing law the requirement that labels should not contain "any statement ... regarding the curative or therapeutic effect ... which is false and fraudulent." However, the government had to prove fraud, which turned out to be difficult (and in fact is still problematic). This amendment did not improve drug products. It only encouraged pharmaceutical companies to be more vague in their advertisements (Temin 1980).

Prescription Versus OTC Drugs

The distinction between prescription and over-the-counter (OTC) drugs is relatively new to the pharmaceutical industry. All nonnarcotic drugs were available OTC prior to World War II. It was not until a drug company unwittingly produced a toxic product that killed over 100 people that the Food and Drug Administration (FDA) was given control over drug safety in the 1938 Federal Food, Drug, and Cosmetic Act (Hunter 1993). The bill had been debated for several years in Congress and showed no promise of passage. Then a pharmaceutical company decided to sell a liquid form of a

TABLE 3.1 Milestones in federal regulations that control drug marketing

Date	Name of Legislation	Cause	Content
1906	Pure Food and Drug	Concern about addiction to patent medicines	Potentially addicting patent medicines required to be labeled
1912	Sherley Amendment	An ineffective cancer remedy	Drug labels could not contain false or fraudulent claims
1938	Federal Food, Drug, and Cosmetic Act	More than one hundred people killed by a sulfa product dissolved in diethylene glycol	Defined what was meant by term *drugs*; gave the FDA authority to regulate new drugs; required new drugs be safe; labels to list ingredients and quantity and explain correct use; created prescription and OTC drugs
1951	Durham-Humphrey Amendment	Concern about public use of OTC drugs	Established criteria for prescription and nonprescription drugs
1962	Kefauver-Harris Amendment	Thalidomide tragedy	Established testing procedure for new drugs; required drug companies to demonstrate safety and effectiveness

sulfa drug (the first antibiotic) and found that the drug would dissolve well in a chemical solvent, diethylene glycol (presently used in antifreeze products). The company marketed the antibiotic as Elixir Sulfanilamide without testing the solvent for toxicity. Under the 1906 Pure Food and Drug Act, the company could not be prosecuted for the toxicity of this form of drug or for not testing the formulation of the drug on animals first. They could only be prosecuted for mislabeling the product on the technicality that *elixir* refers to a solution in alcohol, not a solution in diethylene glycol. Again, it was apparent that the laws in place provided woefully inadequate protection for the public.

The 1938 act differed from the 1906 law in several ways. It defined drugs to include products that affected bodily structure or function even in the absence of disease. Companies had to file applications with the government for all new drugs showing that they were *safe* (not effective, just safe!) for use as described. And the drug label had to include all ingredients and the quantity of each, as well as instructions regarding correct use of the drug and warnings about its dangers.

Prior to passage of the 1938 act, you could go to a doctor and get a prescription for any nonnarcotic drug or go to the pharmacy directly if you had already decided what was needed. The effect of the labeling requirement in the 1938 act was to allow drug companies to create a class of drugs that could not be sold legally without a prescription. It has been suggested that the actions by the FDA were motivated by the frequent public misuse of two classes of drugs developed prior to passage of the 1938 law: sulfa antibiotics and barbiturates. People often took too little of the antibiotics to cure an infection and too much of the barbiturates and became addicted.

The 1938 Food, Drug, and Cosmetic Act allowed the manufacturer to determine whether a drug was to be labeled prescription or nonprescription. The same could be sold as prescription by one company and as OTC by another! After the Durham-Humphrey Amendment was passed in 1951, almost all new drugs were placed in the prescription-only class. The drugs that were patented and marketed after World War II included the potent new antibiotics and the phenothiazine tranquilizers such as Thorazine. The FDA and the drug firms thought these were potentially too dangerous to sell OTC. The Durham-Humphrey Amendment established the criteria, which are still used today, for determining if a drug should be classified as prescription or nonprescription. Basically, if a drug

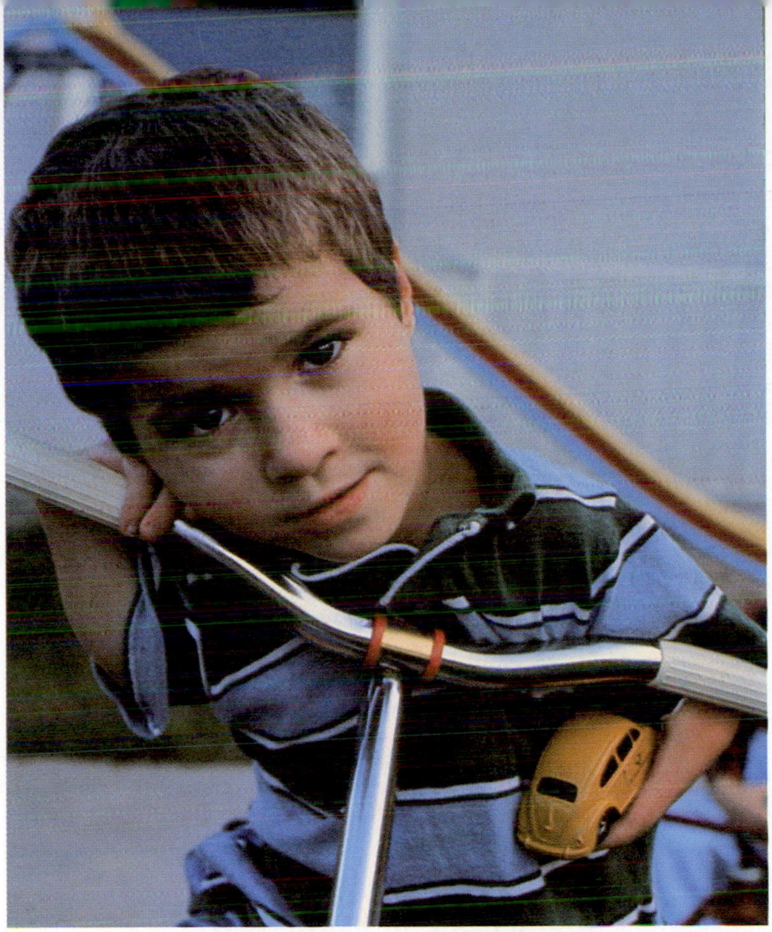

Characteristic limb deformities caused by thalidomide.

does not fall into one of the following three categories, it is considered nonprescription:

1. The drug is habit forming.
2. The drug is not safe for self-medication because of its toxicity.
3. The drug is a new drug that has not been shown to be completely safe.

Senator Kefauver's hearings, which began in 1959, initially were concerned with the enormous profit margins earned by drug companies because of the lack of competition in the market for new, patented drugs. Testimony by physicians revealed that an average doctor in clinical practice often was not able to evaluate accurately the efficacy of the drugs he or she prescribed. The 1938 law did not give the FDA authority to supervise clinical testing of drugs; consequently, the effectiveness of drugs being sold to the public was not being determined. Both the Kefauver and Harris Amendments in the House were intended to deal with this problem but showed no likely signs of becoming law until the **thalidomide** tragedy occurred.

Thalidomide was used in Europe and distributed on a small scale in the United States as a sedative for pregnant women. There are two approximately 24-hour intervals early in pregnancy when thalidomide can alter the development of the arms and legs of an embryo. If a woman takes thalidomide on one or both of these days, the infant could be born with abnormally developed arms and/or legs (called **phocomelia,** from the Greek words for *flippers,* or "seal-shaped limbs").

Although standard testing probably would not have detected this congenital effect of thalidomide

THALIDOMIDE a sedative drug that, when used during pregnancy, can cause severe developmental damage to the fetus

PHOCOMELIA a birth defect; impaired development of the arms or legs or both

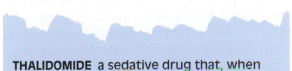

and the tragedy would likely have occurred anyway, these debilitated infants stimulated passage of the 1962 Kefauver and Harris Amendments. They strengthened the government's regulation of both the introduction of new drugs and the production and sale of existing drugs. The amendments required, for the first time, that drug manufacturers demonstrate the efficacy as well as the safety of their drug products. The FDA was empowered to withdraw approval of a drug that was already being marketed. In addition, the FDA was to regulate and evaluate drug testing by pharmaceutical companies and mandate standards of good drug-manufacturing policy.

The Rising Demand for Effectiveness in Medicinal Drugs

To evaluate the effectiveness of the over 4,000 drug products that were introduced between 1938 and 1962, the FDA contracted with the National Research Council to do the Drug Efficacy Study. This investigation started in 1966 and ran for three years. The council was asked to rate drugs as either effective or ineffective. Although the study was supposed to be based on scientific evidence, this often was not available, and so conclusions were sometimes founded on the clinical experience of the physicians on each panel; this was not always reliable information.

A legal challenge resulted when the FDA took an "ineffective" drug off the market and the manufacturer sued. This finally forced the FDA to define what constituted an adequate and well-controlled investigation. Adequate, documented clinical experience was no longer satisfactory proof that a drug was safe and effective. Each new drug application now had to include information about the drug's performance in comparison to that of a carefully defined control group. The drug could be compared with (1) a placebo, (2) another drug known to be active based on previous studies, (3) the established results of no treatment, or (4) historical data on the course of the illness without the use of the drug in question. In addition, a drug marketed before 1962 could no longer be "grandfathered in." If the company could not prove the drug had the qualifications to pass the post-1962 tests for a new drug, it was considered a new, unapproved drug and could not legally be sold.

Regulating the Development of New Drugs

The amended Federal Food, Drug, and Cosmetic Act in force today requires that all new drugs be registered with and approved by the FDA. The FDA is mandated by Congress to (1) ensure the rights and safety of human subjects during clinical testing of experimental drugs; (2) evaluate the safety and efficacy of new treatments based on test results and information from the sponsors (often health-related companies); (3) compare potential benefits and risks to determine if a new drug should be approved and marketed (Hunter et al. 1993). Because of FDA regulations, all pharmaceutical companies must follow a series of steps when seeking permission to market a new drug (see Figure 3.2).

Regulatory Steps for New Prescription Drugs

Step 1: Preclinical Research and Development A chemical must be synthesized and identified as having potential value in the treatment of a particular condition or disease. The company interested in marketing the chemical as a drug must run a series of tests on at least three animal species. Careful records must be kept of side effects, absorption, distribution, metabolism, excretion, and the dosages of the drug necessary to produce the various effects. **Carcinogenic, mutagenic,** and **teratogenic** variables are tested. The dose–response curve must be determined along with potency, and then the risk and benefit of the substance must be calculated (see Chapter 4). If the company still believes there is a market for the

CARCINOGENIC able to cause cancer

MUTAGENIC able to cause mutation (alter genes)

TERATOGENIC able to cause abnormal development of the fetus

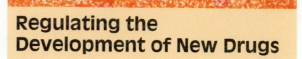

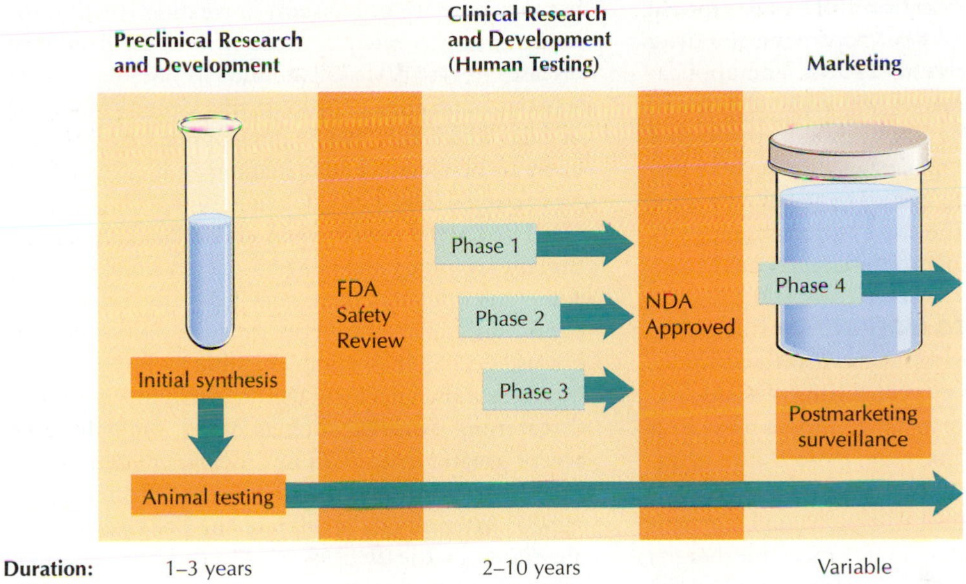

FIGURE 3.2 The steps required by the FDA for reviewing a new drug

substance, it will forward the data to the FDA to obtain an investigational new drug (IND) number for further tests.

Step 2: Clinical Research and Development

Animal tests provide some information, but ultimately, tests must be done on the species for which the potential drug is intended, the human. These tests usually follow three phases (Simonsen 1993). Phase 1 is called the *initial clinical stage.* Small numbers of volunteers (usually 20 to 100), both healthy people and patients in free clinics, are used to establish drug safety and dose range for effective treatment and to examine side effects. Formerly, much of this research was done on prison inmates, but because of bad publicity and the possibility of coercion, fewer prisoners are used today. Medical students, paid college student volunteers, and volunteers being treated at free clinics are more often used after obtaining "informed consent." All the data are collected, analyzed, and sent to the FDA for approval before beginning the next phase of human subject testing.

Phase 2 testing is called the *clinical pharmacological evaluation stage.* The effects of the drug are tested to eliminate investigator bias and to determine side effects and the effectiveness of the treatment. Because the safety of the new drug has not been thoroughly established, a few patients (100–300 volunteers) with the medical problem the drug is intended to treat are used for these studies. Statistical evaluation of all this information is done before proceeding with phase 3 testing.

Phase 3 is the *extended clinical evaluation.* By this time, the pharmaceutical company has a good idea of drug effectiveness as well as dangers. The drug can be offered safely to a wider group of participating clinics and physicians, who cooperate in administration of the potential drug—when medically appropriate—to thousands of volunteer patients who have given informed consent.

This stage makes the drug available on a wide experimental basis. Sometimes, by this point, there has been publicity about the new drug, and people with the particular disease for which the drug was developed may actively seek out physicians licensed to experiment with it.

During phase 3 testing, safety checks are made and any side effects are noted that might show up as more people are exposed to the drug. After the testing program is over, careful analysis is made of the effectiveness, side effects, and recommended dosage. If there are sufficient data to demonstrate the drug is safe and effective, the company will submit a New Drug Application (NDA) as a formal request that the FDA consider approving the drug for marketing (Hunter et al. 1993). The application usually comprises many thousands of pages of data and analysis, and the FDA must sift through it and decide whether the risks of using the drug justify its potential benefits. The FDA usually calls for additional tests before the drug is determined safe and effective and granting permission to market it.

Step 3: Permission to Market At this point, the FDA can allow the drug to be marketed under its patented name. It may cost \$200 to \$500 million and take up to 12 years to develop a new drug in the United States (Simonsen 1993). The situation is similar elsewhere, although in some European countries, the clinical evaluations are less stringent and require less time. Once the drug is marketed, it continues to be closely scrutinized for adverse effects. This postmarketing surveillance is often referred to as *phase 4* and is important, because in some cases negative effects may not show up for a long time. For example, it was determined in 1970 that diethylstilbestrol (DES), when given to pregnant women to prevent miscarriage, causes an increased risk of a rare type of vaginal cancer in their daughters when these children entered their teens and young adult years. The FDA subsequently removed from the market the form of DES that had been used to treat pregnant women. As described earlier, the thalidomide tragedy resulted in passage of the law that gave the FDA this authority.

Exceptions: Special Drug-Marketing Laws

There is continual concern that the process used by the FDA to evaluate prospective drugs is laborious and excessively lengthy. Recently, an amendment was passed to accelerate the evaluation of urgently needed drugs. The so-called fast-track rule has been applied to testing of certain drugs used for the treatment of rare cancers, AZT (zidovudine) for the treatment of AIDS (the review process only required two years; Hunter et al. 1993), and other similar drugs. As a result, they have reached the market after a much reduced testing program.

A second amendment, the Orphan Drug Law, allows drug companies to receive tax advantages if they develop drugs that are not very profitable because they are only useful in treating small numbers of patients, such as those who suffer from rare diseases. A rare disease is defined as one that affects less than 200,000 people in the United States or one for which the cost of developing a drug is not likely to be recovered by marketing it (*Drug Facts and Comparisons* 1991).

The federal government and the FDA are continually refining the system for evaluating new drugs in order to assure that new effective therapeutic substances can be made available for clinical use as soon as it is safely possible. Some of these modifications reflect the fact that patients with life-threatening diseases, such as AIDS, are willing to accept greater drug risks in order gain faster access to potentially useful medications (Hunter et al. 1993). Attempts to accelerate the drug review are illustrated by the *Prescription Drug User Fee Act* of 1992. Under this law fees are paid by the FDA-regulated pharmaceutical companies to support additional FDA reviewers in order to decrease the average review time for drugs that will treat life-threatening and serious diseases from an average of two years to approximately one year ("A Speedier FDA," 1992).

The Regulation of Nonprescription Drugs

As already mentioned, the Durham-Humphrey Amendment to the Food, Drug, and Cosmetic Act made a distinction between prescription and nonprescription (OTC) drugs and required the FDA to regulate OTC marketing. In 1972, the FDA initiated a program to evaluate the effectiveness and safety of the nonprescription drugs on the market and to ensure that they included appropriate labeling (for more details, see Chapter 14). Each so-called active ingredient in the OTC medications was reviewed by a panel of drug experts, including physicians, pharmacologists, and pharmacists. Based on the recommendations of these panels, the ingredients were placed in one of the following three categories:

I. Generally recognized as safe and effective for the claimed therapeutic indication
II. Not generally recognized as safe and effective or unacceptable indications
III. Insufficient data available to permit final classification

By 1981, the panels made initial determinations on over 700 ingredients in more than 300,000 OTC drug products and submitted more than 60 reports to the FDA.

In the second phase of the OTC drug review, the FDA evaluated the panels' findings and submitted a tentative adoption of the panels' recommendations (after revision, if necessary), following public comment and scrutiny. After a period of time and careful consideration of new information, the agency issued a final ruling and classification of the ingredients under consideration.

The Effects of the OTC Review on Today's Medications The review process for OTC ingredients has had a significant impact on the public's attitude about OTC products and their use (both good and bad) in self-medication. It was apparent from the review process that many OTC drug ingredients did not satisfy the requirements for safety and effectiveness. In fact, in 1990 alone, the FDA banned 223 uses of nonprescription drug ingredients, ruling that the ingredients were ineffective against problems ranging from acne to swimmer's ear. Consequently, it is almost certain that, in the future, there will be fewer active ingredients in OTC medicines, but these drugs will be safer and more effective than ever before. In addition, with heightened public awareness, greater demand has been brought to bear on the FDA to make better drugs available to the public for self-medication. In response to these pressures, the FDA has adopted a **switching policy,** which allows it to review prescription drugs and evaluate their suitability as OTC products. The following criteria must be satisfied if a drug is to be switched:

1. The drug has been marketed by prescription for at least three years.
2. Use of the drug has been relatively high during the time it was available as a prescription drug.
3. Adverse drug reactions are not alarming, and the frequency of side effects has not increased during the time the drug was available to the public.

Since this policy was instituted, approximately 50 to 60 drugs have been switched to OTC status, and many more are being considered. Eventually a total of 200–250 ingredients are likely to be considered for switching.

In general, this switching policy has been well received by the public. In fact, 65% of the switched ingredients have ranked first or second in their drug categories within the first five years of being switched (Siegelman 1990). The medical community and the FDA are generally positive about OTC switches, as well. There are some concerns, however, that more effective drug products will lead to increased abuse or misuse of OTC products.

William E. Gilbertson, director of the FDA's division of OTC drug evaluation, feels that the agency needs to proceed cautiously with switches and place greater emphasis on adequate labeling and education to assure that consumers have sufficient information to use OTC products safely and effectively. "Most assuredly, making more drugs available will put an added burden on consumers in terms of benefit/risk decisions. In that regard, the ways we disseminate OTC information will be important" (Siegelman 1990).

The Regulation of Drug Advertising

Much of the public's knowledge and impressions about drugs, especially those available OTC, come from advertisements. It is difficult to ascertain the amount of money currently spent by the pharmaceutical industry to promote its products. Because of the intense competition between OTC drugs, it is likely that up to 15 to 20% of the dollar sales for these products is spent on advertising to the general public and equals a sum of approximately $10 billion annually. For prescription drugs, it is likely that the costs of advertising, promoting, and marketing exceeds $10 billion annually (Woolsey 1994).

There is no doubt that these promotional efforts by pharmaceutical manufacturers have tremendous impact on the drug-purchasing habits of the general public and health professionals. Not surprisingly, drug use based on misleading or false

SWITCHING POLICY an FDA policy allowing the change of suitable prescription drugs to OTC status advertising claims rather than facts can result in unsatisfactory drug therapy and can be extremely dangerous (Woolsey 1994). Regulations governing the advertising of nonprescription drugs are set and enforced by the Federal Trade Commission. These rules are less stringent than those for prescription medicines.

Prescription Advertising The economics of prescription drugs is unique because a second party, the health professional, dictates what the consumer, the patient, will purchase. There have been recent efforts by pharmaceutical companies to advertise medications directly to the public. Direct consumer advertising of prescription drugs has experts concerned that patients will put pressure on physicians to prescribe inappropriately. For example, in 1992 more than $100 million was spent by pharmaceutical companies for public advertising (TV, newspapers, magazines, and so on) of nicotine patches for people trying to quit smoking. Because of advertising, it is argued by medical experts that many consumers perceive the patches as a quick cure for their tobacco dependence and ignore the fact that they only work as part of a serious behavior modification program. Critics claim this lack of consumer understanding led to incorrect use of the patches and has resulted in fatal heart attacks (Hwang 1992). However, the vast majority of prescription drug promotion is directed at the health professional and controlled by the FDA. The approaches employed by manufacturers to encourage health professionals to prescribe their products include advertising in prestigious medical journals, direct mail advertising, and some radio and television advertising. All printed and audio materials distributed by drug salespeople are controlled by advertising regulations from the FDA. Perhaps the most effective sales approach is having drug representatives personally visit health professionals; this tactic is harder to regulate.

Unfortunately, many health professionals rely on drug company salespeople for the so-called latest scientific information concerning drugs and their effects. Although these representatives of the drug industry can provide an important informational service, it is essential that health professionals remember that these people make a living by selling their products, and often their information is biased accordingly (Woolsey 1994).

Many people in and out of the medical community have questioned the ethics of drug advertising and marketing in the United States and are concerned about the negative impact that deceptive promotion has on target populations (Woolsey 1994). One of the biggest problems in dealing with misleading or false advertising is defining such deception. Probably the best guideline for such a definition is summarized in the Wheeler-Lea Amendment to the Federal Trade Commission Act:

> The term *false advertisement* means an advertisement, other than labeling, which is misleading in a material respect; and in determining whether any advertisement is misleading, there shall be taken into account not only representations ... but the extent to which the advertisement fails to reveal facts.

Tough questions are being asked as to how much control should be exerted over the pharmaceutical industry to protect the public without excessively infringing on the rights of these companies to promote their goods. The solutions to these problems will not be simple; however, efforts to keep drug advertisements accurate, in good taste, and informative are worthwhile and will be necessary if the public is expected to make rational decisions about drug use.

Federal Regulation and Quality Assurance

No matter what policy is adopted by the FDA and other drug-regulating agencies, there will always be those who criticize their efforts and complain that they do not do enough or that they do too much. The FDA has been blamed for being excessively careful and requiring too much testing before new drugs are approved for marketing; on the other hand, when new drugs are released and cause serious side effects, the FDA is condemned for being sloppy in its control of drug marketing.

What is the proper balance, and what do we, as consumers, have the right to expect from government? These are questions each of us should ask, and we have a right to share our answers with government representatives.

On the other hand, regardless of our individual feelings, it is important to understand that the current (and likely future) federal regulations do not assure drug safety or effectiveness for everyone. Too many individual variables alter the way each of us responds to drugs, making such universal assurances impossible. Federal agencies can only deal with general policies and make general decisions. For example, what if the FDA determines that a given drug is reasonably safe in 95% of the population and effective in 70%? Are these acceptable figures, or should a drug be safe in 99% and effective in 90% before it is suitable for general marketing? What of the 5 or 1% of the population who will be adversely affected by this drug? What rights do they have to be protected?

There are no simple answers to these questions. Federal policies are compromises that assume that the clinician who prescribes the drug and/or the patient who buys and consumes it will be able to identify when use of that drug is inappropriate or threatening. Unfortunately, sometimes drug prescribing and drug consuming are done carelessly and unnecessary side effects occur or the drug does not work. The questions surface again: Are federal drug agencies doing all they can to protect the public? Should the laws be changed?

It is always difficult to predict the future, especially when it depends on fickle politicians and erratic public opinion. Nevertheless, with the dramatic increase in new and better drugs being available to the public, it is not likely that federal or state agencies will diminish their role in regulating drug use. Now more than ever, the public demands safer and more effective drugs. This public attitude will likely translate into even greater involvement by regulatory agencies in issues of drug development, assessment, and marketing.

Another reason for increased regulation in the future is that many of the larger pharmaceutical companies have become incredibly wealthy. Several of the most profitable companies have become subsidiaries of powerful corporations that are driven more by profit margins than philanthropic interests. In such an environment, governmental agencies are essential to assure that the rights of the public are protected. Only a fool would desire a return to the early days of federal policies based on "buyer beware" principles.

Drug Abuse and the Law

The laws that govern the development, distribution, and use of drugs in general and drugs of abuse in particular are intertwined. There are, however, some unique features concerning the manner in which federal agencies deal with the drugs of abuse that warrant special consideration. A summary of drug abuse laws in the U.S. is shown in Table 3.2, and a section on the development of laws and enforcement agencies appears in Appendix 3.1.

Coffee, tea, tobacco, alcohol, marijuana, hallucinogens, depressants (such as barbiturates), and narcotics have been subject to a wide range of controls, from none to rigid. Islamic countries have instituted severe penalties, such as strangulation for smoking tobacco or opium, and strict bans on alcohol. In other countries, these substances have been legal or prohibited, depending on the political situation and the desires of the population. Historically, laws have been changed when so many people demanded access to a specific drug of abuse that it would have been impossible to enforce a ban (as in the revocation of Prohibition) or because the government needed tax revenues that could be raised by selling the drug (one argument for legalizing drugs of abuse today).

The negative experiences that Americans had at the turn of the century with addicting substances such as opium led to the Harrison Act of 1914. This was the first legitimate effort by the federal government to regulate and control the production, importation, sales, purchase, and distribution of addicting substances. The Harrison Act served as the foundation and reference for subsequent laws directed at regulating drug abuse issues.

Today, the ways in which law enforcement agencies deal with substance abuse are largely determined by the Comprehensive Drug Abuse Prevention and Control Act of 1970. This act divided substances with abuse potential into categories based on the degree of their abuse potential and their clinical usefulness. The classifications are referred to as *Schedules* and range from I to V. Schedule I substances have high abuse potential and no currently approved medicinal use; they can-

TABLE 3.2 Federal laws for the control of narcotic and other abused drugs

Date	Name of Legislation	Summary of Coverage and Intent of Legislation
1914	Harrison Act	First federal legislation to regulate and control the production, importation, sale, purchase, and free distribution of opium or drugs derived from opium
1922	Narcotic Drug Import and Export Act	Intends to eliminate the use of narcotics except for medical and other legitimate purposes
1924	Heroin Act	Makes it illegal to manufacture heroin
1937	Marijuana Tax Act	Provides controls over marijuana similar to the Harrison Act over narcotics
1942	Opium Poppy Control Act	Prohibits growing opium poppies in the United States except under license
1951	Boggs Amendment to the Harrison Narcotics Act	Establishes severe mandatory penalties for conviction on narcotics charges
1956	Narcotics Control Act	Intends to impose very severe penalties for those convicted of narcotics or marijuana charges
1965	Drug Abuse Control Amendments (DACA)	Adopts strict controls over amphetamines, barbiturates, LSD, and similar substances with provisions to add new substances as the need arises
1966	Narcotic Addict Rehabilitation Act (NARA)	Allows treatment as an alternative to jail
1968	DACA Amendments	Provides that sentence may be suspended and record be erased if not convicted for another violation for one year
1970	Comprehensive Drug Abuse Prevention and Control Act	Replaces or updates all other laws concerning narcotics and dangerous drugs
1972	Drug Abuse Office and Treatment Act	Establishes $1.1 billion over three years to combat drug abuse and start treatment programs
1973	Methadone Control Act	Places controls on methadone licensing
1973	Heroin Trafficking Act	Increases penalties for traffickers and makes bail procedures more stringent
1973	Alcohol, Drug Abuse, and Mental Health Administration (ADAMHA)	Consolidates NIMH, NIAAA, and NIDA under ADAMHA
1973	Drug Enforcement Administration (DEA)	Bureau of Narcotics and Dangerous Drugs is remodeled to become the DEA
1974 and 1978	Drug Abuse Prevention, Control, and Treatment Amendments	Extends the 1972 law
1978	Alcohol and Drug Abuse Education Amendments	Sets up Office of Alcohol and Drug Abuse Education in the Department of Education; more emphasis on drug abuse in rural areas and on coordination at the federal–state level
1980	Drug Abuse Prevention, Treatment, and Rehabilitation Amendments	Extends prevention education and rehabilitation programs
1984	Drug Offenders Act	Sets up special program for offenders and organizes treatment
1986	Analogue (Designer Drug) Act	Makes illegal the use of substances similar in effects and structure to substances already scheduled
1988	Anti–Drug Abuse Act	Establishes the Office of the National Drug Control Policy to oversee all federal policies regarding research about and control of drugs of abuse
1992	ADAMHA Reorganization Act	Transfers three institutes of ADAMHA (NIDA, NIAAA, and NIMH) to NIH, and incorporated ADAMHA's services program into the new Substance Abuse and Mental Health Services Administration (SAMHSA)

CSA Schedule	Drugs	Quantity	First Offense	Second Offense
I & II	Methamphetamine Heroin LSD Cocaine and cocaine base Potent narcotics (Fentanyl)	Low quantities	Maximum: 40 years/$2 million	Maximum: life/$4 million
		High quantities	Maximum: life/$4 million	Maximum: life/$8 million
III	All	Any quantity	Maximum: 5 years/$250,000	Maximum: 10 years/$500,000
IV	All		Maximum: 3 years/$250,000	Maximum: 6 years/$500,000
V	All		Maximum: 1 year/$100,000	Maximum: 2 years/$200,000

FIGURE 3.3 Federal trafficking penalties *Source:* "Drugs of Abuse," p. 9. Courtesy of the Drug Enforcement Administration, U.S. Government Printing Office, Washington, DC., 1988.

not be prescribed by health professionals. Schedule II drugs also have high abuse potential but are approved for medical purposes and can be prescribed, with restrictions. The distinctions between Schedule II through V substances are the likelihood of abuse occurring and the degree to which the drugs are controlled by governmental agencies. The least addictive and least regulated of the substances of abuse are classified as Schedule V (see Appendix 3.1 for more details).

Factors in Controlling Drug Abuse

Three principal issues influence laws on drug abuse:

1. If a person abuses a drug, should he or she be treated as a criminal or as a sick person inflicted with a disease?
2. How is the user (supposedly the victim) distinguished from the pusher (supposedly the criminal) of an illicit drug, and who should be more harshly punished—the person that creates the demand for the drug or the person who satisfies the demand?
3. Are the law and associated penalties effective deterrents against drug use or abuse, and how is effectiveness determined?

In regard to the first issue, drug abuse may be considered both an illness and a crime. It is a psychiatric disorder, an abnormal functional state, when a person is compelled (either physically or psychologically—see Chapter 4) to continue using the drug (American Psychiatric Association 1994). It is a crime when the law, reflecting social opinion, has made abuse of the drug illegal. Health issues are clearly involved because uncontrolled abuse of almost any drug can lead to physical and/or psychological damage. Because the public has to pay for health care costs or societal damage, laws are created and penalties implemented to prevent or correct drug abuse problems. (See Figure 3.3 on federal trafficking penalties.)

Concerning the second issue, drug laws have always been more lenient to the *user* than to the *seller* of a drug of abuse. Actually, it is often hard to separate user from pusher, as many drug abusers engage in both activities. Because huge profits are often involved, some people may not use the drugs they peddle and are only pushers; the law tries to deter use of drugs by concentrating on these persons but has questionable success. Organized crime is involved in major drug sales, and these "drug rings" have proven hard to destroy.

In regard to the third issue, all available evidence indicates that, in the United States, criminal law has only limited success in deterring drug abuse. Even though there were signs that the use of illicit drugs declined from 1985–1992, since then, use of illicit drugs has leveled off. During 1992, approximately 27% of twelfth-graders used an illicit drug; marijuana was used by 22%, LSD by

5.6%, and cocaine by 3.1% (Johnston 1993). The total number of Americans using illegal drugs in 1992 has been estimated by the National Household Survey on Drug Abuse to be 11.4 million ("National Household Survey" 1993). It is clear that the drug abuse problem is far from being resolved, and many feel that some changes should be made in how we deal with this problem.

Recent efforts to control illegal drugs have been principally through **interdiction** of supply. In fact, in 1992 interdiction received more than 60% of the total congressional appropriations for drug control (Millstein 1993a), despite the fact that this approach has not been particularly effective. For example, the *Houston Chronicle* investigated the impact of a $2 billion radar and surveillance system designed to detect and apprehend air drug smugglers. During the five months of the study in 1991, none of the 2,500 major drug cases in the Southwest was a direct result of the Custom's Service Air Interdiction Program (Associated Press 1992a). Although it is true that seizures of large caches of illicit drugs seem to be reported routinely in the national press, there is no indication that the availability of drugs has diminished substantially. One can argue that, as long as a strong demand for these psychoactive agents exists, demand will be satisfied if the price is right. Even if interdiction is successful in reducing the supply of one drug of abuse, if demand persists it usually will be replaced by another with similar abuse potential (for example, substitution of amphetamines for cocaine—see Chapter 10).

Demand Reduction

Other approaches based on education should be emphasized in order to eliminate the demand for the drugs of abuses (Fitzpatrick 1992). This objective is not easily achieved. Drug abuse is a complex and very individual problem, with many causes and aggravating factors. Even so, experience has taught us that prevention and demand reduction is a better strategy and, in the long run, less costly than interdiction or the criminal justice system (Goldstein 1994). The following are some suggestions as to how demand can be reduced (Halloway 1991; Fitzpatrick 1992):

INTERDICTION the policy of cutting off or destroying supplies of illicit drugs

1. Reduction of demand by youth must be the top priority of any prevention program if it is to provide a long-term solution. To achieve this requires stabilizing defective family structures, implementing school programs that create an antidrug attitude, establishing a drug-free environment, and promoting resistance training to help youth avoid drug involvement. In addition, youth should be encouraged to be involved in alternative activities that can substitute for drug-abusing activity.

2. Replacement therapy has also shown to be a useful approach to weaning the individual on drugs of abuse. The most common example of this strategy is the use of the narcotic methadone to treat the heroin addict (see Chapter 9). Use of methadone prevents the cravings and severe withdrawal routinely associated with breaking the heroin habit. Unfortunately, most heroin addicts insist that they be maintained on methadone indefinitely. Even though methadone is easier to control and is less disruptive than heroin, one drug addiction has been substituted for another, which draws criticism.

A second example of the replacement approach is the use of Valium-type (benzodiazepines) drugs to treat the alcoholic (see Chapter 6). The benzodiazepines diminish the severe withdrawal responses (both physical and psychological) that occur in the alcohol-dependent person who has abruptly stopped drinking. The amount of benzodiazepine can be gradually decreased, minimizing withdrawal problems.

A similar approach has been advocated for cocaine addiction (see Chapter 10). The use of antidepressants (particularly desipramine) diminishes the intense cravings that cocaine-dependent people experience as they try to give up the habit (Gawin et al. 1989).

Replacement therapy certainly is not the entire answer to all drug abuse problems, but it often can provide a window of opportunity for behavioral modification so that a long-term solution to the abuse problem is possible.

3. Education about drug abuse must be carefully designed and customized for the population or group to be targeted. For example, education based on scare tactics is not likely to dissuade adolescents from experimenting with drugs. Adolescents are at a point in their lives when they feel invincible, and graphically depicting the potential health consequences of drug and alcohol abuse has little impact. A discussion about the nature of addiction and the addiction process is more likely to influence their attitudes. Adolescents need to understand why people use drugs to appreciate the behavior patterns in themselves. Other important topics that should be discussed are how the drugs abuse work and why they lead to dependence. To complement drug education, adolescents also should be taught coping strategies that include proper decision making and problem solving (see Chapter 15).

4. Attitudes toward drug abuse and its consequence must be changed. The drug use patterns of many people, both young and old, are strongly influenced by peers. If people believe that drug abuse is glamorous and contributes to acceptance by friends and associates, the incidence of drug abuse will continue to be high. In contrast, if the prevailing message in society is that drug abuse is unhealthy and not socially acceptable, the incidence will be much less. Some of this message is perhaps being heard: there was a dramatic decline in demand for cocaine in the United States from 1987 to 1990 (see Chapter 10).

Drug Laws and Deterrence

As previously discussed, drug laws often do not serve as a satisfactory deterrent against the use of illicit drugs. People have used and abused drugs for thousands of years despite governmental restrictions. It is very likely they will continue to do so (Balabanova et al. 1992), despite stricter laws and greater support for law enforcement.

As the amount of addiction increased during the mid-1960s, many ill-conceived programs and laws were instituted as knee-jerk reactions, with little understanding about the underlying reasons for the rise in drug abuse. Unpopular restrictive laws rarely work to reduce the use of illicit drugs. Even as laws become more restrictive, there usually is little impact on the level of addiction; in fact, in some cases addiction problems actually have increased. For example, during the restrictive years of the 1960s and 1980s, drugs were sold everywhere to everyone—in high schools, colleges, and probably in every community. In the 1980s especially, increasingly large volumes of drugs were sold throughout the United States. Billions of dollars were paid for those drugs. Although no one knows precisely how much was exchanged, it likely approached $80 to $100 billion a year for all illegal drugs, of which the two biggest categories were an estimated $30 billion for cocaine and $24 billion for marijuana. In fact, it has been claimed that for some states such as California and Oregon, marijuana is the single largest cash crop.

Because of the large sums of money involved, there has been corruption at all levels. Notorious examples include the loss of millions of dollars of contraband heroin and cocaine held as evidence in police vaults in New York City, as well as other cities and towns throughout the country; the indictment of a number of detectives in the homicide division of the Miami police department for selling drugs and taking large bribes; and the claim that there were direct links between drug dealers and the governments of Panama, Colombia, and Bolivia. Some law enforcement agencies have said that drugs are the largest export item from these countries. It is known that Miami has been the key point of entry into the United States for both cocaine and marijuana and that money is "laundered" in businesses set up as fronts.

Other problems associated with the implementation of drug laws are the insufficient number of law enforcement personnel and inadequate detention facilities; consequently much drug traffic goes unchecked. In addition, the judiciary system gets so backlogged that many cases never reach court. Plea bargaining is almost the rule in order to clear the court docket. Often dealers and traffickers are back in business the same day they are arrested. This seriously damages the morale of law enforcers, legislators, and average citizens.

It is estimated that there are nearly 1 million drug-related arrests each year. This is a tremendous cost to society in terms of damaged lives and family relationships; being arrested for drug-related crime seriously jeopardizes the opportunity of a normal life. Drug taking is closely tied to societal problems, and it will remain a problem unless society provides more meaningful experiences to those most susceptible to drug abuse. Improved education and increased support should be given to preteens, because that is the age when deviant behavior starts. In cases where drug education programs have been successful in involving students, the amount of drug taking and illegal activity seems to have decreased (see Chapter 16).

The Costs of Drug Addiction to Society

Society pays a high price for drug addiction. Many of the costs are immeasurable, for example, broken homes, illness, shortened lives, and loss of good minds to industry and professions. The dollar costs are also great. The **National Institute on Drug Abuse (NIDA)** has estimated that the typical narcotic habit costs the user $100 a day or more to maintain, depending on location, availability of narcotics, and other factors. Assuming that a heroin addict has a $100-a-day habit, this addict would need about $36,000 a year just to maintain the drug supply. It is impossible for most addicts to get this amount of money legally, so many resort to criminal activity to support their habits.

Most crimes related to drugs involve theft of personal property—primarily burglary and shoplifting—and less commonly, assault and robbery (mugging). It is estimated that a heroin addict has to steal three to five times the actual cost of the drugs to maintain the habit. This means that he or she would have to steal about $100,000 a year. A number of addicts resort to pimping and prostitution. No accurate figures are available on the cost of drug-related prostitution, although some law enforcement officials have estimated that prostitutes take in a total of $10 to $20 billion a year. It has also been estimated that nearly one out of every three or four prostitutes in major cities has a serious drug dependency.

Another significant concern is the recent increases in clandestine laboratories throughout the country that are involved in synthesizing or processing illicit drugs. Such laboratories produce amphetaminelike drugs, heroinlike drugs, **"designer" drugs**, and LSD and process other drugs of abuse such as cocaine. The **Drug Enforcement Administration (DEA)** reported 184 laboratories seized in 1981 and that increased to 647 in 1987. The reasons for such dramatic increases relate to the enormous profits and relatively low risk associated with these operations. As a rule, clandestine laboratories are fairly mobile, relatively crude (often operating in a kitchen, basement, or garage), and operated by individuals with only elementary chemical skills. Because of a lack of training, the chemical procedures are done crudely, resulting in adulterants and impure products. Such contaminants can be very toxic, causing severe harm or even death to the unsuspecting user (Soine 1989).

The costs to society continue after addicts are caught because it takes from $50 to $100 a day to incarcerate each of them. To support programs like methadone maintenance costs much less. New York officials estimate that methadone maintenance cost about $2,000 a year per patient. Some outpatient programs, such as those in Washington, D.C., claim a cost as low as $5 to $10 a day (not counting cost of staff and facilities), which is much less than the cost of incarceration.

A more long-term effect of drug abuse that has substantial impact on society is the medical and psychological care often required by addicts as a consequence of disease resulting from their drug habit. Particularly noteworthy are the communicable diseases spread because of needle sharing within the drug-abusing population, such as AIDS (acquired immune deficiency syndrome) and

NIDA the National Institute on Drug Abuse, the principal federal agency responsible for directing drug abuse-related research

"DESIGNER" DRUGS illicit drugs that are chemically modified so they are not considered illegal but that retain abusive properties

DEA the Drug Enforcement Administration, the principal federal agency responsible for enforcing drug abuse regulations hepatitis (Millstein 1993). Because of its poor prognosis, AIDS is the most publicized of these diseases. In the United States, 25% of the nearly 100,000 AIDS cases as of June 1992 were intravenous (IV) drug users (see Chapter 15). The AIDS virus in this population appears to be transmitted in small amounts of contaminated blood left on shared needles. The likelihood of contracting AIDS in the drug-abusing population correlates with the frequency of injection and the amount of needle sharing (Booth et al. 1989). Care for these AIDS patients lasts from months to years in intensive care units at a cost of billions of dollars to the public. Some social workers have advocated that new, uncontaminated needles be made available to drug addicts free of charge to prevent the spread of AIDS by contaminated needles. Others argue against this approach, complaining that such a policy encourages abuse of drugs through the more dangerous IV route (Goldstein 1994).

Also of great concern is drug abuse by women during pregnancy. There is no longer doubt that some psychoactive drugs can have profound, permanent effects on a developing fetus. The best documented is fetal alcohol syndrome (FAS), which can affect the offspring of alcoholic mothers (see Chapter 8). It is likely that use of cocaine and amphetamine-related drugs can also cause irreversible congenital changes when used during pregnancy (see Chapter 10). All too often, the affected offspring of addicted mothers become the responsibility of welfare organizations at great cost to social services programs.

Drugs and Crime

There is a long-established close association between drug abuse and criminality. The hypotheses for this association range between (1) criminal behavior develops as a means to support addiction, and (2) criminality is inherently linked to the user's personality and occurs independently of drug use (Kokkevi et al. 1993). Part of the reason for the controversy about the relationship between criminal activity and drug abuse is that conflicting studies have been conducted in different cultures, employing different methods, focusing on different addictive drugs and examining recruit samples from different settings (that is, treatment versus criminal justice systems).

However, there is no doubt that drug-related crimes are overwhelming our judicial system: in 1992 approximately one-third of the prison population was incarcerated due to drug-related criminal activity compared to only 7% in 1980 (Associated Press 1994). In addition, it is clear that the production, merchandising, and distribution of illicit drugs has become a worldwide operation worth hundreds of billions of dollars (Goldstein 1994). These enormous profits have attracted organized crime both in the United States and abroad and all too frequently even corrupted law enforcement agencies (McShane 1994). For such operations, drugs mean incredible wealth and power. For example, in 1992 Pablo Escobar was recognized as a drug kingpin and leader of the cocaine cartel in Colombia, and acknowledged as one of the world's richest men and Colombia's most powerful man (Wire Services 1992). With his drug-related wealth, Escobar literally financed a private army in order to conduct a personal war against the government of Colombia (Associated Press 1993a) and until his death in 1993 was a serious threat to his country's stability. Such power can be very dangerous and destructive to individuals and even to entire societies.

Violence takes its toll at all levels as rival gangs fight to control their "turf" and associated drug operations. Innocent bystanders often become unsuspecting victims of the indiscriminate violence. For example, a Roman Catholic cardinal was killed on 24 May 1993, when a car he was riding inadvertently drove into the middle of a drug-related shootout between traffickers at the international airport in Guadalajara, Mexico. Five other innocent bystanders also were fatally wounded (Associated Press 1993b). Others are injured or even killed by drug users who, while under the influence of drugs commit violent criminal acts (see Case in Point).

Dealing with Drug-Related Crimes How can society best deal with drug-related crime and associated problems? Because of the diverse nature of the problem and the perpetrators, there is no simple solution. Consequently, a portion of the addict population would be heavily involved in crime regardless of their drug activity, while others

Case in Point

Prosecution of Crimes Committed Under Drug Influence

In 1988, Charles McCovey walked into a video store in Kearns, Utah, gun in hand, with the intent of committing robbery. During the crime, McCovey shot and killed Anna Holmes, the pregnant mother of four. The victim's premature baby was delivered by caesarean section following the homicide and died two years later from complications of the early birth. McCovey was apprehended soon after the crime and was tried for first-degree murder. Witnesses claimed that McCovey senselessly murdered Holmes. According to their testimony, the victim did nothing to provoke or oppose the murderer; McCovey unexpectedly turned his gun on Holmes and fired.

What appeared to be a tragic case of senseless homicide was complicated by the fact that the suspect was a chronic drug user. In fact, at the time of the crime, he was under the influence of methamphetamine, alcohol, and perhaps cocaine. At the trial, the defense attorney argued that Charles McCovey "did not do anything more than try to commit a robbery"; the firing of the gun was unintentional and caused by the effects of the drugs. The jury believed the defense and convicted McCovey on lesser second-degree murder charges. Instead of the death penalty, McCovey was given two 5-years-to-life sentences for aggravated robbery and second-degree murder. Was the sentence for McCovey appropriate?

commit crimes because of their need to acquire drugs. A third group consists of professional criminals who deal in drugs as a "business venture" and engage in such activity solely because of the profits (Kokkevi et al. 1993). The strategy for dealing with the crimes committed by each of these types should be different. Treatment for drug dependence will likely reduce the criminal behavior of those addicts who commit illegal acts in order to obtain money for support of their drug habits; however, this approach would have little impact on members of organized crime involved in drug trafficking or on individuals with underlying deviant behavior.

Despite the motive for the drug-related criminal act, the ultimate fate of an apprehended perpetrator is determined to a large extent by "constitutional protections." Thus, the most common defense used in drug-related criminal proceedings is the individual liberty guarantee based on the Bill of Rights, the Fourteenth Amendment to the U.S. Constitution, and additional individual liberty guarantees in states' constitutions. The defenses most commonly used in drug cases are

- Pharmacological duress ("the drug made me do it")
- The right to privacy
- The freedom of religion
- Cruel and unusual punishment
- Double jeopardy
- Insanity

The law works for the protection of the individual, and it often works more smoothly for those who can pay for the best legal assistance. It is difficult for the average citizen and criminal justice worker to see a guilty person released on a technicality. Nevertheless, the system is based on the assumption that it is better to err in releasing some violators than to imprison someone who is innocent. The following are the Articles of the Bill of

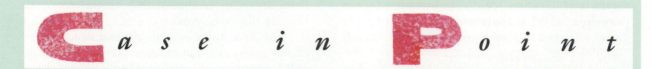

Rights and the Fourteenth Amendment of the Constitution, which have played a major role in criminal defenses for drug prosecutions:

Amendment 1 states that "Congress shall make no law . . . prohibiting the free exercise of religion or abridging the freedom of speech." This has been the basis for allowing the Native American Church to use peyote (see Chapter 12).

Amendment 4 guarantees the right to be secure in your own home, sometimes called *the right to privacy*, and to have protection against unauthorized search and seizure. This amendment is the basis for many successful drug defenses. Legal authorities cannot search someone's home without just cause but must have a search warrant or other permission to do so. If a person is stopped while driving a car, the car is searched, and a hidden drug is found, this is not admissible as evidence unless the officer can demonstrate that there was a reason, such as unsafe driving, to stop the driver.

Amendment 5 stipulates that a person cannot be charged twice for the same crime and once released, cannot be recharged for the same crime. This is sometimes called the *due process amendment* because it further says that you cannot be deprived of life, liberty, or property without due process of law.

Amendment 8 is the cruel and unusual punishment limitation. Sentences that are clearly out of line with the norm for the times can be successfully appealed.

Amendment 14 provides each person equal protection under the law. This amendment also guarantees due process.

The insanity defense is used in some drug criminal proceedings. The Fifth and Fourteenth Amendments provide due process, but people are excluded from criminal responsibility if they carried out the act as a result of insanity or the inability to tell right from wrong (as when under the influence of a drug). The American Psychiatric Association has declared that drug addiction is a nonpsychotic mental disorder, so people can claim they are not able to control their actions; at the same time, they must show they were insane at the time of the crime, which is difficult. Addicts are often given leniency if they agree to enroll in treatment or rehabilitation programs. If a person commits a serious crime while under the influence of the drug, the defense is much more complex. The claim that crimes were committed under the influence of alcohol, cocaine, amphetamines, or other behavior-altering substances has, on occasions, resulted in diminished sentences for the defendant.

Future Considerations in Drug Abuse Regulation

During the Republican administrations of Ronald Reagan and George Bush (1980–1992), the official policy of the federal government included a "get tough" attitude about drug abuse. Slogans such as "Just say no" and "War on Drugs" reflected the frustration of a public that had been victimized by escalating crime (many of which were drug related); personally touched by drug tragedies in families, at work, or with associates and friends; and economically strained by dealing with the cost of the problem. It is no wonder that, in 1989 and 1990, drug abuse was viewed as the number one problem in this country by the majority of its citizens (see description of the Anti-Drug Abuse Act of 1988 in Appendix 3.1). Consequently, from 1989 to 1991, the National Institute on Drug Abuse dramatically increased its budget directed at improving education and treatment programs in communities and schools. In addition, new research money was earmarked for identifying the causes of abuse and new therapeutic approaches (Halloway 1991).

How has the "War on Drugs" gone? Although during the final three years of the Bush administration more than $32 billion was spent to combat drug abuse and associated problems, many critics complain that this war goes badly and at best a stalemate has resulted (Knight-Ridder News Service 1992b). Defenders of Bush's policies for 1989–1992 claim:

1. Overall drug use dropped 13% and cocaine use decreased 35%.
2. Federal seizures of cocaine increased approximately 10% (from 99 metric tons in 1989 to 108 in 1991).

3. Drug arrests were up.
4. The capacity of treatment centers increased.

Those who attack the policies of the Bush administration claim (Associated Press 1992b; Knight-Ridder News Service 1992a):

1. During Bush's administration, 3 million Americans became addicted to cocaine or heroin and a million addicts were unable to get treatment.
2. Because their mothers used addicting drugs during pregnancy, 900,000 babies were born drug dependent.
3. The incidence of drug overdoses dipped temporarily, but then returned to the pre-1989 level.
4. Approximately 72,000 murders (highest of any three-year period in American history) occurred during the "War on Drugs," and most of the homicides were drug related.
5. increased cocaine seizures were offset by increased production despite the "Andean Strategy" of interdiction designed to choke off South American sources of this drug.
6. Comprehensive antidrug education was only available to about 50% of the nation's schoolchildren, and almost none of the states require drug education at every grade level.

The lack of a well-established victory, inconsistencies in drug laws (see Case in Point), and the resulting frustration to both governmental agencies and the general public likely will lead to revised drug policies. In addition, because of enormous governmental budget deficits, diminished money for dealing with drug abuse problems are likely; consequently, creative, less expensive strategies will have to be developed to replace the expensive and often ineffectual approaches. As new approaches for old problems are sought, some issues not yet discussed merit scrutiny.

Drug Legalization Debate

The persistence of the drug abuse problem and the high cost in dollars and frustration of waging the "War on Drugs" helps to energize the ongoing debate of legalizing the use of drugs of abuse (see Crosscurrents). It is argued that legalizing substances of abuse would eliminate law enforcement as a major factor in the control of drug abuse; consequently, if consumption and sale of these substances are decriminalized, individuals would decide for themselves whether or not to buy and use these addicting drugs, much as they already do for alcohol and tobacco. Proponents of legalization are no longer limited to *libertarians* and so-called *academic intellectuals,* but more and more include representative of a distressed law enforcement system. For example, discontented judges whose courts are swamped with drug cases, and police officers who spend much of their on-duty time trying to trap and arrest every drug dealer and user on the street are publicly declaring that the drug laws are wasteful and futile. Even notable public figures such as former secretary of state George Schultz, Nobel Laureate economist Milton Friedman, and the surgeon general for the Clinton administration, Joycelyn Elders (Buckley 1994) claim that laws against drugs of addiction have been as ineffective as Prohibition against alcohol (Knight-Ridder News Service 1992b; Wilson 1993; Kearns 1993). Although it is true that laws against the use and distribution of drugs of addiction, according to the FBI, have resulted in a doubling of drug-related arrests since 1981 (of 1.08 million drug arrests in 1990, 68% were for possession, not selling [Knight-Ridder News Service 1992b]), there are plenty of people ready to replace those dealers imprisoned. Proponents claim that drug legalization would

1. Remove governmental involvement from issues that unnecessarily deprive individuals of their freedom of choice (Nadelman 1993)
2. Eliminate dealers' high profit margin by removing the illegality, which drives up the cost of illicit drugs
3. Reduce drug-related violence by taking drug trade out of the hands of criminals
4. Relieve law enforcement costs by eliminating the backlog of drug-related court cases and reduce populations in overcrowded prisons (35% of which are for drug-related crimes (Knight-Ridder News Service 1992b; Nadelman 1993)
5. Eliminate unfair drug-related laws, which are often accused of being inequitable and biased by racial and socioeconomical factors

Case in Point

Often severe prison sentences are mandated by law for what appears to be relatively minor first-time offenders; for example,

1. Nicole Richardson, age 20, despite having no previous criminal record, was sentenced to 10 years in prison for distributing LSD in Mobile, Alabama. Judge Alex Howard, Jr., imposed the sentence reluctantly, describing it a "total miscarriage of justice."
2. Kathy-Ann Tannis, a 21-year-old mother with no previous arrest record, received a mandated 10-year prison term in Newark, New Jersey, for conviction as a drug courier. U.S. District Judge Alfred M. Wolin declared the sentence excessively harsh but claimed he had no choice.

These are but two examples of drug-related convictions in the United States that have received mandatory sentences declared excessive by the very judges forced to impose the decision. Are harsh mandated drug laws, such as those illustrated here, justified, and are they effective in preventing illicit use of drugs?

Source: Gary Cohn. "Judges Wince at Mandatory Drug-Sentencing Law." *Salt Lake Tribune* 246 (27 June 1993): A6, 7.

6. Allow governments to regulate and tax drugs of addiction in the same manner as alcohol and tobacco; monies generated by such taxes could be used for drug treatment programs
7. Change the official perspective of drug addiction from that of a criminal activity requiring punitive action, to that of a health problem requiring therapeutic action (Nadelman 1993)
8. Help to identify addicts and heavy drug abusers who require treatment; such people may be more likely to submit themselves for therapy if they are confident that no punitive action will be taken against them
9. Reduce the spread of diseases, such as AIDS and hepatitis, associated with the drug abuse lifestyle
10. Allow regulation of purity and quality of the drug products (Kalant 1992) to eliminate the dangers of contaminants and additives often found in illegal substances (Nadelman 1993)

Despite some of the compelling arguments for legalization of drugs of addiction, the majority of law enforcement professionals, politicians, federal agencies and medical associations oppose legalization of some or all drugs of abuse. In addition, polls indicate most voters object to legalization or decriminalization of illicit drugs (Knight-Ridder News Service 1992b). Their opposition to legalization is based on the following concerns (Goldstein 1994; Wilson 1993; Kalant 1992; Goldstein and Kalant 1990):

1. It will increase drug abuse due to greater availability. Once legitimized, substances such as marijuana, narcotics, and even cocaine may be merchandised and sold like cigarettes and beer.
2. It will increase use due to decreased cost.
3. It will increase use due to perceived social approval that is inherent with legalization.

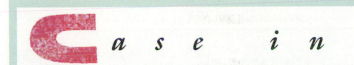

CROSSCURRENTS

As discussed in this chapter, a continual controversy relates to the effectiveness of the judiciary system to curtail problems associated with drug abuse. Two extreme positions on this issue are represented by the following statements:

1. Laws prohibiting the use of drugs of abuse are unrealistic, problematic, and should be abolished.
2. Laws prohibiting the use of drugs of abuse are necessary and need to be rigidly enforced if we are to win the "War on Drugs."

Choose a side and support your decision with arguments based on the information found in the text and other authoritative sources.

Many "law-abiding" people avoid the use of illicit drugs of abuse because they do not want "trouble with the law."

4. It will increase costs to society due to greater medical and social problems resulting from greater availability and increased use. The two most frequently abused substances, alcohol and tobacco, are both legal and readily available. These two substances cause much greater medical, social, and personal problems than all the illicit drugs of abuse combined.

Although arguments for both sides warrant consideration, extreme policies are not likely to be implemented; instead a compromise will most probably be adopted. For example, some areas of compromise include (Kalant 1992) the following:

1. *Selective legalization.* Eliminate harsh penalties for those drugs of abuse that are the safest, and least likely to cause addiction, such as marijuana.
2. *Control substances of abuse by prescription or through specially approved outlets.* Have the availability of the illegal drugs controlled by physicians and trained clinicians, rather than by law enforcement agencies.
3. *Discretionary enforcement of drug laws.* Allow greater discretion by judicial systems for prosecution and sentencing of those who violate drug laws. Such decisions would be based on perceived criminal intent.

Drug Testing

In response to the demand by society to stop the spread of drug abuse and its adverse consequences, drug testing has been implemented in some situations to detect drug users (Catlin et al. 1992). The drugs of abuse most frequently tested are marijuana, cocaine, amphetamines, narcotics, sedatives, phencyclidine (PCP), and anabolic steroids. Drug testing is mandatory for some professions where public safety is a concern (such as airline pilots, railroad workers, law enforcement employees, medical personnel; see box) or for employees of some organizations and companies as part of general policy (such as military, many federal agencies, some private companies). Drug testing is also mandatory for participants in sports at all levels, in high school, college, international, and professional competition (Catlin et al. 1992) in order to prevent unfair advantages that might result from the pharmacological effects of these drugs and to discourage the spread of drug abuse in the athlete population (see Chapter 15). Drug testing is also

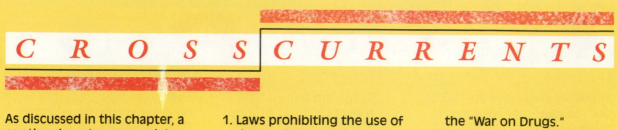

Here and Now

Drug Testing to Assure Public Safety

Federal law mandates that transportation workers routinely undergo testing for drugs, including alcohol. As part of "Operation Roadblock" (a railroading red signal that means "Stop immediately!"), drug testing has caused a decline in positive drug tests from 6% in 1988 to 3.2% in 1991. This program was in response to a 1987 tragedy caused by an engineer of a Conrail freight train in Maryland who missed a warning signal while under the influence of marijuana. The accident killed 16 and injured more than 170 passengers (Bryson 1992).

used routinely by law enforcement agencies to assist in the prosecution of those believed to violate drug abuse laws. Finally, drug testing is used by health professionals to assess the success of drug abuse treatment; that is, to determine if a dependent patient is diminishing drug use or has experienced a relapse in drug abuse habits.

Drug testing to identify drug offenders is usually accomplished by analyzing body fluids, in particular urine, although other approaches (such as analysis of expired air for alcohol) are also used. To understand the accuracy of these tests, several factors should be considered (Catlin et al. 1992).

1. *Testing must be standardized and conducted efficiently.* In order to reliably interpret testing results, it is essential that fluid samples be collected, processed, and tested using standard procedures. Guidelines for proper testing procedures have been established by federal regulatory agencies as well as scientific organizations. Deviations from established protocols can result in false positives (test indicates a drug is present when none was used), false negatives (test is unable to detect a drug that is present), or inaccurate assessments of drug levels.

2. *Sample collection and processing must be done accurately and confidentially.* In many cases, drug testing can have punitive consequences (for example, athlete's can't compete; employees are fired if results are positive). Consequently, drug users often attempt to outsmart the system. Some individuals have attempted to avoid submitting their own drug-containing urine for testing by filling specimen bottles with "clean" urine from artificial bladders hidden under clothing or in the vagina or by introducing "clean" urine into their own bladders just before the collection (Catlin et al. 1992). To confirm the legitimacy of the specimen, it often is necessary to have the individual strip and the urine collection witnessed directly by a trustworthy observer. To assure that tampering not occur with the fluid specimens and confidentially be maintained, samples should be immediately coded and the movement of each sample from site to site during analysis should be documented and confirmed.

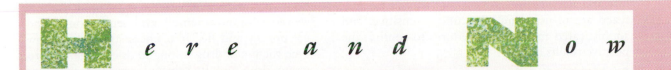

Just as it is important that testing identify those who are using drugs, it is also important that those who have not used drugs not be wrongfully accused. To avoid false positives, all samples that are positive in the screening tests (these are usually fast and inexpensive procedures) should be analyzed again, using more accurate, sensitive, and sophisticated analytical procedures to confirm the positive results.

3. *Confounding factors can be inadvertently or deliberately present that interfere with the accuracy of the testing.* For example, normal dietary consumption of pastries containing poppy seeds is sufficient to cause a positive urine test for the narcotic morphine. The use of bicarbonate alkalinizes the urine and increases the rate of elimination of some drugs, such as methamphetamine, and thereby diminishes the likelihood of a positive test (Catlin et al. 1992). Excessive intake of fluid, or the use of diuretics, increases the volume of urine formed and decreases the concentration of drugs, making them more difficult to detect.

The dramatic increase in drug testing since 1985 has caused experts to question the value of this process in dealing with drug abuse problems. Unfortunately, drug testing often is linked exclusively to punitive consequences, such as disqualification from athletic competition, loss of job, or even fines and imprisonment. Use of drug testing in such negative ways likely does little to diminish the number of drug abusers or their personal problems. However, it is important to recognize that drug-testing programs can also have positive consequences by identifying drug users who require professional care. After being referred for drug rehabilitation, the offender can also be monitored by drug testing to confirm the desired response to therapy. In addition, tests can identify those individuals who put others in jeopardy because of their drug abuse habits as they perform tasks that are dangerously impaired by the effects of these drugs (for example, airline pilots, train engineers, truck drivers, and so forth).

The widespread application of drug testing to control the illicit use of drugs in the general population would be extremely expensive, difficult to enforce, and almost certainly ineffective. In addition, such indiscriminate testing would likely be viewed as an unwarranted infringement on individual privacy and declared unconstitutional. However, the use of drug testing to discourage inappropriate drug use in selected crucial professions, which directly impact public welfare, appears to be publicly tolerated and has been shown to be effective (Bryson 1992). Even so, it is probably worthwhile to periodically revisit the issue of drug testing and analyze its benefits and liabilities relative to "public safety" and "individual privacy" issues.

Pragmatic Drug Policies

Several principles for a pragmatic drug policy emerge from a review of past drug policies and an understanding of the drug-related frustrations of today. First, it is essential that government develops programs that are consistent with the desires of the majority of the population. Second, due to the lack of success and high cost of efforts to prevent illicit drugs from reaching the market, it is logical to de-emphasize interdiction and stress programs that reduce demand. Third, government and society need to better understand the role of law in its efforts to reduce drug addiction. Antidrug laws by themselves do not eliminate drug problems, and can even create significant social difficulties (for example, the Prohibition laws against all alcohol use). However, used properly and selectively, laws can reinforce and communicate expected social behavior and values (for example, laws against public drunkenness or driving a vehicle under the influence of alcohol). Finally, programs should be implemented that more effectively employ "public consensus" to campaign against drug abuse. For example, antismoking campaigns demonstrate the potential success of such programs that alter drug abuse behavior. Similar approaches can be used to change public attitudes about drugs through education without moral judgments and crusading tactics (Kalant 1992).

Appendix

Appendix 3.1: The Development and Administration of Drug Abuse Laws

The History of Drug Abuse Laws

The Harrison Narcotics Act Several of the important drug laws described were passed in the United States for such ugly and irrelevant reasons as anti-Chinese sentiment. These had a significant impact on the use of opiates and other drugs legally defined as narcotics. In 1909, Congress passed the Smoking Opium Exclusion Act, which forbade the importation of opium for nonmedical use; however, it permitted the use and manufacture of opium for nonmedical use. By 1914, it was still possible to purchase opiates legally in the form of patent medicines or to smoke opium (provided you were a white American) in some states (28 had state laws against smoking opium).

For some time, the United States had been attempting to improve trade relations with China. The Harrison Narcotics Act was passed as much to impress the Chinese government that the United States was willing to regulate opiate use and help China control its serious opium addiction problem as to address the opiate addiction problem in the United States. *Collier's* and also *Harper's Magazine* had helped to create public pressure for antidrug legislation by publishing articles about the use of "dope," vividly illustrated with pictures and cartoons of opium dens and drug abuse. In 1914, there were an estimated 200,000 addicted Americans; as many as 1 person in 400 was an opium addict.

The Harrison Act was a tax bill, rather than a drug regulatory bill. It controlled dispensing and dealing in narcotics. All dealers in narcotics—such as physicians, veterinarians, and dentists—were required to register with the Bureau of Internal Revenue, which was to enforce the law. The medical groups were upset and felt that their freedom to prescribe had been compromised.

U.S. Supreme Court Decisions on Narcotics In 1919, the Supreme Court ruled in the Webb case that it was illegal to give drugs to an addict simply to prevent withdrawal. In the Behrman case in 1922, the Court ruled that it was unlawful to use drugs for a cure program.

The Narcotic Drugs Import and Export Act of 1922 This legislation limited imports to crude opium and coca leaves for medical purposes. Also called the Jones-Miller Act, it doubled penalties for dealing in narcotics to a $5,000 fine and 10 years in prison. It further specified conviction for mere possession of illegal drugs.

The Heroin Act of 1924 This law made it illegal to manufacture heroin or to process the drug for any purpose other than government-controlled research.

Federal Narcotics Hospitals In 1928, over one-third of all prisoners in the United States were serving sentences for drug-related offenses. Nearly half were convicted for use of two drugs, mescaline and marijuana, which were classified as narcotics at the time. In 1929, the federal government authorized the establishment of two narcotics hospitals, or treatment facilities: one at Lexington, Kentucky, which opened in 1935, and the other at Fort Worth, Texas, which opened in 1938. They were closed in the early 1970s, partly because the associated programs had been shown to be ineffectual. Of the patients addicted to narcotics, over 90% were using the same drug within six months after they were released, and only 5% remained drug free over an extended period of time. With the advent of methadone and outpatient treatment, it was decided that the centers were no longer needed.

The Marijuana Tax Act As will be described in the chapter on marijuana (Chapter 13), this plant was the center of controversy in the early 1930s because of the increasing use of it for smoking. In 1937, after a strong publicity campaign by papers and magazines, the Marijuana Tax Act was passed, providing controls over marijuana similar to those of the Harrison Act on narcotics. A tax was levied on all transactions connected with marijuana. The law was never very effective, and gradually, use of marijuana became more widespread. In 1969, the Supreme Court ruled the punishment for non-payment of the tax was unconstitutional because of self-incrimination. (It was comparable to the leading question "When did you stop beating your wife?") Marijuana was still controlled by federal narcotics laws and was legally (although not pharmacologically) considered a narcotic until 1971.

The Opium Poppy Control Act In 1942, this law was passed to license the growing of opium poppies in the United States because supplies from abroad had been cut off by World War II. Opium was necessary for use in medicine. There was also a demand for poppy seeds, which were used in baked goods. There is no opium in the seeds, which are sterilized so they are unable to germinate and produce opium poppies.

The Boggs Amendment This legislation was passed in 1951 as an amendment to the Harrison Narcotics Act; it established minimum mandatory sentences for all narcotic and marijuana offenses. This was the beginning of a new program of hardline control of addictive drugs and of marijuana.

The Narcotics Drug Control Act of 1956 In 1955, a report by a subcommittee of the Senate Judiciary Committee stated that drug addiction was responsible for 50% of crime in urban areas and 25% of all reported crimes. It was also reported that Communist China planned to demoralize the people of the United States by encouraging drug addiction. In view of the subcommittee's report, Congress passed an even tougher law, the Narcotic Drug Control Act of 1956. This act imposed very stiff penalties for narcotics and marijuana use. It prohibited suspended sentences, probation, or parole for all narcotic offenses except a first conviction for possession. Under the law, a convicted seller or distributor of illegal narcotics was to be sentenced to prison. In most federal cases, an individual who possessed over a few ounces of narcotics or marijuana was assumed to be a "pusher" and was treated as such. This law also provided for execution of a "pusher" selling heroin to a person under age 18.

The Single Convention Treaty This agreement replaced and consolidated parts of eight previous international agreements on narcotics. Sponsored by the United Nations World Health Organization, it became effective in 1964, although the U.S. Senate did not ratify participation until 1967 because it thought parts of the treaty were weaker than an earlier 1953 treaty. This treaty regulated the production, manufacture, import, export, trade, distribution, use, and possession of products from the opium poppy, coca plant, and cannabis plant. It did not regulate depressant, stimulant, and hallucinogenic drugs. Signatory parties were required to phase out quasimedical use of opium smoking (within 15 years of signing), coca leaf chewing, and the nonmedical use of cannabis (within 25 years of signing). In order to legalize marijuana in the United States, it would be necessary to abrogate this treaty, which could be done by announcing the intent to withdraw from it six months in advance.

The Drug Abuse Control Amendments (DACA) of 1965 In the early 1960s, the use of illegal drugs rose sharply, and a shift in the types of drugs being used took place. Large numbers of people were experimenting with drugs that altered mood and state of consciousness. Along with these new drugs came a rash of "bad trips," medical complications, and drug emergency cases. Publicity on adverse reactions caused by these new varieties of "street" drugs roused the public to bring pressure on Congress for controls. By the end of 1965, Congress had passed a new series of laws, the Drug Abuse Control Amendments (DACA).

These laws, which excluded narcotics and marijuana, brought three classes of drugs under federal control: (1) amphetamines, (2) barbiturates, and (3) a group of drugs that had a potential for abuse because of their psychedelic or hallucinogenic effects. For the first time, lysergic acid and lysergic acid amide were placed in a controlled-substance group because LSD could easily be made from them. However, the DACA laws did allow the use of peyote by members of the Native American Church in their religious ceremonies.

Some of the key regulations in the 1965 amendments were

1. No prescription for these drugs could be filled or refilled after six months from date of issue or refilled more than five times.
2. Manufacturers had to keep records of sales for three years.
3. Penalties for violation of the regulations ranged from up to one year and a $1,000 fine

for a first offense to up to three years and a $10,000 fine for a second offense. Penalties were much more severe for selling to anyone under 21 years of age.

In 1968, an amendment to the DACA established that the sentence was to be suspended for a first conviction. If there was no conviction in the one-year probationary interlude, the first conviction was to be erased from the record.

The Narcotic Addict Rehabilitation Act (NARA) This act passed in 1966 and gave states the opportunity to put pressure on addicts to go through treatment programs or go to jail. The law allowed reduction of a sentence if progress could be shown in treatment and rehabilitation.

The Comprehensive Drug Abuse Prevention and Control Act of 1970 This act was passed by Congress in 1971. President Nixon had proposed a broader education, research, and rehabilitation program to be covered by new drug laws, but after a great deal of political hassling, Congress made it primarily a law enforcement bill, with some provision for treatment and education. This act did the following:

1. Expanded community mental health centers and the Public Health Service Hospitals for drug abusers and authorized drug education workshops and material for professional workers and public schools
2. Set up a Commission on Marijuana and Drug Abuse to study certain drugs for two years and to submit a report and make recommendations
3. Excluded alcohol and tobacco from the group of drugs under study
4. Determined that there would be no mandatory federal sentence for a first offense of illegal possession of any controlled drugs and decreed that the possible sentences could be a year's imprisonment and/or a $5,000 fine or one year's probation (if probation was not violated, the conviction was erased from the person's record, first offense only)
5. Determined that any person over 18 selling drugs to anyone under 21 should receive twice the first offense penalty and three times the penalty for a second or subsequent offense
6. Decreed that any individual caught selling as part of a group of five or more (considered a drug ring) may receive a penalty of at least 10 years and not more than a $100,000 fine for the first offense; a second offense had a penalty of not less than 20 years and not more than a $200,000 fine or life imprisonment
7. Divided drugs with actual or relative potential for abuse into five categories called *Schedules:*
   a. Schedule I substances have a high potential for abuse and have no currently accepted medical use in treatment in the United States (currently include heroin, LSD, peyote, MDMA "Ecstasy," marijuana).
   b. Schedule II substances have a high potential for abuse, with severe psychic dependence potential. They have some currently accepted medical uses in the United States, but their availability is tightly restricted. Currently, amphetamines, raw opium, morphine, methadone, cocaine, and pentobarbital are in this category.
   c. Schedule III substances have less potential for abuse than those in groups I or II, and they have current medical use in the United States. They have low to moderate potential for physical addiction but a high potential for psychological dependence. Examples of Schedule III drugs include limited quantities of certain opioid drugs, some depressants such as glutethimide (Doriden), paregoric, certain barbiturates (except those listed in another schedule), and more recently, the anabolic steroids (testosterone type).
   d. Schedule IV drugs have low potential for abuse relative to drugs in Schedule III, have a currently accepted medical use in the United States, and have a limited potential for psychological or physical addiction compared to Schedule III drugs. Phenobarbital, chloral hydrate, diazepam (Valium), and other benzodiazepines and propoxyphene (Darvon) are in this schedule.
   e. Schedule V substances have a low poten-

TABLE 3.3 Regulatory requirements

CSA Schedule	Registration	Recordkeeping	Distribution Restrictions	Dispensing Limits
I	Required	Separate	Order Forms	Research use only
II	Required	Separate	Order Forms	R_X: written; no refills
III	Required	Readily retrievable	Records required	R_X: written or oral; with medical authorization, refills up to 5 in 6 months
IV	Required	Readily retrievable	Records required	R_X: written or oral; with medical authorization, refills up to 5 in 6 months
V	Required	Readily retrievable	Records required	OTC (R_X drugs limited to M.D.'s order)

Source: Drugs of Abuse, 1989, p. 9. Courtesy of the Drug Enforcement Administration. Washington, DC: U.S. Government Printing Office.

tial for abuse relative to Schedule IV drugs and have a currently accepted medical use in the United States. Abuse of this class of drugs may lead to limited physical or psychological dependence relative to Schedule IV drugs. Lomotil and small amounts of codeine in cough preparations and analgesics are included in Schedule V.

Prescription orders can be written for drugs in Schedules II through IV only by health professionals who are especially licensed by the Drug Enforcement Administration (DEA). Some Schedule V drugs may be distributed without prescription by a pharmacist, subject to state regulation. See Table 3.3 for regulatory requirements for each level of scheduling.

The Methadone Control Act In 1972, the Food and Drug Administration released methadone to be used in treatment of opiate addiction. It had only been used experimentally up to that time. Because of poor administration and coordination of some early methadone maintenance programs, abuse of the drug on the street had increased. The Methadone Control Act of 1973 put controls on dispensing and monitoring methadone to help keep the drug off the streets.

The Heroin Trafficking Act of 1973 This law tightened penalties for traffickers so that bail making could not be continually abused.

The Alcohol and Drug Abuse Education Amendments In 1978, several amendments set up an Office of Alcohol and Drug Abuse Education in the Office of Education. These laws gave more emphasis to drug abuse in rural areas and helped to coordinate federal, state, and local programs in education and prevention training.

In 1980, the Drug Abuse Prevention, Treatment, and Rehabilitation Amendments updated and funded further efforts in prevention education, as well as new programs in rehabilitation. This law was followed by the Drug Offenders Act of 1984 and the Alcohol and Drug Abuse Amendments of 1986, both of which reorganized rehabilitation programs for both alcohol and drugs of abuse. The Controlled Substances Analogue Enforcement Act of 1986 set guidelines to control the growing problem of designer drugs flooding some markets.

The Drug Abuse Office and Treatment Acts Starting with the increased publicity on drug use by servicepeople in Vietnam, new policies were formed to try to control the situation and try new treatment techniques that had never been funded before. In 1972, the Drug Abuse Office and Treatment Act was signed; in 1974 and 1978, amendments were made to improve the law. This law has financially supported treatment slots for addicts including many methadone clinics and experimental programs (discussed in Chapter 16).

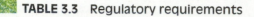

At the same time, the funds given to the Veterans Administration (VA) hospitals were greatly increased to handle addiction in the military. All military branches became more attentive to drug problems and initiated drug information and treatment programs. One significant advance was the recognition of alcoholism as a drug problem. The military had largely ignored alcoholism previously, even though it was visible and common. The VA hospitals began to devote more effort to the specific treatment of alcoholism than to problems caused by all other drugs.

The Analogue (Designer Drug) Act of 1986 This act makes illegal any substance that is similar in structure or psychological effect to any substance already scheduled, providing it is manufactured, processed, or sold with the intention that it will be consumed by humans (Controlled Substances Analogue Enforcement Act, 1986, 21 U.S.C. 802 [32] and 813).

The Anti–Drug Abuse Act of 1988 This legislation was a result of the so-called "War on Drugs" declared by President Reagan and supposedly continued by President Bush. The original act authorized a total of $2.7 billion for federal, state, and local drug law enforcement, school-based drug prevention efforts (from preschool through high school), and drug abuse treatment, with a special emphasis on intravenous drug abusers at high risk for AIDS. It supported a new research intended to identify the reasons for drug abuse behavior and more effective ways to treat the abuser. The specific result of this act was the creation of the Office of National Drug Control Policy, which was to oversee all federal policies relating to drug abuse (Schuster 1989). In 1990, the total estimated money directed by this office for drug law enforcement and criminal justice was $6.5 billion (Halloway 1991).

The federal laws controlling drug use and attempting to prevent drug abuse are summarized in Table 3.2. It is certain that new laws will be passed in the future with the intent of solving problems caused by drug abuse.

Federal Agencies with Drug Abuse Missions

Drug Enforcement Administration (DEA) Because of the unique problems of drug abuse, Congress, in 1930, authorized the establishment of the Bureau of Narcotics in the Treasury Department to administer the relevant laws. This agency remained in the Treasury Department until 1968, when it became part of a new group in the Justice Department, the Bureau of Narcotics and Dangerous Drugs. Harry Anslinger served as head of the bureau for over 30 years, from its creation until 1962 when he retired. Anslinger was an agent during the Prohibition, and later, as head of the bureau, he played an important role in getting marijuana outlawed by the federal government. In 1973, the Bureau of Narcotics and Dangerous Drugs became the Drug Enforcement Administration (DEA). Today, the DEA has the responsibility of infiltrating and breaking up illegal drug traffic in the United States, as well as controlling the use of Scheduled substances.

Special Action Office for Drug Abuse Prevention (SAODAP) In 1971, President Nixon set up a temporary agency, SAODAP, to initiate short-term and long-term planning of programs and to coordinate anti–drug abuse programs with the states so that proper funding procedures and policies were followed. This office was in the White House and was intended to advise the president. One of the major reasons for establishing such an office was the initial report of a high heroin addiction rate in returning Vietnam veterans. This program was supposed to fight the increase in addiction in the United States. SAODAP was abolished, as planned, with most of its education, research, treatment, and rehabilitation functions going to a new agency, the National Institute on Drug Abuse (NIDA). An expert on the staff of advisors to the president, the domestic policy staff, assumed the duties of advising the president on drug related matters and drug abuse programs. The advisor was to keep track of budgets for drug programs and coordinate policy with law enforcement groups. Under the Reagan administration, further changes were proposed. A pattern of federal policy was established; that is, control and management of drug programs in the United States change with each new "crisis."

Alcohol, Drug Abuse, and Mental Health Administration (ADAMHA) In 1973, a new agency was formed after the Department of Health, Education, and Welfare Secretary Weinberger stripped the alcohol and drug abuse sections from the

National Institute of Mental Health (NIMH). This action formed the National Institute of Alcohol Abuse and Alcoholism (NIAAA) and the NIDA (see previous section). NIAAA, NIDA, and NIMH were under the agency ADAMHA (Alcohol, Drug Abuse and Mental Health Administration). This shuffling and redesign was part of federal attempts to bring the post–Vietnam War heroin crisis under control and address the perennial problems of alcoholism and dependence on other drugs. The mission of NIAAA and NIDA was and still is to coordinate both clinical and basic research involved directed at drugs of abuse. Today, these institutes support 80–90% of all drug dependence research conducted in the United States. During fiscal year 1993, these institutes controlled budgets of $330 (NIDA) and $180 (NIAAA) million (*FASEB* Newsletter 1992, 4).

As of October 1, 1992, ADAMHA was reorganized and both NIDA and NIAAA officially became Institutes of the National Institutes of Health (NIH) as mandated by the ADAMHA Reorganization Act of 1992 (Greenhouse 1992).

The Substance Abuse and Mental Health Services Administration (SAMHSA) With passage of the ADAMHA Reorganization Act of 1992, the services programs of NIDA, NIAAA, and NIMH were incorporated into the newly created SAMHSA. This agency was given the lead responsibility for prevention and treatment of addictive and mental health problems and disorders. Their overall mission is to reduce the incidence and prevalence of substance abuse and mental disorders by ensuring the best therapeutic use of scientific knowledge and improving access to high-quality, effective programs (*SAMHSA Bulletin* 1992).

State Regulations There have always been questions regarding the relative responsibilities of state versus federal laws and their respective regulatory agencies. In general, the U.S. form of government has allowed local control to take precedence over national control. Because of this historic attitude, states were the first to pass laws to regulate the abuse or misuse of drugs. Federal laws developed later, after the federal government gained greater jurisdiction over the well-being and lives of the citizens and it became apparent that, due to interstate trafficking, national drug abuse problems could not be effectively dealt with on a state-by-state basis. Some early state laws banned the use of smoking opium, regulated the scale of various psychoactive drug substances, and in a few instances, set up treatment programs. However, these early legislative actions made no effort to *prevent* drug abuse. Drug abuse was controlled to a great extent by social pressure rather than by law. It was considered morally wrong to be an alcoholic or an addict to opium or some other drug.

The drug laws in 1932 varied considerably from state to state, so the National Conference of Commissioners on Uniform State Laws set up the Uniform Narcotic Drug Act (UNDA), which was later adopted by nearly all states. The UNDA provided for the control of possession, use, and distribution of opiates and cocaine. In 1942, marijuana was included as a narcotic.

In 1967, the Food and Drug Administration proposed the Model Drug Abuse Control Act and urged the states to adopt it on a uniform basis. This law extended controls over depressant, stimulant, and hallucinogenic drugs similar to the 1965 federal law. Many states set up laws based on this model.

The federal Controlled Substances Act of 1970 stimulated the National Conference of Commissioners to propose a new Uniform Controlled Substances Act (UCSA). The UCSA permits enactment of a single state law regulating the illicit possession, use, manufacture, and dispensing of controlled psychoactive substances. At this time, most states have enacted the UCSA or modifications of it.

Today, state law enforcement of drug statutes does not always reflect federal regulations, although for the most part, the two statutory levels are harmonious. For example, marijuana in small amounts for personal use is only considered an act of minor misconduct in Alaska or Oregon but is considered a Schedule I substance by federal regulatory agencies (as of this writing). Consequently, as long as this substance is used inside the state boundaries of Alaska or Oregon for personal use only, there is little likelihood of prosecution. However, the more severe federal laws are invoked whenever use of this illicit substance involves interstate issues (such as being transported across state boundaries).

Review Questions

1. What are the disadvantages of having the FDA be excessively thorough in its assessment of safety and effectiveness for newly developed drugs?
2. What are the problems when a society has unrealistic expectations concerning drug regulation by its government?
3. Why did the Kefauver and Harris Amendments of 1962 represent a basic change in the governmental philosophy regarding drug regulation?
4. What are principal advantages and disadvantages of the procedures used by the FDA to evaluate new drugs for marketing?
5. What are the principal advantages and disadvantages to switching prescription drugs to OTC status?
6. How tightly should the federal government regulate advertising for both prescription and nonprescription drugs? Justify your answers.
7. Would decriminalization of illicit drug use increase or decrease related social problems? Justify your answer.
8. What constitutes the so-called War on Drugs? What changes need to be made if this "war" is to be won?

Key Terms

patent medicines
thalidomide
phocomelia
carcinogenic
mutagenic
teratogenic
switching policy
interdiction
NIDA
"designer" drugs
DEA

Summary

1. Developed societies, such as that found in the United States, have evolved to believe that they have the right to protect themselves from the damaging impact of drug use and abuse. Consequently, governments, including that of the United States, have passed laws and implemented programs to prevent social damage from inappropriate drug use. In addition, such societies have come to expect that drugs be effective.
2. The patent medicines of the late 1800s and early 1900s demonstrated to the public the problems of insufficient regulation of the drug industry. These often ineffective products were promoted as cures for every kind of illness. In addition, patent medicines were often poorly made and contained dangerous and sometimes addicting ingredients. Because of these dangers, drug regulation evolved that formed the foundation of U.S. drug laws.
3. Both opium and cocaine have long histories of use and abuse in many societies. Both substances were included in early patent medicines and extolled as miracle drugs that could cure an array of medical disorders. Both drugs were also found to cause severe dependence when used over the long term and ironically were frequently promoted as cures for drug addiction. After going through a period of fascination with these drugs in the late 1800s, the American public became aware of their addicting properties and pressured the government into becoming more involved in regulating patent medicines and other drug products. These concerns led to the Pure Food and Drug Act of 1906 and ultimately the

Harrison Act of 1914. These experiences helped to shape public and government awareness toward regulation of all types of drugs but most particularly those with abuse properties, such as opium and cocaine.

4. The 1906 Pure Food and Drug Act was not a strong law, but it required manufacturers to include on labels the amounts of alcohol, morphine, opium, cocaine, heroin, or marijuana extract in each product. This was the first real attempt to make consumers aware of the actual contents in the drug products they were consuming and help them make educated decisions about using these substances. This act also prohibited misrepresentation and marked the beginning of involvement by the government in drug manufacturing and promotion.
5. The 1938 Federal Food, Drug, and Cosmetic Act gave the Food and Drug Administration control over drug safety. This act was passed following a deadly tragedy that killed over 100 people who consumed an antibiotic product containing diethylene glycol as a solvent. The act required drugs to be safe (although not necessarily effective) and that all ingredients, quantities, instructions for use, and warnings be included on the labels. This legislation allowed drug companies to create the prescription and nonprescription classes of drugs and also served as the basis for most subsequent drug legislation that regulates the distribution and use of both prescription and nonprescription drugs.
6. The 1951 Durham-Humphrey Amendment to the Food, Drug, and Cosmetic Act made a formal distinction between prescription and nonprescription drugs. This amendment required all new drugs to be placed, at least temporarily, in the prescription category. In addition, it established the criteria still used today for determining into which category a drug should be classified.
7. The Kefauver-Harris Amendments of 1962 resulted from the thalidomide incident. Although the objectives of these amendments have little to do with issues directly related to the thalidomide problem in pregnancy, this tragedy convinced the public and government that greater control of the drug industry was necessary. This legislation required manufacturers to demonstrate both efficacy and safety of their products and established the testing procedures that would be necessary before the FDA would approve a drug for marketing.
8. All new drugs to be considered for marketing must be first tested for safety on three species of animals. Following these initial tests, if the drug is favorably reviewed by the FDA, it is given investigational new drug (IND) status and authorized to be used for human testing. In phase I, the *initial clinical phase,* the drug is given to small numbers of healthy volunteers in order to determine side effects and the manner in which the body responds to the drug. Phase 2 is called the *clinical pharmacological evaluation stage* and assesses the clinical effectiveness of the drug in a few patients with the disorder the drug is intended to treat. Phase 3 is the *extended clinical evaluation.* The drug is given to a wide range of volunteer patients with the condition that the drug is to treat. During this phase, thousands of patients receive the drug and its effectiveness and safety are determined. After completing these phases of review, the FDA assesses the data and determines if the drug should be allowed to be marketed for use.
9. There is concern that the process used by the FDA to evaluate drugs is not versatile enough to address all of the public's drug requirements. Attempts have been made to deal with special needs or take care of special groups in society. The "fast-track" rule is an amendment to accelerate the evaluation of new drugs with obvious therapeutic action. Another special provision made by the FDA, the Orphan Drug Law, provides provisions and tax incentives to pharmaceutical companies to develop and test drugs to be used in the treatment of rare diseases.

   The "Prescription Drug User Fee Act" of 1992 was passed to help fund the accelerated processing of new drugs being tested for marketing.
10. In 1972, the FDA initiated a program to assure that all OTC drugs were safe and effective. Special panels were selected to evaluate the safety and effectiveness of over 700 OTC drug ingredients. Each of these ingredients was classified as follows: category I, those

found to be safe and effective and approved for OTC use; category II, those either ineffective or unsafe and removed from OTC medicinal products; and category III, those for which there was insufficient information to make a decision.

11. The FDA is committed to making more effective drugs available OTC in response to public demand for greater self-treatment opportunities and reduced health care costs. The *switching policy* allows the FDA to review prescription drugs and evaluate their suitability as OTC products.
12. Three of the principal factors that influence laws on drug abuse are (a) Should drug abusers be treated as criminals or patients? (b) How can drug users and drug pushers be distinguished? (c) What types of laws and programs are effective deterrents against drug abuse?
13. The Harrison Act of 1914 was a principal piece of legislation in defining drug abuse and preventing its occurrence. Specifically, the Harrison Act attempted to regulate the production, importation, sale, purchase, and distribution of addicting substances, such as opium.
14. There is controversy as to how to best reduce substance abuse. A principal strategy by governmental agencies to achieve this objective is interdiction; the majority of money used to fight drug abuse is spent on trying to stop and confiscate drug supplies. Experience has proven that it is impossible to eliminate access to drugs of abuse and that interdiction is rarely effective. In order to reduce drug abuse, demand for these substances must be diminished. The youth must be a top priority in any substance abuse program. Young people should be educated that drug abuse is undesirable. Treatment should be provided that enables drug addicts to stop their habits with minimal discomfort. Finally, education should be used to change attitudes toward drug abuse and its consequences. Potential drug abusers need to be convinced that substance abuse is personally and socially damaging and unacceptable.
15. Society pays a high price for drug addiction and dependence. Drug addiction disrupts and traumatizes individuals, families, communities, and countries. The costs are measured in billions of dollars used for treating drug emergencies, caring for family members, rehabilitating users, enforcing laws, and paying for the effects of drug-related crimes. Other costs of drug abuse, not less significant but more difficult to quantify, include personal suffering, emotional trauma, and permanent damage done to lives.
16. Crime and drug addiction are strongly linked. The enormous profits of drug trafficking attract hardened criminals and organized crime. Our courts and prisons have been overwhelmed due to current, sometimes unfair, drug laws. The way the judicial system deals with illicit drug use needs to be re-evaluated. Legalization of drugs and drug testing are controversial issues that require close scrutiny. Clearly, if we are to be successful in the "War on Drugs," we need to be practical and creative.

References

Adams, S. H. "The Great American Fraud." *Collier's* 36, no. 5 (1905): 17–18; no. 10 (1905): 16–18; no 16 1906): 18–20.

Aldrich, M. and R. Barker. "Historical Aspects of Cocaine Use and Abuse." In *Cocaine: Chemical, Biological, Clinical, Social and Treatment Aspects*, edited by S. Mule. Cleveland, OH: CRC Press, 1976.

"A Speedier FDA." *American Druggist* (November 1992), p. 13.

American Psychiatric Association. *Diagnostic and Statistical Manual*, 4th ed. [DSM-IV], A. Frances, chairperson, 175–272. Washington, DC: American Psychiatric Association, 1994.

Associated Press. "Program to Fight Drug Smuggling

Costs U.S. a Lot, Produces Little." *Salt Lake Tribune* 244 (17 August 1992a): A-1.

Associated Press. "The War over the War on Drugs Puts White House on the Defensive." *Salt Lake Tribune* 244 (11 September 1992b): A-4.

Associated Press. "Drug Lord Vows to Lead Army Against Bogota." *Salt Lake Tribune* 245 (19 January 1993a): A-2.

Associated Press. "Mexican Cardinal, Six Others Killed in Cross-Fire as Drug Battles Erupt in Guadalajara." *Salt Lake Tribune* 246 (25 May 1993b): A-1.

Associated Press. "U.S. Prisons Lock Up Record as Inmate Populations Escalate 300% Since 1980." *Salt Lake Tribune* 248 (2 June 1994): A-1.

Austin, G. A. "Perspectives on the History of Psychoactive Substance Use." NIDA Research Issues no. 24. Washington, DC: U.S. Department of Health, Education, and Welfare, 1978.

Balabanova, S., F. Parsche, and W. Pirsig. "First Identification of Drugs in Egyptian Mummies." *Naturwissenschaften* 79 (1992): 358.

Booth, R., et al. "A Tale of Three Cities: Risk Taking Among Intravenous Drug Users." In *Problems of Drug Dependence*. NIDA Research Monograph Series no 95. Washington, DC: U.S. Department of Health, Education, and Welfare, 1989.

Bryson, R. "Railroads Try to Derail Drug Abuse." *Salt Lake Tribune* 244 (9 June 1992): D-5.

Buckley, B. "Pharmacists Offer Their Views on Reimbursement, Illicit Drugs, Suicide." *Pharmacy Times* (4 April 1994): 43–44.

Catlin, D., D. Cowan, M. Donike, D. Fraisse, H. Oftebro, and S. Rendic. "Testing Urine for Drugs." *Journal of Automated Chemistry* 14 (1992): 85–92.

Drug Facts and Comparisons. St. Louis: Lippincott, 1991.

FASEB [Federation of American Societies for Experimental Biology] *Newsletter* 25 (March 1992): 4.

Fitzpatrick, P. "Drug Abuse Education: Opportunity to Serve." *Pharmacy Times* (October 1992): 100–104.

Gawin, F., D. Allen, and B. Humbleston. *Archives of General Psychiatry* 46 (1989): 322.

Goldstein, A. "Lessons from the Street." *In Addiction from Biology to Drug Policy*. New York: Freeman, 1994.

Goldstein, A., and H. Kalant. "1990 Drug Policy: Striking the Right Balance." *Science* (Washington, DC) 249 (1990): 1513–21.

Greenhouse, S. "NIDA Becomes Part of NIH Under Recent ADAMHA Reorganization." *NIDA Notes* (September–October 1992): 1.

Halloway, M. "R_x for Addiction." *Scientific American* (March 1991): 95–103.

Holmstedt, B. "Historical Survey." In *Ethnopharmacological Search for Psychoactive Drugs*, edited by D. H. Efron. Public Health Service Publication no. 1645. Washington, DC: U.S. Government Printing Office, 1967.

Hunter, J. R., D. L. Rosen, and R. DeChristoforo. "How FDA Expedites Evaluation of Drugs." *Welcome Trends in Pharmacy*. [Health Education Technologies, New York, NY] (January 1993): 2–9.

Hwang, S. "Nicotine Patch Reignites Fight over Drug Ads." *Wall Street Journal* 73 (30 June 1992): B-1.

Johnston, L. *University of Michigan National High School Senior Survey*. Ann Arbor: University of Michigan, 1993.

Kalant, H. "Formulating Policies on the Non-Medical Use of Cocaine." In *Cocaine: Scientific and Social Dimensions*, Ciba Foundation Symposium 166. New York: Wiley, 1992. 261–76.

Kearns, R. "Legalize Drugs? Elders Speaks Firestorm." *Salt Lake Tribune* 247 (9 December 1993): A-18.

Knight-Ridder News Service. "Experts Call War on Drugs a $32 Billion Stalemate." *Salt Lake Tribune* 244 (21 September 1992a): A-3.

Knight-Ridder News Service. "Time to Make Drugs Legal? Many Say Yes." *Salt Lake Tribune* 244 (11 July 1992b): A-1, A-2.

Kokkevi, A., J. Liappas, V. Boukouvala, V. Alevizou, E. Anastassopoulou, and C. Stefanis. "Criminality in a Sample of Drug Abusers in Greece." *Drug and Alcohol Dependence*, 31 (1993): 111–21.

McShane, L. "Cops Are Crooks in N.Y.'s 30th Precinct." *Salt Lake Tribune* 248 (18 April 1994): A-5.

Millstein, R. "Remarks on the Status of NIDA." Made at the 55th Annual Scientific Meeting of the College on Problems of Drug Dependence, Toronto, Canada, 12 June 1993.

Morgan, H. W. "The Therapeutic Revolution." In *Drugs in America, A Social History, 1800–1980*. Syracuse, NY: Syracuse University Press, 1981.

Nadelman, E. A. "America's Drug Problem: A Case for Decriminalization." In *Taking Sides*, edited by Raymond Goldberg, 4–14. Guilford, CT: Dushkin, 1993.

"National Household Survey." *Salt Lake Tribune* 246 (24 June 1993): A-4.

SAMHSA Bulletin. CMHS Office of Public Affairs, Rm 13C-05, 5600 Fishers Lane, Rockville, MD 20857, 1992.

Schuster, C. "Implication for Research of the 1988 Anti-Drug Abuse Act." In *Problems of Drug Dependence*. NIDA Research Monograph Series no. 95. Washington, DC: U.S. Department of Health, Education, and Welfare, 1989.

Scott, J. M. *The White Poppy: A History of Opium*. New York: Funk & Wagnalls, 1969.

Siegelman, S. "The Coming Wave of R_x-to-OTC

Switches." *American Druggist* (August 1990): 37–42.

Simonsen, L. "Medicines in Development Keep Older Americans Healthy, at Home, Longer." *Pharmacy Times* 59 (1993): 81–85.

Temin, P. *Taking Your Medicine: Drug Regulation in the United States.* Cambridge, MA: Harvard University Press, 1980.

Wallace, I., D. Wallechinsky, and A. Wallace. "Dr. Freud's Magic Nose Powder." *Parade Magazine* (20 September 1981).

Wilson, J. Q., "Against the Legalization of Drugs." In *Taking Sides,* edited by Raymond Goldberg, 15–25. Guilford, CT: Dushkin, 1993.

Wire Services. "Cocaine Kingpin Escapes After Bloody Shootout." *Salt Lake Tribune* 244 (23 July 1992): A-1.

Woolsey, R. "A Prescription for Better Prescriptions." *Issues in Science and Technology* (Spring 1994): 59–66.

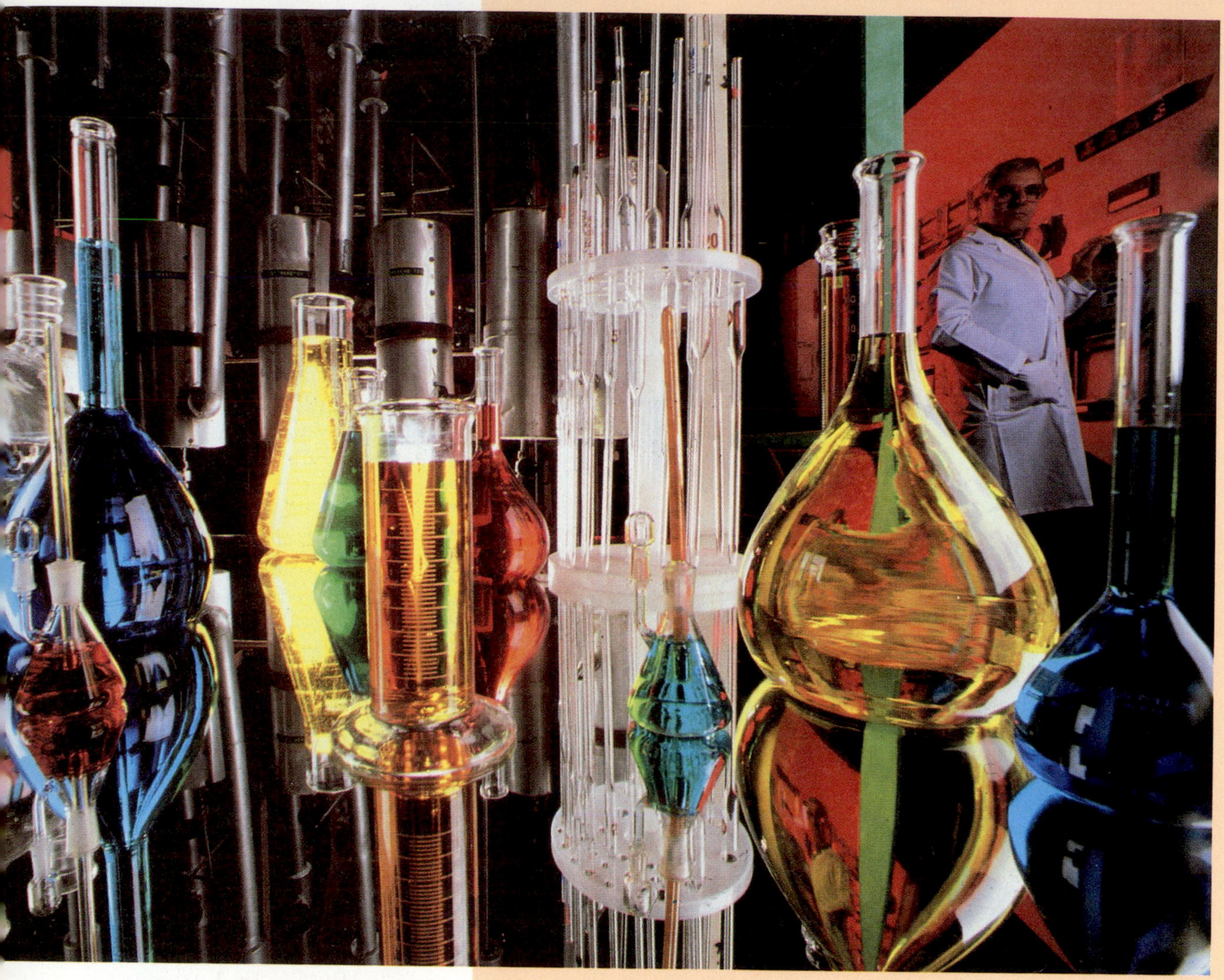

Chapter 4

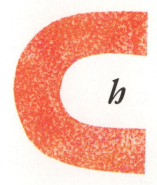

DID YOU KNOW THAT . . .

- The same dose of a drug does not have the same effect on everyone.
- In high-enough doses, almost any drug or substance can be toxic.
- 65% of the strokes among young Americans are related to cigarette, cocaine, or amphetamine use.
- Use of some drugs can dramatically enhance the effects of others.
- The form in which a drug is taken can influence the effect it has.
- Many drugs are unable to pass from the blood into the brain.
- Most drugs cross the placental barrier from the mother to the fetus.
- Physical dependence is characterized by withdrawal effects when use of the drug is stopped.
- Tolerance to one drug can often cause tolerance to other similar drugs; this is called *cross-tolerance*.
- Placebos can have significant effects in relieving symptoms such as pain.
- The body produces endorphins, which have effects like narcotics.
- Psychological dependence on a drug often leads to drug abuse.
- Hereditary factors may predispose some individuals to becoming psychologically dependent on drugs with abuse potential.

How and Why Drugs Work

LEARNING OBJECTIVES

On completing this chapter, you will be able to

1 Describe some of the common unintended drug effects.
2 Explain why the same dose of a drug may affect individuals differently.
3 Explain the difference between potency and toxicity.
4 Describe the concepts of a drug's margin of safety and therapeutic index.
5 Identify and give examples of additive, antagonistic, and potentiation (synergistic) drug interactions.
6 Identify the pharmacokinetic factors that can influence the effects caused by drugs.
7 Cite the physiological and pathological factors that influence drug effects.
8 Explain the significance of the blood–brain barrier to psychoactive drugs.
9 Define *threshold dose, plateau effect,* and *cumulative effect.*
10 Discuss the role of the liver in drug metabolism and the consequences of this process.
11 Define *biotransformation.*
12 Describe the relationships among tolerance, withdrawal, rebound, physical dependence, and psychological dependence.

continued

Healthy People 2000

Reduce drug-related deaths to no more than three per 100,000 people.

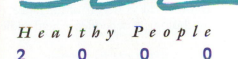

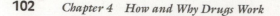

LEARNING OBJECTIVES

13 Discuss the significance of placebos in responding to drugs.

14 Describe drug craving and how it affects drug abuse.

Many people believe that life's physical and emotional problems can be resolved merely by taking the right drug. Although it is true that medications are very important in the treatment of almost every type of physical and psychiatric disease, this simplistic attitude causes unrealistic expectations that may lead to dangerous, even fatal, responses. For example, drug addiction and dependence are often the result of being excessively reliant on drugs for answers to medical and psychological problems. Obviously, not every person who inappropriately uses drugs becomes a drug addict, nor are patients who use drugs as prescribed by the doctor immune from becoming physically and mentally dependent on their medication. In fact, because of individual variability, there is no way to accurately predict which drug users will or will not have drug problems such as addiction and dependence

In this chapter we consider the factors that account for the variability of drug responses. We discuss how the body responds to drugs and why some drugs work while others do not. First we review the general effects of drugs, both intended and unintended. The dose–response relationship is addressed next, followed by a discussion of drug interaction. The section on pharmacokinetic factors considers how drugs are introduced, distributed, and eliminated from the body, along with physiological and pathological variables that modify drug effects. The last sections in the chapter consider the concepts of tolerance, physical versus psychological dependence, and addiction.

The Intended and Unintended Effects of Drugs

When physicians prescribe drugs, their objective is usually to cure or relieve symptoms of a disease. However, frequently drugs cause unintended effects that neither the physician nor the patient expected.

The intended responses produced by a drug are called *main effects,* whereas those that are unintended are called *side effects.* The distinction between main and side effects depends on the therapeutic objective. A response that is considered unnecessary or undesirable in one situation may, in fact, be the intended effect in another. For example, antihistamines found in many over-the-counter (OTC) drugs have an intended main effect of relieving allergy symptoms, but they often cause annoying drowsiness as a side effect. However, these antihistamines are also included in OTC sleep aids, where their sedating action is the desired main effect because it encourages sleep in people suffering from insomnia.

Side effects can influence many body functions and occur in any organ (see Figure 4.1). The following are basic kinds of side effects that can result from drug use:

Nausea or vomiting. Almost any drug can cause an upset stomach; in fact, with some medications, such as aspirin, this is a common complaint.

Changes in mental alertness. Some medications can cause sedation and drowsiness

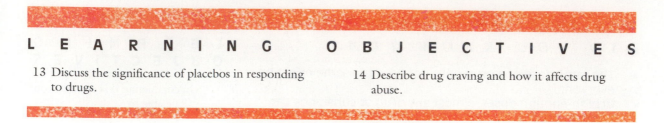

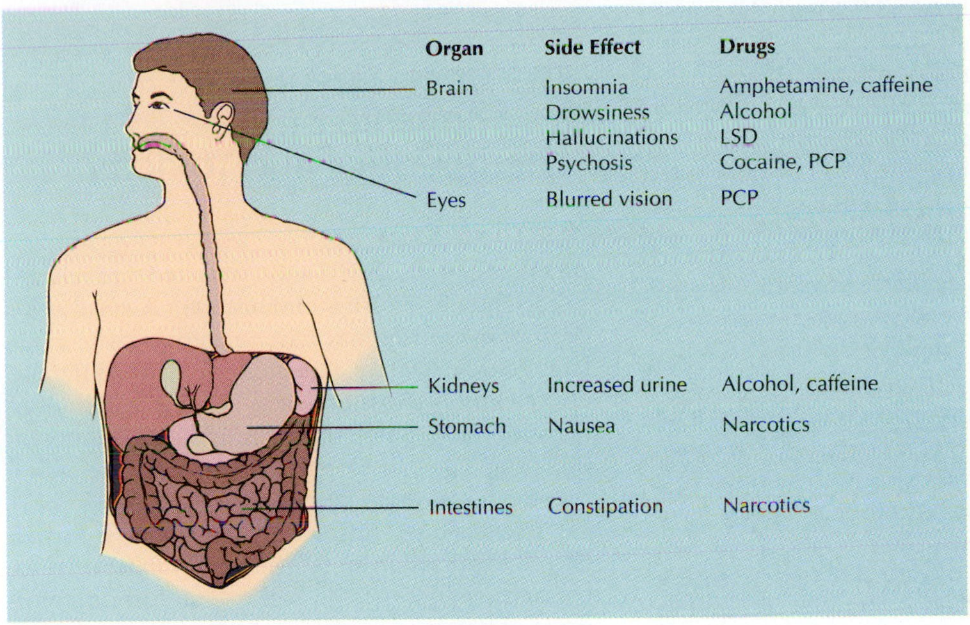

Organ
Side Effect
Drugs
Brain
Insomnia
Drowsiness
Hallucinations
Psychosis
Amphetamine, caffeine
Alcohol
LSD
Cocaine, PCP
Eyes
Blurred vision
PCP
Kidneys
Increased urine
Alcohol, caffeine
Stomach
Nausea
Narcotics
Intestines
Constipation
Narcotics

FIGURE 4.1 Common side effects with drugs of abuse. Almost every organ or system in the body can be unintentionally altered by the effects of substances of abuse.

(for example, antihistamines in OTC allergy medications) or nervousness and insomnia (for example, caffeine in OTC stay-awake products).

Dependence. This phenomenon compels people to continue using a drug because they want to achieve a desired effect or they fear unpleasant reaction, called **withdrawal,** that occurs when the drug is discontinued. Dependence has been associated with such apparently benign OTC drugs as nasal decongestant sprays and laxatives, as well as more potent drugs such as alcohol (see Chapters 7 and 8), narcotics (see Chapter 9), and stimulants (see Chapter 10).

Allergic reactions (hypersensitive reactions or sensitization). Allergic reactions occur when the body becomes sensitized to a drug and attempts to destroy and dispose of it. During an allergic reaction, the body produces antibodies that bind to the drug, causing tissue reactions and possible cell damage. The results of these events can include

1) Skin rashes, swelling, and pain
2) Hives, itching, and sweating
3) *Angioneurotic edema,* an accumulation of fluid in the soft tissue of the face, resulting in swelling of the eyes, cheeks, and lips
4) Shock (anaphylactic type) or even death
5) Delayed reactions, which occur 7 to 14 days after exposure to the drug and include hives, arthritis, fever, and damage to internal organs such as the heart and kidneys

Changes in cardiovascular activity. Many drugs that are available OTC or by prescription, or are used illicitly, can alter the

WITHDRAWAL unpleasant effects that occur when use of a drug is stopped activity of the heart and change the state of the blood vessels. These changes can cause the heart to beat faster, slower, or in irregular patterns (called *arrhythmias*) and can dilate (enlarge) or constrict (shrink) arteries and veins. The result of these side effects includes changes in blood pressure, fainting, heart attacks, and strokes.

This partial list of side effects demonstrates the types of risk involved whenever any drug (prescription, nonprescription, or illicit) is used. Consequently, before taking a drug, whether for therapeutic or recreational use, you should understand the potential disadvantages it poses and determine if the benefits justify the risks. For example, it is important to know that morphine is a good drug for relieving severe pain, but it also depresses breathing and retards intestinal activity, causing constipation. Likewise, amphetamines are used to suppress appetite, but they also increase blood pressure and stimulate the heart. Cocaine is a good local anesthetic but can cause tremors or even seizures. The greater the danger of using a drug, the less likely the benefits will warrant its use.

Adverse effects to drugs of abuse are particularly troublesome in the United States. Studies have suggested that 20% of the total hospital costs in this country are due to medical care for the health damage caused by alcohol, tobacco, and other drugs of abuse. Other statistics illustrating the major negative health impact of adverse unintended effects caused by drugs of abuse include the following ("Trends, Policy and Research," 1993):

- Patients who abuse alcohol, tobacco, and other drugs are hospitalized twice as long as other patients with the same diagnosis.
- Seventy-five percent of the chronic pancreatitis (damaged pancreas) cases in the United States are due to alcohol abuse.
- Sixty-five percent of the strokes among young Americans are related to cigarette, cocaine, or amphetamine use.
- Youth under 15 years old are hospitalized three to four times longer, regardless of their illness, if they have an alcohol, tobacco, or other drug problem.
- More than 50 percent of the pediatric AIDS cases are the result of parental use of drugs of abuse.

The Dose–Response Relationship of Therapeutics and Toxicity

All effects, both desired and unwanted, are related to the amount of drug administered. A small concentration of drug may have one effect, whereas a larger dose may have a greater effect or a different effect entirely. Because there is some correlation between the response to a drug and the quantity of the drug dose, it is possible to calculate *dose–response* curves (see Figure 4.2).

Once a dose–response curve for a drug has been determined in an individual, it can be used to predict how that person will respond to different doses of the drug. For example, the dose–response curve for user B in Figure 4.2 shows that 600 mg of aspirin will only relieve 50% of his or her headache. However, it is important to understand that not everybody responds the same to a given dose of drug. Thus, in Figure 4.2 while 600 mg of aspirin gives 50% relief from a headache for user B, it relieves 100% of the headache for user A and none of the headache for user C.

This variability in response makes it difficult to predict the precise drug effect from a given dose. Consequently, a physician will sometimes prescribe a drug with the warning that, if any side effect occurs or if the drug does not work, the prescription will be changed. Such caution is important because without doing a dose–effect curve for every drug user it is very difficult to know precisely how an individual will respond to a drug dosage.

Many factors can contribute to the variability in drug responses. One of the most important is tolerance, or reduced response over time to the same dosage, an effect that is examined carefully in a later section. Other factors include the size of the person, stomach contents if the drug is taken by mouth, different levels of enzymatic activity in the liver (which changes the drug by metabolism), acidity of the urine (which affects rate of drug elimination), the time of day, and the state of a person's health. Multiple interacting factors such as these make it difficult to calculate accurately the final drug effect for any given individual.

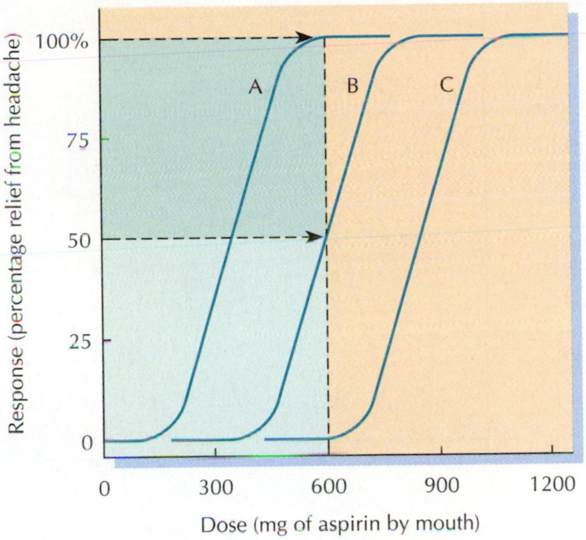

FIGURE 4.2 Dose–response curve for relieving a headache with aspirin in three users. User A is the most sensitive and has 100% headache relief at a dose of 600 mg. User B is the next sensitive and gets 50% headache relief with a 600-mg dose. The least sensitive is user C: with a 600-mg dose user, C has no relief from a headache.

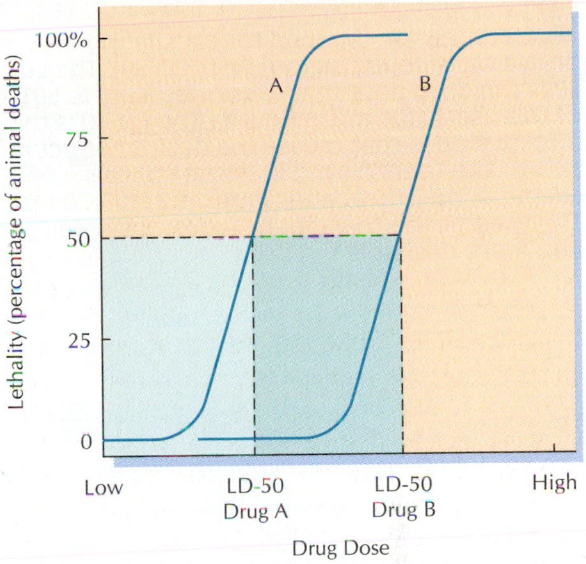

FIGURE 4.3 Dose–response curve for lethal drug doses. The lethal dose for 50% of the animals (LD-50) is found by extending vertical lines from the point of 50% lethality to the "Drug Dose" line. Graphs such as this make it possible to compare lethality between drugs. In this example, drug A is more lethal than drug B because its LD-50 is lower.

Toxicity and Effectiveness

Even though the ways in which individuals respond to drugs vary, it is important to compare, as accurately as possible, therapeutic and toxic doses. For new drugs being considered for marketing, this is done by extensive testing on three species of animals before humans are tested. The animal testing is accomplished by administering a wide range of drug dosages and assessing toxicity by determining the lethal dose. From the results, calculations of the lethal dose (LD) for 50% of the test animals are made. This dose, also called the *LD-50,* is found by plotting the dose against the percentage of lethality.

Such information is important in assessing the safety, or risk, of new drugs and provides important dosage information that can be used for human testing. In addition, the concept of LDs (lethal doses) also is useful in assessing the risk of illicit use of drugs of abuse and the likelihood of life-threatening effects. Figure 4.3 is a typical graph showing the lethality curves of two drugs given to laboratory animals.

After determining the LD-50 of a new drug, the pharmacologist will lower the dose while evaluating the therapeutic (intended) response to the drug. Using this approach, the therapeutically effective dose (ED) in 50% of the animals, the *ED-50,* can be determined and compared to the LD-50 (see Figure 4.4). The difference between the ED-50 and LD-50 represents the margin of drug safety. The wider the margin of safety, or the greater the difference between therapeutic and toxic doses, the more desirable the drug.

Potency Versus Toxicity

Most of us know that some drugs of abuse are more dangerous than others. For example, it is common knowledge that abuse of the narcotic

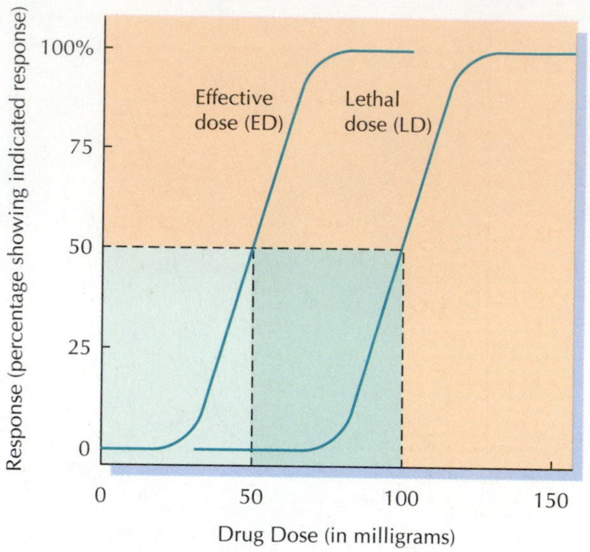

FIGURE 4.4 Method for calculating a drug's *therapeutic index* (LD-50/ED-50). The LD-50 is the drug dose that causes lethality in 50% of the users (100 mg in figure). The ED-50 is the effective dose that causes the desired effect in 50% of the users (50 mg in figure). In this example, the *therapeutic index* is 2 (100/50 = 2). The greater the *therapeutic index*, the safer and more desirable the drug.

drug heroin is more likely to be lethal than abuse of another narcotic drug, codeine. One of the important features that makes heroin more dangerous than codeine is its high potency. **Potency** is a way of expressing how much of a drug is necessary to cause an effect, whether it be desired or toxic. The smaller the dose required to achieve a drug action, the greater the drug potency. For example, in Figure 4.3, drug B is less potent than drug A when considering death as the measured effect. In other words, it takes more of drug B to get the same lethal response as from drug A. Thus, using the example of the narcotic drugs, if drug B represented codeine, drug A would represent heroin.

The concept of potency also can be used to describe a drug's ability to cause a therapeutic effect. More potent medications require lower doses to be effective. Obviously, knowledge of a drug's potency is essential if it is to be used properly and safely.

Toxicity is the capacity of a drug to upset or even destroy normal body functions. Toxic compounds are often called *poisons,* although almost any compound—including sugar, table salt, aspirin, and vitamin A—can be toxic at sufficiently

TABLE 4.1 A simple classification for comparing toxic potency

Classification	Description	Example
Extremely toxic	LD-50 is greater than 1 mg per kilogram body weight	Fentanyl (narcotic)
Highly toxic	LD-50 is 1 to 50 mg per kilogram body weight	Heroin (narcotic) Cocaine (stimulant)
Moderately toxic	LD-50 is 50 to 100 mg per kilogram body weight	Codeine (narcotic)
Slightly toxic	LD-50 is 0.1 to 5 g per kilogram body weight	Caffeine (stimulant) Valium (depressant)

Here and Now

Fatal Consequences of Potent Synthetic Narcotics

The issues of potency and toxicity are particularly important when dealing with new drugs of abuse that are being created in clandestine laboratories and then sold on the "streets." Some of these new pharmacological creations are referred to as "*designer*" *drugs* and are unexpectedly potent. For example, derivatives of the commonly used narcotic pain reliever fentanyl (see Chapter 9) have been reported to be many times more potent than heroin. One such drug, alpha methylfentanyl, has been sold on the "streets" since 1982 as an illicit synthetic heroin. This drug actually has a potency 3,000 to 5,000 times greater than that of heroin, and if mistakenly taken as heroin by a narcotic addict, a lethal dose can easily be administered (Henderson 1988). From 1985 to 1990, such mistakes resulted in scores of fatal narcotic overdoses in the United States.

high doses. If a foreign chemical is introduced into the body, it may disrupt the body's normal functions. In many instances, the body can compensate for this disruption, perhaps by metabolizing and rapidly eliminating the chemical, and little effect is noted. Sometimes the delicate balance is altered and the person becomes sick or even dies. If the body's functional balance is already under stress from the disease, the introduction of a drug may have a much more serious effect than in a healthy person who can adjust to its toxicity.

A drug with high potency often is toxic even at low doses, so the amount given must be carefully measured and the user closely monitored; if caution is not taken, serious damage to the body or death can occur (see box). Very potent drugs that are abused, such as heroin, are particularly dangerous because they are often consumed by unsuspecting users who are ignorant of the drug's extreme toxicity. Potency depends on many factors, such as absorption of the drug, its distribution in the body, individual metabolism, the form of excretion, the rate of elimination, and its activity at the site of action.

A simple classification system that is sometimes used to compare the toxic potency of drugs is shown in Table 4.1.

POTENCY the amount of drug necessary to cause an effect

TOXICITY the capacity of a drug to do damage or cause adverse effects in the body

MARGIN OF SAFETY the range in dose between the amount of drug necessary to cause a therapeutic effect and a toxic effect

Margin of Safety

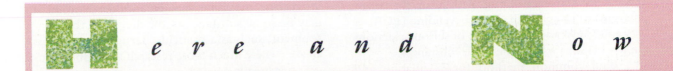

An important concept for developing new drugs for therapy, as well as for assessing the probability of serious side effects for drugs of abuse, is called the **margin of safety.** The margin of safety is determined by the difference between the doses necessary to cause the intended (therapeutic or recreational) effects and the toxic unintended effects. The larger the margin of safety, the less likely that serious adverse side effects will occur when using the drug to treat medical problems or even when abusing it. Drugs with relatively narrow margins of safety, such as phencyclidine (PCP) or cocaine, have a very high rate of serious reactions in populations who abuse these substances.

One common method for calculating and comparing the margin of safety for drugs is the **therapeutic index** (see Figure 4.4 for details). One way to calculate the index is by dividing the lethal dose of a drug by its therapeutic dose. The higher the therapeutic index, the safer and more desirable is the drug.

There is no such thing as the perfect drug that goes right to the target, has no toxicity, produces no side effects, and can be removed or neutralized when not needed. Unfortunately, most effective drugs are potentially dangerous if the doses are high enough. Pharmacologists refer to a perfect drug as a "magic bullet"; so far, we have no "magic bullets." Even relatively safe drugs available over the counter can cause problems for some prospective users. Not surprisingly, all drugs of abuse can cause very serious side effects especially when self-administered by users unfamiliar with the potential toxicities of these substances. The possibility that adverse effects will occur should always be considered before using any drug.

Drug Interaction

A drug's effects can be dramatically altered when other drugs are also present in the body: this is known as *drug interaction*. A typical example of multiple drug use is in treatment of the common cold. Because of the many cold-related symptoms, the sufferer may consume an assortment of pain relievers, antihistamines, decongestants, and anti-cough medications all at the same time.

Multiple drug use can create a serious medical problem because many drugs influence the actions of other drugs (Brenner 1994). Even physicians may be baffled by unusual effects when multiple drugs are consumed. Frequently, drug interactions are misdiagnosed as symptoms of a disease. Such errors in diagnosis can lead to inappropriate treatment and serious health consequences. Complications can arise that are dangerous, even fatal. The interacting substance may be another drug, or it may be some substance in the diet or in the environment, such as a pesticide. Drug interaction is an area where much more research and public education is greatly needed.

Depending on the effect on the body, drug interaction may be categorized into three types: *additive, antagonistic (inhibitory)*, and *potentiative (synergistic)*.

Additive Effects

Additive interactions are the combined effects of drugs taken concurrently. An example of an additive interaction results from using aspirin and acetaminophen (the active ingredient in Tylenol) at the same time. The pain relief provided is equal to the sum of the two analgesics, which could be achieved by a comparable dose of either drug alone. Thus, if a 300-mg tablet of Bayer aspirin were taken with a 300-mg tablet of Tylenol, the relief would be the same as if two tablets of either Bayer or Tylenol were taken instead.

Antagonistic (Inhibitory) Effects

An antagonistic drug effect occurs when one drug cancels or blocks the effect of another. For example, if a person takes antihistamines to reduce nasal congestion, he or she may be able to antagonize some of the drowsiness often caused by these drugs by using a central nervous system (CNS) stimulant such as caffeine.

It is likely that drug abusers who use two drugs at the same time often are trying to antagonize the unpleasant side effects of the first drug by administering the second. It has been reported that as many as 90 percent of those currently abusing cocaine also use alcohol (Grant and Harford 1990). The combined use of these two drugs is a major factor in drug-related problems and death in emergency rooms (Drug Abuse Warning Network

THERAPEUTIC INDEX the toxic dose divided by the therapeutic dose; used to calculate margin of safety

SYNERGISM the ability of one drug to enhance the effect of another; potentiation

TABLE 4.2 Common interactions with substances of abuse

Drug	Combined with	Interaction
Sedatives		
Valium, Halcion	Alcohol, barbiturates	Increase sedation
Stimulants		
Amphetamines, cocaine	Insulin	Decrease insulin effect
	Antidepressants	Cause hypertension
Narcotics		
Heroin, morphine	Barbiturates, Valium	Increase sedation
	Anticoagulant	Increase bleeding
	Antidepressants	Cause sedation
	Amphetamines	Increase euphoria
Tobacco		
Nicotine	Blood pressure medication	Elevate blood pressure
	Amphetamines, cocaine	Increase cardiovascular effects
Alcohol	Cocaine	Produces cocaethylene, which enhances euphoria and toxicity

1988). Nevertheless, it appears that some users may coadminister these drugs in order to antagonize the disruptive effects of alcohol with the stimulant action of the cocaine (Higgins et al. 1992).

Potentiative (Synergistic) Effects

The third type of drug interaction is known as *potentiation,* or **synergism.** Potentiation occurs when the effect of a drug is enhanced due to the presence of another drug or substance. This other substance may, in turn, stimulate or inhibit specific body enzymes that increase the duration and/or potency of the effects of the first drug. A common example is the combination of alcohol and Valium. It has been estimated that as many as 3,000 people die each year from mixing alcohol with CNS depressants such as Valium. Alcohol, like barbiturates, is a CNS depressant. When depressants are taken together, CNS functions become impaired and the person becomes groggy. A person in this state may forget he or she has taken the pills and repeat the dose. The combination of these two depressants (or other depressants, such as antihistamines) can depress the CNS to the point where vital functions such as breathing and heartbeat are severely impaired.

Although the mechanisms of interaction among CNS depressants are not entirely clear, it is likely that these drugs enhance each others' direct effects on inhibitory chemical messengers in the brain (see Chapter 5). In addition, interference by alcohol with liver-metabolizing enzymes also contributes to the potentiation that occurs between alcohol and some depressants, such as barbiturates (Jaffe 1990).

Dealing with Drug Interactions

Although many drug effects and interactions are not very well understood, it is important to be aware of them. Increasing amounts of evidence indicate that many of the drugs and substance we deliberately consume will interact and produce unexpected and sometimes dangerous effects (see Table 4.2). It is alarming to know that many of the foods we eat and some chemical pollutants also interfere with and modify drug actions. Pesticides, traces of hormones in meat and poultry, traces of metals in fish, nitrites and nitrates from fertilizers, and wide range of chemicals—some of which are used as food additives—have been shown, under certain conditions, to interact with some drugs.

As the medical community has become aware of the frequent complications arising from multiple drug use, efforts have been made to reduce the incidence as well as the severity of the problem. It is essential that the public be educated about interactions most likely to occur with drugs that are prescribed, self-administered legitimately (for example, OTC drugs), or recreationally (for example, drugs of abuse). People need to be aware that OTC drugs are as likely to cause interaction problems as prescription drugs; consequently, drug combinations should be used with caution. If there is any question concerning the possibility of drug interaction, people should talk to their physicians, pharmacists, or other health care providers. Also, if a patient is being effectively treated by a drug for a medical problem and the drug is suddenly no longer effective or the effects become exaggerated, the possibility of interference by another drug being jointly consumed should be considered.

Drug interaction is a major problem in drug abusing populations, as well. Most abusers are multiple drug *(polydrug)* users with little concern for the dangerous interactions that could occur. It is common for drug abusers to combine multiple CNS depressants to enhance their effects or a depressant with a stimulant to titrate a CNS effect (to determine the smallest amount that can be taken to achieve the desired "high") or to experiment with a combination of stimulants, depressants, and hallucinogens just to see what happens. The effects of such haphazard drug mixing are impossible to predict, difficult to treat in emergency situations, and all too frequently fatal.

Pharmacokinetic Factors That Influence Drug Effects

Although it is difficult to predict precisely how any single individual will be affected by drug use, the following major factors represent different major aspects of the body's response and should be considered when attempting to anticipate a drug's effects.

1. How does the drug enter the body? (administration)
2. How does the drug move from the site of administration into the body's system? (absorption)
3. How does the drug move to various areas in the body? (distribution)
4. How and where does the drug produce its effects? (activation)
5. How is the drug inactivated, metabolized, and/or excreted from the body? (biotransformation and elimination)

These issues relate to the **pharmacokinetics** of a drug and are important considerations when predicting the body's response.

Forms and Methods of Taking Drugs

Drugs come in many forms. The form in which a drug is administered may influence the rate of passage into the bloodstream from the site of administration and consequently its efficacy. The ways that drugs may be compounded and introduced onto or into the body are summarized in Table 4.3.

The means of introducing the drug into the body will also affect how quickly the drug enters the bloodstream and is distributed to the site of action, as well as how much will ultimately reach its target and exert an effect (Mathias 1994). The principal forms of drug administration include oral ingestion, inhalation, injection, topical application, and implantation.

Oral Ingestion One of the most common and convenient ways of taking a drug is orally. This type of administration usually introduces the drug into the body by way of the stomach or intestines.

Following oral administration, it is difficult to control the amount of drug that reaches the site of action, for three reasons:

1. The drug must enter the bloodstream after

PHARMACOKINETICS the study of factors that influence the distribution and concentration of drugs in the body

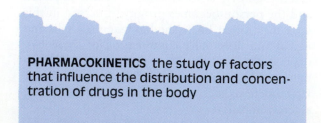

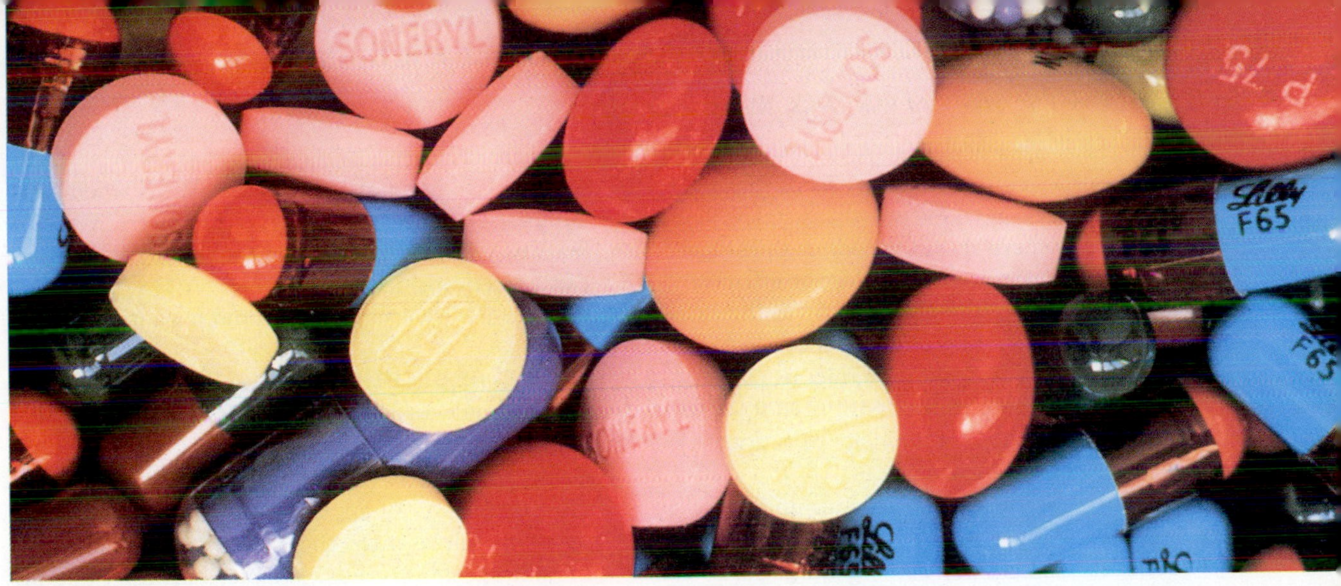

Drugs to be taken orally may be packaged as tablets or capsules

passing through the wall of the stomach or intestines without being destroyed or changed to an inactive form. From the blood the drug must diffuse to the target area and remain there in sufficient concentration to have an effect.

2. Materials in the gut, such as food, may interfere with the passage of some drugs through the gut lining and thus prevent drug action. For example, food in the stomach interferes with the absorption of alcohol; thus, when eating, more alcohol can be consumed without having a significant effect.
3. The liver might metabolize orally ingested drugs too rapidly, before they are able to have an effect. The liver is the major detoxifying organ in the body, which means it removes chemicals and toxins from the blood and usually

TABLE 4.3 Common drug forms

Category	Types	Description
Solutions	Waters	Volatile oils in water
	Syrups	Sugar + water + flavoring
	Elixirs	Sugar + water + flavoring + alcohol
Suspensions	Emulsions	Fat globules in water
	Magma	Finely ground particles in water
Topicals	Liniments	Drug mixtures in oil, water, or alcohol
	Lotions	Mild liquid preparations
	Ointments	Fatty or oily preparations
Solids	Powders	Fine particles
	Tablets	Compressed powders
	Pills	Powders held together by honey or candy
	Capsules	Drugs in gelatin containers
	Enteric coated	Protect capsule in stomach
	Sustained release	Released over a period of time
	Suppositories	Inserted into anus or vagina

changes them into an inactive form that is easy for the body to excrete. This function is essential to survival, but it creates a problem for the pharmacologist developing effective drugs. It is especially problematic in the case of oral administration because the substances absorbed from the digestive tract usually go to the liver before being distributed to other parts of the body and their site of action.

Inhalation Some drugs are administered by inhalation. The lungs have large beds of capillaries, so chemicals capable of crossing membranes can enter the blood as rapidly as intravenous injection and can be equally as dangerous (Mathias 1994). Ether, chloroform, and nitrous oxide anesthetics are examples of drugs that are therapeutically administered by inhalation. Nicotine from tobacco smoke and even cocaine, methamphetamine, and heroin, are drugs of abuse that can be inhaled as smoke. One serious problem with inhalation is the potential for irritation to the mucous membrane lining of the lungs; another is that the drug may have to be continually inhaled to maintain the concentration necessary for an effect.

Injection Some drugs are given by injection: intravenously (IV), intramuscularly (IM), or subcutaneously (SC). A major advantage of administering drugs by IV is the speed of action; the dosage is delivered rapidly and directly, and often less drug is needed because it reaches the site of action quickly. This method can be very dangerous if the dosage is calculated incorrectly. Additionally, impurities in injected materials may irritate the vein; this is a particular problem in the drug abusing population, where needle sharing frequently occurs. The injection itself injures the vein by leaving a tiny point of scar tissue where the vein is punctured. If repeated injections are administered into the same area, the elasticity of the vein is gradually reduced, causing the vessel to collapse.

Intramuscular injection can damage the muscle directly if the drug preparation irritates the tissue or indirectly if the nerve controlling the muscle is damaged. If the nerve is destroyed, the muscle will degenerate (atrophy). A subcutaneous injection may kill the skin at the point of injection if a particularly irritating drug is administered. Another danger of drug injections occurs when contaminated needles are shared by drug users. This has become a serious problem in the spread of dangerous infectious diseases such as AIDS (acquired immune deficiency syndrome) and hepatitis.

Topical Application Those drugs that readily pass through surface tissue such as the skin, the lining of the nose, and the mouth can be applied topically, for systemic (whole-body) effects. Although most drugs do not appreciably diffuse across these tissue barriers into the circulation, there are notable exceptions. For example, a product to help quit smoking (Nicoderm) can be placed on the skin; the drug passes through the skin and enters the body to prevent tobacco craving and withdrawal. Another example of a topical drug is the controversial substance (not FDA approved) DMSO (dimethylsulfoxide), which often is used by athletes or sometimes trainers to treat inflammation of athletic injuries. After applying DMSO to the skin at the site of an injury, the drug quickly passes through the skin into the circulation and within a few minutes is secreted into the saliva, causing a distinctive taste and smell of garlic.

Implantation Administering drugs orally, by inhalation, or via injection is usually satisfactory; however, the concentration of the drug increases rapidly and then declines in the blood, ranging between too much and too little, neither of which is desirable. Implantable drug delivery devices are being used to provide a more constant, steady release of a variety of drugs. With such devices, a person is exposed to lower total doses of drugs and need not be concerned about when to take the drug.

An example of an implantable drug delivery system is the subdermal hormonal implant Norplant, a contraceptive made available in the United States in 1990. This contraceptive consists of multiple silastic (a permeable plastic) capsules, which are placed beneath the skin under the arm. Norplant slowly and consistently releases a progestin-type female hormone (levonorgestrel), which reliably prevents pregnancy in more than 99 percent of the users. The effectiveness of this product continues for approximately five years (*Drug Facts and Comparisons* 1994).

Distribution of Drugs in the Body and Time–Response Relationships

Following administration (regardless of the mode), most drugs are distributed throughout the body in the blood. The circulatory system consists of many miles of arteries, veins, and capillaries and includes 5 to 6 liters of blood. Once a drug enters the bloodstream, by passing across thin capillary walls, it is rapidly diluted and carried to organs and other body structures. It requires approximately one minute for the blood, and consequently the drugs that are in it, to circulate completely throughout the body.

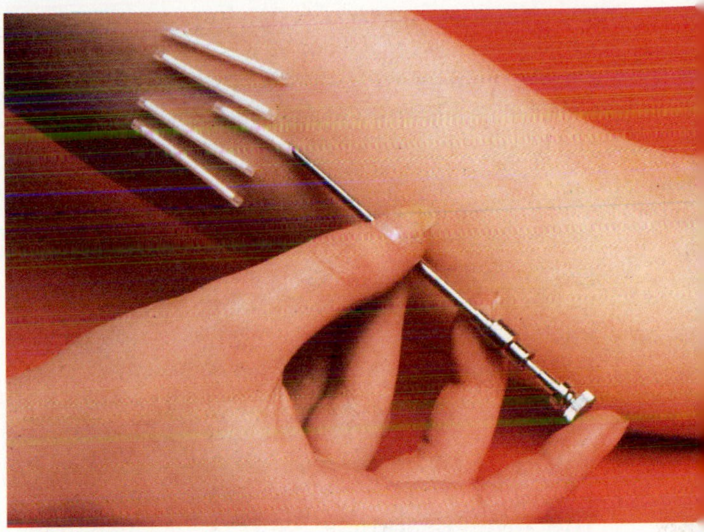

Implantable drug-delivery devices provide steady release of drugs.

Factors Affecting Distribution Drugs have different patterns of distribution depending on their chemical properties such as

- Their ability to pass across membranes and through tissues
- Their molecular size (large versus small molecules)
- Their solubility properties (do they dissolve in water or in fatty—oily—solutions?)
- Their tendency to attach to proteins and tissues throughout the body

These distribution-related factors are very important because they determine whether a drug can pass across tissue barriers in the body and reach the site of their action. By preventing the movement of drugs into organs or across tissues, these barriers may interfere with drug activity and limit the therapeutic usefulness of a drug if they do not allow it to reach its site of action. Such barriers may also be protective by preventing entry of a drug into a body structure where it can cause problems. Two of the principal biological barriers in the body are the **blood–brain barrier** and the placental barrier.

Because of its continual state of high activity, the brain requires about 20% of the body's blood in order to satisfy its nutrient and oxygen needs. The blood is carried to the nerve cells of the brain in a vast network of thin-walled capillaries. Drugs that are soluble in fatty (oily) solutions are most likely to pass readily through the capillaries into brain tissue. Most psychoactive drugs, such as the drugs of abuse, are able to pass across the blood–brain barrier with little difficulty. However, many water-soluble drugs cannot pass across the fatty capillary wall; such drugs are not likely to affect the brain.

A second biological barrier, the placenta, prevents the transfer of certain molecules from the mother to the fetus. A principal factor that determines passage of substances across the placental barrier is molecular size. Large molecules do not usually cross the placental barrier, while smaller molecules do. Because most drugs are relatively small molecules, they usually cross from the maternal circulation into the fetal circulation; thus most drugs (including the drugs of abuse) taken by a woman during pregnancy get into the fetus.

Required Doses for Effects Most drugs do not take effect until a certain amount has been administered and a crucial concentration has reached the site of action in the body. The smallest amount of a drug needed to elicit a response is called its **threshold.**

BLOOD–BRAIN BARRIER selective filtering between the cerebral blood vessels and the brain

THRESHOLD the minimum drug dose necessary to cause an effect

The effectiveness of some drugs may be calculated in a *linear* (straight-line) fashion, which means that the more drug taken, the more drug distributes throughout the body and the greater the effect. However, many drugs have a maximum effect they can cause, regardless of dose; this is called the **plateau effect.** OTC medications, in particular, have a limit on their effects. For example, nonprescription analgesics such as aspirin can be effective in treating mild to moderate pain, but regardless of dose, aspirin will not relieve severe pain. Other drugs may cause distinct or opposite effects, depending on the dose. For example, low doses of alcohol may act like a stimulant, whereas high doses usually cause sedation.

The Time–Response Factors An important time–response factor is the time that has elapsed since a drug was administered and the onset of the effect. The delay in effect after administering a drug often relates to the time required for the drug to distribute from the site of administration to the site of action. Consequently, the closer a drug is placed to the target area, the faster the onset of action.

The drug response is often classified as immediate, short term, or **acute**, referring to the response after a single dose. The response can also be **chronic,** or long term, usually associated with repeated doses. The intensity and quality of a drug's acute effect may change considerably within a short period of time. For example, the main intoxicating effects of a larger dose of alcohol generally peak in less than one hour and then gradually taper off. In addition, an initial stimulating effect by alcohol may later change to sedation and depression.

The effects of long-term, or chronic, use of some drugs can be quite different from their short-term, or acute, use. The administration of small doses may not produce any apparent, immediate, detrimental effect, but chronic use of the same drug (frequent use over a long time) may cause prolonged effects that are not apparent until years later. Although there is little evidence to show any immediate damage or detrimental response to short-term use of small doses of tobacco, there is evidence that its chronic use has damaging effects on heart and lung functions. Because of these long-term consequences, research on tobacco and its effects often continues for years, making it difficult to link specific diseases or health problems with use of this substance. Thus, the results of tobacco research are often disputed by tobacco manufacturers with vested financial interests in the substance and its public acceptance.

Another important time factor that influences drug responses is the interval between multiple administrations. If sufficient time for drug metabolism and elimination does not occur between doses, a drug can accumulate within the body. This buildup of drug due to relatively short dosing intervals is referred to as a **cumulative effect.** Because of the resulting high concentrations of drug in the body, unexpected prolonged drug effects or toxicity can occur when multiple doses are given.

Inactivation and Elimination of Drugs from the Body

Immediately following drug administration, the body begins to eliminate the substance in various ways. The time required to remove half of the original amount of drug administered is called the **half-life** of the drug. The body will eliminate either the drug directly without altering it chemically or (in most instances) after the drug has been metabolized (chemically altered) or modified. The process of changing the chemical or pharmacological properties of a drug by metabolism is called **biotransformation. Metabolism** usually (but not always) makes it possible for the body to inactivate, detoxify, and excrete drugs and other chemicals. Pharmacologists must consider how these natural systems will eliminate drugs and what the resulting breakdown products will be before implementing any drug treatment.

The liver is the major organ that metabolizes drugs in the body. It is a complex biochemical laboratory with hundreds of enzymes that continuously synthesize, modify, and deactivate biochemical substances such as drugs. The healthy liver is also capable of metabolizing many of the chemicals naturally occurring in the body (such as hormones). After the liver enzymes metabolize a drug (the resulting chemicals are called **metabolites**), the products usually pass into the urine or feces for final elimination. Drugs and their metabolites can appear in other places as well, such as sweat, saliva, or expired air.

The rate at which liver enzymes metabolize some substances can be increased under certain conditions. This increased rate is referred to as liver **enzyme induction** and can occur if a particular drug is taken repeatedly over a period of time. Barbiturates, opiates, and other depressants can all cause liver enzyme activity to increase, which in turn increases the body's capacity to remove the drug and clear it from the body more rapidly. However, enzymes are seldom totally specific; this means that other drugs that are metabolized by the same enhanced enzymes will also be metabolized at an accelerated rate. Increased liver enzyme activity can more rapidly inactivate a drug and cause tolerance. This means that the same dose of a drug becomes less effective with continued use due to increased metabolism. Liver enzyme induction is responsible for tolerance to many drugs of abuse and causes the drug addict to escalate the dose to compensate for the lost effects.

The kidneys are probably the next most important organ for drug elimination because they remove metabolites and foreign substances from the body. The kidneys constantly filter substances in the blood. It is estimated that the kidneys filter nearly 200 liters of fluid from the blood each day. The rate of excretion of some drugs by the kidneys can be altered by making the urine more acidic or more alkaline. For example, nicotine and amphetamines can be cleared faster from the body by making the urine slightly more acidic, and salicylates and barbiturates can be cleared faster by making it more alkaline. Such techniques are used in emergency rooms and can be useful in the treatment of drug overdosing.

The body may eliminate small portions of drugs through perspiration and exhalation. About 1% of consumed alcohol is excreted in the breath and thus may be measured with a breathalyzer; this technique is used by police officers in evaluating suspected drunk drivers. Most people are aware that consumption of garlic will change body odor because garlic is excreted through perspiration. Some drugs are handled in the same way. The mammary glands are modified sweat glands, so it is not surprising that many drugs are concentrated and excreted in milk during lactation, including antibiotics, nicotine, barbiturates, caffeine, and alcohol. Excretion of drugs in a mother's milk can be of particular concern during nursing, as the excreted drugs can be consumed by and have an effect on the infant.

PLATEAU EFFECT the maximum drug effect, regardless of dose

ACUTE immediate or short-term effects after taking a single drug dose

CHRONIC long-term effects, usually after taking multiple drug doses

CUMULATIVE EFFECT the buildup of a drug in the body after multiple doses taken at short intervals

HALF-LIFE the time required for the body to eliminate and/or metabolize half of a drug dose

BIOTRANSFORMATION the process of changing the chemical properties of a drug, usually by metabolism

METABOLISM chemical alteration of drugs by body processes

METABOLITES chemical products of metabolism

ENZYME INDUCTION an increase in the metabolic capacity of an enzyme system

Physiological Variables That Modify Drug Effects

As previously mentioned, individuals' responses to drugs can vary greatly, even when the same doses are administered in the same manner. This variability can be especially troublesome when dealing with drugs that have a narrow margin of safety. Many of these variables reflect differences in the pharmacokinetic factors just discussed and are associated with diversity in body size, composition, or functions and include the following:

Age—Changes in body size and makeup occur throughout the aging process, from infancy to old age. Changes in the rates of drug absorption, biotransformation, and elimination also occur as a consequence of getting older. As a general rule, young children and elderly people should be administered low drug doses (calculated as drug quantity per weight) due to immature or compromised body processes.

Gender—Variations in drug responses due to gender usually relate to differences in body size, composition, or hormones (male versus female types; for example, androgens versus estrogens). However, most clinicians find many more similarities than differences between males and females relative to their responses to drugs.

Pregnancy—During the course of pregnancy, unique factors must be considered when administering drugs. For example, the physiology of the mother changes as the fetus develops and puts additional stress on organ systems, such as the heart, liver, and kidneys. This increased demand can make the woman more susceptible to the toxicity of some drugs. In addition, as the fetus develops, it can be very vulnerable to drugs with **teratogenic** (causing abnormal development) properties. Consequently, it is usually advisable to avoid taking any drugs during pregnancy, if possible.

Pathological Variables That Modify Drug Effects

Individuals with diseases or compromised organ systems need to be particularly careful when taking drugs. Some diseases can damage or impair organs that are vital for appropriate and safe responses to drugs. For example, hepatitis (inflammation and damage to the liver) interferes with the metabolism and disposal of many drugs, resulting in a longer duration of drug action and increased likelihood of side effects. Similar concerns are associated with kidney disease, which causes compromised renal activity and diminished excretion capacity. Because many drugs affect the cardiovascular system (especially drugs of abuse, such as stimulants, tobacco, and alcohol), patients with a history of cardiovascular disease (heart attack, stroke, hypertension, or abnormal heart rhythm) need to be particularly careful when using drugs. They should be aware of those medicines that stimulate the cardiovascular system, especially those that are self-medicated, such as OTC decongestants. These drugs should either be avoided or only used under the supervision of a physician.

Adaptive Processes and Drug Abuse

The body strives to establish and maintain balance in its physiological and mental functions: such balance is necessary for optimal functioning of all organ systems including the brain, heart, lungs, gastrointestinal tract, liver, and kidneys. Sometimes drugs interfere with the activity of the body's systems and compromise their normal workings. These drug-induced disruptions can be so severe that they can even cause death. For example, stimulants can dangerously increase the heart rate and blood pressure and cause heart attacks while CNS depressants can diminish brain activity, resulting in unconsciousness and a loss of breathing reflexes.

To protect against potential harm, the organ systems of the body can adjust to disruption. Of particular relevance to drugs of abuse are adaptive processes known as **tolerance** and **dependence** (both psychological and physical types) and the related phenomenon of *withdrawal* (see Figure 4.5).

Tolerance and dependence are closely linked, most likely to result from multiple drug exposures, and thought to be caused by similar mechanisms. Tolerance occurs when the response to the same dose of a drug decreases with repeated use (Goldstein 1994). Increasing the dose can usually compensate for tolerance to a drug of abuse. For the most part, the adaptations that cause the tolerance phenomenon are also associated with altered physical and psychological states that lead to dependence. These altered states reflect the efforts of the body and brain to re-establish balance in the continual presence of a drug. The user develops dependence in the sense that if the drug is no longer taken, the systems of the body become overcompensated and unbalanced, causing unpleasant effects known as *withdrawal* (a type of *rebound*). In general, withdrawal symptoms are opposite in nature to the direct effects of the drug that caused the dependence (Goldstein 1994). Thus, dependence on CNS depressants tends to result in excitatory-type of withdrawal symptoms during abstinence, and the opposite is true for CNS stimulant dependence.

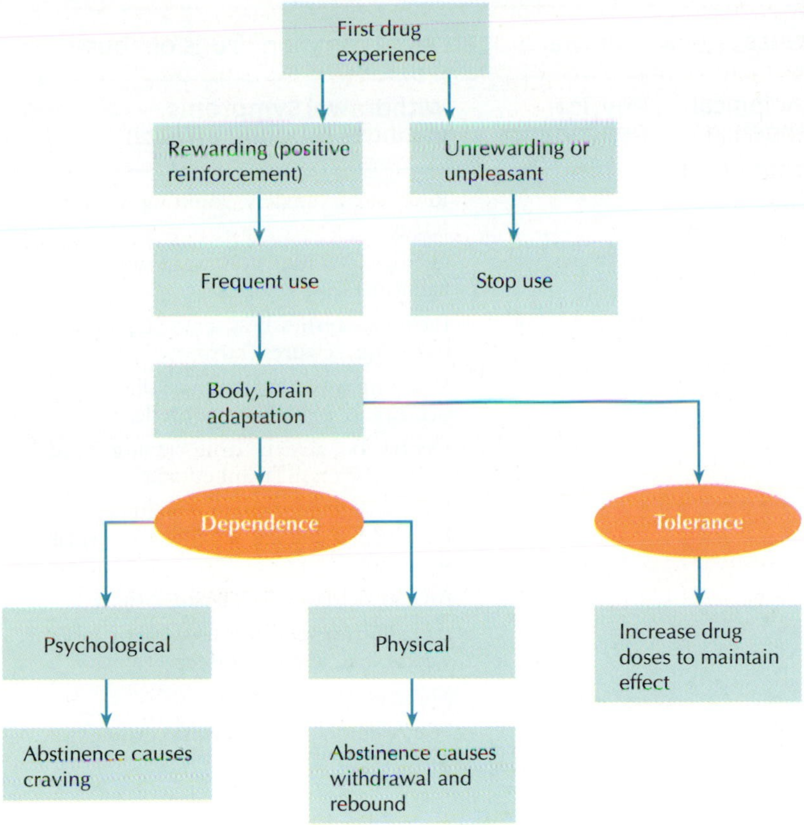

FIGURE 4.5 The relationship and consequences of adaptive processes to drug use. The processes discussed in the text are highlighted in the figure.

Although tolerance, dependence, and withdrawal are all consequences of adaptation by the body and its systems, they are not inseparably joined processes. It is possible to become tolerant to a drug without developing dependence and vice versa (see Table 4.4). The following sections provide greater detail about these very important adaptive drug responses.

TERATOGENIC something that causes physical defects in the fetus

TOLERANCE changes causing decreased response to a set dose of a drug

DEPENDENCE the physiological and psychological changes or adaptations that occur in response to the frequent administration of a drug

Tolerance to Drugs

The extent of tolerance and the rate at which it is acquired depends on the drug, the person using the drug, and the dosage and frequency of administration. Some drug effects may be reduced more rapidly than others when drugs are used frequently. Tolerance to effects that are rewarding or reinforcing often causes users to increase the dosage. Sometimes, abstinence from a drug can reduce tolerance when use of the drug is renewed.

The body does not necessarily develop tolerance to all effects of a drug equally. For example, with repeated use a moderate degree of tolerance develops to most effects of alcohol and barbiturates. A heavy drinker may be able to consume two or three times the alcohol tolerated by an occasional drinker. Little tolerance develops, however, to the lethal toxicity of these drugs. A heavy user of sedatives is just as susceptible to death by overdose as a nontolerant person, even though the

TABLE 4.4 Tolerance, dependence, and withdrawal properties of common drugs of abuse

Drug	Tolerance	Psychological Dependence	Physical Dependence	Withdrawal Symptoms (includes rebound effects)
Barbiturates	++	++	+++	Restlessness, anxiety, vomiting, tremors, seizures
Alcohol	++	++	+++	Cramps, delirium, vomiting, sweating, hallucinations, seizures
Benzodiazepines	+	++	++	Insomnia, restlessness, nausea, fatigue, twitching, seizures (rare)
Narcotics (heroin)	+++	++	+++	Vomiting, sweating, cramps, diarrhea, depression, irritability, gooseflesh
Cocaine, amphetamines	+[a]	+++	++	Depression, anxiety, drug craving, need for sleep ("crash"), anhedonia
Nicotine	+	+	+	Highly variable, craving, irritability, headache, increased appetite, abnormal sleep
Caffeine	+	+	+	Anxiety, lethargy, headache, fatigue
Marijuana	+	+	+	Irritability, restlessness, decreased appetite, weight loss, abnormal sleep
LSD	++	+	–	Minimal
PCP	+	+	+	Fear, tremors, some craving, problems with short memory

[a]Can sensitize.

Note: +++ Intense; ++ Moderate; + Some; – Not significant

heavy user has been forced to increase doses to maintain the relaxing effects of the drug. In contrast, frequent use of opiate narcotics such as morphine can cause profound tolerance, even to the lethal effects of these drugs. Heavy users have been known to use with relatively few problems up to 10 times the amount that will kill a nonuser. Obviously, the mechanism that causes death by CNS depressants such as alcohol and sedatives is different from that associated with narcotics.

The exact mechanisms by which the body becomes tolerant to different drug effects are not completely understood, but as mentioned earlier, may be related to those that cause dependence (Goldstein 1994). Several processes have been suggested. Drugs such as barbiturates stimulate the body's production of metabolic enzymes, primarily in the liver, and cause drugs to be inactivated and eliminated faster. This is called *drug disposition tolerance*. In addition, there is evidence that a considerable degree of CNS tolerance to some drugs develops independently of changes in the rate of metabolism or excretion. This is called *pharmacodynamic tolerance* and reflects the adaptation of drug target sites in nervous tissue, so that the effect of the same concentration of drug decreases. A person tolerant to alcohol, for example, can be relatively unaffected by several glasses of wine, resulting in a high level of alcohol in the blood. This situation may be due to some general molecular adaptation to the drug at the level of the individual nerve cell or caused by a specific brain response to counteract the sedating effects and maintain normal function (a counterbalancing excitatory system is enhanced to compensate for the depression caused by the alcohol).

Another type of drug response that can appear to be tolerance but is a learned adjustment is called *behavioral compensation*. Drug effects that are troubling may be compensated for or hidden by the drug user. Thus, alcoholics learn to speak and walk slowly to compensate for the slurred speech and stumbling gait they usually experience. To an observer, it might appear as though the pharmacological effects of the drug are diminished, but they are actually unchanged. Consequently, this type of adaptation is not a true form of tolerance.

Other Tolerance-Related Factors The tolerance process can affect drug responses in several ways. We have discussed the effect of tolerance to diminish the action of drugs and cause the user to compensate by increasing the dose. The following are examples of two other ways that the tolerance process can influence drug responses.

Reverse Tolerance (Sensitization) Under some conditions, a response to a drug is elicited that is the opposite of tolerance. This is known as **reverse tolerance,** or sensitization. When sensitized, a drug user will have the same response to a lower dose of a drug than he or she did to the initial, higher dose. This seems to occur in users of marijuana, and some hallucinogens, as well as amphetamines and cocaine (Drew and Glick 1990).

Although explanations of reverse tolerance are still unclear, some researchers believe that it depends on how often and how much of the drug is consumed. It has been speculated that this heightened response to drugs of abuse may reflect adaptive changes in the nervous tissues (target site of these drugs). The reverse tolerance that occurs with cocaine use may be responsible for the psychotic effects or the seizures caused by chronic use of this drug (Jaffe 1990).

Cross-Tolerance Development of tolerance to a drug sometimes can cause tolerance to other similar drugs: this phenomenon, known as *cross-tolerance,* may be due to altered metabolism resulting from chronic drug use. For example, a heavy drinker will usually exhibit tolerance to barbiturates, other depressants, and anesthetics because the alcohol has induced (stimulated) his or her liver metabolic enzymes. Cross-tolerance might also occur among drugs that cause similar pharmacological actions; for example, if adaptations have occurred in nervous tissue that cause tolerance to one drug, such changes might also result in tolerance to other similar drugs that exert their effects by interacting with that same nervous tissue site. This type of cross-tolerance has been shown to develop among some of the hallucinogens, such as LSD, mescaline, and psilocybin.

Drug Dependence

Drug dependence can be associated with either physiological or physchological adaptations. Physical dependence reflects changes in the way organs and systems in the body respond to a drug, while psychological dependence is caused by changes in attitudes and expectations. In both types of dependence, there is a need (either physical or emotional) for the drug to be present in order for the body or the mind to function properly.

Physical Dependence In general, the drugs that cause physical dependence also cause a condition called the **rebound effect,** which is a form of drug withdrawal. This is sometimes known as the *paradoxical effect* because the symptoms associated with rebound are nearly opposite to the direct effects of the drug. For example, a person taking barbiturates or benzodiazepines will be greatly depressed physically but on withdrawal becomes irritable, hyperexcited, nervous, and generally shows symptoms of extreme stimulation of the nervous system, even life-threatening seizures. All this constitutes the rebound effect.

Physical dependence may develop with high-intensity use of such common drugs as alcohol, barbiturates, and other CNS depressants. However, with moderate, intermittent use of these drugs, most people do not become physically dependent. Those who do become physically

REVERSE TOLERANCE an enhanced response to a given drug dose; opposite of tolerance

REBOUND EFFECT a form of withdrawal; paradoxical effects that occur when a drug has been eliminated from the body dependent experience damaged social and personal skills and relationships and impaired brain and motor functions. By contrast, potent opiate narcotics also tend to induce pronounced tolerance and physical dependence demonstrated by their intense withdrawal effects, but usually the dependence has little impact on daily activities and social interactions in chronic narcotic users. As long as users have undisturbed access to narcotics, they can often function normally in their personal and professional lives (Kreek 1983). The reason for the difference in the impact of physical dependence on CNS depressants and narcotics is not clear.

Withdrawal symptoms resulting from physical dependency can be prevented by administering a sufficient quantity of the original drug or one with similar pharmacological activity. The latter case, in which different drugs can be used interchangeably to prevent withdrawal symptoms, is called *cross-dependence*. For example, barbiturates and other CNS depressants can be used to treat the abstinence syndrome of the chronic alcoholic. Another example is the use of methadone, a long-acting narcotic, to treat withdrawal from heroin. Such therapeutic strategies allow the substitution of safer and more easily managed drugs for dangerous drugs of abuse and play a major role in treatment of drug dependency.

Psychological Dependence The World Health Organization (WHO) states that **psychological dependence** instills a feeling of satisfaction and psychic drive that requires periodic or continuous administration of the drug to produce a desired effect or to avoid psychological discomfort. This sense of dependence usually leads to repeated self-administration of the drug in a fashion described as abuse. This type of dependence may be found independent of or associated with physical dependence. Psychological dependence does not produce the physical discomfort, rebound effects, or life-threatening consequences that can be associated with physical dependence. Even so, psychological dependence does produce intense craving and strong urges that frequently lure former drug abusers back to their habits of drug self-administration. In many instances, psychological aspects may be more significant than physical dependence in maintaining chronic drug use. Thus, the major problem with opiate dependence is not the physical aspects because withdrawal can be successfully achieved in a few weeks; rather, strong urges often cause a return to chronic narcotic use because of psychological dependence.

How is psychological dependence thought to develop? If the first drug trial is rewarding, a few more rewarding trials will follow until drug use becomes a conditioned pattern of behavior. Continued positive psychological reinforcement with the drug leads, in time, to primary psychological dependence. Primary psychological dependence, in turn, may lead to uncontrollable compulsive abuse of any psychoactive drug in certain susceptible people and cause physical dependence. The degree of drug dependence is contingent on the nature of the psychoactive substance, the quantity used, the duration of use, and the characteristics of the person and his or her environment. It is often not possible to draw a sharp line between use and abuse when it comes to developing dependence. There are many shades of gray between the drug user and the drug addict.

Even strong psychological dependence on some psychoactive substances does not necessarily result in injury or social harm. For example, typical dosages of mild stimulants such as coffee usually do not induce seriously harmful reactions. Even though the effects on the central nervous system are barely detectable by a casual observer, strong psychological dependence on mild stimulants like tobacco and caffeine-containing beverages may develop; however, the fact that their dependence does not typically induce antisocial behavior distinguishes them from most of the forms of dependence–producing drugs.

Psychological Factors

The general effect of most drugs is greatly influenced by a variety of psychological and environmental factors. Unique qualities of an individual's personality, his or her past history of drug and social experience, attitudes toward the drug, expectations of its effects, and motivation for use are extremely influential (see Case in Point). These

Case in Point

Researchers Probe Which Comes First, Drug Abuse or Antisocial Behavior?

A study conducted by the University of Colorado School of Medicine and directed by Thomas Crowley, a psychiatrist, asked 51 troubled substance-abusing boys ages 14 to 19 how and when their antisocial behavior began. All the boys were diagnosed with conduct disorders and were enrolled in a Denver residential drug abuse treatment improvement program. Seventy-seven percent of the boys claimed to have engaged in their antisocial behavior (including stealing, truancy, fighting, arson, property destruction, cruelty to people or animals, lying, and running away) 1 to 13 years before regular drug use (Swan 1993). What are the implications of these findings for dealing with drug abuse offenders?

factors are often referred to collectively as the person's **mental set.** The *setting,* or total environment, in which a drug is taken may also modify its effect.

The set and setting are particularly important in influencing the responses to psychoactive drugs (drugs that alter the functions of the brain). For example, ingestion of LSD, a commonly abused hallucinogen, can cause pleasant, even spiritual-like experiences in comfortable, congenial surroundings. In contrast, when the same amount of LSD is consumed in hostile, threatening surroundings, the effect can be frightening, taking on a nightmarish quality.

The Placebo Effect

The psychological factors that influence responses to drugs, independent of their pharmacological properties, are known as **placebo effects.** The word *placebo* is derived from Latin and means "I shall please." The placebo effect is most likely to occur when an individual's mind-set is susceptible to suggestion. A placebo drug is a pharmacologically inactive compound that the user thinks causes some therapeutic change.

In certain persons and/or in particular settings, a placebo substance may have surprisingly powerful consequences (Sherman 1992). For example, a substantial component of most pain is perception. Consequently, placebos administered as pain relievers and promoted properly can provide dramatic relief. Therefore, in spite of what appears to be a drug effect, the placebo is not considered a pharmacological agent because it does not directly alter any body functions by its chemical nature.

The bulk of medical history may actually be a history of confidence in the cure—a history of placebo medicine—because many effective cures of the past have been shown to be without relevant

PSYCHOLOGICAL DEPENDENCE dependence that results because a drug produces pleasant mental effects

MENTAL SET the collection of psychological and environmental factors that influence an individual's response to drugs

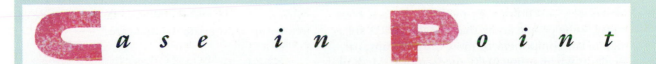

PLACEBO EFFECTS effects caused by suggestion and psychological factors, not the pharmacological activity of a drug

pharmacological action, suggesting that their effects were psychologically mediated. In fact, even today, some people argue that placebo effects are a significant component of most drug therapy, particularly when using OTC medications. Medical researchers currently are investigating so-called psychological cures, attempting to identify which factors contribute to this interesting phenomenon. It is important when testing new drugs for effectiveness that drug experiments be conducted in a manner that allows a distinction between pharmacological and placebo effects. This can usually be done by treating with the real drug or a placebo that appears like the drug and by comparing the responses to both treatments.

In some situations, perhaps placebos, or the power of suggestion, activate endogenous systems that help relieve medical problems or associated symptoms (Sherman 1992). This is most likely the explanation for the effectiveness of placebos against pain. A family of *peptides* (called *endorphins*) produced by the body has action similar to morphine and other opiate narcotics (Hughes 1975). The endorphins, among other things, are potent endogenous analgesics (substances that block pain) that provide the means for the body to defend itself against the debilitating effects of extreme pain. Research has shown that placebos cause the release of the endorphins to control pain. Other placebo effects may have similar biochemical basis in that they cause the release of endogenous substances that influence the body's functions and alter the course of disease.

Some factors that make placebos effective include the following:

1. A positive attitude by the health provider
2. The idea that more is always better; thus two capsules are better than one
3. The patient's perspective—for example, that injections are more effective than just taking tablets
4. Color—a large brown, purple, or red pill is more effective than a white one
5. Taste—a bad-tasting substance is more active than a neutral-tasting one (Evans 1977)

The clinician who is aware of such psychological issues can use them to therapeutic benefit. In fact, placebos have been advocated as an aid to help wean some patients from drug addiction (Sherman 1992). The clinician who chooses to ignore these placebo-related factors often meets with frustration and therapeutic failure in spite of rendering appropriate medical care.

Addiction and Abuse: The Significance of Dependence

The term *addiction* has many meanings. It is often used interchangeably with *dependence,* either physiological or psychological; other times, it is used synonymously with the term *drug abuse* (*drug addiction*).

The traditional model of the addiction-producing drug is based on opiate narcotics and requires the individual to develop tolerance and both physical and psychological dependence. This model often is not satisfactory because only a few commonly abused drugs seem to fit its parameters. It is clearly inadequate for many other drugs that can cause serious dependency problems but have little tolerance, even with extended use (see Table 4.4).

Because it is difficult to assess the contribution of physical and psychological factors to drug dependency, it becomes difficult to determine if all psychoactive drugs truly cause drug addiction. To alleviate confusion, it has been suggested that the term *dependence* (either physical or psychological) be used in place of *addiction*. However, because of its acceptance by the public, the term *addiction* is not likely to disappear from general use.

There has been speculation that the only means by which drug dependence can be eliminated from society is to prevent exposure to those drugs that have potential abuse liability. Because some drugs are such powerful, immediate reinforcers, it is feared that rapid dependence (psychological) will occur when anyone uses them. Although it may be true that most people, under certain conditions, could become dependent on some drug with abuse potential, in reality, most people who have used psychoactive drugs do not develop significant psychological or physical dependence. For example, approximately 87% of those who use alcohol experience minimal personal injury and social consequences. Of those who have

CROSSCURRENTS

An often debated issue relates to the role of hereditary and environmental factors as causes in drug abuse. The following represent two extreme positions:

1. Abuse of drugs, such as alcohol, tends to run in families, suggesting that inherited traits are the most important factors to determining drug abuse susceptibility.
2. Anyone can become dependent on drugs if the circumstances are right, suggesting that environment is the most important factor for determining drug abuse susceptibility.

In this chapter we have introduced you to factors that determine the variability in drug response. Select one of the positions listed here and discuss how these factors can explain your position.

used stimulants, depressants, or hallucinogens for illicit recreational purposes, only 10 to 20% become dependent (Jaffe 1990).The following sections discuss some possible reasons for the variability.

Hereditary Factors

Why some people readily develop dependence on psychoactive drugs and others do not is not well understood. One factor may be heredity, which predisposes some people to drug abuse (see Crosscurrents). For example, studies of identical and fraternal twins have revealed that there is greater similarity in the rate of alcoholism for identical than for fraternal twins if alcohol abuse begins before the age of 20 years (McGue et al. 1992). Because identical twins have 100% of their genes in common while fraternal twins share only 50%, these results suggest that genetic factors can be important in determining the likelihood of alcohol dependence (Schuckit 1987). It is possible that similar genetic factors contribute to other types of drug dependence, as well.

Drug Craving

Frequently, a person who becomes dependent develops a powerful, uncontrollable desire for drugs during or after withdrawal from heroin, cocaine, alcohol, nicotine, or other addicting substances: this desire for drugs is known as **craving.** Because researchers do not agree as to the nature of craving, there does not exist a universally recognized scientific definition nor an accepted method to measure this psychological phenomenon. Some drug abuse experts claim that craving is the principal cause of drug abuse while others believe that it is not a cause but a side effect of drugs that cause dependence. Craving is often assessed by (1) questioning patients about the intensity of their drug urges; (2) measuring physiological changes such as increases in heart and breathing rates, sweating, and subtle changes in the tension of facial muscles; and (3) determining patients' tendency to relapse into drug-taking behavior (Swan 1993).

There is evidence that at least two levels of craving can exist. For example, cocaine users experience an acute craving when using the drug itself, but the ex-cocaine abuser can have chronic cravings that are triggered by familiar environmental cues that elicit positive memories of cocaine's reinforcing effects.

Although it is not likely that craving itself causes drug addiction, it is generally believed that if pharmacological or psychological therapies could be devised that reduce or eliminate drug craving, that treatment of drug dependence would be more successful. Thus, many researchers are attempting to identify drugs or psychological strategies that interfere with the development and expression of the craving phenomenon.

Other Factors

If a drug causes a positive effect in the user's view, it is much more likely to be abused than if it causes an aversive experience (see Figure 4.5). Perhaps genetic factors influence the brain or personality so that some people find taking drugs an enjoyable experience (at least initially), while others find the effects very unpleasant and uncomfortable (**dysphoric**). Other factors that could also contribute significantly to drug use patterns include (1) peer pressure (especially in the initial drug experimentation); (2) home, school, and work environment (Mello and Griffith 1987); and (3) mental state. It is estimated that 20 to 30% of those who abuse drugs, particularly stimulants, are attempting to self-medicate some form of mental disorder; for example, the stimulant cocaine is frequently used to self-treat depression (Weiss et al. 1989; Pagliaro et al. 1992). Consequently, it is not surprising that one of the most frequently used treatments for cocaine abuse is the antidepressant desipramine (Kosten 1989).

It is difficult to identify all the specific factors that influence the risk of drug abuse for each individual. (Some of the possible influences are discussed in Chapter 2.) If such factors could be identified, treatment would be improved and those at greatest risk for drug abuse could be determined and informed of their vulnerability.

It has been suggested by some that the CNS limbic system (that part of the brain that controls mood; see Chapter 5) is affected by many of the drugs of abuse in such a way that it rewards the user and reinforces the drug abuse pattern (Jaffe 1990). More specifically, evidence suggests that all the readily abused drugs increase the activity of some CNS systems that use the messenger substance dopamine (Koob and Bloom 1988; Uhl et al. 1993). (This is discussed in greater detail in Chapter 5.) If this is true, perhaps drugs that affect dopamine in the brain may be useful for treatment of many drug abuse problems. Many researchers are currently investigating this possibility. However, because of the tremendous diversity, it is not likely that there exists a single *magic bullet* solution for all cases of drug abuse. But, it is likely that the more we understand about how and why the body responds to drugs of abuse, the more successful we will be in preventing or satisfactorily treating this major social and personal problem.

DYSPHORIC characterized by unpleasant mental effects; the opposite of euphoric

Review Questions

1. What is the significance of drug "potency" for therapeutic use and abuse of drugs?
2. How can drug interactions be both detrimental and beneficial? Give examples of each.
3. Why would a drug with a relatively narrow "margin of safety" be approved by the FDA for clinical use?
4. What are possible explanations for the fact that you (for example) may require twice as much of a drug to get an effect as does your friend?
5. What significance would the "blood–brain" barrier have on drugs with abuse potential?
6. Contrary to your advice, a friend is going to spend $20 on a "cocaine buy." What significance will the pharmacokinetic concepts of threshold, half-life, cumulative effect, and "biotransformation" have on your friend's drug experience?
7. How would the factors of tolerance, physical dependence, rebound, and psychological dependence affect a chronic heroin user?
8. Why would the lack of physical dependence on LSD for some drug abusers make it preferred over cocaine, which does cause physical dependence?

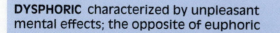

Key Terms

withdrawal
potency
toxicity
margin of safety
therapeutic index
synergism
pharmacokinetics
blood–brain barrier
threshold
plateau effect
acute
chronic
cumulative effect
half-life
biotransformation
metabolism
metabolites
enzyme induction
teratogenic
tolerance
dependence
reverse tolerance
rebound effect
psychological dependence
mental set
placebo effects
dysphoric

Summary

1. All drugs have intended and unintended effects. The unintended effects of drugs can include effects such as nausea, altered mental states, dependence, a variety of allergic responses, and changes in the cardiovascular system.
2. Many factors can affect the way an individual responds to a drug: dose, inherent toxicity, potency and pharmacokinetic properties such as the rate of absorption into the body, the way it is distributed throughout the body, and the manner and rate it is metabolized and eliminated. The form the drug is in as well as the manner in which it is administrated can also affect the response to a drug.
3. *Potency* is determined by the amount of a drug necessary to cause a given effect. *Toxicity* is the ability of the drug to adversely affect the body. A drug that is very toxic is very potent for causing a harmful effect.
4. A drug's *margin of safety* relates to the difference in the drug doses that cause a therapeutic or a toxic effect; the bigger the difference, the greater the margin of safety. The *therapeutic index* is a method to quantify the margin of safety; a large therapeutic index is desirable.
5. *Additive* interactions occur when the effects of two drugs are combined; for example, the analgesic effects of aspirin plus acetaminophen are additive. *Antagonistic* effects occur when the effects of two drugs cancel; for example, the stimulant effects of caffeine tend to antagonize the drowsiness caused by antihistamines. *Synergism* (potentiation) occurs when one drug enhances the effect of another; for example, alcohol enhances the CNS depression caused by Valium.
6. Pharmacokinetic factors include absorption, distribution, biotransformation, and elimination of drugs.
7. Many physiological and pathological factors can alter the response to drugs. For example, age, gender, and pregnancy are all factors that should be considered when making drug decisions. In addition, some diseases can alter the way in which the body responds to drugs. Medical conditions associated with the liver, kidneys, and cardiovascular system are of particular concern.
8. In order for psychoactive drugs to influence the brain and its actions, they must pass through the blood–brain barrier. Many of these drugs are fat soluble and able to pass through capillary walls from the blood into the brain.
9. The *threshold dose* is the minimum amount of a drug necessary to have an effect. The *plateau effect* is the maximum effect a drug can have, regardless of dose. The *cumulative effect* is the buildup of drug concentration in the body due to multiple doses taken within short intervals.
10. The liver is the primary organ for metabolism of drugs and many natural occurring substances in the body, such as hormones. By altering the molecular structure of drugs, the metabolism usually inactivates drugs and makes them easier to eliminate through the

kidneys. Liver function can sometimes be stimulated (*induction*) or inhibited (*tolerance*). These changes affect the rate at which some drugs are metabolized.

11. *Biotransformation* is the process that alters the molecular structure of a drug. Metabolism contributes to biotransformation.
12. Drug tolerance causes a decreased response to a given dose of a drug. It can be caused by increasing metabolism and elimination of the drug by the body or by a change in the systems or receptors that are affected by the drug.
13. *Physical dependence* is characterized by the adaptive changes that occur in the body due to the continual presence of a drug. These changes are often chemical in nature and reduce the response to the drugs and cause *tolerance*. If drug use is stopped after physical dependence has occurred, the body finds itself overcompensated, causing a *rebound* response. Rebound effects are similar to the *withdrawal* that occurs because drug use is stopped for an extended period. *Psychological dependence* occurs because drug use is rewarding, bringing euphoria, increased energy, relaxation, or causing craving.
14. Suggestion can have a profound influence on a person's drug response. Health problems with significant psychological aspects are particularly susceptible to the effects of placebos. An example is pain. Because much of pain is related to its perception, a placebo can substantially relieve pain discomfort. This placebo effect may relate to the release of a natural pain-relieving substance, such as endorphins. Other placebo responses may likewise be due to the release of endogenous factors in the body.
15. A powerful, uncontrollable desire (*craving*) for drugs can occur with chronic use of some drugs of abuse. Although craving by itself may not cause drug addiction, if it can be eliminated treatment of substance abuse is more likely to be successful.

References

Brenner, L., "How Common Is Counseling?" *American Druggist* (January 1994): 40.

Drug Abuse Warning Network (DAWN). "National Institute on Drug Abuse: Annual Data 1987" (NIDA Series no. 7, DHHS Publication no. ADM 88-1584). Washington, DC: U.S. Government Printing Office, 1988.

Drug Facts and Comparisons. St. Louis: Lippincott, 1994.

Evans, F. J. "The Power of a Sugar Pill." In *Ethical Issues in Modern Medicine,* edited by R. Hunt and J. Arras. Palo Alto, CA: Mayfield, 1977.

Goldstein, A. In *Addiction from Biology to Drug Policy.* New York: Freeman, 1994.

Grant, B., and S. Harford. "Concurrent and Simultaneous Use of Alcohol with Cocaine. Results of National Survey." *Drug and Alcohol Dependence* 25 (1990): 97–104.

Henderson, G. "Designer Drugs: Past History and Future Prospects." *Journal of Forensic Sciences* 33 (1988): 569–75.

Hughes, J. "Isolation of an Endogenous Compound from the Brain with Pharmacological Properties Similar to Morphine." *Brain Research* 88 (1975): 295–308.

Jaffe, H. "Drug Addiction and Drug Abuse." In *The Pharmacological Basis of Therapeutics,* 8th ed., edited by A. Gilman, T. Rall, A. Nies, and P. Taylor. New York: Plenum, 1990.

Koob, G., and F. Bloom. "Cellular and Molecular Mechanisms of Drug Dependence." *Science* 242 (1988): 715–23.

Kosten, T. "Pharmacotherapeutic Interventions for Cocaine Abuse: Matching Patients to Treatments." *Journal of Nervous and Mental Disease* 177 (July 1989): 379–89.

Kreek, M. *Health Consequences Associated with the Use of Methadone.* NIDA Treatment Research Monograph Series No. 83. Washington, DC: U.S. Department of Health, Education, and Welfare, 1983.

Mathias, R. "Smoking Drugs Creates New Dangers." *NIDA Notes* 9 (February–March 1994): 6.

McGue, M., R. Pickens, and D. Svikis. "Sex and Age Effects on the Inheritance of Alcohol Problems: A Twin Study." *Journal of Abnormal Psychology* 101 (January 1992): 3–17.

Mello, K., and R. Griffith. "Alcoholism and Drug Abuse: An Overview." In *Psychopharmacology: The Third Generation of Progress,* edited by H. Meltzer. New York: Raven Press, 1987.

Pagliaro, L., L. Jaglalsingh, and A. Pagliaro. "Cocaine Use and Dependence." *Canadian Medical Association Journal* 147 (1992): 1636.

Schuckit, M. "Biology of Risk for Alcoholism." In *Psychopharmacology: Third Generation of Progress,* edited by H. Meltzer. New York: Raven Press, 1987.

Sherman, M. "The Placebo Effect." *American Druggist* (January 1992): 39–42.

Swan, N. "Despite Advances, Drug Craving Remains an Elusive Research Target." *NIDA Notes* (May–June 1993): 1–4.

"Trends, Policy and Research." *Prevention Pipeline* [Center for Substance Abuse Prevention] (November–December 1993): 27.

Uhl, G., K. Blum, E. Noble, and S. Smith. "Substance Abuse Vulnerability and D-2 Receptor Genes." *Trends in Neurological Sciences* 16 (1993): 83–87.

Weiss, R., M. Griffin, and S. Mirin. "Diagnosing Major Depression in Cocaine Abuser: The Use of Depression Rating Scales." *Psychiatry Research* 28 (1989): 335–43.

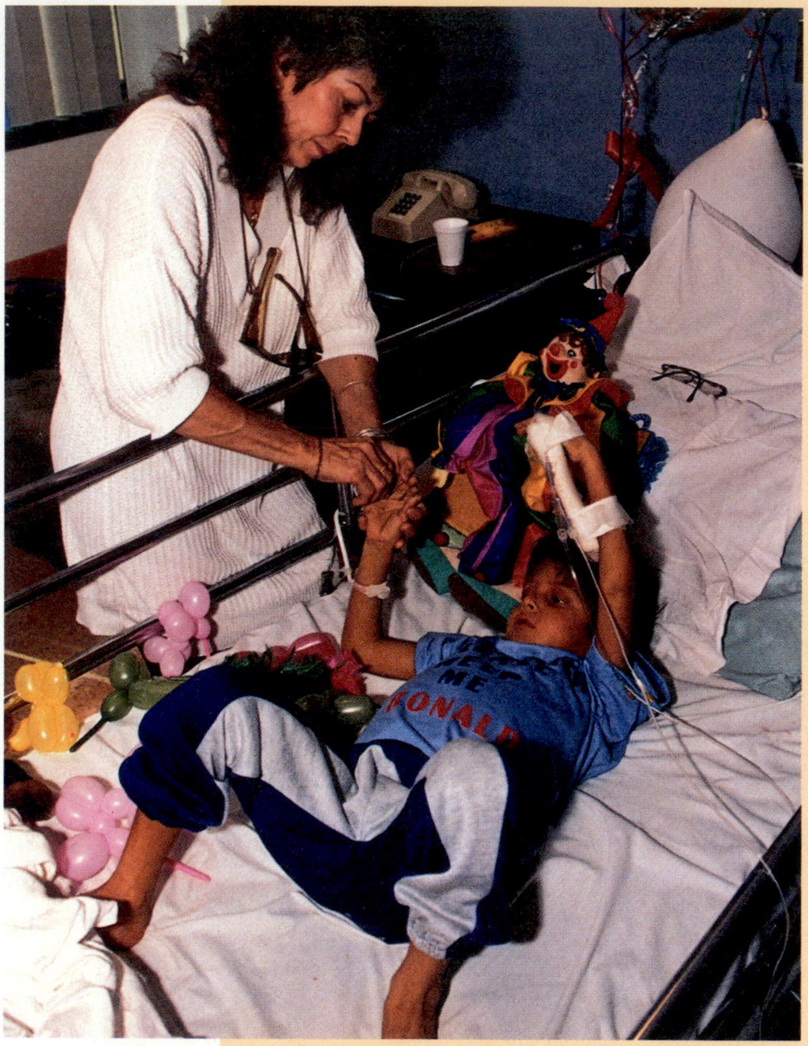

Chapter 5

DID YOU KNOW THAT . . .

- The brain is composed of over 10 billion neurons that communicate with each other by releasing chemical messengers called *neurotransmitters.*
- Many drugs exert their effects by interacting with specialized protein regions in cell membranes called *receptors.*
- Some natural chemicals, produced by the body, have the same effect as narcotic drugs; these chemicals are called *endorphins.*
- Drugs that affect the neurotransmitter dopamine usually alter both mental state and motor activity.
- The pleasant sensations that encourage continual use of most drugs of abuse are due to stimulation of dopamine activity in the limbic system.
- The hypothalamus is the principal brain region for control of endocrine systems.
- The anabolic steroids often abused by athletes are chemically related to testosterone, the male hormone.
- Anabolic steroids are considered controlled drugs by the Drug Enforcement Administration (DEA) and have been classified as Schedule III substances.

Homeostatic Systems and Drugs

LEARNING OBJECTIVES

On completing this chapter, you will be able to

1. Explain the similarities and differences between the nervous and endocrine systems.
2. Describe how a neuron functions.
3. Describe the role of receptors in mediating the effects of hormones, neurotransmitters, and drugs.
4. Distinguish between receptor agonists and antagonists.
5. Describe the different features of the principal neurotransmitters.
6. Outline the principal components of the central nervous system, and explain their general functions.
7. Identify which brain areas are most likely to be affected by drugs of abuse.
8. Distinguish between the sympathetic and parasympathetic nervous systems.
9. Identify the principal components of the endocrine system.
10. Explain how and why anabolic steroids are abused and what health impact that abuse has.

Healthy People 2000

Increase to at least 75% the proportion of primary care providers who screen for alcohol and other drug use problems and provide counseling and referral as needed.

Why is the body susceptible to the influence of drugs and other substances? Part of the answer is that the body is constantly adjusting and responding to its environment in order to maintain internal stability or equilibrium. This delicate process of dynamic adjustments—homeostasis—is necessary to optimize body functions and essential for survival. These continual compensations help to maintain physiological and psychological balances and are mediated by the release of endogenous regulatory chemicals (such as neurotransmitters and hormones). Many drugs exert intended or unintended effects by altering the activity of these substances, which changes the function of nervous or endocrine systems. For example, all drugs of abuse profoundly influence mental states by altering the chemical messages of the neurotransmitters in the brain, and some alter endocrine function by affecting the release of hormones. By understanding the mechanisms of how drugs alter these body processes, we are able to recognize drug benefits and risks and devise therapeutic strategies to deal with ensuing problems.

This chapter is divided into two sections. The first is a brief overview section to introduce the reader to the basic concepts of how the body is controlled by nervous and endocrine homeostatic systems and why drugs influence the elements of these systems. The second section is intended for readers who desire a more indepth understanding of the anatomical, physiological, and biochemical basis of these homeostatic functions. In this section the elements of the nervous system are discussed in detail followed by an examination of its major divisions: the central, peripheral and autonomic nervous systems. The components and operation of the endocrine system are discussed in specific relation to drugs. The use of steroids is given as an example.

HOMEOSTASIS maintenance of internal stability; often biochemical in nature

NEURON specialized nerve cells that make up the nervous system

AXON an extension of the neuronal cell body along which electrochemical signals travel

NEUROTRANSMITTERS chemical messengers released by neurons

RECEPTOR a special region in a membrane that is activated by natural substances or drugs to alter cell function

PSYCHOACTIVE drugs that affect mood or alter the state of consciousness

Section I Overview of Homeostasis and Drug Actions

The body continuously adjusts to both internal and external changes in the environment. To cope with these adjustments, the body systems have elaborate self-regulating mechanisms. The name given to this compensatory action is **homeostasis,** which refers to the maintenance of internal stability or equilibrium. For example, homeostatic mechanisms control the response of the brain to changes in the physical, social, and psychological environment, as well as regulate physiological factors such as body temperature, metabolism, nutrient utilization, and organ functions. The two principal systems that help human beings maintain homeostasis are the nervous system and the endocrine system. They are often referred to, respectively, as the *coordinating* and *regulating* systems. They greatly influence each other and work together closely.

Introduction to Nervous Systems

All nervous systems consist of specialized nerve cells called **neurons.** The neurons are responsible for conducting the homeostatic functions of the brain and other nervous systems by receiving and sending information. The transfer of messages by neurons includes chemical and electrical processes that consist of the following steps (see Figure 5.1):

- The *receiving region* of the neuron is affected by a chemical message that either excites (causes the neuron to send its own message)

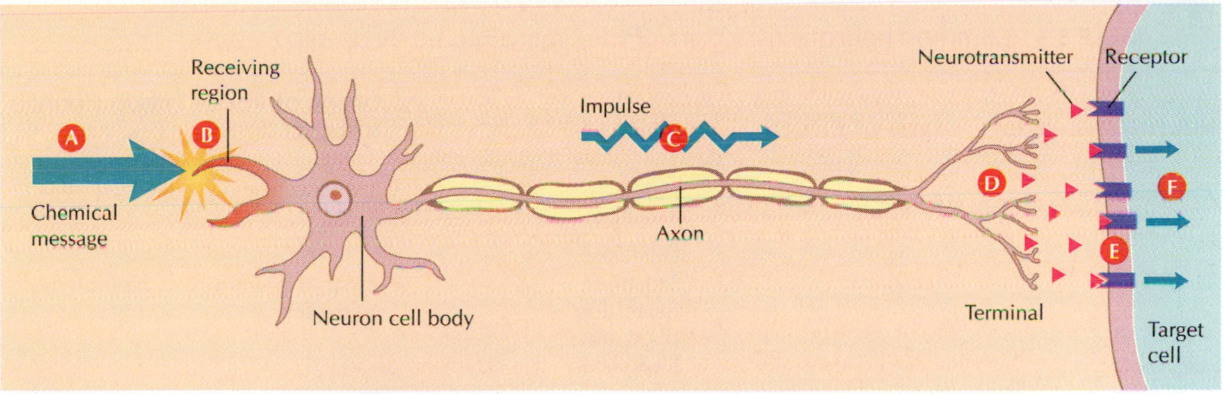

FIGURE 5.1 The process of sending messages by neurons. The receiving region (B) of the neuron is activated by an incoming message (A) near the neuronal cell body. The neuron sends an electricity-like impulse down the axon to its terminal (C). The impulse causes the release of neurotransmitter from the terminal to transmit the message to the target (D). This is done when the neurotransmitter molecules activate the receptors on the membranes of the target cell (E). The activated receptors then cause a change in intracellular functions to occur (F).

or inhibits (prevents the neuron from sending a message).

- If the message is excitatory, an impulse (much like electricity) moves from the receiving region of the neuron, down its wirelike processes (called **axons**) to the *sending region* (called the *terminal*). When the electricity-type impulse reaches the terminal, chemical messengers called **neurotransmitters** are released.
- The neurotransmitters travel very short distances and attach to specialized and specific *receiving proteins* called **receptors** on the outer membranes of their target cells.
- Activation of receptors by their associated neurotransmitters causes a change in the activity of the target cell. The target cells can be other neurons or cells that make up organs (such as heart, lungs, kidneys, and so on), muscles, or glands.

Neurons are highly versatile and, depending on their functions, can send discrete excitatory or inhibitory messages to their target cells. Neurons are distinguished by the type of neurotransmitter they release to send their messages. The neurotransmitters represent a wide variety of chemical substances that are classified according to their functional association as well as their ability to stimulate or inhibit the activity of target neurons, organs, muscles, and glands. This is discussed in greater detail in Section II of this chapter for those readers desiring more information. An example of a common neurotransmitter used by neurons in the brain to send messages is the substance *dopamine*. When released from neurons associated with the *pleasure center* in the brain, dopamine causes substantial euphoria by activating its receptor on target neurons (Goldstein 1994). This is relevant to drugs of abuse because some of these substances are addicting due to their ability to stimulate dopamine release from these neurons (for example, amphetamine or cocaine) and thus cause pleasant euphoric effects in the user. In fact, recent research suggests that activation of this dopamine system may account for the addicting potential of most drugs of abuse (Uhl et al. 1993).

It is important to understand that many of the effects of **psychoactive** drugs (which alter the mental functions of the brain), such as the drugs of abuse, are due to their ability to alter the neurotransmitters associated with neurons. Some of the most likely transmitter messenger systems to be affected by drugs of abuse are listed in Table 5.1 and are discussed in greater detail in the next section.

TABLE 5.1 Common neurotransmitters of the brain affected by drugs of abuse

Neurotransmitter	Type of Effect	Major CNS Changes	Drugs of Abuse That Influence (drug action)
Dopamine	Inhibitory–excitatory	Euphoria Agitation Paranoia	Amphetamines, cocaine (activate)
GABA	Inhibitory	Sedation Relaxation Drowsiness Depression	Alcohol, Valium-type, barbiturates (activate)
Serotonin	Inhibitory	Sleep Relaxation Sedation	LSD (activate)
Acetylcholine	Excitatory–inhibitory	Mild euphoria Excitation Insomnia	Tobacco, nicotine (stimulate)
Endorphins	Inhibitory	Mild euphoria Block pain Slow respiration	Narcotics (activate)

Introduction to Endocrine Systems

The endocrine system consists of secreting glands (for example, adrenal, thyroid, and pituitary) that produces biochemical agents called **hormones** (for example, adrenaline, steroids, insulin, and sex hormones). These substances are information-transferring molecules and are usually secreted into the bloodstream and carried by the blood to all the organs and tissues of the body. Hormones affect selected tissues that are designed to receive the information (see Figure 5.2). They may stimulate new tissue growth, affect the body's metabolism, assist in storage of nutrients, depress the activity of cells, or act in many other ways necessary to maintain homeostasis.

Hormones may be highly selective with regard to the cells or organs they influence, or they may be very general and influence the whole body. The endocrine system, more or less, sets the limits for proper functioning of the nervous system. Because hormones are carried in the blood, the action of the endocrine system is much slower and usually more generalized than that of the nervous system. The interpretation of the chemical messages of hormones in the various parts of the body is quite complex and is only now being deciphered by scientists.

Although hormones and neurotransmitters are distributed differently, there are many similarities between these two chemical systems. For example, both are released from cells that are appropriately stimulated, both exert their effects by activating receptors on target cells, and in some cases, the same substance can be used as both a neurotransmitter and a hormone (for example, adrenaline). Because of these similarities, it is not surprising that drugs that affect neurotransmitter systems, such as the substances of abuse, can also alter the hormones. Thus, besides causing release of brain transmitters such as dopamine, amphetamines also cause a dramatic release of adrenaline. The endocrine actions of the drugs of abuse may contribute to their adverse side effects.

Also of relevance to the topics of this text is the trend in the United States to abuse hormone-like substances themselves. This is a major problem

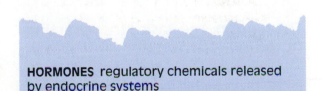

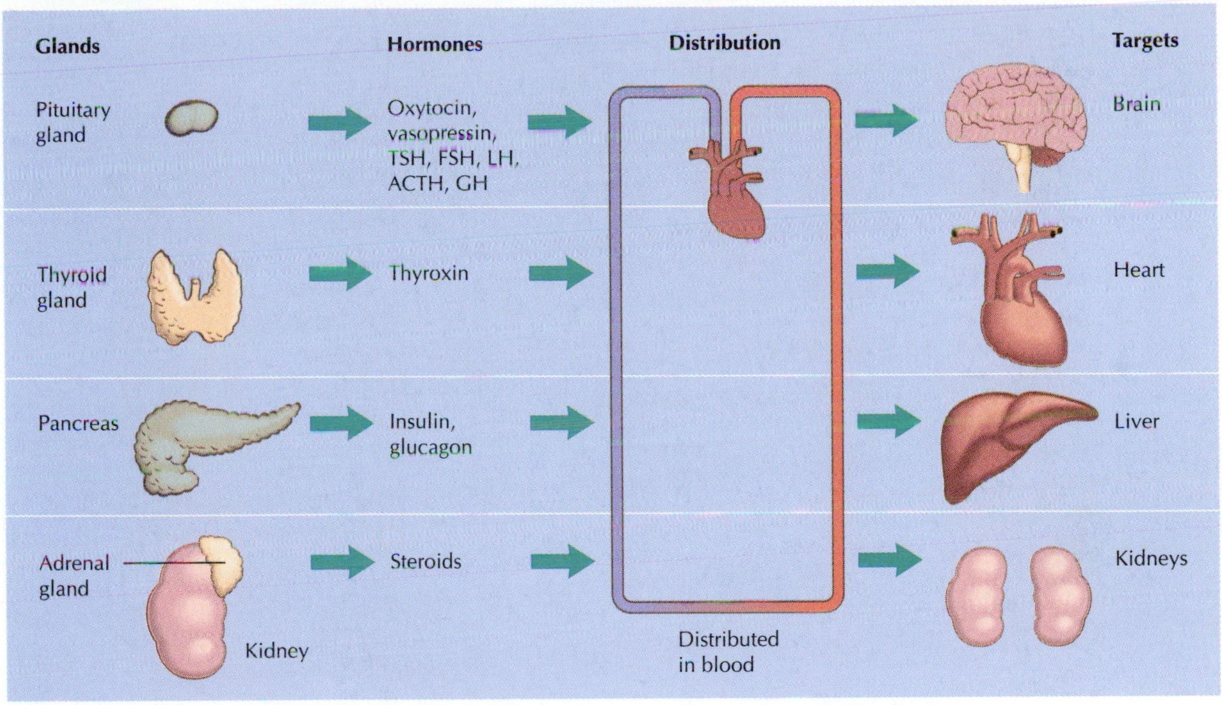

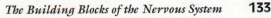

FIGURE 5.2 Components of the endocrine system

among athletes. Of particular concern is the abuse of anabolic steroids to stimulate muscle growth and enhance competitive performance. Use and effects of the steroids and other hormone-related drugs are detailed in the second section of this chapter and in Chapter 15.

Section II Comprehensive Explanation of Homeostatic Systems

For those readers who desire a more thorough understanding of the consequences of drug effects on the homeostatic systems of the body, this section provides greater details about the anatomical and physiological nature and biological arrangements of the nervous and endocrine systems. Because drugs of abuse are most likely to exert their psychoactive effects on neurons and their receptor targets, the nervous system is presented first and in greater depth, followed by a less detailed description of endocrine function.

The Building Blocks of the Nervous System

The nervous system is composed of the brain, the spinal cord, and all the neurons that connect to the other organs and tissues of the body (see Figure 5.10). It enables people to receive information about

HORMONES regulatory chemicals released by endocrine systems

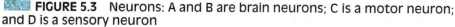

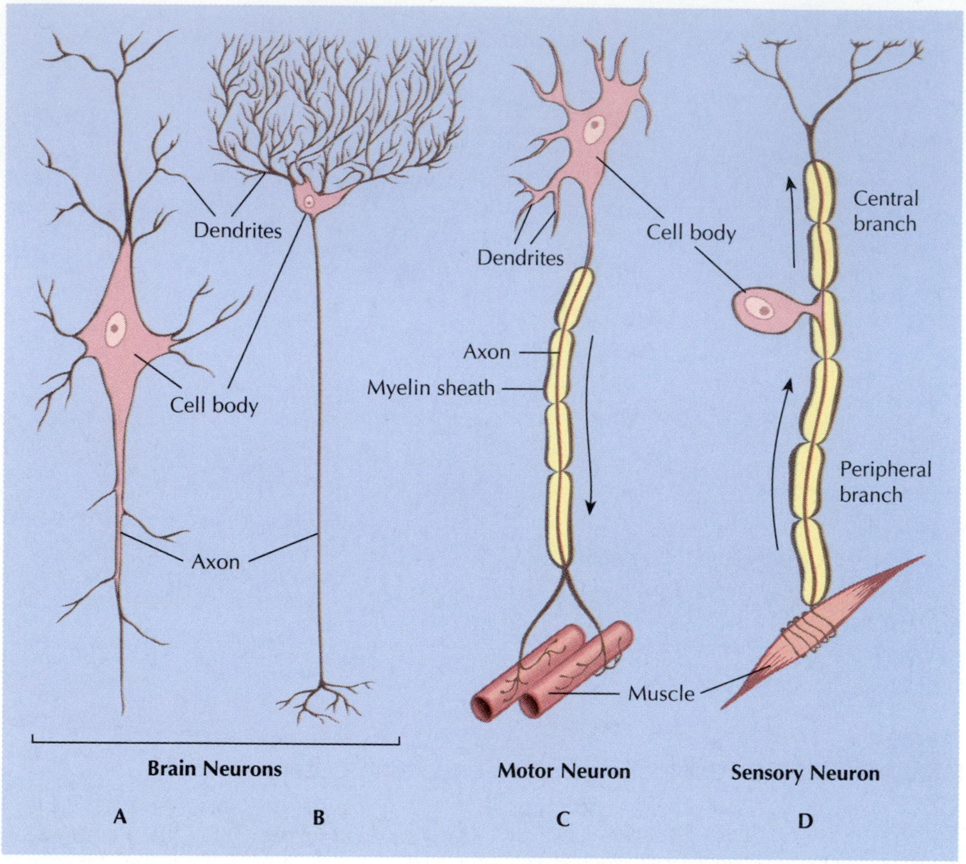

FIGURE 5.3 Neurons: A and B are brain neurons; C is a motor neuron; and D is a sensory neuron

their internal and external environment and to make the appropriate responses essential to survival. Some scientists have said that we know more about the surface of the moon than we do about our nervous system. Although this may be an exaggeration, it indicates our lack of understanding about neurological functions. Considerable money and effort are currently being dedicated to explore the mechanisms whereby the nervous system functions and processes information. New and exciting discoveries are frequently reported.

The Neuron: The Basic Structural Unit of the Nervous System

The building block of the nervous system is the nerve cell, or neuron. Each neuron in the central nervous system (brain and spinal cord) is in close proximity with other neurons, forming a complex network. There are over 10 billion neurons in the human brain, each of which is composed of similar parts (see Figure 5.3), although they may differ in some structural aspects depending on their location and function. Neurons do not form a continuous network. They always remain separate, never actually touching, although they are very close. The point of communication between one neuron and another is called a **synapse.** The gap (called the **synaptic cleft**) between neurons at a synapse may be only 0.00002 millimeter, but it is essential for proper functioning of the nervous system (see Figure 5.4).

The neuron has a cell body with a nucleus and receiving regions called **dendrites,** which are short, treelike branches that pick up information from the environment and surrounding neurons.

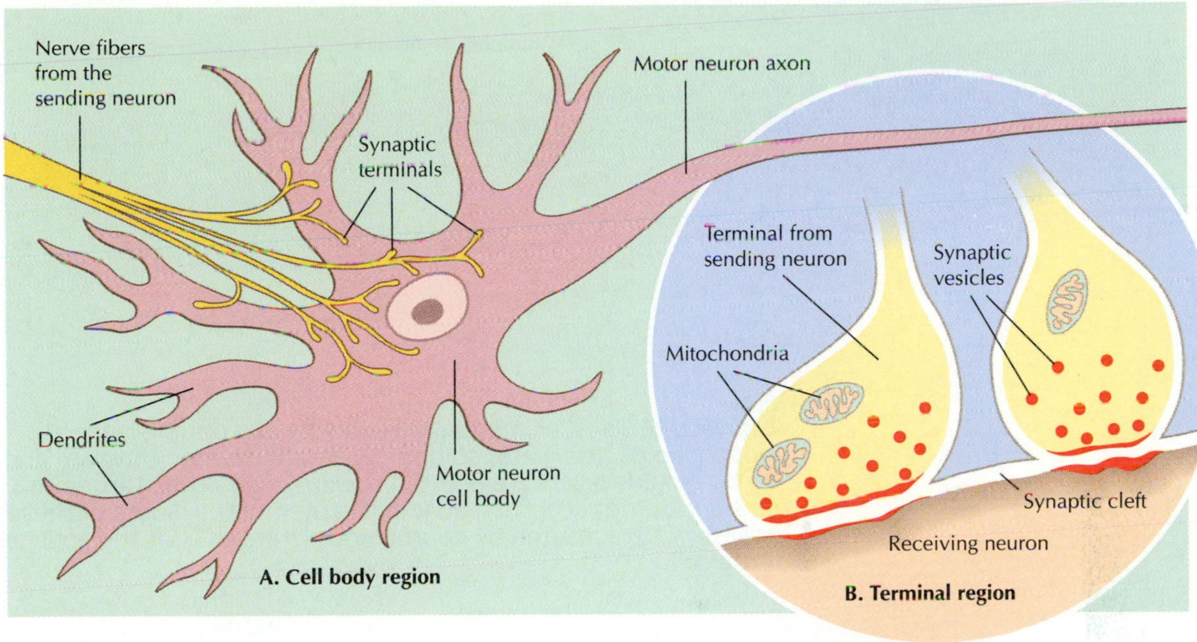

FIGURE 5.4 (A) Each neuron may have many synaptic connections. They are designed to deliver short bursts of a chemical transmitter substance into the synaptic cleft, where it can act on the surface of the receiving nerve cell membrane. Before release, molecules of the chemical neurotransmitter are stored in numerous vesicles, or sacs. (B) A closeup of the synaptic terminals, showing the synaptic vesicles and mitochondria. Mitochondria are specialized structures that help supply the cell with energy. The gap between the synaptic terminal and the target membrane is the synaptic cleft.

The axon of a neuron is a threadlike extension that receives information from the dendrites near the cell body, in the form of an electrical impulse; then, like an electrical wire, it transmits the impulse to the cell's terminal. This electrical information is usually a series of pulses, each with an amplitude of about 0.10 volt and lasting 0.001 to 0.002 seconds. Some axons may be quite long; for example, some extend from the spinal cord to the toes.

The electrical impulses are normally not affected by drugs directly because they are generated by the neuron cell membrane. However, a few drugs (for example, local anesthetics such as lidocaine) can influence information processing by acting on and changing the cell membrane and interfering with impulse transmission.

As discussed, at the synapse information is transmitted chemically to the next neuron as shown in Figure 5.1. A similar synaptic arrangement also exists at sites of communication between neurons and target cells in organs, muscles, and glands; that is, neurotransmitters are released from the message-sending neurons and activate receptors located in the membranes of message-receiving target cells.

There are two types of synapses: (1) the ex-

SYNAPSE site of communication between a message-sending neuron and its message-receiving target cell

SYNAPSE CLEFT a minute gap between the neuron and target cell, across which neurotransmitters travel

DENDRITES short branches of neurons, that receive transmitter signals

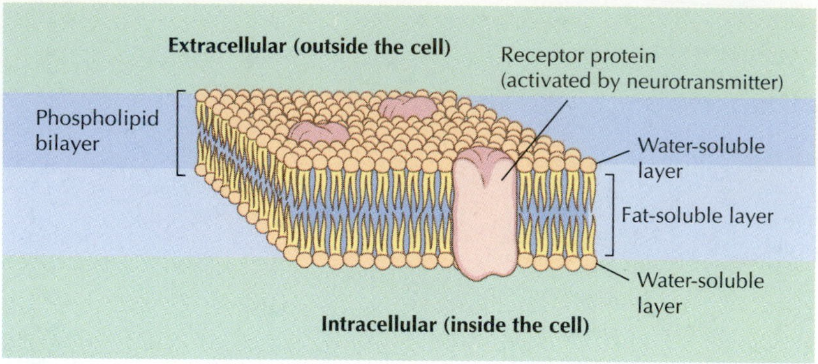

FIGURE 5.5 Cell membranes consist of a double layer of phospholipids. The water-soluble layers are pointed outward and the fat-soluble layers are pointed toward each other. Large proteins, including receptors, float in the membrane. Some of these receptors are activated by neurotransmitters to alter the activity of the cell.

citatory synapse, which initiates an impulse in the receiving neuron when stimulated and causes release of neurotransmitters, or increases activity in the target cell; and (2) the inhibitory synapse, which diminishes the likelihood of an impulse in the receiving neuron or reduces the activity in other target cells. A receiving neuron or target cell may have many synapses connecting it to neurons and their excitatory or inhibitory information (see Figure 5.4, part A). The final cellular activity is a summation of these many excitatory and inhibitory synaptic signals.

The Nature of Drug Receptors

Receptors are special proteins located in the membranes of receiving neurons and other target cells (see Figure 5.5). These receptors help regulate the activity of cells in the nervous system and throughout the body. These are selective protein sites on specific cells that react to endogenous messenger substances (chemicals produced and released within the body), such as neurotransmitters and hormones. These receptors serve to process the complex information each cell receives as it attempts to maintain metabolic constancy, or homeostasis, and fulfill its functional role. Many drugs used therapeutically and almost all drugs of abuse exert their effects on the body by directly or indirectly interacting (either to activate or antagonize) with these receptors.

The discovery of receptors that interact with specific drugs has led to some interesting results. For example, there are opiate receptors (sites of action by narcotic drugs, such as heroin and morphine) naturally present in the animal brain (Snyder 1977). Why would the brain have receptors for opiate narcotics, which are plant chemicals? This discovery suggested the existence of internal (endogenous) neurotransmitter substances in the body that normally act at these receptor sites. This led to the discovery that the body produces its own opiates, the **endorphins** (Goldstein 1994). Specific receptors have also been found for other drugs such as the central nervous system (CNS) depressant Valium and the active ingredient in marijuana. Because of these discoveries, it is speculated that endogenous substances exist that mimic the effects of Valium and marijuana and help provide natural sedation and relaxation for the body (Izquierdo 1989; Swan 1993). Presently, several research laboratories are attempting to identify the natural chemical messengers that normally act at the Valium (referred to as the *benzodiazepine receptor*) and marijuana (called the *cannabinoid receptor*) sites of activity.

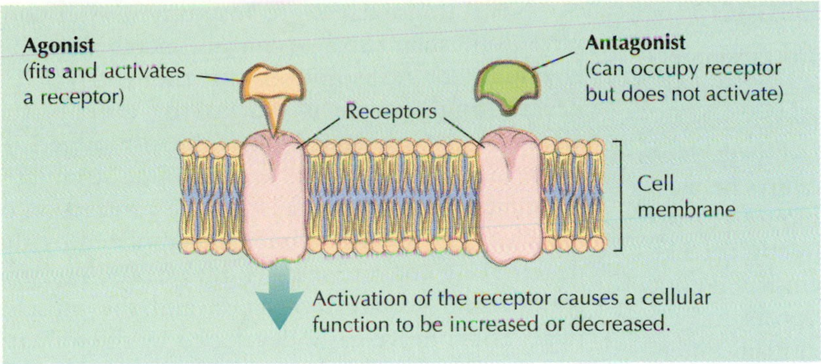

FIGURE 5.6 Interaction of agonist and antagonist with membrane receptor. When this receptor is occupied and activated by an agonist, it can cause cellular changes.

Much remains unknown about how receptors respond to or interact with drugs. However, using molecular biology techniques, many of these receptors have been found to initiate a cascade of linked chemical reactions, which can change intracellular environments, resulting in either activation or inactivation of cellular functions. For example, within the target cell are secondary chemical messengers that pick up the signal from the receptor and convert it into cellular changes, altering genes (chromosome expression), enzyme functions, or energy stores (Linder and Gilman 1992). Cyclic adenosine monophosphate (cAMP) and G proteins are two of these secondary messengers. It is not known how many secondary messengers actually exist in the body, but they play an essential role in the chain of events that convert neurotransmitter signals into some cellular change.

Receptors that have been isolated and identified are protein molecules; it is believed that the shape of the protein is essential in regulating a drug's interaction with a cell. If the drug is the proper shape and size and has a compatible electrical charge, it may substitute for the endogenous messenger substance and activate the receptor protein by causing it to change its shape, or conformation. This process is like a "lock-and-key" arrangement, with only certain shapes of chemicals (the keys) being able to interact and activate a receptor (the "lock") (Goldstein 1994).

ENDORPHINS neurotransmitters that have narcoticlike effects

AGONISTIC a type of substance that activates a receptor

ANTAGONISTIC a type of substance that blocks a receptor

Agonistic and Antagonistic Effects on Drug Receptors

A drug may have two different effects on a receptor when interaction occurs: **agonistic** or **antagonistic.** As shown in Figure 5.6, an agonistic drug interacts with the receptor and produces some type of cellular response, whereas an antagonistic drug interacts with the receptor but prevents that response. By analogy, using the lock-and-key model, a key can be used to open a lock (agonistic effect), whereas another key that fits in the lock but does not work can jam it (antagonistic effect).

An agonistic drug mimics the effect of a substance (such as a neurotransmitter) that is naturally produced by the body and interacts with the receptor to cause some cellular change. For example, narcotic drugs are agonists that mimic the endorphins and activate opiate receptors. An antagonist has the opposite effect: it inhibits the sequence of metabolic events that a natural substance or an agonist drug can stimulate, without initiating an effect itself. Thus, a drug called *naloxone* is an antagonist at the opiate receptors and blocks the effects of narcotic drugs as well as the effects of the naturally occurring endorphins.

Neurotransmitters: The Messengers

Many drugs affect the activity of neurotransmitters by altering their synthesis, storage, release, or deactivation. By acting at the synthesis, storage, release, or deactivation steps, a drug may modify or block information transmitted by these neurochemical messengers. Thus, by altering the amount of neurotransmitter, such drugs can indirectly act like agonists and antagonists even though they do not directly change neurotransmitter receptors.

Experimental evidence shows that many different neurotransmitters exist, although much remains to be learned abut their specific functions. These biochemical messengers are released from specific neurons. Some of the best understood transmitters include acetylcholine, norepinephrine, epinephrine, dopamine, serotonin, gamma-aminobutyric acid (GABA), and substance P (a peptide). Each neurotransmitter affects only its specific receptors; all neurotransmitters differ in shape and do not fit into other receptor configurations (Kandel et al. 1991). Drugs can also affect these receptors if they are sufficiently similar in shape to the neurotransmitters. Figure 5.7 summarizes some of the important features about the common neurotransmitters.

Acetylcholine Large quantities of acetylcholine (ACh) are found in the brain; however, ACh was first identified as a neurotransmitter outside of the central nervous system. It is synthesized in the neuron by combining molecules of choline (provided by diet and also manufactured in the body) and acetyl CoA (a product of glucose metabolism). Acetylcholine is one of the major neurotransmitters in the autonomic portion of the peripheral nervous system (which will be discussed later in the chapter).

Neurons that respond to ACh are distributed throughout the brain. Depending on the region, ACh can have excitatory or inhibitory effects. The receptors activated by acetylcholine have been divided into two main subtypes based on the response to two drugs derived from plants: muscarine and nicotine. Muscarine (a substance in mushrooms that causes mushroom poisoning) and similarly acting drugs activate **muscarinic** receptors. Nicotine, whether experimentally administered or inhaled by smoking tobacco, stimulates **nicotinic** receptors.

Neurotransmitters are inactivated after they have done their job by removal, metabolism (by enzymes), or reabsorption into the neuron. If a deactivating enzyme is blocked by a drug, the effect of the transmitter may be prolonged or intensified. For example, acetylcholine stimulates nicotinic receptors that cause strong contraction of muscles. The acetylcholine is metabolized by the deactivating enzyme acetylcholinesterase into the choline and acetate molecules, and the muscles relax. Some nerve gases developed by the military for chemical warfare purposes block the acetylcholinesterase enzyme. The target receptors in the presence of these drugs continue to be stimulated because the ACh is not metabolized. This continual firing of electrical impulses causes muscle paralysis due to the persistent muscle contraction.

Catecholamines **Catecholamines** comprise the neurotransmitter compounds norepinephrine, epinephrine, and dopamine, and have similar chemical structures. Neurons that synthesize catecholamines convert the amino acids phenylalanine or tyrosine to dopamine. In some neurons, dopamine is further converted to norepinephrine, and finally to epinephrine.

Unlike acetylcholine, after acting at their receptors most of the catecholamines are taken back up into the neurons that released them, to be used over again; this is called *reuptake*. There is also an enzymatic breakdown system that metabolizes the catecholamines to inactive compounds. The reuptake process and the activity of metabolizing enzymes, especially monoamine oxidase (MAO), can be greatly affected by some of the drugs that are discussed. If these deactivating

MUSCARINIC a receptor type activated by ACh; usually inhibitory

NICOTINIC a receptor type activated by ACh; usually excitatory

CATECHOLAMINES a class of biochemical compounds, including the transmitters norepinephrine, epinephrine, and dopamine

SYMPATHOMIMETIC agents that mimic the effects of norepinephrine or epinephrine

Acetylcholine
Chemical type: Choline product
Location: CNS—Basal ganglia, cortex, reticular activating system
PNS—Neuromuscular junction, parasympathetic system
Action: Excitatory and inhibitory

Norepinephrine
Chemical type: Catecholamine
Location: CNS—Limbic system, cortex, hypothalamus, reticular activating system, brain stem, spinal cord
PNS—Sympathetic nervous system
Action: Usually inhibitory; some excitation

Epinephrine
Chemical type: Catecholamine
Location: CNS—Minor
PNS—Adrenal glands
Action: Usually excitatory

Dopamine
Chemical type: Catecholamine
Location: CNS—Basal ganglia, limbic system, hypothalamus
Action: Usually inhibitory

Serotonin (S-HT)
Chemical type: Tryptophan-derivative
Location: CNS—basal ganglia, limbic system, brain stem, spinal cord, cortex
Other—Gut, platelets, cardiovascular
Action: Inhibitory

GABA
Chemical type: Amino acid
Location: CNS—basal ganglia, limbic system, cortex
Action: Inhibitory

Substance P
Chemical type: Peptide (small protein)
Location: CNS—basal ganglia, hypothalamus, brain stem, spinal cord
Other—Gut, cardiovascular system
Action: Excitatory

Key: CNS—Central nervous system
PNS—Peripheral nervous system

FIGURE 5.7 Features of common neurotransmitters

enzymes are blocked, the concentration of norepinephrine and dopamine may build up in the brain, causing a significantly increased effect. Cocaine, for example, prevents the reuptake of norepinephrine and dopamine in the brain, resulting in continual stimulation of neuron catecholamine receptors until the transmitters are depleted. The eventual depletion of catecholamines may result in depression, or the "crash" that occurs after high doses of cocaine are used.

Norepinephrine and Epinephrine Although norepinephrine and epinephrine are structurally very similar, their receptors are selective and do not respond with the same intensity to either transmitter or to **sympathomimetic** drugs. Just as the receptors to acetylcholine can be separated into muscarinic and nicotinic types, the norepinephrine and epinephrine receptors are separated into the categories of alpha and beta. Receiving cells may have alpha- or beta-type receptors or both. When both types of receptors are activated, the response to one is usually stronger and dominates the response to the other. Epinephrine and norepinephrine differ mainly in the ratio of their effectiveness in stimulating alpha and beta receptors. Norepinephrine acts predominantly on alpha receptors and has little action on beta receptors.

The antagonistic (blocking) action of many drugs that act on these catecholamine receptors can be selective for alpha, whereas others block only beta receptors. This distinction can be therapeutically useful. For example, beta receptors tend to stimulate the heart, while alpha receptors constrict blood vessels; thus, a drug that selectively affects beta receptors can be used to treat heart ailments without altering the state of the blood vessels.

Dopamine As has been discussed, dopamine is also a catecholamine transmitter that is particularly influenced by drugs of abuse (Koob 1992; Uhl et al. 1992; Uhl et al. 1993). Most drugs that elevate mood, have abuse potential, or cause psychotic behavior in some way enhance the activity of dopamine, particularly in brain regions associated with limbic structures (areas that regulate mood and mental states; see Uhl et al. 1992). In addition, dopamine is an important transmitter in controlling movement and fine muscle activity, as well as endocrine functions. Thus, drugs that affect dopamine neurons can alter all these functions.

Serotonin Serotonin (5-hydroxytryptamine, or 5HT) is synthesized in neurons and elsewhere (for example, gastrointestinal tract and platelet-type blood cells) from the dietary source of tryptophan. Tryptophan is one of the essential amino acids, meaning that humans do not have the ability to synthesize it and must obtain it through diet. Normally, about 2% of the tryptophan in the diet is converted to serotonin. Like the catecholamines, serotonin is degraded by the enzyme monoamine oxidase; thus, drugs that alter this enzyme affect levels of not only the catecholamines but also serotonin.

Serotonin is also found in the upper brain stem, which connects the brain and the spinal cord (see Figure 5.8). Axons from serotonergic neurons are distributed throughout the entire central nervous system. Serotonin, for the most part, inhibits action on its target neurons. One important role of the serotonergic neurons is to prevent overreaction to various stimuli, which can cause aggressiveness, excessive motor activity, exaggerated mood swings, insomnia, and abnormal sexual behavior. Serotonergic neurons also help regulate the release of hormones from the hypothalamus.

Alterations in serotonergic neurons, serotonin synthesis, and degradation have been proposed to be factors in mental illness and contribute to the side effects of many drugs of abuse. In support of this hypothesis is the fact that drugs such as psilocybin and LSD, which have serotonin-like chemical structures, are frequently abused because of their hallucinogenic properties and can cause psychotic effects.

Major Divisions of the Nervous System

The nervous system can be divided into two major components: the central (CNS) and peripheral (PNS) nervous systems. The CNS consists of the brain and spinal cord (see Figure 5.8), which receive information through the input nerves of the PNS. This sensory information allows the CNS to evaluate the specific status of all organs and the general status of the body. After receiving and processing this information, the CNS reacts by regulating muscle and organ activity through the output nerves of the PNS (Kelly and Dodd 1991).

The PNS is comprised of neurons whose cell bodies or axons are located outside of the brain or spinal cord. The PNS consists of input and output nerves to the CNS. The PNS input to the brain and spinal cord conveys sensory information such as pain, pressure, and temperature, while its output activities are separated into somatic types (control of voluntary muscles) and autonomic types (control of unconscious functions, such as essential organ and gland activity).

The Central Nervous System

The human brain is an integrating (information-processing) and storage device unequaled by the most complex computers. Not only can it handle a great deal of information simultaneously from the senses, but it can evaluate and modify the response to the information rapidly. Although the brain weighs only 3 pounds, with over 10 billion neurons it has the potential to perform a multitude of functions. For our purposes, we will discuss those parts of the brain most likely to be influenced by psychoactive drugs: (1) the reticular activating system, (2) the basal ganglia, (3) the limbic system, (4) the cerebral cortex, and (5) the hypothalamus.

The Reticular Activating System The reticular activating system (RAS) is an area of the brain that receives input from all the sensory systems as well as from the cerebral cortex. The RAS is at the junction of the spinal cord and the brain, and it has a vast network of multiple synaptic neurons

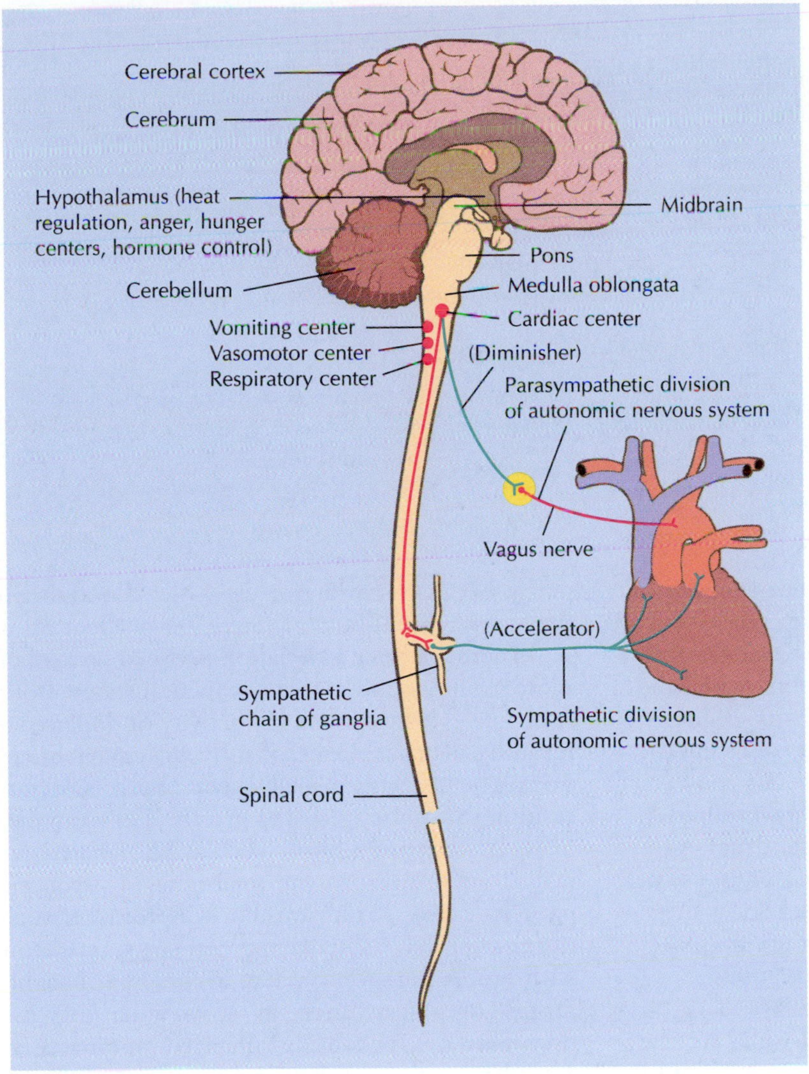

FIGURE 5.8 Functional components of the central and autonomic nervous systems

extending throughout the brain (see Figure 5.9). Because of this complex, diffuse network, the RAS is very susceptible to the effects of drugs. The RAS is sensitive to the effects of LSD, potent stimulants such as cocaine and amphetamines, and CNS depressants such as alcohol and barbiturates.

One of the major functions of the RAS is to control the brain's state of arousal (sleep versus awake). Arousal is especially linked to activity in the cerebral cortex. If the cortex is not aroused, it cannot handle input from the sensory system. The RAS is stimulated by sensory input and will initiate its own impulses to the cerebral cortex, which becomes alert if the impulses are of sufficient intensity or cause alarm. After the cortex is activated, the person is awake, and the nervous system is active and ready to receive and process further stimuli from the environment. The RAS can also filter out distracting stimuli, allowing the person to concentrate intently, even to the point of being unaware of severe injury until the immediate, pressing situation is over.

Norepinephrine and acetylcholine are important neurotransmitters in the RAS. High levels of

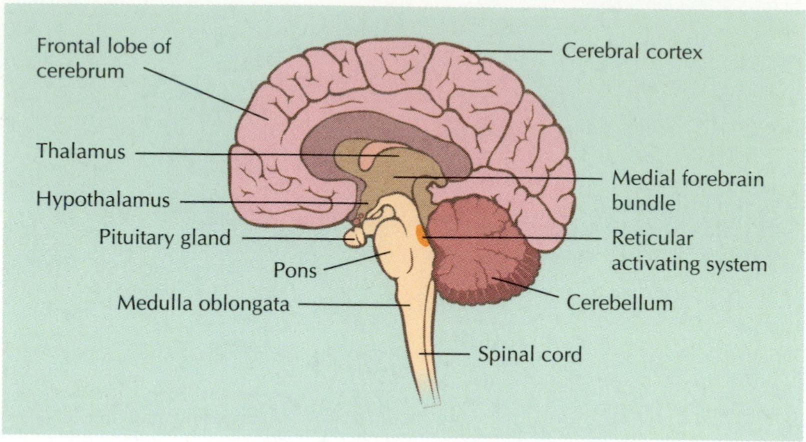

FIGURE 5.9 Sagittal section of the brain, showing major CNS structures

epinephrine, norepinephrine, or sympathomimetic drugs activate both the RAS and the cerebral cortex. Because of their effects on these transmitters, compounds like amphetamines increase the response of the RAS and diminish its ability to screen out nonessential stimuli, thus confusing the system with exaggerated sensations. In contrast, drugs that block the actions of another transmitter, acetylcholine, called **anticholinergic** drugs, suppress RAS activity, causing sleepiness. Thus, use of antihistamines, which have anticholinergic activity, often causes annoying drowsiness; they are sometimes used as sleep aids in OTC medications.

The Basal Ganglia The basal ganglia are the primary centers for involuntary and fine-tuning of motor function involving, for example, posture and muscle tone. Two important neurotransmitters in the basal ganglia are dopamine and acetylcholine. Damage to neurons in this area may cause Parkinson's disease, the progressive yet selective degeneration of the main dopaminergic neurons in the basal ganglia. This process results in an imbalance between dopamine and acetylcholine. The imbalance in these transmitters interferes with regulation of muscle activity by the brain and causes the person to be debilitated, with postural rigidity, tremors, and a decrease in facial expressiveness. Parkinson's disease may be treated with the drug L-DOPA, which is converted to dopamine in the brain and replenishes the depleted stores of this transmitter. Dopamine itself is not used in therapy, partly because it will not cross the blood–brain barrier and reach the area where it is needed.

There is a close association between control of motor abilities and control of mental states. Both functions rely heavily on the activity of dopamine-releasing neurons. Consequently, drugs that affect dopamine activity usually alter both systems, resulting in undesired side effects. For example, heavy use of tranquilizers (such as Thorazine, Stelazine, and so on) in the treatment of psychotic patients causes Parkinson-like symptoms. If such drugs are given daily over several years, problems with motor functioning may become permanent. Drugs of abuse, such as stimulants, increase dopamine activity, causing enhanced motor activity as well as psychotic behavior.

The Limbic System The limbic system includes an assortment of linked brain regions located near and including the hypothalamus (see Figure 5.9). Besides the hypothalamus, the limbic structures include the thalamus, medial forebrain bundle, and front portion of the cerebral cortex. Functions of the limbic and basal ganglia structures are inseparably linked; often, drugs that affect one system also affect the other.

The primary roles of limbic brain regions include regulating emotional activities (such as fear, rage, and anxiety), memory, modulation of basic hypothalamic functions (such as endocrine activity), and activities such as mating, procreation, and caring for the young. In addition, reward centers are also believed to be associated with limbic structures. It is almost certain that the mood-elevating effects of even the narcotic opiates (such as heroin) are mediated by the limbic systems of the brain.

Recent studies in laboratory animals have shown that most stimulant drugs of abuse (such as amphetamines and cocaine) are self-administered through a cannula surgically placed into limbic structures (such as the medial forebrain bundle and frontal cerebral cortex). This is done by linking injection of the drug into the cannula with a lever press by the animal (Koob and Bloom 1988). It is thought that euphoria or intense "highs" associated with these drugs are due to their effects on these brain regions. Some of the limbic system's principal transmitters include dopamine, norepinephrine, and serotonin; dopamine activation appears to be the primary reinforcement that accounts for the abuse liability of most drugs (Koob and Bloom 1988; Uhl et al. 1993).

The Cerebral Cortex The unique features of the human cerebral cortex gives humans a special place among animals. The cortex is a layer of gray matter made up of nerves and supporting cells that almost completely surrounds the rest of the brain and lies immediately under the skull (see Figure 5.9). It is responsible for the interpretation of incoming information and for the initiation of voluntary motor behavior. The center for speech and areas for perception of sensation from all parts of the body are located in this cortex.

The cerebral cortex can be divided into receiving areas, output areas, and association areas. The receiving areas obtain input from the various senses such as touch, pain, sight, smell, and sound. Drugs that affect the electrical activity, the receptors, the connecting neurons, or the synapses in the pathways from the site of sensory activation to the cortex will thus affect the response of the individual to that stimulus. Consequently, many psychoactive drugs, such as psychedelics, dramatically alter the perception of sensory information by the cortex and cause hallucinations that result in strange behavior.

The part of the cortex that has developed most in the evolutionary process is called the *association cortex*. In large part, the ratio of association cortex to cerebral cortex is a good index of the extent to which an animal functions independently of the environment; that is, the larger the association cortex, the more independent the animal. The association areas do not directly receive input from the environment, nor do they directly initiate output to the muscles or the glands. The association areas may store memories or control complex behaviors. Some psychoactive drugs disrupt the normal functioning of these areas and thereby interfere with an individual's ability to deal with complex issues.

The Hypothalamus The hypothalamus (see Figures 5.8 and 5.9) is located near the base of the brain. It integrates information from many sources and serves as the CNS control center for the autonomic nervous system and many vital support functions. It is also the primary point of contact between the nervous and the endocrine systems. Because the hypothalamus controls the autonomic nervous system, it is also responsible for maintaining homeostasis in the body and participates in functions mediated by the limbic system (discussed earlier).

It is now known that most of the body's hormones are regulated, in part, by the hypothalamus. If a hormone level drops below a certain point, a signal is sent from the hypothalamus to the appropriate gland (such as adrenal, thyroid, sex glands, and so on), which releases the needed hormone.

Because the hypothalamus has many blood vessels, drugs are quickly carried in the blood to this region. The rate at which drugs affect the hypothalamus depends on how these compounds pass across the blood–brain barrier. Because of the vital regulatory role of the hypothalamus, drugs that alter its function can have a major impact on systems that control homeostasis. The catecholamine transmitters are particularly important in regulating the function of the hypothalamus; thus, most drugs of abuse that alter the activity of norepinephrine and dopamine are likely to alter the activity of this brain structure.

ANTICHOLINERGIC agents that antagonize the effects of acetylcholine

The Autonomic Nervous System

Although the cell bodies of the neurons of the autonomic nervous system (ANS) are located within the brain or spinal cord, their axons project outside of the CNS to involuntary muscles, organs, and glands; thus the ANS is considered part of the peripheral nervous system. The ANS is an integrative, or regulatory, system that does not require conscious control (that is, you do not have to think about it). It is usually considered primarily a motor or output system. A number of drugs that cannot enter the CNS because of the blood–brain barrier are able to affect the ANS only. The ANS is divided into two functional components, the sympathetic and the parasympathetic nervous systems. Both systems send neurons to most visceral organs and to smooth muscles, glands, and blood vessels (see Figure 5.10).

The two components of the ANS generally have opposite effects on an organ or its function. The working of the heart is a good example of sympathetic and parasympathetic control (see Figure 5.8). Stimulation of the parasympathetic nervous system slows the heart rate, whereas stimulation of the sympathetic nerves accelerates it. These actions constitute a constant biological check-and-balance, or regulatory system. Because the two parts of the ANS work in opposite ways much of the time, they are considered physiological antagonists. These two systems control most of the internal organs, the circulatory system, and the secretory (glandular) system. The sympathetic system is normally active at all times; the degree of activity varies from moment to moment and from organ to organ. The parasympathetic nervous system is organized mainly for limited, focused activity and usually conserves and restores energy rather than expends it. For example, it slows the heart rate, lowers blood pressure, aids in absorption of nutrients, and is involved in emptying the urinary bladder. Table 5.2 lists the structures and/or functions of the sympathetic and parasympathetic nervous systems and their effects on each other.

The two branches of the autonomic nervous system use two different neurotransmitters. The parasympathetic branch releases acetylcholine at its synapses, whereas the sympathetic neurons release norepinephrine. An increase in epinephrine in the blood or the administration of drugs that mimic norepinephrine cause the body to respond as if the sympathetic nervous system had been activated. As previously mentioned, such drugs are referred to as *sympathomimetics*. Thus, taking amphetamines (which enhances the sympathetic nervous system by releasing norepinephrine and epinephrine) raises blood pressure, speeds up heart rate, slows down motility of the stomach walls, and may cause the pupils of the eyes to enlarge; other so-called "uppers," like cocaine, have similar effects.

Drugs that affect acetylcholine release, metabolism, or its interaction with its respective receptor are referred to as *cholinergic* drugs and can either mimic or antagonize the parasympathetic nervous system according to pharmacological action.

TABLE 5.2 Sympathetic and parasympathetic control

Structure or Function	Sympathetic	Parasympathetic
Heart rate	Speeds up	Slows
Breathing rate	Speeds up	Slows
Stomach wall	Slows motility	Increases
Skin blood vessels (vasomotor function)	Constricts	Dilates
Iris of eye	Constricts (pupil enlarges)	Dilates
Vomiting center	Stimulates	N/A

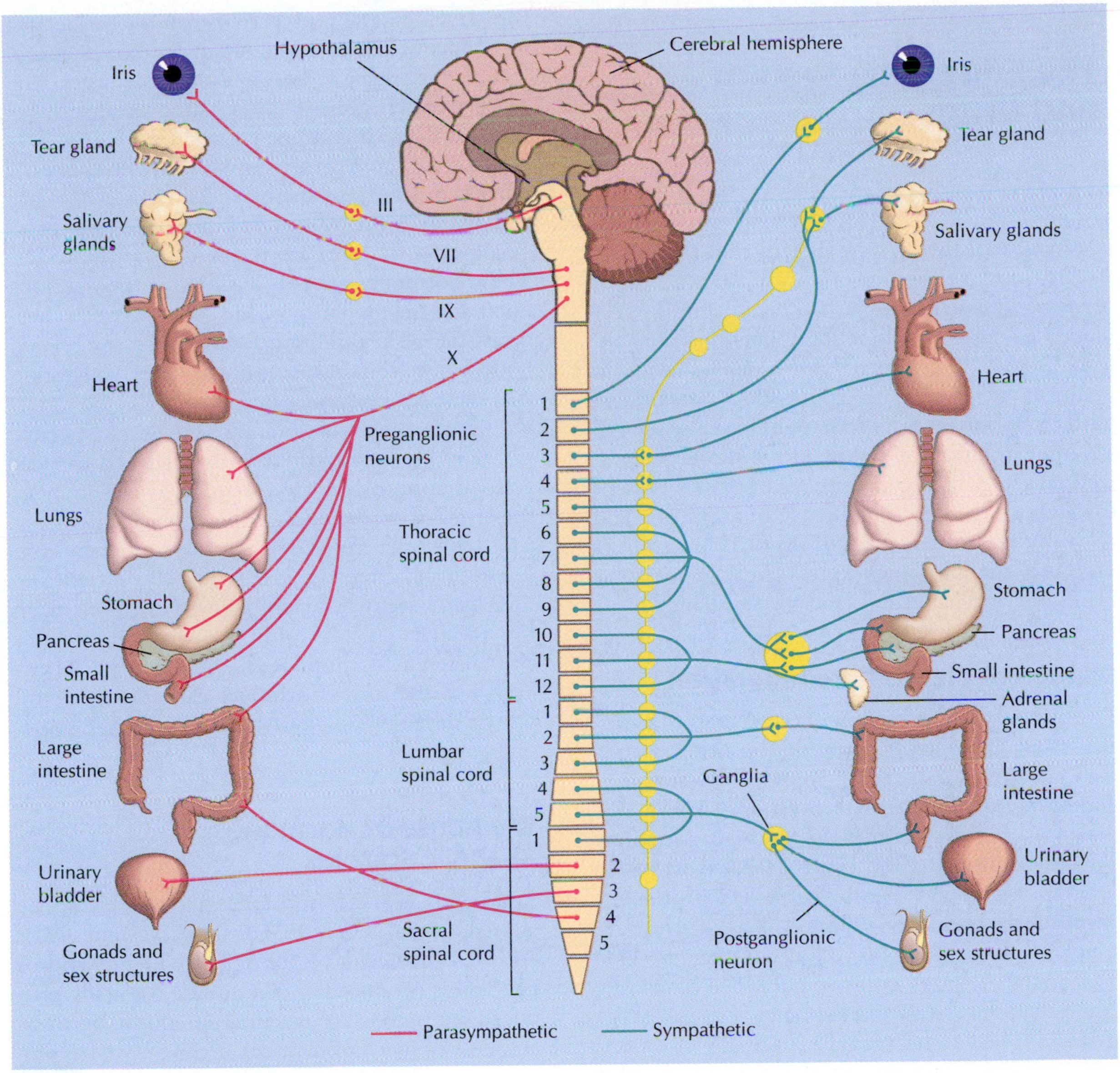

FIGURE 5.10 Pathways of the parasympathetic and sympathetic nervous systems and the organs affected

The Endocrine System and Drugs

As explained earlier in this chapter, the endocrine system consists of glands, which are ductless (meaning that they secrete directly into the bloodstream) and release chemical substances called *hormones.* These hormones are essential in the regulation of many vital functions, including metabolism, growth, tissue repair, and sexual behavior, to mention just a few. In contrast to neurotransmitters, hormones tend to have a slower onset and a longer duration of action with a more generalized target. Although a number of tissues present throughout the body are capable of producing and releasing hormones, three of the principal sources of these chemical messengers are the pituitary gland, the adrenal glands, and the sex glands.

Endocrine Glands and Regulation

The pituitary gland is often referred to as the *master gland.* It controls many of the other glands comprising the endocrine system by releasing regulating factors and growth hormone. The hypothalamus, besides controlling the brain functions already mentioned, helps control the activity of the pituitary gland and thereby has a very prominent effect on the endocrine system.

The adrenal glands are located near the kidneys and are divided into two parts: the outer surface, called the *cortex,* and the inner part, called the *medulla.* The adrenal medulla is actually a component of the sympathetic nervous system and releases adrenaline (another name for *epinephrine*) during sympathetic stimulation. The hormones released by the adrenal cortex are called *corticosteroids,* or frequently just *steroids.* Steroids help the body to respond appropriately to crises and stress. In addition, small amounts of male sex hormones, called *androgens,* are also released by the adrenal cortex. The androgens produce **anabolic** effects that increase the retention and synthesis of proteins, causing increases in the mass of tissues such as muscles and bones.

Sex glands are responsible for the secretion of male and female sex hormones that help regulate the development and activity of the respective reproductive systems. The organs known as *gonads* include the female ovaries and the male testes. The activity of the gonads is regulated by hormones released from the pituitary gland (see Figure 5.9) and, for the most part, is suppressed until puberty. After activation, estrogens and progesterones are released from the ovaries and the androgens (principally testosterone) are released from the testes. These hormones are responsible for the development and maintenance of the secondary sex characteristics. They influence not only sex-related body features but also emotional states, suggesting that these sex hormones enter the brain and significantly affect the functioning of the limbic systems.

For the most part, drugs prescribed to treat endocrine problems are intended as replacement therapy. For example, diabetic patients suffer from a lack of insulin from the pancreas, so therapy consists of insulin injections. Patients who suffer from dwarfism have insufficient growth hormone from the pituitary gland; thus, growth hormone is administered to stimulate normal growth. However, because some hormones can affect growth, muscle development, and behavior, they are sometimes abused.

The Abuse of Hormones: Anabolic Steroids

Androgens are the hormones most likely to be abused in the United States (Burke and Davis 1992). Testosterone is the primary natural androgen and is produced by the testes. Naturally produced androgens are essential for normal growth and development of male sex organs as well as secondary sex characteristics such as male hair patterns, voice changes, muscular development, and fat distribution. The androgens are also necessary for appropriate growth spurts during adolescence (*Drug Facts and Comparisons* 1994). Accepted therapeutic use of the androgens is usually for replacement in males with abnormally functioning testes. In such cases, the androgens are administered before puberty and for prolonged periods during puberty, to stimulate proper male development.

There is no question that androgens have an impressive effect on development of tissue (Griggs et al. 1989); in particular, they cause pronounced growth of muscle mass and a substantial increase in

Case in Point

The Risks of Nonmedical Use of Anabolic Steroids

A 37-year-old nonsmoking weight lifter was rushed to an emergency room with chest pains, sweating, and shortness of breath, which began midway through his lifting exercises. Although he had a negative medical history, he had used anabolic steroids off and on for seven years. A physical exam revealed normal blood pressure, but his EKG suggested a heart attack accounted for his symptoms (Ferenchick and Adelman 1992). Do you think knowledge about cases such as this would discourage nonmedical use of anabolic steroids by most athletes? Explain your response.

body weight in young men with deficient testes function. Because of these effects, androgens are classified as **anabolic** (able to stimulate the conversion of nutrients into tissue mass) **steroids** (they are chemically similar to the steroids).

In addition, many athletes and trainers have assumed that, in very high doses, androgens can also enhance muscle growth above that achieved by normal testicular function. Based on this assumption, male and female athletes as well as nonathletes who are into body building have been attracted to these drugs in hopes of enlarging muscle size and improving their athletic performances as well as their physiques. Although the androgens might cause some of the desired anabolic effects, they also cause unwanted sex changes: evidence is mounting that they can also cause undesirable changes in liver, reproductive system, skin, cardiovascular system, and psychological makeup of the user (Burke and Davis 1992; Ferenchick and Adelman 1992; *Drug Facts and Comparisons* 1994; Pope and Katz 1991). (See the Case in Point box). The abuse of anabolic steroids by athletes is discussed in greater detail in Chapter 15.

ANABOLIC chemicals able to convert nutrients into tissue mass

ANABOLIC STEROIDS compounds chemically like the steroids that stimulate production of tissue mass

In the 1950s weight lifters started using androgens to build muscle mass and increase strength as well as improve their physiques. Today, steroid use is widespread throughout all sports, at all levels of competition, and among all ages. Concern about the use of steroids has grown as publicity about the problem has increased.

Neither the short- nor long-term effects of androgen abuse are yet understood. Although it is clear that, in both women of all ages and boys, use of the androgens increases muscle mass, their effects on mature men are not so apparent. Nonetheless, many anecdotal stories are told in locker rooms of athletes who experienced dramatic increases in muscle size and strength because of steroid use. Certainly, such testimonials have enhanced the demand for these hormones, whether obtained legally or illegally (Wilson 1990).

The risks caused by androgens are not well understood either. Most certainly, the higher the doses and the longer the use, the greater the potential damage these drugs can do to the body. However, not everyone is convinced that steroid

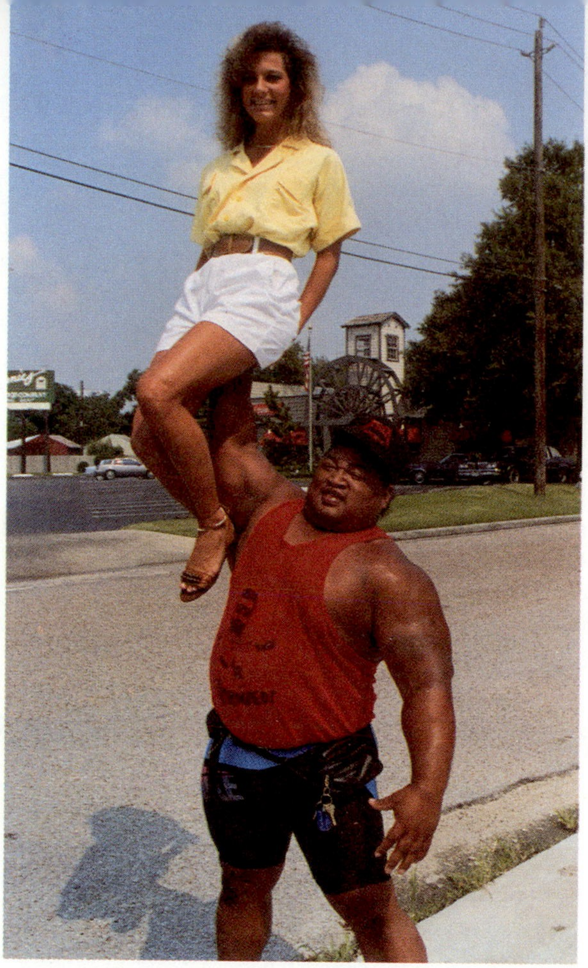

Anthony Clark became the first teenager to bench press 600 pounds in national teenage power lifting competition, and set a 1,025-pound squat world record in 1988.

use is dangerous and should be outlawed (see Crosscurrents). Some professional sports trainers even claim that low-dose, intermittent use can enhance athletic performance while causing no health risk (*Morning Edition* 1991).

Several studies have demonstrated that anabolic hormones particularly affect the limbic structures of the brain. Consequently, these drugs can cause excitation and a sense of superior strength and performance in some users. These effects, coupled with increased aggressiveness, could encourage continual use of these drugs. Other CNS effects, however, may be disturbing to the user. Symptoms that may occur include uncontrolled rage (referred to as "roid rage"), headaches, anxiety, insomnia, and perhaps paranoia (*Drug Facts and Comparisons* 1994; Pope and Katz 1991).

The medical community has become very concerned about the inappropriate use of androgens. Attempts have been made to prevent abuse by implementing education programs, drug screening, and associated penalties when rules are violated. To help prevent abuse, anabolic steroids were classified as a controlled drug by the Drug Enforcement Administration (DEA). The Anabolic Steroids Control Act of 1990 placed these drugs into Schedule III of the Controlled Substances Act, effective 27 February 1991. The term *anabolic steroid* is defined in this act as "any drug or hormonal substance chemically and pharmacologically related to testosterone (other than estrogens, progestins, and corticosteroids) that promotes muscle growth" (*Federal Register* 1991). This requires anyone who distributes or dispenses anabolic steroids to be registered with the DEA. Persons distributing androgens who are not properly authorized can be imprisoned for not more than five years and be required to pay fines as deemed appropriate. If the offense involves providing drugs to an individual under 18 years of age, the violation is punishable by not more than ten years in prison.

Because of concerns about the effects and detection of anabolic steroids, many athletes are turning to other drugs to enhance their competitive performance by stimulating the endocrine systems. These alternatives include "human growth factor," erythropoietin, and gamma-hydroxybutyrate (GHB), and are discussed in Chapter 15.

Conclusion

All psychoactive drugs affect brain activity by altering the ability of neurons to send and receive messages. Consequently, drugs of abuse exert their addicting effects by stimulating or blocking the activity of CNS neurotransmitters or their receptors. Thus, to understand why these drugs are abused and the nature of their dependence, we need to study how neurons and their neurotransmitter systems function. In addition, many scientists believe that elucidating how substances of abuse affect nervous systems will lead to new and more effective methods for treating drug addiction.

CROSS CURRENTS

Because the abuse of anabolic steroids is a relatively new phenomenon, not much is known about the consequence of its long-term use. Consequently, there is considerable disagreement as to its potential dangers. Consider the following opposing opinions:

1. Routine use of low doses of anabolic steroids by an athlete shouldn't be illegal because no one has proven such treatment is dangerous; besides, such steroid use has been shown to enhance the athletic performance of the user.
2. It is known that high doses of anabolic steroids are dangerous, so even though we don't know the exact effects of long-term low doses, nonmedical use of this drug should be illegal.

Choose a side, and support your argument with factual information from this text and other authoritative sources. (See Chapter 15 for additional information.)

Review Questions

1. How are neurotransmitters and hormones alike, and how are they different?
2. Why is it important for the body to have chemical messengers that can be quickly released and rapidly inactivated?
3. Why are "receptors" so important in understanding the effects of drugs of abuse?
4. Why do many drugs of abuse affect motor behavior?
5. What are some mechanisms whereby a drug of abuse can increase the activity of dopamine transmitter systems in the brain?
6. Some drugs of abuse are described as "sympathomimetics" and some as "anticholinergic": what features distinguish these two pharmacological properties?
7. Was classifying anabolic steroids as Schedule III drugs justified? What do you think will be the long-term consequence of this action?

Key Terms

homeostasis
neurons
axons
neurotransmitters
receptors
psychoactive
hormones
synapse
synaptic cleft
dendrites
endorphins
agonistic
antagonistic
muscarinic
nicotinic
catecholamines
sympathomimetic
somatic nervous system
autonomic nervous system
anticholinergic
anabolic
anabolic steroids

Summary

1. The nervous and endocrine systems help mediate internal and external responses to the body's surroundings. Both systems release chemical messengers in order to achieve their homeostatic functions. These messenger substances are called *neurotransmitters* and *hormones* and exert their functions through receptors. Many drugs exert their effects by influencing these chemical messengers.
2. The neuron is the principal cell type in the nervous system. This specialized cell consists of dendrites, a cell body, and an axon. It communicates with other neurons and organs by releasing neurotransmitters, which can cause either excitation or inhibition at their target sites.
3. The chemical messengers from glands and neurons exert their effects by interacting with special protein regions in membranes called *receptors.* Because of their unique structures, receptors only interact with molecules that have specific configurations. Activation of receptors can initiate a chain of events within cells, resulting in changes in gene expression, enzyme activity, or metabolic function.
4. *Agonists* are substances or drugs that stimulate receptors. *Antagonists* are substances or drugs that attach to receptors and prevent them from being activated.
5. A variety of different substances are used as neurotransmitters by neurons in the body. The classes of transmitters include the catecholamines, serotonin, acetylcholine, GABA, and peptides. These transmitters are excitatory, inhibitory, or sometimes both, depending on which receptor is being activated. Many drugs selectively act to either enhance or antagonize these neurotransmitters and their activities.
6. The central nervous system consists of the brain and spinal cord. Regions within the brain help to regulate specific functions. The hypothalamus controls endocrine and basic body functions. The basal ganglia are primarily responsible for controlling motor activity. The limbic system regulates mood and mental states. The cerebral cortex helps interpret, process, and respond to input information.
7. The limbic system and its associated transmitters, especially dopamine, are a major site of action for the drugs of abuse. Substances that increase the activity of dopamine cause a sense of well-being and euphoria, which encourage psychological dependence.
8. The autonomic nervous system is composed of the sympathetic and parasympathetic systems; neurons associated with these systems release noradrenalin and acetylcholine as their transmitters, respectively. These systems work in an antagonistic fashion to control unconscious, visceral functions such as breathing and cardiovascular activity. The parasympathetic nervous system usually helps conserve and restore energy in the body, while the sympathetic nervous system is continually active.
9. The endocrine system consists of glands that synthesize and release hormones into the blood. Distribution via blood circulation carries these chemical messengers throughout the body, where they act on specific receptors. Some of the principal structures include the pituitary, adrenals, and thyroid glands, as well as the pancreas.
10. Anabolic steroids are structurally related to the male hormone testosterone. They are often abused by both male and female athletes trying to build muscle mass and enhance performance. The continual use of high doses of anabolic steroids can cause annoying and dangerous side effects. The long-term effects of low, intermittent doses of these drugs has not been determined. Because of concern by most medical authorities, anabolic steroids are controlled substances and have been classified as Schedule III substances.

References

Burke, C., and S. Davis. "Anabolic Steroid Abuse." *Pharmacy Times* (June 1992): 35–40.

Drug Facts and Comparisons. St. Louis: Lippincott, 1994.

Federal Register 56 (13 February 1991): 3754.

Ferenchick, G., and S. Adelman. "Myocardial Infarction Associated with Anabolic Steroid Use in a Previously Healthy 37-Year-Old Weight Lifter." *American Heart Journal* 124 (August 1992): 507–08.

Goldstein, A. *Addiction from Biology to Drug Policy,* 15–60. New York: Freeman, 1994.

Griggs, R., W. Kingston, R. Jozetowicz, B. Herr, G. Forbes, and D. Halliday. "Effect of Testosterone on Muscle Mass and Muscle Protein Synthesis." *Journal of Applied Physiology* 66 (1989): 498–503.

Izquierdo, I. "A Game with Shifting Mirrors." *Trends in Pharmacological Sciences* 10 (1989): 473–75.

Kandel, E., J. Schwartz, and T. Jessell, eds. *Principles of Neural Science,* 3d ed. New York: Elsevier, 1991.

Kelly, J., and J. Dodd. "Anatomical Organization of the Nervous System." In *Principles of Neural Science,* 3d ed., edited by E. Kandel, J. Schwartz, and T. Jessell, 273–82. New York: Elsevier, 1991.

Koob, G. "Drugs of Abuse: Anatomy, Pharmacology and Function of Reward Pathways." *Trends in Pharmacologic Sciences* 13 (1992): 177–84.

Koob, G., and F. Bloom. "Cellular and Molecular Mechanisms of Drug Dependence." *Science* 242 (1988): 715–23.

Linder, M., and A. Gilman. "G Proteins." *Scientific American* (July 1992): 56–65.

Morning Edition. "Sports and Drugs" Series on National Public Radio (14 January 1991, 10 A.M.).

Pope, H., and D. Katz. "What Are the Psychiatric Risks of Anabolic Steroids?" *Harvard Mental Health Letter* 7 (April 1991): 8.

Snyder, S. H. "Opiate Receptors in the Brain." *New England Journal of Medicine* 296 (1977): 266–71.

Swan, N. "Researchers Make Pivotal Marijuana and Heroin Discoveries." *NIDA Notes* 8 (September–October 1993): 1.

Uhl, G., K. Blum, E. Noble, and S. Smith. "Substance Abuse Vulnerability and D-2 Receptor Genes." *Trends in Neurological Sciences* 16 (1993): 83–87.

Uhl, G., A. Persico, and S. Smith. "Current Excitement with D-2 Dopamine Receptor Gene Alleles in Substance Abuse." *Archives of General Psychiatry* 49 (1992): 157–60.

Wilson, J. "Androgens." In *The Pharmacological Basic of Therapeutics,* 8th ed., edited by A. Gilman, T. Rall, A. Nies, and P. Taylor. New York: Plenum, 1990.

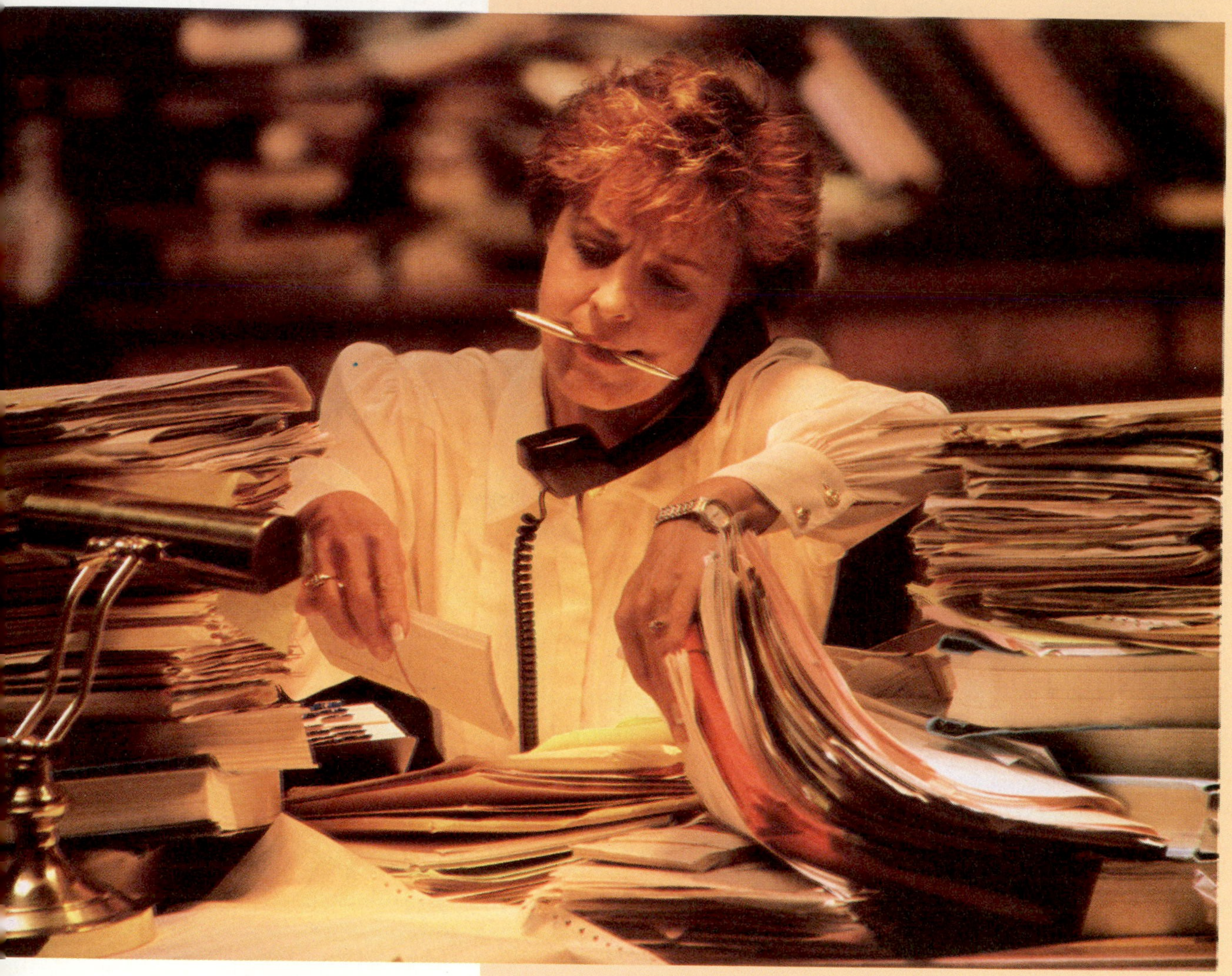

Chapter 6

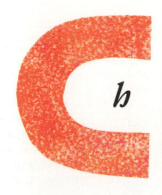

CNS Depressants

Sedative-Hypnotics

Did You Know That . . .

- Alcohol relieves anxiety and stress because of its CNS depressant effects.
- At low doses a CNS depressant relieves anxiety, and at high doses it becomes a sleep aid.
- The Valium-like benzodiazepines are much safer drugs than the barbiturates.
- Benzodiazepines are by far the most frequently prescribed CNS depressant.
- Most people dependent on benzodiazepines get their drugs legally by prescription.
- Long-term users of Valium can experience severe withdrawal symptoms if drug use is stopped abruptly.
- Our bodies probably produce a natural antianxiety substance that is like Valium.
- Antihistamines are the principal active ingredient in OTC sleep aids.
- The illicit use of CNS depressants has substantially decreased in the past 10 to 15 years.
- The short-acting CNS depressants are the most likely to be abused.

Learning Objectives

On completing this chapter, you will be able to

1. Identify the primary drug groups used for CNS depressant effects.
2. Explain the principal therapeutic uses of the CNS depressants and how the effects relate to drug dose.
3. Explain why CNS depressant drugs are commonly abused.
4. Identify the differences and similarities between benzodiazepines and barbiturates.
5. Relate how benzodiazepine dependence usually develops.
6. Describe the differences in effects between short- and long-acting CNS depressants.
7. Explain the current status of methaqualone.
8. Describe the CNS depressant properties of antihistamines, and compare their therapeutic usefulness to that of benzodiazepines.
9. List the four principal types of people who abuse CNS depressants.
10. Identify the basic principles in treating dependence on CNS depressants.

Healthy People 2000

Reduce to less than 35% the proportion of people aged 18 and older who experienced adverse health effects from stress within the past year.

Increase to at least 40% the proportion of worksites employing 50 or more people that provide programs to reduce employee stress.

Central nervous system (CNS) depressants are some of the most widely used and abused drugs in the United States. Why? With low doses they all produce a qualitatively similar "high" by their disinhibitory effects on the brain. In addition, they relieve stress and anxiety and even induce sleep—effects that appeal to many people, particularly those who are struggling with problems and looking for a break, physically and emotionally. However, CNS depressants also can cause a host of serious side effects, including problems with tolerance and dependence. Ironically, many individuals who have become dependent on depressants have obtained them through legitimate means: a prescription given by a physician. In fact, homemakers are often prone to this type of drug abuse. Depressants are also available "on the streets," although this illicit source is not the bulk of the problem.

In this chapter, we briefly review the history of CNS depressants, in terms of both development and use, and then discuss the positive and negative effects these drugs can produce. Each of the major types of depressant drugs are then reviewed in detail: benzodiazepines (Valium-like drugs), barbiturates, and other smaller categories. We conclude with an examination of abuse patterns of depressant drugs, and discuss how drug dependence and withdrawal are treated.

An Introduction to CNS Depressants

Henry (not his real name) lived with his wife and two children. He claimed to be a nonsmoker and denied any use of illegal drugs; however, he did have a history of daily coffee consumption and admitted to occasionally consuming moderate amounts of alcohol. Despite no history of mental illness, his behavior changed over the course of several months—he experienced insomnia, depression, difficulty concentrating, nightmares, irritability, loss of job, and marital discord. His problems culminated one summer afternoon after drinking beer with a friend, when he got into an argument with the manager of his apartment. Acting in an incoherent manner, Henry picked up a kitchen knife and small hand ax from his apartment, proceeded to the manager's office, and tried to chop down the door, while yelling at both the manager and witnesses in the hallway. He was apprehended by police and charged with criminal behavior. When questioned, Henry had no recollection of the incident. A medical history revealed that he had been prescribed Rivotril (a Valium-type CNS depressant) for insomnia and stress as well as Anafranil (an antidepressant that can cause CNS depression or excitation). Psychotherapists concluded that his aberrant personal and criminal behavior were directly caused by the effects of the prescribed CNS depressants in combination with alcohol. Given the conclusions of the clinicians, the city prosecuting attorney offered Henry a plea bargain to reduce the charge to a misdemeanor and a suspended sentence (Pagliaro and Pagliaro 1992).

This actual case study illustrates several reasons why CNS depressants can be problematic. First, in contrast to most other substances of abuse, CNS depressants are usually not obtained illicitly and self-administered but are prescribed under the direction of a physician. Second, use of CNS depressants can cause very alarming, even dangerous, behavior if not monitored closely: most problems associated with these drugs occur due to a lack of professional supervision. Third, several seemingly unrelated drug groups have some ability to cause CNS depression. When these drugs are combined, there can be bizarre and dangerous interactions. Particularly problematic is the combination of alcohol with other CNS depressants. Finally, CNS depressants can cause disruptive personality changes that are unpredictable and sometimes very threatening.

This chapter can help the reader understand the nature of the CNS depressant effects experienced by Henry as well as other important features of these drugs. In addition, the similarities and differences among the commonly prescribed CNS depressant drugs are discussed.

The History of CNS Depressants

Before the era of modern drugs, the most common depressant used to ease tension, cause relaxation, and help people forget their problems was

CROSSCURRENTS

Life can become very stressful due to school, work, and personal problems. It often is difficult to decide when such problems are best handled by counseling or the use of anxiolytic drugs. The following are two extreme views on this dilemma:

1. Excessive anxiety is caused by a chemical imbalance in the brain, and anxiolytic drugs are necessary to restore normal balance and reliably relieve anxiety.
2. Even the safest anxiolytic drugs have significant side effects and should be avoided. To resolve the real cause of the stress, personal and social problems need to be dealt with by professional psychotherapy and counseling.

Choose one of these positions, and support your side with arguments based on the information found in the text and other authoritative sources.

alcohol. These effects no doubt accounted for the immense popularity of alcohol and help explain why this traditional depressant is the most commonly abused drug of all time. (Alcohol is discussed in detail in Chapters 7 and 8.)

Attempts to find CNS depressants other than alcohol that could be used to treat nervousness and anxiety began in the 1800s with the introduction of bromides. These drugs were very popular until their toxicities became known. In the early 1900s, bromides were replaced by barbiturates. Like bromides, barbiturates were initially heralded as safe and effective depressants; however, problems with tolerance, dependence, and lethal overdoses became evident. It was learned that the doses of barbiturates required to treat anxiety also could cause CNS depression, affecting respiration and impairing mental functions. The margin of safety for barbiturates was too narrow, so research for a safer CNS depressant began again.

It was not until the 1950s that the first benzodiazepines were marketed as substitutes for the dangerous barbiturates. Benzodiazepines were originally viewed as extremely safe and free from the problems of tolerance, dependence, and withdrawal that occurred with the other drugs in this category (Mondanaro 1988, 95). Unfortunately, benzodiazepines also have been found to be less than ideal antianxiety drugs. Although relatively safe when used for short periods, long-term use can cause dependence and withdrawal problems much like those associated with their depressant predecessors. These problems have become a major concern of the medical community, which will be discussed in greater detail later in the chapter.

Many of the people who become dependent on CNS depressants such as benzodiazepines began use of the drugs under the supervision of a physician. Some clinicians routinely prescribe CNS depressants for cases of stress, anxiety, or apprehension, without trying nonpharmacological approaches, such as psychotherapy. It is quicker and less troublesome for a clinician to write a prescription to cure emotional problems (hoping that it will resolve itself in time) than to spend time counseling a patient, helping him or her to work out difficulties. This practice sends an undesirable and often detrimental message to patients; that is, CNS depressants are a simple solution to their complex, stressful problems (see Crosscurrents).

Consequently, during the 1970s and 1980s, there was an epidemic of prescriptions for CNS

FIGURE 6.1 Dose-dependent effects of CNS depressants

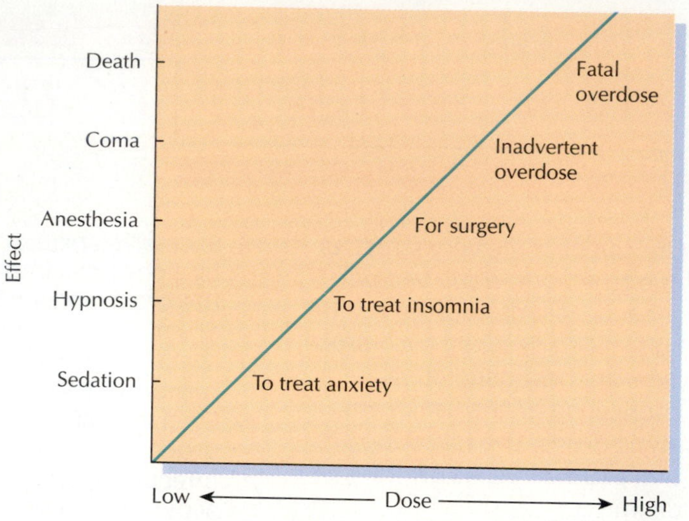

depressants. For example, in 1973 100 million prescriptions were written for benzodiazepines alone. Approximately twice as many women as men were taking these drugs at this time; a similar gender pattern continues today. Many homemakers made CNS depressants a part of their household routine, as described in the lyrics of the rock song "Mother's Little Helper" on the Rolling Stones' album *Flowers:*

> Things are different today
> I hear every mother say
> "Mother needs something today to calm her down"
> And though she's not really ill,
> There's a little yellow pill.
> She goes running for the shelter
> Of her "mother's little helper"
> And it helps her on her way,
> Gets her through her busy day.

As the medical community became more aware of the problem, the use of depressants declined. In 1984, 70 million prescriptions of benzodiazepines were written (Mondanaro 1988), and even fewer were written in 1992 ("Top 200 Drugs of 1992," 1993). Today, efforts are again being made by pharmaceutical companies and scientists to find new classes of CNS depressants that can be used to relieve stress and anxiety without causing serious side effects such as dependence and withdrawal.

The Effects of CNS Depressants: Benefits and Risks

The CNS depressants are a diverse group of drugs that share an ability to reduce CNS activity and diminish the brain's level of awareness. Besides the benzodiazepines, barbituratelike drugs, and alcohol, depressant drugs also include antihistamines and opioid narcotics like heroin (see Chapter 9).

Depressants are usually classified according to the degree of their medical effects on the body. For instance, **sedatives** cause mild depression of the CNS and relaxation. This drug effect is used to treat extreme anxiety and often is referred to as **anxiolytic.** Many sedatives also have muscle-relaxing properties that enhance their relaxing effects.

Depressants are also used to promote sleep. **Hypnotics** (from the Greek god of sleep, Hypnos) are CNS depressants that encourage sleep by inducing drowsiness. Often when depressants are used as hypnotics, they have **amnesiac** effects, as well. As already mentioned, the effects produced by depressants can be very enticing and encourage inappropriate use.

The effects of the CNS depressants tend to be dose dependent (see Figure 6.1). Thus, a larger dose of a sedative may have a hypnotic effect. Often the only difference between a sedative and a hypnotic effect is the dosage. By increasing the dose still further, an anesthetic state can be reached. **Anesthesia** is deep depression of the CNS and is used to achieve a controlled state of uncon-

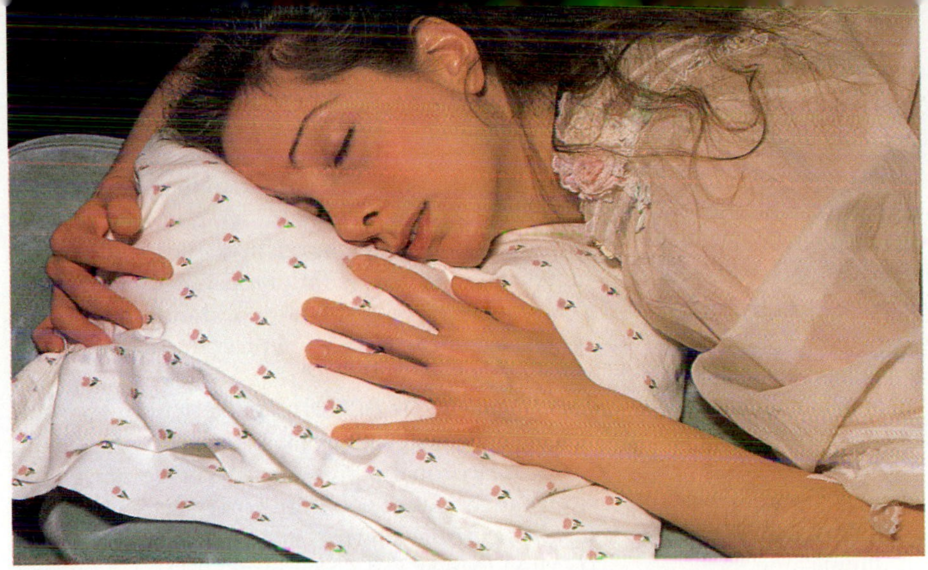

CNS depressants can be used as hypnotics to initiate sleep.

sciousness so a patient can be treated, usually by surgery, in relative comfort and without memory of an unpleasant experience. With the exception of benzodiazepines, if the dose of most of the depressants is increased much more, coma or death will ensue because the CNS becomes so depressed that vital centers controlling breathing and heart activity cease to function properly.

As a group, persistent use of the CNS depressant drugs causes tolerance. Because of the diminished effect due to the tolerance, users of these drugs continually escalate their doses. Under such conditions, the depressants alter physical and psychological states resulting in dependence. The dependence can be so severe that abrupt drug abstinence results in severe withdrawals that include life-threatening seizures (American Psychiatric Association 1994). Because of these dangerous pharmacological features, treatment of dependence on CNS depressants must proceed very carefully (Goldstein 1995). This is discussed in greater detail at the end of this chapter.

It is important to realize that all CNS depressants are not "created equal." Some have wider margins of safety; others have a greater potential for nonmedicinal abuse. These differences are important when considering the therapeutic advantages of each type of CNS depressant. In addition, unique features of the different types of depressants make them useful for treatment of other medical problems. For example, some barbiturates and benzodiazepines are used to treat forms of epilepsy or acute seizure activity, while opioid narcotics are important in the treatment of many types of pain. Some of these unique features will be dealt with in greater detail when the individual drug groups are discussed. The benzodiazepines, barbiturate-like drugs, and antihistamines are dealt with in this chapter. Other CNS depressants, such as alcohol and opiates, are covered in Chapter 7, 8, and 9, respectively.

SEDATIVES CNS depressants used to relieve anxiety, fear, and apprehension

ANXIOLYTICS drugs that relieve anxiety

HYPNOTICS CNS depressants used to induce drowsiness and encourage sleep

AMNESIAC causing the loss of memory

ANESTHESIA a state characterized by loss of sensation or consciousness

Types of CNS Depressants

Benzodiazepines: Valium-Type Drugs

Benzodiazepines are by far the most frequently prescribed CNS depressants for anxiety and sleep. In fact, four of the top-selling prescription drugs in the United States during 1992 were benzodiazepines and included Xanax, Halcion, Ativan, and diazepam ("Top 200 Drugs" 1993). Because of their wide margin of safety (death from an overdose is rare), benzodiazepines have replaced barbiturate-like drugs in use as sedatives and hypnotics ("Halcion and Other Sleeping Pills" 1992; Goldstein 1995). Benzodiazepines were originally referred to as the *minor tranquilizers,* but this terminology erroneously implied that they had pharmacological properties similar to those of antipsychotic drugs (the major tranquilizers), when in fact they are very different. Consequently, the term *minor tranquilizer* is diminishing.

The first true benzodiazepine, *Librium,* was developed for medical use and marketed about 1960; the very popular drug Valium came on the market about the same time. In fact, Valium was so well received that from 1972 to 1978 it was the top-selling prescription drug in the United States. Its popularity continues to this day, as it still ranks in the top 20 of prescribed generic drugs ("Top 200 Drugs" 1993).

Because of dependence problems, the benzodiazepines are now classified as Schedule IV. In recent years, there has been considerable concern that benzodiazepines are overprescribed because of their perceived safety; it has been said, somewhat facetiously, that the only way a person could die from using the benzodiazepines would be to choke on them. The American Medical Association (AMA) and even consumer organizations ("High Anxiety" 1993) have become very concerned about this overconfident attitude toward benzodiazepines and have warned patients and doctors against prolonged and unsupervised administration of these drugs.

Medical Uses Benzodiazepines are used for an array of therapeutic objectives, including the relief of anxiety, treatment of neurosis, muscle relaxation, alleviation of lower-back pain, treatment of some convulsive disorders, induction of sleep (hypnotic), relief from withdrawal symptoms associated with narcotic and alcohol dependence, and induction of amnesia usually for preoperative administration (administered just before or during surgery or very uncomfortable medical procedures).

Mechanisms of Action In contrast to barbiturate-type drugs, which cause general depression of most neuronal activity, benzodiazepines selectively affect those neurons that have receptors for the neurotransmitter gamma-aminobutyric acid (GABA) (Miller and Greenblatt 1992). GABA is a very important inhibitory transmitter in several brain regions: the limbic system, the reticular activating system, and the motor cortex (see Chapter 5). In the presence of benzodiazepines, the inhibitory effects of GABA are increased. Depression of activity in these brain regions likely accounts for the ability of benzodiazepines to alter mood (a limbic function), cause drowsiness (a reticular activating system function), and relax muscles (a cortical function). The specific GABA-enhancing effect of these drugs explains the selective CNS depression caused by benzodiazepines.

Of considerable interest is the observation that these Valium-like drugs act on specific receptor sites that are linked to the GABA receptors in the CNS. As yet, no endogenous substance has been identified that naturally interacts with this so-called benzodiazepine site. However, it is very likely that a natural benzodiazepine does exist that activates this same receptor population and serves to reduce stress and anxiety by natural means. Several laboratories are attempting to locate an endogenous benzodiazepinelike substance (Miller and Greenblatt 1992).

Types Because benzodiazepines are so popular and thus profitable, new related drugs are routinely being released into the pharmaceutical market. Currently, approximately 14 benzodiazepine compounds are available in the United States.

Benzodiazepines are distinguished primarily by their duration of action (see Table 6.1). As a general rule, the short-acting drugs are used as hypnotics to treat insomnia, thus allowing the user to awake in the morning with few aftereffects (such as a hangover). The long-acting benzodiazepines tend to be prescribed as sedatives, giving prolonged relaxation and relief from persistent

REM SLEEP the restive phase of sleep associated with dreaming

PARADOXICAL an unexpected effect

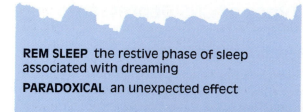

TABLE 6.1 Half-lives of various benzodiazepines

Drug	Half-Life (hours)
Alprazolam (Xanax)	12–15
Chlordiazepoxide (Librium)	5–30
Clonazepam (Klonopin)	18–50
Clorazepate (Tranxene)	30–100
Diazepam (Valium)	20–80
Flurazepam (Dalmane)	2–4
Halazepam (Paxipam)	14
Lorazepam (Ativan)	10–20
Midazolam (versed)	1–12
Oxazepam (Serax)	5–20
Prazepam (Centrax)	30–100
Quazepam (Doral)	39
Temazepam (Restoril)	10–17
Triazolam (Halcion)	1.5–5.5

Source: Adapted from G. McEvoy, ed. *American Hospital Formulary Service Drug Information*. Bethesda, MD: American Society of Hospital Pharmacists, 1994.

anxiety (Woods et al. 1992). Some of the long-acting drugs can exert a relaxing effect for up to two to three days. One of the reasons for the long action in some benzodiazepines is that they are converted by the liver into metabolites that are as active as the original drug. For example, Valium (diazepam) has a half-life of 20 to 80 hours and is converted by the liver into several active metabolites, including oxazepam (which itself is marketed as a therapeutic benzodiazepine—see Table 6.1).

Side Effects Reported side effects of benzodiazepines are drowsiness, lightheadedness, lethargy, impairment of mental and physical activities, skin rashes, nausea, diminished libido, irregularities in the menstrual cycle, blood cell abnormalities, and increased sensitivity to alcohol and other CNS depressants (McEvoy 1994). In contrast to barbiturate-type drugs, only very high doses of benzodiazepines have a significant impact on respiration. There are actually few verified instances of death resulting from overdose of benzodiazepines alone. Almost always, serious suppression of vital functions occurs when these drugs are combined with other depressants, most often alcohol (Woods et al. 1992).

There is no clear evidence of permanent, irreversible damage to neurological or other physiological processes, even with long-term benzodiazepine use (Woods et al. 1992). Benzodiazepines have less effect on **REM sleep** (rapid eye movement, the restive phase) than do barbiturates. Consequently, sleep under the influence of benzodiazepines is more likely to be restful and satisfying. However, prolonged use of hypnotic doses of benzodiazepines may cause rebound increases in REM sleep and insomnia when the drug is stopped.

On rare occasions, benzodiazepines can have **paradoxical** effects, producing unusual responses such as nightmares, anxiety, irritability, sweating, and restlessness (McEvoy 1994). Bizarre, uninhibited behavior—such as extreme agitation with hostility, paranoia, and rage—may occur as well. One such case was reported in 1988 in Utah. A 63-year-old patient who was taking Halcion (a relatively short-acting benzodiazepine) murdered her 87-year-old mother. The suspect claimed that the murder occurred because of the effects of the drug and that she was innocent of committing a crime. Her defense was successful, and she was acquitted of murder. After her acquittal, the woman initiated a $21 million lawsuit against Upjohn Pharmaceuticals for marketing Halcion, which she claimed is a dangerous drug. The lawsuit was settled out of court for an undisclosed amount ("British Spark" 1991).

Concerns of "consumer health groups" that Halcion causes unacceptable "amnesia, confusion, paranoia, hostility and seizures" (Reuters News Service 1992) has prompted the FDA to closely evaluate this benzodiazepine. Despite the fact that several other countries have banned Halcion, the FDA concluded that its benefits outweigh the reported risk; however, the FDA also concluded that "In no way should this [the FDA's conclusion] suggest that Halcion is free of side effects (see Case in Point). It has long been recognized and emphasized in Halcion's labeling that it is a potent drug that produces the same type of adverse effects as other CNS sedative hypnotic drugs" ("New Halcion Guidelines" 1992). Although the FDA did not require that Halcion be

Case in Point

The FDA is expected to watch over the safety of drug consumers in the United States, but sometimes it decides that the demands of public interest groups are not in the best interest of the people of this country. For example, the short-acting benzodiazepine, Halcion, has come under fire for causing psychiatric side effects and was removed from the market in the United Kingdom and 17 other countries. Concern in this country caused consumer health groups and clinicians to demand that the FDA place an immediate ban on this sleeping pill, which is made by Upjohn Company. However, the FDA declared that it believed the benefits of Halcion outweighed the risks and this drug likely was no more dangerous than other drugs in its category ("Halcion and Other Sleeping Pills" 1992). Because of this FDA decision, Halcion continued to be sold by prescription in the United States. Was the FDA response to concerns about Halcion appropriate, and how sensitive should the FDA be to such complaints by consumer health organizations?

withdrawn, it did negotiate changes in the labeling and package inserts with Halcion's manufacturer, the Upjohn Company. These changes emphasize appropriate Halcion use in treatment of insomnia and additional information about side effects, warnings, and dosage. As a result of these concerns, the sales of Halcion plummeted from being the eighteenth largest-selling prescription drug in 1987 to eighty-third in 1992.

There is no obvious explanation for these strange benzodiazepine-induced behaviors, although it is possible that, in some people, the drugs mask inhibitory centers of the brain and allow expression of antisocial behavior that is normally suppressed and controlled.

Related concerns have also been made public about another very popular benzodiazepine, Xanax. In 1990 Xanax became the first drug approved for the treatment of panic disorder (repeated, intense attacks of anxiety that can make life unbearable). Reports that long-term use of Xanax can cause severe withdrawal effects and a stubborn dependency on the drug ("High Anxiety" 1993) have raised public concerns about use of benzodiazepines in general. For example, how many people are severely dependent on these CNS depressants? What is the frequency of side effects such as memory impairment, serious mood swings, and cognitive problems? And how many patients currently using the benzodiazepines would be better served with nondrug psychotherapy? Clearly, use of the benzodiazepines to relieve acute stress or insomnia can be beneficial, but these drugs should be prescribed at the lowest dose possible and for the shortest time possible.

Tolerance, Dependence, Withdrawal, and Abuse As with most CNS depressants, frequent, chronic use of benzodiazepines can cause tolerance, dependence (both physical and psychological), and withdrawal (McEvoy 1994). However, such side effects are usually not as severe as those of most other depressants and occur only after using the drugs for prolonged periods (Woods et al. 1992). In addition, for most people the effects of the benzodiazepines are not viewed as reinforcing; thus, compared to other depressants, such as the barbiturates, the benzodiazepines are not especially addicting (Woods et al. 1992).

Withdrawal can mimic the condition for which the benzodiazepine is given; for example, with-

Here and Now

Valium: From Therapeutics to Abuse

A woman who had been abandoned as a child was then left by her husband for another woman. To deal with the emotional trauma and her sense of being unwanted, the patient was prescribed Valium. Over the next few years, the stress in her life continued unabated, due to frequent periods of unemployment and associated financial difficulties as well as serious problems with her children. The patient became dependent on Valium and continued to use it daily for 15 years. This drug had been the only therapy for this woman's emotional problems during the entire period. Because of concern about drug dependence, psychotherapy was attempted to help the patient deal with her continuing problems. With counseling, she was weaned from the Valium and eliminated her benzodiazepine dependence (Mondanaro 1988).

drawal symptoms can include anxiety or insomnia. In such cases, the clinician may be fooled into thinking that the underlying emotional disorder is still present, and may resume drug therapy without realizing that the patient has become drug dependent. In situations where users have consumed high doses of benzodiazepine over the long term, more severe, even life-threatening withdrawal symptoms may occur (Goldstein 1995); depression, panic, paranoia, and convulsions have been reported (see Table 6.2). Severe withdrawal can often be avoided by gradually weaning the patient from the benzodiazepine (Hays 1992).

It is very unusual to find nontherapeutic drug-seeking behavior in a patient who has been properly removed from benzodiazepines, unless that individual already has a history of drug abuse. Research has shown that when benzodiazepines

TABLE 6.2 Abstinence symptoms that occur when long-term users of benzodiazepines abruptly stop taking the drug

Duration of Abstinence	Symptoms
1–3 days	Often no noticeable symptoms
3–4 days	Restlessness, agitation, headaches, problems in eating, and inability to sleep
4–6 days	The preceding symptoms plus twitching of facial and arm muscles and feeling of intense burning in the skin
6–7 days	The preceding symptoms plus seizures

Source: G. McEvoy, ed. *American Hospital Formulary Service Drug Information,* 1333–1339. Bethesda, MD: American Society of Hospital Pharmacists, 1991.

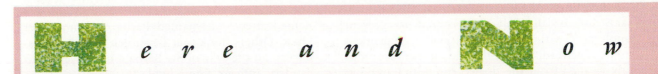

are the primary drug of abuse, these CNS depressants are usually self-administered to prevent unpleasant withdrawal symptoms in dependent users. If benzodiazepine-dependent users are properly weaned from the drugs, and withdrawal has dissipated, there is no evidence that craving for the benzodiazepines occurs (Woods et al. 1992). In general, people do not consider use of the benzodiazepines particularly pleasant (Woods et al. 1992). An exception to this conclusion appears to be former alcoholics. Many people with a history of alcoholism find the effects of benzodiazepines rewarding; consequently, nearly 21% of prior alcoholics use benzodiazepines chronically (Woods et al. 1992).

Long-term use of benzodiazepines (periods longer than three to four months) to treat anxiety or sleep disorders has not been shown to be therapeutically useful for most patients. Even so, this is a common indiscriminate practice and has been suggested by some clinicians to be responsible for the largest group of prescription drug-dependent people in the United States (see Here and Now). Possibly as many as 1 million people in the United States continue to take benzodiazepines because they have become physically dependent through such inappropriate use (Mondanaro 1988, 100).

Benzodiazepines are commonly used as a secondary drug of abuse and combined with illicit drugs (Woods et al. 1992). For example, narcotic users frequently combine benzodiazepines with weak heroin to enhance the narcotic effect. It is very common to find heroin users who are dependent on depressants as well as narcotics (Jaffe 1990).

Another frequent combination is the use of benzodiazepines with stimulants such as cocaine. Some addicts claim that this combination enhances the pleasant effects of the stimulant and reduces the "crashing" that occurs after using high doses. (More is said about benzodiazepine abuse later in this chapter.)

Barbiturates

Barbiturates are defined as "barbituric acid derivatives used in medicine as sedatives and hypnotics." Barbituric acid was synthesized by A. Bayer (of aspirin fame) in Germany in 1864. The reason for choosing the name *barbituric acid* is not known. Some have speculated that the compound was named after a girl named Barbara whom Bayer knew. Others think that Bayer celebrated his discovery on the Day of St. Barbara in a tavern that artillery officers frequented. (St. Barbara is the patron saint of artillery men.)

The first barbiturate, barbital (Veronal), was used medically in 1903. The names of the barbiturates all end in *-al,* indicating a chemical relationship to barbital, the first one synthesized.

Historically, barbiturates have played an important role in therapeutics because of their effectiveness as sedative-hypnotic agents, routinely used in the treatment of anxiety, agitation, and insomnia. However, because of their narrow margin of safety and their abuse liability, barbiturates have been largely replaced by safer drugs such as the benzodiazepines.

Uncontrolled use of barbiturates can cause a state of acute or chronic intoxication. Initially, there may be some loss of inhibition, euphoria, and behavioral stimulation, a pattern often seen with moderate consumption of alcohol. When taken to relieve extreme pain or mental stress, barbiturates may cause delirium and other side effects that can include nausea, nervousness, rash, and diarrhea. The person intoxicated with barbiturates may have difficulty thinking and making judgments, may be emotionally unstable, may be uncoordinated and unsteady when walking, and may slur speech (not unlike the drunken state caused by alcohol).

When used for their hypnotic properties, barbiturates cause an unnatural sleep. The user awakens feeling tired, edgy, and quite unsatisfied, most likely because barbiturates markedly suppress the REM phase of sleep. (As discussed earlier, REM sleep is necessary for the refreshing renewal that usually accompanies a good sleep experience.) Because benzodiazepines suppress REM sleep (as do all CNS depressants) less severely than barbiturates, use of benzodiazepines as sleep aids is generally better tolerated.

Continued misuse of barbiturate drugs has a cumulative toxic effect on the CNS that is more life threatening than misuse of opiates. In large doses or in combination with other CNS depressants, barbiturates may cause death from respiratory or cardiovascular depression. Because of this toxicity, barbiturates have been involved in many

TABLE 6.3 Classifications of common barbiturates

Classification	Duration of Pharmacological Effect	Drug
Ultrashort acting	¼ to 3 hours	Thiopental (Pentothal)
Short acting	3 to 6 hours	Amobarbital (Amytal) Pentobarbital (Nembutal) Secobarbital (Seconal)
Intermediate acting	6 to 12 hours	Butabarbital (Butisol)
Long acting	12 to 24 hours	Phenobarbital (Luminal)

drug-related deaths, accidental and suicidal. Repeated misuse induces severe tolerance of and physical dependence on these drugs. Discontinuing use of a short-acting barbiturate (see Table 6.3) in people who are using large doses can cause dangerous withdrawal effects such as life-threatening seizures. Table 6.4 summarizes the range of effects of barbiturates and other depressants on the mind and body.

Concern about the abuse potential of barbiturates has caused the federal government to include some of these depressants in the Controlled Substance Act. Consequently, the short-acting barbiturates, such as pentobarbital and secobarbital, are Schedule II drugs, while the long-acting barbiturates, such as phenobarbital, are less rigidly controlled as Schedule IV.

Effects and Medical Uses Barbiturates have many pharmacological actions. They depress the activity of nerves and skeletal, smooth, and cardiac muscles and impact the CNS in several ways, ranging from mild sedation to coma, depending on the dose. At sedative or hypnotic dosage levels, only the CNS is significantly affected. Higher anesthetic doses cause slight decreases in blood pressure, heart

TABLE 6.4 Effects of barbiturates and other depressants on the body and mind

	Body	Mind
Low dose ↓	Drowsiness	Decreased anxiety, relaxation
	Trouble with coordination	Decreased ability to reason and solve problems
	Slurred speech	
	Dizziness	Difficulty in judging distance and time
	Staggering	
	Double vision	Amnesia
	Sleep	
	Depressed breathing	Brain damage
	Coma (unconscious and cannot be awakened)	
	Depressed blood pressure	
High dose	Death	

rate, and flow of urine. The metabolizing enzyme systems in the liver are important in inactivating barbiturates; thus, liver damage may result in exaggerated responses to barbiturate use. In addition, barbiturates can also induce increased liver enzyme activity, which accelerates the metabolism and shortens the action of other drugs (Harvey 1980). Because of the complex effect on drug-metabolizing enzymes, caution must be taken whenever using barbiturates with other medication.

Low doses of barbiturates relieve tension and anxiety, effects that give several barbiturates substantial abuse potential. It is not surprising that the clinical use of the barbiturates has diminished dramatically in recent years. The side effects of barbiturates are extensive and severe. They lack selectivity and safety; they have a substantial tendency for tolerance, dependence, withdrawal, and abuse; and they cause problems with drug interaction. Thus barbiturates have been replaced by benzodiazepines in most treatments; however, they are still included in a number of combination products for the treatment of an array of medical problems, such as gastrointestinal disorders, hypertension, asthma, and pain (Rall 1990). Their use in such preparations is very controversial. The long-acting phenobarbital is still frequently used for its CNS depressant activity to alleviate or prevent convulsions in some epileptic patients and seizures caused by strychnine, cocaine, and other stimulant drugs. Thiopental (Pentothal) and other ultrashort- and short-acting barbiturates are used as anesthesia for minor surgery and as preoperative anesthetics in preparation for major surgery.

Mechanism of Action and Elimination The precise mechanism of action for barbiturates is unclear. Like benzodiazepines, barbiturates likely interfere with activity in the reticular activating system, the limbic system, and the motor cortex. However, in contrast to benzodiazepines, barbiturates do not seem to act at a specific receptor site; they probably have a general effect on the activity of certain neurons due to effects on calcium and chloride (elements necessary for normal activity in many neurons). These changes in calcium and chloride appear to enhance the activity of the inhibitory transmitter GABA. Because benzodiazepines also increase GABA activity (but in a more selective manner), these two types of drugs have overlapping effects. Because the mechanisms whereby they exert their effects are different, it is not surprising that these two types of depressants also have different pharmacological features.

Like the benzodiazepines, barbiturates can be classified in terms of duration of action (see Table 6.3). In general, the more fat soluble the barbiturate is, the more easily it enters the brain, the faster it will act, and the more potent it will be as a depressant. Barbiturates are eliminated through the kidneys at varying rates. The rate of removal depends primarily on how quickly the barbiturate is metabolized in the liver to a fat-insoluble metabolite. Excretion of barbiturates is faster when the urine is alkaline, which can be manipulated to treat barbiturate poisoning.

Because barbiturates are not completely removed from the body overnight, even the short-acting ones used for insomnia can cause subtle distortions of mood and impaired judgment and motor skills the following day (Julien 1992). The user may have mild withdrawal symptoms such as hyperexcitability, nausea, and vomiting even after short-term use (Harvey 1980). The long-acting barbiturates such as phenobarbital are metabolized more slowly and cause an extended drug hangover.

The fat solubility of barbiturates is also an important factor in the duration of their effects. Barbiturates that are the most fat soluble move in and out of body tissues (such as the brain) rapidly and are likely to be shorter acting. Fat-soluble barbiturates also are more likely to be stored in fatty tissue; consequently, the fat content of the body can influence the effects on the user. Because women have a higher body–fat ratio than men, their reaction to barbiturates may be slightly different.

Tolerance and Dependence The development of tolerance is usually necessary for true physical dependence to occur. Two types of tolerance result when barbiturates are taken repeatedly at short intervals:

1. Enzyme stimulation increases metabolism of the barbiturate, which means an increase in the average dose is required to achieve the same pharmacological effect.
2. Neurons in the CNS adapt to the barbiturate; this response can also result in cross-tolerance to other CNS depressants and causes barbitu-

TABLE 6.5 Details on the most frequently abused barbiturates

Drug	Nicknames	Dose and Description	Effects
Amobarbital (Amytal)	Blues, blue heavens, blue devils	65- or 200-mg blue capsule	Moderately rapid action; duration of 3 to 6 hours; takes 15 to 30 minutes for effect.
Pentobarbital (Nembutal)	Nembies, yellow jackets, yellows	30- or 100-mg yellow, 50-mg orange-and white capsule	Short acting; dose of 30 to 50 mg is usually sufficient to induce sleep; for true hypnosis, as little as 100 mg is sufficient for a 6- to 8-hour period of fretful sleep without much hangover; will cause euphoria and excitation at first, so it is abused.
Phenobarbital (Luminal)	Purple hearts	Purple tablet	A long-acting barbiturate particularly well suited for treatment of epilepsy. Daily doses of 60–250 mg are routinely used in adults. Because of its long action, it is not often abused.
Secobarbital (Seconal)	Reds, red devils, red birds, Seccy	50-, 100-mg red capsule	Short acting with a prompt onset of action; usually lasts under 3 hours and is commonly abused to produce intoxication and euphoria by blocking inhibitions.
Tuinal (50% amobarbital and 50% secobarbital)	Tooeys, double-trouble, rainbows	50-, 100-, 200-mg capsule, blue body with red-orange cap	Results in a rapidly effective, moderately long-acting sedative; sedative dose is around 50 mg; hypnotic dose is 100 to 200 mg.

Note: A fatal overdose from each commonly used barbiturate is usually about 10 times the hypnotic dose. Death is from respiratory failure.

rate addicts to become resistant to other general depressants, including alcohol.

Development of physical dependence on barbiturates is a relatively slow process, requiring weeks or months of use before withdrawal symptoms occur during drug abstinence. Doses of 200 milligrams (mg) to 400 mg of pentobarbital or secobarbital can be taken daily for a year with little or no physical dependence. Daily doses of between 400 mg and 600 mg for more than one month are required to induce withdrawal symptoms when the drug is discontinued (Smith et al. 1979).

Withdrawal from barbiturates after dependence has developed causes hyperexcitability because of the rebound of depressed neural systems. Qualitatively (but not quantitatively), the withdrawal symptoms are similar for all sedative-hypnotics (Goldstein 1995).

Table 6.5 gives details on the barbiturates abused most frequently.

Other CNS Depressants

While benzodiazepines and barbiturates are by far used most frequently to produce CNS depressant effects, many other agents, representing an array of distinct chemical groups, can similarly reduce brain activity. Although the mechanisms of action might be different for some of these drugs, if any CNS depressants (alcohol included) are combined, they will interact in a synergistic manner and can suppress respiration in a life-threatening manner. Thus, it is important to avoid such mixtures if possible. Even some over-the-counter (OTC) products such as cold and allergy medications contain drugs with CNS depressant actions.

Nonbarbiturate Drugs With Barbiturate-Like Properties This category of depressants that are not barbiturates but act like them includes several drugs that are chemically unrelated but produce CNS depression effects. They all cause substantial tolerance, physical and psychological dependence, and withdrawal symptoms. The therapeutic safety of these CNS depressants is more like that of barbiturates than benzodiazepines; consequently, like barbiturates, these agents have been replaced by the safer and easier-to-manage benzodiazepines.

Because these drugs have significant abuse potential, they are restricted much like other CNS depressants. In this group of depressants, methaqualone is a Schedule II drug; glutethimide and methyprylon are Schedule III drugs; chloral hydrate and ethchlorvynol are Schedule IV drugs. The basis for the classification is the relative potential for physical and psychological dependence. Abuse of Schedule II drugs may lead to severe or moderate physical dependence or high psychological dependence, and abuse of Schedule III drugs may cause moderate physical and psychological dependence. Schedule IV drugs are considered much less likely to cause either type of dependence.

Chloral Hydrate Chloral hydrate, or "knockout drops," has the unsavory reputation of being a drug that is slipped into a person's drink to make him or her unconscious. The combination of chloral hydrate and alcohol was given the name "Mickey Finn" on the waterfront of the Barbary Coast of San Francisco when sailors were in short supply. As legend has it, the name of one of the bars dispensing unwanted knockout drops was Mickey Finn's. An unsuspecting man would have a friendly drink and wake up as a crew member on an outbound freighter to China.

It takes about 30 minutes for chloral hydrate (Noctec) to take effect. It is metabolized to trichloroethanol, which is the active hypnotic agent. Alcohol accelerates the rate of conversion and potentiates the CNS depressant effect. Chloral hydrate does not depress the CNS as much as a comparable dose of barbiturates. It is a good hypnotic, but it has a narrow margin of safety. Chloral hydrate is a stomach irritant, especially if given repeatedly and in fairly large doses. Addicts may take enormous doses of the drug; as with most CNS depressants, chronic, long-term use of high doses will cause tolerance and physical dependence (Rall and Schleifer 1990).

Ethchlorvynol Ethchlorvynol (Placidyl) is a short-acting sedative-hypnotic drug. It causes side effects in some people, such as facial numbness, blurred vision, nausea, dizziness, gastric upset, and skin rash. Abusers may take up to 4 grams (g) a day. A dose of 10 to 25 g can cause death. Chronic high-dose use causes the development of tolerance and physical as well as psychological dependence. Because of synergistic interaction, use of ethchlorvynol and ethanol together can be potentially lethal. Due to its rapid, but short action, Placidyl is sometimes found as a "street" drug.

Glutethimide Glutethimide (Doriden) is another example of a barbiturate-like drug that has been abused and causes severe withdrawal symptoms. Doriden causes side effects similar to those of Placidyl. In addition, it induces blood abnormalities in sensitive individuals, such as a type of anemia and abnormally low white cell counts. In children, the drug may cause paradoxical excitement (unusual agitation and stimulation). Nausea, fever, increased heart rate, and convulsions occasionally occur in patients who have been taking this sedative regularly in moderate doses. The sedative dose for adults is 125 to 250 mg one to three times a day. As a hypnotic, the dose is usually 250 to 500 mg at bedtime.

Doriden seems to have a smaller margin of safety than barbiturates. Continual use causes tolerance and physical dependence. Doriden was used more commonly as a "street" drug before it was definitely proven to be addictive and tighter controls were instituted.

Methyprylon Methyprylon (Noludar) is a short-acting nonbarbiturate that is used as a sedative and hypnotic. Its effects are similar to those of Doriden, and it is capable of causing tolerance, physical dependence, and addiction much like barbiturates. Death has occurred during untreated withdrawal. Dosage for sedation is 50 to 100 mg three or four times a day. For inducing sleep, the dosage is usually 200 to 300 mg.

Methaqualone Few drugs have become so popular so quickly as methaqualone. It is a barbiturate-like sedative-hypnotic that was introduced in India in the 1950s as an antimalarial agent. Its sedative properties, however, were soon discovered. It was available in the United States as Quaalude, Mequin, and Parest.

After several years of "street" abuse, methaqualone was classified as a Schedule II drug. Since 1985, methaqualone has not been manufactured in the United States because of adverse publicity. It is interesting to note, however, that large amounts of illegal methaqualone are still imported into the United States from Colombia, Mexico, and Canada. It is referred to by "street" names such as *Ludes, Sopors,* or *714s.*

In humans, methaqualone accumulates in fatty tissue and readily enters the brain, like barbiturates. Also like barbiturates, methaqualone stimulates the activity of some metabolizing enzymes in the liver and may therefore induce tolerance. Common side effects are fatigue, dizziness, anorexia, nausea, vomiting, diarrhea, sweating, dryness of the mouth, depersonalization, headache, and paresthesia of the extremities (a pins-and-needles feeling in the fingers and toes). Hangover is frequently reported.

The standard hypnotic dose of methaqualone is 150 to 300 mg, whereas the average dose for daytime sedation is 75 mg three to four times daily. Coma may occur if a dose of 2 g is taken. During coma, methaqualone does not cause as marked a depression of heartbeat and respiration as do barbiturates. Doses between 8 and 20 g can be fatal; lower doses can be fatal if methaqualone is taken with alcohol or other sedative-hypnotics because of potentiation of the CNS depression. Mild overdosage causes an excessive CNS depression much like that from barbiturates. Severe overdoses can cause delirium, restlessness, muscle spasms, and even convulsions (Harvey 1980).

High doses of methaqualone can cause psychological and physical dependence and dangerous withdrawal symptoms when drug use is stopped. People who have taken 600 to 3,000 mg of methaqualone daily experience insomnia, abdominal cramps, headaches, anorexia, and nightmares when drug use is discontinued. Severe grand mal (major motor) convulsions may occur after withdrawal from high doses; the symptoms are similar to the delirium tremens that occur during withdrawal from alcohol.

Antihistamines Antihistamines are drugs used in both nonprescription and prescription medicinal products. The most common uses for antihistamines are to relieve the symptoms associated with the common cold, allergies, and motion sickness (see Chapter 14). Although frequently overlooked, many antihistamines cause significant CNS depression and are used both as sedatives and hypnotics. For example, the agents hydroxyzine (Visteril) and promethazine (Phenergan) are prescribed for their sedative effects, while diphenhydramine is commonly used as an OTC sleep aid.

The exact mechanism of CNS depression caused by these agents is not totally known but appears to relate to their blockage of acetylcholine receptors in the brain (they antagonize the muscarinic receptor types). This **anticholinergic** activity (see Chapter 5) helps cause relaxation and sedation and can be viewed as a very annoying side effect when these drugs are being used to treat allergies or other problems.

Therapeutic Usefulness and Side Effects. Antihistamines are viewed as relatively safe agents with some annoying but rarely dangerous side effects. In comparison with other more powerful CNS depressants, antihistamines do not appear to cause significant physical or psychological dependence or addiction problems, although drugs with anticholinergic activity are sometimes abused, especially by children and teenagers (Carlini 1993). However, tolerance to antihistamine-induced sedation occurs quite rapidly. Reports of significant cases of withdrawal problems when use of the antihistamines is stopped are rare. This may be due to the fact that these agents are used as antianxiety drugs for only minor problems and for short periods of time (often only for a single dose).

One significant problem with antihistamines is

ANTICHOLINERGIC antagonizing the activity of acetylcholine receptors the variability of responses they produce. Different antihistamines work differently on different people. Usually therapeutic doses will cause decreased alertness, relaxation, slowed reaction time, and drowsiness. But it is not uncommon for some individuals to be affected in the opposite manner; that is, an antihistamine can cause restlessness, agitation, and insomnia. There are even cases of seizures caused by toxic doses of antihistamine, particularly in children (Farrison and Rall 1990). Other annoying side effects of antihistamines relate to their anticholinergic effects, including dry mouth, constipation, and inability to urinate. These factors probably help to discourage the abuse of these drugs.

Even though antihistamines are relatively safe in therapeutic doses, they can contribute to serious problems if combined with other CNS depressants. Because of this potentially dangerous interaction, patients who have been prescribed other sedative-hypnotics should be aware of consuming drugs that contain antihistamines. For example, many OTC cold, allergy, antimotion, and sleep aid products contain antihistamines and should be avoided by patients using the potent CNS depressants.

Patterns of Abuse with CNS Depressants

The American Psychiatric Association considers dependence on CNS depressants a psychiatric disorder. According to its widely used *Diagnostic and Statistical Manual of Mental Disorders (DSM-IV)*, (American Psychiatric Association 1994), "substance dependence disorder" is present when three of the following criteria are satisfied at any time in a 12-month period:

1. Person needs greatly increased amounts of the substance to achieve the desired effect or experiences a markedly diminished effect with continued use of the substance.
2. Characteristic withdrawal occurs when drug use is stopped which encourages continued use of the substance to avoid the unpleasant effects.
3. Substance is consumed in larger amounts over a longer period of time than originally intended.
4. Person shows persistent desire or repeated unsuccessful efforts to decrease or control substance use.
5. A great deal of time is spent obtaining and using the substance or recovering from its effects.
6. All daily activities revolve around the substance—important social, occupational, or recreational activities are given up or reduced because of substance use.
7. Person withdraws from family activities and hobbies to use the substance privately or spend more time with substance-using friends.
8. Person continues use of substance despite recognizing it causes social, occupational, legal or medical problems.

A review of the previous discussion about the properties of CNS depressants reveals that severe dependence on these drugs can satisfy all these *DSM-IV* criteria; thus, according to the American Psychiatric Association, dependence on CNS depressants is classified as a form of mental illness.

The AMA (American Medical Association 1965) has characterized those types of people who are most inclined to abuse CNS depressants:

1. Those who seek sedative effects to deal with emotional stress, trying to escape from problems they are unable to deal with. Sometimes, these individuals are able to persuade clinicians to administer depressants for their problems; other times, they self-medicate with depressants that are obtained illegally.
2. Those who seek the excitation that occurs, especially after some tolerance has developed; instead of depression, they feel exhilaration and euphoria.
3. Those who try to counteract the unpleasant effect or withdrawal associated with other drugs of abuse, such as some stimulants, LSD, and other hallucinogens.
4. Those who use sedatives in combination with other depressants drugs such as alcohol and heroin. Alcohol plus a sedative gives a faster "high" but can be dangerous because of the multiple depressant effects and synergistic interaction. Heroin users often resort to

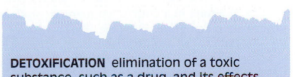

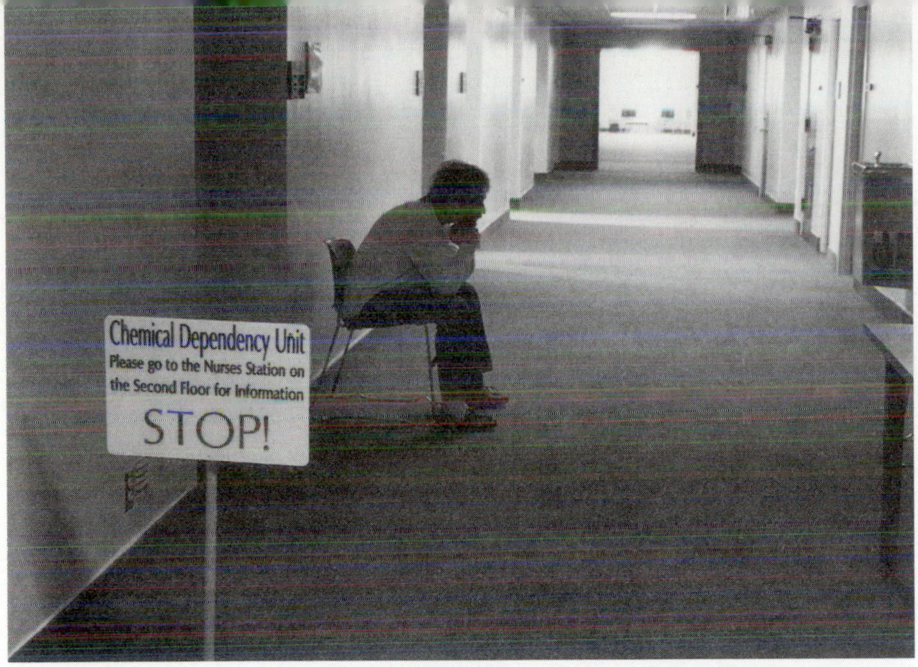

Detoxification of patients dependent on CNS depressants can be very unpleasant and even life-threatening.

barbiturates if their heroin supply is compromised.

As mentioned earlier, depressants are commonly abused in combination with other drugs (Goldstein 1995). In particular, opioid narcotic users take barbiturates, benzodiazepines, and other depressants to augment the effects of a weak batch of heroin or a rapidly shrinking supply. Chronic narcotic users also claim that depressants help to offset tolerance to opioids, thereby requiring less narcotic to achieve a satisfactory response by the user. It is not uncommon to see joint dependence on both narcotics and depressants.

Another common use of depressants is by alcoholics to soften the withdrawal from ethanol or to help create a state of intoxication without the telltale odor of alcohol. It is interesting that similar strategies are also used therapeutically to help detoxify the alcoholic. For example, long-acting barbiturates or benzodiazepines are often used to wean an alcohol-dependent person. Treatment with these depressants helps to reduce the severity of withdrawal symptoms, making it easier and safer for alcoholics to eliminate their drug dependence.

In general, those who chronically abuse the CNS depressants prefer (1) the short-action barbiturates, such as pentobarbital and secobarbital, (2) the barbiturate-like depressants, such as or glutethimide, methyprylon, and methaqualone; (3) the faster-acting benzodiazepines, such as diazepam (Valium), alprazalam (Xanax), or lorazepam (Ativan). However, most nonabusing people do not find the benzodiazepines particularly reinforcing (Woods et al. 1992).

Dependence on sedative-hypnotic agents can develop insidiously. Often a long-term patient has been treated for persistent insomnia or anxiety with daily exposures to a CNS depressant. When an attempt to withdraw the drug is made, the patient becomes agitated, unable to sleep, and severely anxious; a state of panic may be experienced when deprived of the drug. These signs are frequently mistaken for a resurgence of the medical condition being treated and are not recognized as part of a withdrawal syndrome to the CNS depressant. Consequently, the patient is restored to his or her supply of CNS depressant, and the symptoms of withdrawal subside. Such conditions generally lead to a gradual increase in dosage as tolerance to the sedative-hypnotic develops. The patient becomes severely dependent on the depressant, both physically and psychologically, and the drug habit becomes an essential feature in the user's daily routines. Only after severe dependence has developed does the clinician often realize what has taken place. The next stage is the unpleasant task of trying to wean the patient from the drug (**detoxification**) with as little discomfort as possible.

DETOXIFICATION elimination of a toxic substance, such as a drug, and its effects

TABLE 6.6 Prevalence of abuse of CNS depressants for twelfth-graders

Year	1980	1985	1990	1991	1992
Any Illicit Drug	37.2%	29.7%	17.2%	16.4%	14.4%
Barbiturates	2.9	2.0	1.3	1.4	1.1
Methaqualone	3.3	1.0	0.2	0.2	0.4
Other Depressants (including benzodiazepines)	3.1	2.1	1.2	1.4	1.0

Source: L. Johnston. *Seniors Drug Abuse Survey.* Lansing: University of Michigan, 1993.

Because of the similarities between alcohol and barbiturate-like drugs, it is common to see individuals who abuse both types of depressants. One of the dangers is that these people use both drugs together. Due to the synergism that exists between CNS depressants in general, such a mixture can severely suppress respiration and cardiovascular function, often with deadly consequences (Goldstein 1995). Knowledge of this dangerous interaction is quite common among the drug-using population; consequently, many suicide attempts are made by self-administering high doses of barbiturate-like drugs with a chaser of ethanol.

As with other drugs of abuse, the prevalence of illicit CNS depressant use has declined (see Table 6.6). However, in 1990 CNS depressant drugs, such as the benzodiazepines and barbiturates, were involved in approximately 15% of the total deaths and 15% of the total U.S. emergency room episodes due to drug overdoses (Drug Abuse Warning Network [DAWN] 1991).

At this point, an explanation is in order regarding statistics of drug use: You will note that, throughout this book, figures that report trends in drug use are usually based on samples of high school and college students—namely, teenagers and young adults. The primary reason for this is that studies based on older populations are often not done or delayed. It is difficult to survey large groups of adults in a controlled manner; student groups are much more accessible. This is true for a lot of social science research.

You could argue whether student groups are in fact representative of society as a whole. Can findings about drug use among teens and young adults be extrapolated in this manner? It is a legitimate question. We argue that such findings are representative in the sense that they probably predict future drug use. Research has shown that patterns of drug use established in youth will likely be maintained later in life. Thus, current trends in drug use by society's youngest members have significant long-term implications.

Treatment for Withdrawal

All sedative-hypnotics, including alcohol and benzodiazepines, can produce physical dependence and a barbiturate-like withdrawal syndrome if taken in sufficient dosage over a long-enough period. Withdrawal symptoms include anxiety, tremors, nightmares, insomnia, anorexia, nausea, vomiting, seizures, delirium, and maniacal activity.

The duration and severity of withdrawal depends on the particular drug taken. With short-acting depressants—such as pentobarbital, secobarbital, and methaqualone—withdrawal symptoms tend to be more severe. They begin 12 to 24 hours after the last dose and peak in intensity between 24 and 72 hours later. Withdrawal from longer-acting depressants—such as phenobarbital, diazepam, and chlordiazepoxide—develops more slowly and is less intense; symptoms peak on the fifth to eighth day (Jaffe 1990).

Not surprisingly, the approach to detoxifying a person dependent on a sedative-hypnotic depends on the nature of the drug itself (that is, to which category of depressants it belongs), the severity of the dependence, and the duration of action of the drug. The general objectives of detoxification are to eliminate drug dependence (both physical and psychological) in a safe manner while minimizing discomfort. Having achieved these objectives, it is hoped that the patient will be able to remain free of dependence on all CNS depressants.

Often the basic approach for treating severe dependence on sedative-hypnotics is substitution of either pentobarbital or the longer-acting phenobarbital for the offending, usually shorter-acting, CNS depressant. Once substitution has occurred, the long-acting barbiturate dose is gradually reduced. Using a substitute is necessary because abrupt withdrawal for a person who is physically dependent can be dangerous and cause life-threatening seizures. This substitution treatment uses the same rationale as the treatment of heroin withdrawal by methadone replacement. Detoxification also includes supportive measures such as vitamins, restoration of electrolyte balance, and prevention of dehydration. The patient must be watched closely during this time because he or she will be apprehensive, mentally confused, and unable to make logical decisions (Jaffe 1990).

If the person is addicted to both alcohol and barbiturates, the phenobarbital dosage must be increased to compensate for the double withdrawal. Many barbiturate addicts who go to a hospital for withdrawal are also dependent on heroin. In such cases, the barbiturate dependence should be dealt with first because the associated withdrawal can be life threatening. Detoxification from any sedative-hypnotic should be done under close medical supervision, most often in a hospital (Jaffe 1990).

It is important to remember that elimination of physical dependence does not necessarily result in a cure. The problem of psychological dependence can be much more difficult to deal with. If an individual is abusing a CNS depressant because of emotional instability, personal problems, or a very stressful environment, eliminating physical dependence alone will not solve the problem. Drug dependence is likely to recur because the cause of the problem has not been addressed. These types of patients require intense psychological counseling and must be trained to deal with their problems in a more constructive and positive fashion. Without such psychological support, benefits from detoxification will only be temporary, and therapy will ultimately fail.

Review Questions

1. Why have benzodiazepine drugs replaced the barbiturates as the sedative-hypnotic drugs most prescribed by physicians?
2. Which features of CNS depressants give them abuse potential?
3. Why is long-term use of the benzodiazepines more likely to cause dependence than short-term use?
4. Why are some physicians careless when prescribing benzodiazepines for patients suffering from severe anxiety?
5. Currently sleep aid products are available over the counter. Should the FDA also allow sedatives to be sold without a prescription? Support your answer.
6. Are there any real advantages to using barbiturates as sedatives or hypnotics? Should the FDA remove them from the market?
7. What types of people are most likely to abuse CNS depressants? Suggest ways to help these people avoid abusing these drugs.
8. What dangers are associated with treating individuals who are severely dependent on CNS depressants?

Key Terms

sedatives
anxiolytics
hypnotics
amnesiac
anesthesia
REM sleep
paradoxical
anticholinergic
detoxification

Summary

1. Several unrelated drug groups cause CNS depression, but only a few are actually used clinically for their depressant properties. The most frequently prescribed CNS depressants are benzodiazepines including drugs such as Valium, Xanax, and Halcion. Barbiturates once were popular but, because of their severe side effects, they are not used by most clinicians. Much like barbiturates, drugs such as chloral hydrate, glutethimide, and methaqualone are little used today. Finally, some antihistamines, such as diphenhydramine, hydroxyzine, and promethazine, are still occasionally used for their CNS depressant effects.
2. The clinical value of CNS depressants is dose dependent. At low doses, these drugs relieve anxiety and promote relaxation (sedatives). At higher doses, they can cause drowsiness and promote sleep (hypnotics). At even higher doses, some of the depressants cause anesthesia and are used for patient management during surgery.
3. Because CNS depressants help to relieve anxiety and reduce stress, they are viewed as desirable by many people. But if used frequently over long periods, they can cause tolerance that leads to dependence.
4. The principal reason benzodiazepines have replaced barbiturates in the treatment of stress and insomnia is that benzodiazepines have a greater margin of safety and are less likely to alter sleep patterns. Benzodiazepines enhance the GABA transmitter system in the brain, while the effects of barbiturates are less selective. Even though benzodiazepines are safer than barbiturates, dependence and significant withdrawal problems can result if the drugs are used indiscriminately.
5. Often benzodiazepine dependence occurs with patients who suffer stress or anxiety disorders and are under a physician's care. If the physician is not careful and the cause of the stress is not resolved, drug treatment can drag on for weeks or months. After prolonged therapy, tolerance develops to the drug, so that when benzodiazepine use is stopped, withdrawal occurs, which itself causes agitation. What is really a rebound response to the drug might appear as the effects of emotional stress, so use of benzodiazepine is continued until the patient becomes severely dependent.
6. The short-acting CNS depressants are preferred for treatment of insomnia. These drugs help the patient get to sleep and then are inactivated by the body; when the user awakes the next day, he or she is less likely to experience residual effects than with long-acting drugs. The short-acting depressants are also preferred for abuse because of their relatively fast and intense effects. In contrast, the long-acting depressants are better suited to treating persistent problems such as anxiety and stress. The long-acting depressants are also used to help wean dependent people from their use of the short-acting compounds such as alcohol.
7. Although at one time very popular, methaqualone is no longer legally available in the United States due to abuse problems. Even so, methaqualone continues to be found in the "streets" because it is smuggled across the Mexican and Canadian borders into the United States.
8. Many antihistamines cause sedation and drowsiness due to their anticholinergic effects. Several of these agents are useful for short-term relief of anxiety and are available in OTC sleep aids. The effectiveness of these CNS depressants is usually less than that of benzodiazepines. Because of their anticholinergic actions, antihistamines can cause some annoying side effects and are not likely to be used for long periods; thus, dependence or abuse rarely develops.
9. The people most likely to abuse CNS depressants include individuals who (a) use drugs to relieve continual stress; (b) paradoxically feel euphoria and stimulation from depressants; (c) use depressants to counteract the unpleasant effects of other drugs of abuse, such as stimulants; and (d) combine depressants with alcohol and heroin to potentiate the effects.
10. The basic approach for treating dependence

on CNS depressants is to detoxify in a safe manner while minimizing discomfort. This is achieved by substituting a long-acting barbiturate or benzodiazepine, such as phenobarbital or Valium, for the offending CNS depressant. The long-acting drug causes less severe withdrawal symptoms over a longer period of time. The dependent person is gradually weaned from the substitute drug until depressant free.

References

American Medical Association (AMA), Committee on Alcoholism and Addiction, Dependence on Barbiturates and Other Sedative Drugs. *JAMA* 193 (1965): 673–77.

American Psychiatric Association. "Substance Related Disorders." In *Diagnostic and Statistical Manual of Mental Disorders,* 4th ed. *[DSM-IV],* Allen Frances, chairperson, 175–272. Washington, DC: American Psychiatric Association, 1994.

"British Spark U.S. Debate by Banning Halcion Sales." *Salt Lake Tribune* (3 October 1991): A-2.

Carlini, E. "Preliminary Note: Dangerous Use of Anticholinergic Drugs in Brazil." *Drug and Alcohol Dependence* 32 (1993): 1–7.

Crabtree, B. "Substance Use Disorders." In *Pharmacotherapy, A Pathophysiological Approach,* edited by J. DiPiro, 697–713. New York: Elsevier, 1989.

DAWN (Drug Abuse Warning Network). Series 1, no. 10-A and 10-B, NIDA, DHHS Publication no. (ADM) 90-1839 and 90-1840. Washington, DC: U.S. Government Printing Office, 1991.

Goldstein, A. "Pharmacological Aspects of Drug Abuse." In *Remington's Pharmaceutical Sciences,* 19th ed., edited by A. R. Gennaro. Easton, PA: 1995.

"Halcion and Other Sleeping Pills." *Wellness Letter* 8 (July 1992): 3.

Harvey, S. C. "Hypnotics and Sedatives." In *The Pharmacological Basis of Therapeutics,* 6th ed., edited by A. Gilman, L. Goodman, and A. Gilman. New York: Macmillan, 1980.

Hays, R. "Drug Abuse in General Practice." *Medical Journal of Australia* 156 (1992): 782–84.

"High Anxiety." *Consumer Reports* (January 1993): 19–24.

Jaffe, J. "Drug Addiction and Drug Abuse." In *The Pharmacological Basis of Therapeutics,* 8th ed., edited by A. Gilman, T. Rall, A. Nies, and P. Taylor. New York: Pergamon, 1990.

Julien, R. "General Nonselective Central Nervous System Depressants." In *A Primer of Drug Action,* 6th ed., 51–70. New York: Freeman, 1992.

McEvoy, G., ed. *American Hospital Formulary Service Drug Information.* Bethesda, MD: American Society of Hospital Pharmacists, 1994.

Miller, L., and D. Greenblatt. "Neurochemistry of the Benzodiazepines." In *Drugs of Abuse and Neurobiology,* edited by Ronald Watson, 175–83. Ann Arbor, MI: CRC Press, 1992.

Mondanaro, J. *Chemically Dependent Women.* Lexington, MA: Lexington Books/Heath, 1988.

"New Halcion Guidelines." *American Druggist* (January 1992): 14.

Pagliaro, L., and A. Pagliaro. "Drug Induced Aggression." *Medical Psychotherapist* (Newsletter of the American Board of Medical Psychotherapists) 8 (Fall 1992): 1.

Rall, T., and S. Schleifer. "Drugs Effective in the Therapy of the Epilepsies." In *The Pharmacological Basis of Therapeutics,* 8th ed., edited by A. Gilman, T. Rall, A. Nies, and P. Taylor. New York: Pergamon, 1990.

Reuters News Service. "Consumer Group Calls Halcion Dangerous, Urges Immediate Ban." *Salt Lake Tribune* 244 (23 July 1992): A-8.

Smith, D. E., D. R. Wesson, and R. B. Seymour. "The Abuse of Barbiturates and Other Sedative-Hypnotics." In *Handbook on Drug Abuse,* edited by R. I. DuPont, A. Goldstein, and J. H. O'Donnell. Washington, DC: National Institute on Drug Abuse/U.S. Department of Health, Education, and Welfare, 1979.

"Top 200 Drugs of 1992." *Pharmacy Times* (April 1993): 30–32.

Woods, J., J. Katz, and G. Winger. "Benzodiazepines: Use, Abuse and Consequences." *Pharmacological Reviews* 44 (1992): 155–323.

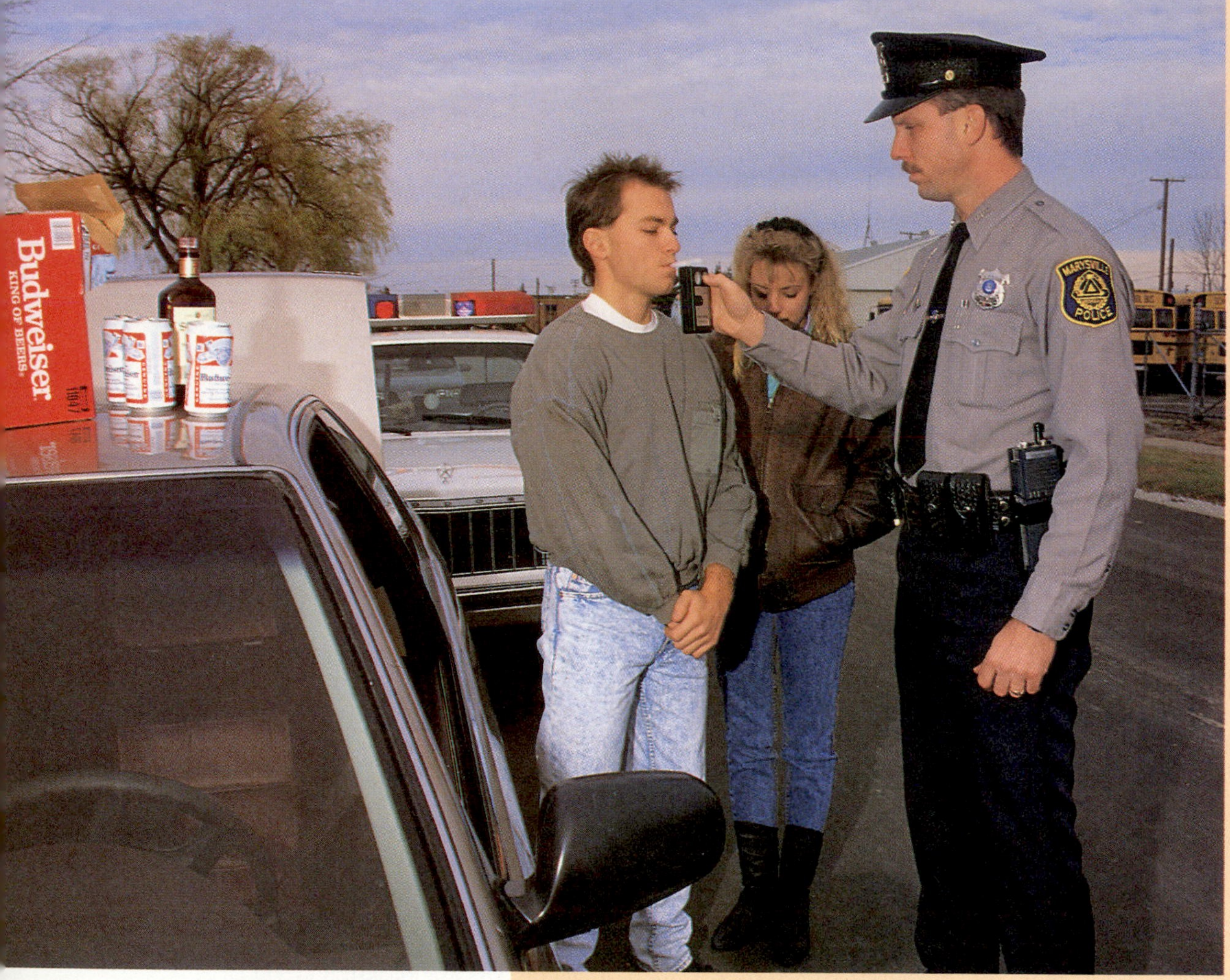

Chapter 7

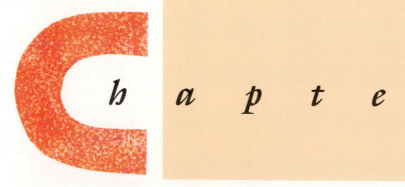

Alcohol

Pharmacological

Effects

DID YOU KNOW THAT . . .

- The Egyptians had breweries over 6,000 years ago.
- Ethyl alcohol is fit for human consumption and is found in alcohol beverages; other alcohols are poisonous to humans.
- The first recorded beer brewery was in existence in 3700 B.C.
- In some communities, malt liquors are called "liquid crack."
- Woman reach a higher blood alcohol level than men even when consuming the same amount of alcohol.
- Alcohol used in combination with other drugs (polydrug use) ranks first as the most frequently reported drug in medical emergencies and deaths.
- The lethal level of alcohol is between 0.4 and 0.6% by volume in the blood.
- Fetal alcohol syndrome (FAS) is characterized by facial deformities, growth deficiencies, and mental retardation.
- The liver metabolizes alcohol at a slow and constant rate unaffected by the amount ingested.
- Among alcoholics, liver disorders are the most common causes of death.

LEARNING OBJECTIVES

On completing this chapter, you will be able to

1. Explain why alcohol is a drug.
2. Identify three types of poisonous alcohols and name the fourth type, which is used in alcoholic beverages.
3. Explain the concepts of absorption, distribution, and elimination.
4. Describe the factors that affect the concentration of alcohol in the blood.
5. Name the short-term physical effects of drinking alcohol at low and moderate doses.
6. Name the possible physical effects of prolonged heavy alcohol consumption.
7. Describe fetal alcohol syndrome and its effects.
8. Explain how prolonged consumption of alcohol affects the brain and nervous system, liver, digestive system, blood, cardiovascular system, sexual organs, endocrines, kidneys, mental disorder and damage to the brain, and the fetus.

Healthy People 2000

Reduce the proportion of high school seniors and college students engaging in recent occasions of heavy drinking of alcoholic beverages to no more than 28% of high school seniors and 32% of college students.

Increase to at least 20 the number of states that have enacted statutes to restrict promotion of alcoholic beverages that is focused principally on young audiences.

In this chapter and the next, we will be looking at alcohol. This chapter focuses on how from a pharmacological perspective alcohol affects the body. The next chapter, as indicated by its title, studies the social effects of this drug; mainly, the effects and consequences of alcohol on our social life.

As a licit drug, alcohol is not only extensively promoted socially through advertising, but more importantly, drinking is perceived as normal. Given the popularity of this drug, as recently shown by the 1993 National Household Survey on Drug Abuse that 83% of the U.S. population has used alcohol in 1992 (National Institute on Drug Abuse [NIDA] 1993), this chapter focuses on the many adverse effects of alcohol on the human body. Overall, *this chapter provides the reader with a foundation on which to develop a largely pharmacological understanding of alcohol as a drug.* We hope that such an understanding of how this drug affects the various organ systems of the body will lead to more responsible use and less abuse of alcohol.

Alcohol as a Drug

Alcohol (more precisely designated as **ethanol**) is a natural product of fermentation, an extremely popular social beverage and the second most widely used and abused of all the psychoactive drugs (next to caffeine). Alcohol is a central nervous system depressant that is considered a *psychoactive* substance because it affects both brain and body functions. This drug is also an addictive drug in that it may produce a physical and behavioral dependence. ("Centerpiece" 1993). Tradition and attitude play a powerful role in the use patterns of this substance, but the typical consumer rarely appreciates the diversity of pharmacological effects caused by alcohol, the drug. The pharmacological action of alcohol accounts for both its pleasurable and CNS effects as well as its hazards to health and public safety.

ETHANOL the consumable type of alcohol that is the psychoactive ingredient in alcoholic beverages; often called *grain alcohol*

SOCIAL LUBRICANT the belief that drinking (misconceived as safe) that represses inhibitions and strengthens extraversion leads to increased sociability

FERMENTATION the biochemical process in which yeast converts sugar into alcohol

DISTILLATION heating fermented mixtures of cereal grains or fruits in a still to evaporate and be trapped as purified alcohol

Alcohol as a Social Drug

We begin by answering the question posed earlier: Why is alcohol often perceived as an acceptable adjunct to such celebrations as parties, birthdays, weddings, anniversaries, and as a way of relieving stress and anxiety? Social psychologists refer to the perception of alcohol as a ***social lubricant.*** This means that drinking is misconceived as a safe drug promoting conviviality, social interaction, and as an activity that bolsters confidence by repressing inhibitions and strengthening extraversion. Why do many people have to be reminded that alcohol is a drug like tobacco, marijuana, and cocaine? There are four reasons for this misconception: (1) the use of alcohol is legal; (2) through widespread advertising, the media promote the notion that alcohol consumption is as normal as drinking fruit juices and soft drinks; (3) the distribution or the sale of alcoholic beverages is widely practiced; and (4) alcohol use has a very long history, dating back to 30,000 B.C. (Royce 1989, 28).

Impact of Alcohol

Although many consider the effects of alcohol enjoyable and reassuring, the adverse pharmacological impact of this drug is extensive and its effects are associated with more than 100,000 deaths each year in the United States. In 1990, alcohol-related traffic accidents killed more than 22,000 people in this country. At some time during their lives, almost 50% of all Americans will be involved in an alcohol-related traffic accident ("Centerpiece" 1993). The pharmacological effects of alcohol abuse cause severe dependence; disrupt personal, family, social, and professional functioning; and frequently result in multiple illnesses and accidents, violence, and crime. Alcohol consumed during pregnancy can lead to devastating damage to offspring and is the principal cause of mental retardation in newborns. Next to tobacco, alcohol is the leading cause of premature death in America. Experts have estimated that in the United States approximately $136 billion are spent annually dealing with social and health problems resulting from the pharmacological effects of alcohol (Samson and Harris 1992). However, such estimates fall short of assessing the emotional upheaval and human suffering caused by this drug ("Centerpiece" 1993).

Despite all of alcohol's problems, banning access to this drug is not acceptable in our free society. However, it is equally unthinkable to ignore the tremendous negative social impact of this drug. There are no simple answers to this dilemma, yet clearly governmental and educational institutions could do more to protect members of society against the dangers of alcohol. The best weapons we have against the problems of alcohol are education, prevention, and treatment (see Chapter 16).

The Nature and History of Alcohol

Alcohol has been part of human culture since the beginning of recorded history. The technology for alcohol production is ancient. Several basic ingredients and conditions are needed: sugar, water, yeast, and warm temperatures.

The process of making alcohol, called **fermentation,** is a natural one. It occurs in ripe fruit and berries and even in honey that wild bees leave in trees. These substances have sugar and water and are found in warm climates, where yeast spores are transported through the air. Animals such as elephants, baboons, birds, wild pigs, and bees will seek and eat fermented fruit. Elephants under the influence of alcohol have been observed bumping into one another and stumbling around. Intoxicated bees fly an unsteady beeline toward their hives. Birds eating fermented fruit become so uncoordinated that they cannot fly, or if they do, they crash into windows or branches.

Fermented honey, called *mead,* may have been the first alcoholic beverage. The Egyptians had breweries 6,000 years ago; they credited the god Osiris with introducing wine to humans. The ancient Greeks used a large amount of wine and credited the god Bacchus (or Dionysus) with introducing the drink. Today, we use the words *bacchanalia* and *dionysian* to refer to revelry and drunken events. The Hebrews were also heavy users of wine. The Bible mentions that Noah, just nine generations after Adam, made wine and became drunk.

Alcohol is produced by a single-celled microscopic organism, one of the yeasts, which by a metabolic form of combustion breaks down sugar, releasing carbon dioxide and forming water and ethyl alcohol as a waste product. Carbon dioxide creates the foam on a glass of beer and the fizz in champagne. Fermentation continues until the sugar supply is exhausted or the concentration of alcohol reaches the point at which it kills the yeast (12 to 14%). Thus, 12 to 14% is the natural limit of alcohol found in fermented wines or beers.

The **distillation** device, or *still,* was developed by the Arabs around A.D. 800 and was introduced into medieval Europe around A.D. 1250 (see Figure 7.1). By boiling the fermented drink and gathering the condensed vapor in a pipe, a still increases the concentration of alcohol, potentially up to 50% or more. Because distillation made it easier for people to get drunk, it greatly intensified the problem of alcohol abuse. However, even before the arrival of the still, alcoholic beverages had been known to cause problems in heavy users. It had been noticed that some individuals were sensitive to alcoholic beverages and became dependent on them.

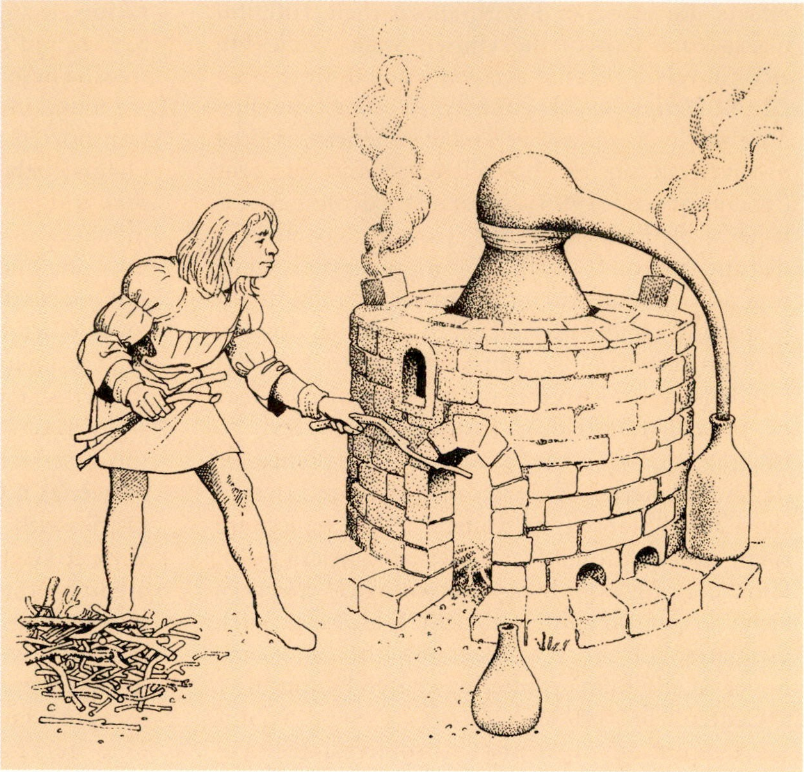

FIGURE 7.1 A medieval still

The Properties of Alcohol

Technically alcohol is a chemical structure that has a hydroxyl group (OH, for one oxygen and one hydrogen atom) attached to a carbon atom. Of the many types of alcohol, several are important in this context. The first is **methyl alcohol** (methanol, or wood alcohol), so called because it is made from wood products. Its metabolites are poisonous. Small amounts (4 ml) cause blindness, affecting the retina, and larger amounts (80 ml to 150 ml) are usually fatal (Ritchie 1980). Methyl alcohol is added to ethyl alcohol (ethanol or grain alcohol, the drinking type) intended for industrial use so that people will not drink it. The mixture known as *denatured alcohol methyl alcohol* is sometimes found added to "bootleg" liquor.

Another type of poisonous alcohol, **ethylene glycol,** is used in antifreeze, and a third type, **isopropyl alcohol,** is commonly used as rubbing alcohol and as an antiseptic (a solution for preventing the growth of micro-organisms). They are also poisonous if consumed. Pure ethyl alcohol (ethanol) is recognized as an official drug in the U.S. pharmacopoeia, although the various alcoholic beverages as such are no longer listed for medical use.

Alcohol can be used as a solvent for other drugs or as a preservative in tinctures and elixirs. It is used to cleanse, disinfect, and harden the skin and to reduce sweating. A 70% alcohol solution is an effective bactericide. However, it should not be used on open wounds because it will dehydrate the injured tissue and make damage worse. Since it cools the skin by evaporation, alcohol-saturated sponges are commonly used to reduce fever. Alcohol may be used as a solvent for the irritating oil in poison ivy and may prevent the formation of rash if used quickly enough after contact. Alcohol may be deliberately injected in or near nerves to treat severe pain; it causes local anesthesia and deterioration of the nerve. For the elderly or convalescent who enjoys it, a drink of ethanol before meals may appear to improve appetite and digestion (Ritchie 1980). In small amounts, ethanol alcohol is used by many physicians as a CNS depressant or sedative for convalescent and geriatric patients.

In all alcoholic beverages—beer, wine, liqueurs or cordials, and distilled spirits—the psychoactive agent is the same: ethanol. The concentration of alcohol is usually about 4% by volume in U.S. beers; 4 to 7% in wine coolers; 10 to 12% in table wines; 17 to 20% in cocktail and dessert wines, such as sherries; 22 to 50% in liqueurs; and 40 to 50% (80 to 100 proof) in distilled spirits. The amount of alcohol is expressed either as a percentage by volume or in the older proof system, based on the military assay method. To make certain that they were getting a high alcohol content in the liquor, the British military would place a sample on gunpowder and touch a spark to it. If the alcohol content was over 50%, it would burn and ignite the gunpowder. This was "proof" that there was at least 50% alcohol. If the distilled spirits were "under proof," the water content would prevent the gunpowder from igniting. The percentage of alcohol volume is one-half the proof number. For example, 100-proof whiskey has a 50% alcohol content.

In addition, alcoholic beverages contain a variety of other chemical constituents, some of which come from the original grains, grapes, and other fruits and some of which come from added flavorings or colorings. Other constituents are produced during fermentation, distillation, or storage. These nonalcoholic constituents, called **congeners,** contribute to the effects of certain beverages, either directly affecting the body or affecting the rate at which the alcohol content is absorbed into the blood. Congeners are oils and other alcohols that exist in alcoholic beverages; some congeners are very toxic. Only small amounts of congeners are found when alcohol is formed. Beers and wines contain organic compounds, minerals, and salts, none that are toxic. The higher-molecular-weight alcohols, or fusel oils, are toxic, but usually found in such low concentrations that there is no appreciable hazard. Vodka and gin tend to have lower concentrations of congeners than whiskeys and rum.

The Physical Effects of Alcohol

How does alcohol work in the body? Figure 7.2 graphically illustrates how alcohol is absorbed into the body. The body is affected by alcohol in two ways. First, alcohol has direct contact with the mouth, esophagus, stomach, and intestine, acting as an irritant and an **anesthetic** (blocking sensitivity to pain). Second, alcohol influences almost every organ system in the body after entering the bloodstream. Alcohol diffuses into the blood rapidly after consumption by passing (absorption process) through gastric and intestinal walls. Once the alcohol is in the small intestine, its absorption is largely independent of the presence of food, unlike the stomach, where food retards absorption.

The effects of alcohol on the human body depend on the amount of alcohol in the blood or BAC (blood alcohol concentration). This concentration largely determines behavioral and physical responses to alcoholic beverages. On the behavioral side, the drinking situation, the drinker's mood, and his or her attitude and previous experience with alcohol all contribute to the reaction to drinking. People have individual patterns of psychological functioning that may affect their reactions to alcohol, as well. For instance, the time it takes to empty the stomach may be either slowed down or speeded up by anger, fear, stress, nausea, and the condition of the stomach tissues.

The blood alcohol level produced depends on the presence of food in the stomach, the rate of alcohol consumption, the concentration of the

METHYL ALCOHOL wood alcohol or methanol

ETHYLENE GLYCOL alcohol used as antifreeze

ISOPROPYL ALCOHOL rubbing alcohol, sometimes used as an anesthetic

CONGENERS nonalcoholic substances found in alcoholic beverages

ANESTHETIC a drug that blocks sensitivity to pain

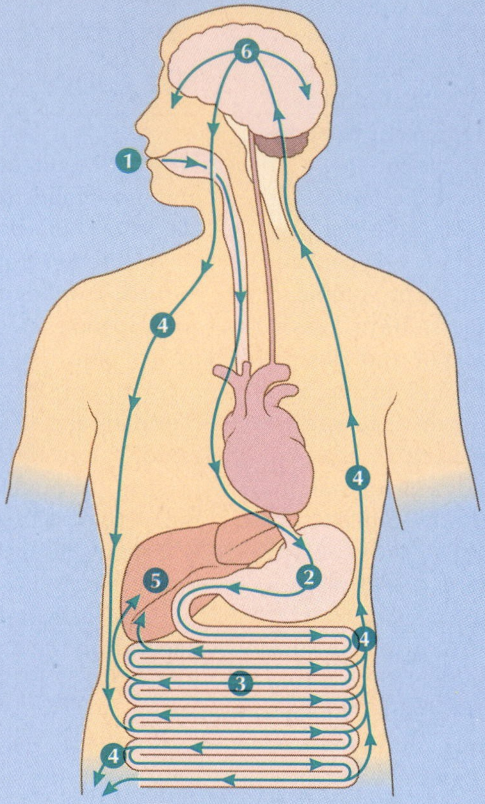

1. Mouth.—Alcohol is drunk.
2. Stomach.—Alcohol goes right into the stomach. A little of the alcohol goes through the wall of the stomach and into the bloodstream. But most of the alcohol goes down into the small intestine.
3. Small intestine.—Alcohol goes from the stomach into the small intestine. Most of the alcohol then goes through the walls of the intestine and into the bloodstream.
4. Bloodstream.—The bloodstream then carries the alcohol to all parts of the body, such as the brain, heart, and liver.
5. Liver.—As the bloodstream carries the alcohol around the body, it carries it through the liver too. The liver changes the alcohol to water, carbon dioxide, and energy. The process is called *oxidation*. The liver can oxidize (change into water, carbon dioxide, and energy) only about one-half ounce of alcohol an hour. This means that until the liver has time to oxidize all of the alcohol, the alcohol keeps on passing through all parts of the body, including the brain.
6. Brain.—Alcohol goes to the brain almost as soon as it is drunk. The bloodstream carries it there. Alcohol keeps passing through the brain until the liver has had time to change (oxidize) all the alcohol into carbon dioxide, water, and energy.

FIGURE 7.2 How alcohol is absorbed in the body *Source:* National Institute on Alcohol Abuse and Alcoholism. *Alcohol Health and Research World.* Washington, DC: U.S. Department of Health and Human Services, 1988.

alcohol, and the drinker's body composition. Fatty foods, meat, and milk slow the absorption of alcohol, allowing more time for its metabolism and reducing the peak concentration in the blood. When alcoholic beverages are taken with a substantial meal, peak blood alcohol concentrations (BACs) may be as much as 50% lower than they would have been had the alcohol been consumed by itself. When large amounts of alcohol are consumed in a short period, the brain is exposed to higher peak concentrations. Generally, the more alcohol in the stomach, the greater the absorption rate. There is, however, a modifying effect of very strong drinks on the absorption rate. The absorption of drinks stronger than 100 proof is inhibited. This may be due to blocked passage into the small intestine or irritation of the lining of the stomach, causing mucus secretion, or both.

The presence of congeners in alcoholic beverages also modifies the rate of absorption. High concentrations of congeners slow alcohol absorption. The net result is that the effects of beer and wine are felt more slowly than those of distilled spirits, even when the same amounts of alcohol are consumed. Diluting an alcoholic beverage with water also helps to slow down absorption, but mixing with carbonated beverages increases the absorption rate. The carbonation causes the stomach to empty its contents into the small intestine more rapidly, causing a more rapid "high." The carbonation in champagne has the same effect.

Once in the blood, distribution occurs as the alcohol uniformly diffuses throughout all tissues and fluids, including fetal circulation in pregnant women. Because the brain has a large blood supply, its activity is quickly affected by a high alcohol concentration in the blood. Body composition—the amount of water available for the alcohol to be dissolved in—is a key factor in blood alcohol concentration and distribution. The greater the muscle mass, the lower the blood alcohol concentration that will result from a given amount of alcohol. This is because muscle has more fluid volume than does fat. For example, the blood alcohol level produced in a 180-pound man drinking 4 ounces of whiskey will be substantially lower than that of an equally muscular 130-pound man drinking the same amount over the same period. The heavier man will show fewer effects. A woman of a weight equivalent to a given man will have a higher blood alcohol level because women on average have a higher percentage of fat. Thus, they will be affected more by identical drinks.

Alcoholic beverages have almost no vitamins, minerals, protein, or fat—just large amounts of carbohydrates. Alcohol cannot be used by most cells; it must be metabolized by an enzyme (alcohol dehydrogenase) that is found almost exclusively in the liver. Alcohol provides more calories per gram than carbohydrate or protein and only slightly less than pure fat. Because alcohol does provide calories, the drinker's appetite may be satisfied, and he or she may not eat properly, causing malnutrition. The tolerance developed to alcohol is comparable to that of barbiturates (see Chapter 6). Some people have a higher tolerance for alcohol and can more easily disguise intoxication.

Alcohol and Tolerance

Repeated use of alcohol results in tolerance and in a reduction in many of alcohol's pharmacological effects. As with other psychoactive drugs, tolerance to alcohol encourages increased consumption to regain its effects and can lead to severe physical and psychological dependence (Samson and Harris 1992). Tolerance to alcohol is similar to that seen with CNS depressants, such as the barbiturates and benzodiazepines. It consists of both an increase in the rate of alcohol metabolism (due to induction of metabolizing enzymes—see Chapter 4) and a reduced response by neurons and transmitter systems (particularly those related to the transmitter substance, GABA) to this drug. Development of tolerance to alcohol is extremely variable, allowing some users to consume large quantities of this drug with minor pharmacological effects. The tolerance-inducing changes caused by alcohol can also alter the body's response to other drugs (referred to as *cross-tolerance;* see Chapter 4) and specifically reduce the effects of some other CNS depressants (Sellers and Bendayan 1987).

Many chronic alcohol users learn to compensate for the motor impairments of this drug by modifying their patterns of behavior. These adjustments are referred to as **behavioral tolerance** and are not due to changes in the manner in which alcohol affects the body. Rather, chronic alcohol users learn to modify their motor behavior in order to mask the actions of the drug and avoid the negative consequence of excessive drinking. For example, such individuals may alter and slow their speech, walk more deliberately, or move more cautiously to hide the fact that they have consumed debilitating quantities of alcohol.

Experiencing the Effects of and Metabolizing Alcohol

For the effects of drugs to be experienced, they must reach the brain. Drugs can be administered in the following manners: oral, injection (intravenous, intramuscular, subcutaneous), inhalation, or application to mucous membranes either by mouth or nose (intranasal). After the drug is administered, the body absorbs, distributes, and finally eliminates the drug.

Absorption occurs through the body's circulatory system. In essence, the drug molecules reach the

BEHAVIORAL TOLERANCE compensation of motor impairments by chronic alcohol users through behavioral pattern modification

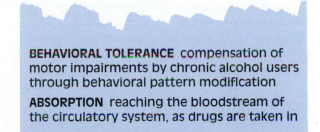

ABSORPTION reaching the bloodstream of the circulatory system, as drugs are taken in

bloodstream when absorption occurs. When drugs are swallowed, often the mouth initially absorbs the drug before entering the stomach. **Distribution** involves a drug entering the bloodstream as it moves to the site of action. Whatever amount of the drug reaches the brain produces and causes the drug effect. Drugs rapidly move throughout the body within seconds. The last process is **elimination.** Both in the absorption and distribution process, the body is affected by the drug. In the last stage, the body exercises control over the drug for elimination purposes. Excretion is a process of removing the drug from the body. Excretion mainly occurs in the lungs, sweat, tears, tissues, saliva, mucus secreted through the nose, bile, urine, and mother's milk (White 1991).

When any drug is taken, the body immediately begins to metabolize it and eventually excrete it. Metabolizing is processing, the breakdown of molecules by enzymes. "About 95% of the alcohol [orally administered] is metabolized by the liver before it is excreted at the rate of about one-third of an ounce of pure alcohol per hour in the normal, healthy individual. The other 5% of the alcohol is excreted unchanged through the lungs and skin, as well as through urine" (Schuckit 1984). The rate of metabolizing or processing alcohol is approximately one can of beer or other single 8–12 ounce alcoholic beverage per hour.

The liver metabolizes alcohol at a slow and constant rate unaffected by the amount ingested. Thus, if 1 can of beer is consumed each hour, the blood alcohol level (BAL) will remain constant without resulting in intoxication. In essence, if 24 cans of beer are consumed—1 per hour—the drinker will never experience alcohol intoxication because the liver is maintaining parity with the alcohol consumed. If however, more alcohol is consumed per hour, the BAC will rise proportionately to the amount of alcohol consumed during short drinking intervals. The liver metabolizes alcohol or any drug at a set pace. Large amounts of alcohol that cannot be metabolized spill over into the bloodstream, increasing the BAC level. Such factors as the presence of food in the stomach, time of day, and tolerance to alcohol slows the rate of alcohol consumption beyond the metabolism occurring. The liver, weighing about 3 pounds, is the most important organ involved in metabolizing drugs. Through its extensive network of enzymes, it metabolizes lipids, carbohydrates, and proteins. This "no nonsense" organ also stores vitamins, iron, and nutrients, and detoxifies such harmful compounds as dyes, food preservatives, pesticides, and drugs.

Polydrug Use

Using alcohol with other drugs is known as **polydrug use.** Mixing alcohol with other types of drugs can intensify intoxication. For example, alcohol combined with other depressant drugs such as barbiturate and benzodiazepine tranquilizers can produce lethal results. Some surveys show that as many as 60% of high school and college students often mix alcohol with marijuana and, to a lesser extent, mix alcohol with marijuana and cocaine (Royce 1989, 6). In a recent report from the National Institute on Drug Abuse, alcohol used in combination with other drugs ranked first in 1985 as the most frequently reported drug in medical emergencies and deaths, accounting for 21,090 emergencies (including deaths) nationwide. In 1990, alcohol in combination with other drugs also ranked first, with cocaine second, as the most frequently reported drugs in emergency rooms, with a combined total of 115,162 cases (National Institute on Drug Abuse [NIDA] 1991).

Short-Term Effects

The impact of alcohol on the central nervous system (CNS) is most similar to that of sedative-hypnotic agents such as barbiturates. Alcohol depresses CNS activity at all doses, producing definable results.

At low to moderate doses, **disinhibition** occurs, which is the loss of conditioned reflexes due to depression of inhibitory centers of the brain. This results from the depression of inhibitory centers in the brain. The effects on behavior are variable and somewhat unpredictable. To a large extent, the social setting and mental state determine the individual's response to such alcohol consumption. For example, alcohol can cause one person to become euphoric, friendly, and talkative but can cause another to become aggressive and hostile. Low to moderate doses also interfere with motor activity, reflexes, and coordination. Often this impairment isn't apparent to the affected person.

In moderate quantities, alcohol slightly increases the heart rate; slightly dilates blood vessels in the arms, legs, and skin; and moderately lowers blood pressure. It stimulates appetite, increases production of gastric secretions, and markedly stimulates urine output.

At higher doses, the social setting has little influence on the expression of depressive actions of the alcohol. The CNS depression incapacitates the individual, causing difficulty in walking, talking, and thinking. These doses tend to induce drowsiness and cause sleep. If large amounts of alcohol are consumed rapidly, severe depression of the brain system and motor control area of the brain occurs, producing uncoordination, confusion, disorientation, stupor, anesthesia, coma, and even death.

The lethal level of alcohol is between 0.4 and 0.6% by volume in the blood. Death is caused by severe depression of the respiration center in the brain stem, although the person usually passes out before drinking this much. Though an alcoholic person may metabolize the drug more rapidly, the alcoholic toxicity level of alcohol stays about the same. In other words, it takes approximately the same amount of alcohol to kill a nondrinker as to kill a drunk. The amount of alcohol required for anesthesia is very close to the toxic level, which is why it would not be a useful anesthetic. See Table 7.1 for a summary of the psychological and physical effects of various blood alcohol concentration levels.

As a rule, it takes as many hours as the number of drinks consumed to sober up completely. Drinking black coffee, taking a cold shower, breathing pure oxygen, and so forth will not hasten the process. Stimulants such as coffee may help keep the drunk person awake but will not improve judgment or motor reflexes to any significant extent. Drinking coffee only produces a wide-awake drunk.

Because of the disinhibition, relaxation, and sense of well-being mediated by alcohol, some degree of psychological dependence often develops, and the use of alcoholic beverages at social gatherings becomes routine. Unfortunately, many people become so dependent on the psychological influences of alcohol that they become compulsive, continually consuming it. These individuals can be severely handicapped because of their alcohol dependence and are often unable to function normally in society. People who have become addicted to this drug are called **alcoholics.**

Because of the psychological effects, physical dependence also results from the regular consumption of large quantities of alcohol. The consequence becomes apparent when ethanol use is abruptly interrupted and withdrawal symptoms result. For example, during abstinence alcohol-dependent individuals can experience periods of rebound hyperexcitability marked by anxiety, agitation, confusion, insomnia, and delirium. The excitation might progress to convulsions and death. Short-term, intermittent episodes of mild to moderate alcohol consumption appear to exert only reversible and transient effects on the CNS. However, the extended use of large quantities of alcohol have been associated with permanent brain damage and dementia (destruction of thinking capabilities).

The Hangover A familiar aftereffect of overindulgence is fatigue combined with nausea, upset stomach, headache, sensitivity to sounds, and ill temper—the hangover ("Centerpiece" 1993). The symptoms are usually most severe many hours after drinking, when little or no alcohol remains in the body. There is no simple explanation for what causes the hangover (other than having had too much to drink). Theories include accumulation of acetaldehyde (a metabolite of ethanol), dehydration of the tissues, poisoning due to tissue deterioration, depletion of important enzyme systems

DISTRIBUTION the movement of a drug in the bloodstream throughout the body

ELIMINATION the final stage, in which the body exercises control over a drug by means of excretion (getting rid of the drug)

POLYDRUG USE using other types of drugs with alcohol

DISINHIBITION the loss of conditioned reflexes due to depression of inhibitory centers of the brain

ALCOHOLIC a person who is addicted to alcohol

TABLE 7.1 Psychological and physical effects of various blood alcohol concentration levels

Number of Drinks[a]	Blood Alcohol Concentration	Psychological and Physical Effects
1	0.02–0.03%	No overt effects, slight mood elevation
2	0.05–0.06%	Feeling of relaxation, warmth; slight decrease in reaction time and in fine muscle coordination
3	0.08–0.09%	Balance, speech, vision, hearing slightly impaired; feelings of euphoria, increased confidence; loss of motor coordination
	0.10%	Legal intoxication in most states; some have lower limits
4	0.11–0.12%	Coordination and balance becoming difficult; distinct impairment of mental faculties, judgment
5	0.14–0.15%	Major impairment of mental and physical control; slurred speech, blurred vision, lack of motor skills
7	0.20%	Loss of motor control—must have assistance in moving about; mental confusion
10	0.30%	Severe intoxication; minimum conscious control of mind and body
14	0.40%	Unconsciousness, threshold of coma
17	0.50%	Deep coma
20	0.60%	Death from respiratory failure

Note: For each hour elapsed since the last drink, subtract 0.015% blood alcohol concentration, or approximately one drink.

[a] One drink = one beer (4% alcohol, 12 oz.) or one highball (1 oz. whiskey).

Source: Modified from data given in Ohio State Police Driver Information Seminars and the National Clearinghouse for Alcohol and Alcoholism Information, 5600 Fishers Lane, Rockville, MD 85206.

needed to maintain routine functioning, an acute withdrawal (or rebound) response and metabolism of the congeners in alcoholic beverages.

The body loses fluid in two ways through alcohol's **diuretic** action: (1) the water content, such as in beer, will increase the volume of urine, and (2) the alcohol depresses the center in the hypothalamus of the brain that controls release of a water conservation hormone (antidiuretic hormone). With less of this hormone, urine volume is further increased. Thus, after drinking heavily, especially the highly concentrated forms of alcohol, the person is thirsty. However, this by itself does not explain the symptoms of hangover.

The type of alcoholic beverage you drink may influence the hangover that results. Some people are more sensitive to particular congeners than others. For example, some drinkers have no problem with white wine but an equal amount of some red wine will give them a hangover. Whiskeys, scotch, and rum may cause worse hangovers than vodka or gin, given equal amounts of alcohol, because vodka and gin have fewer congeners. There is little evidence that mixing different types of drinks per se causes a worse hangover. What is more likely is that more than the usual amount of alcohol is consumed because of trying a variety of drinks.

A common technique for treating a hangover is to take a drink of the same alcoholic beverage that caused the hangover. This is called "taking the

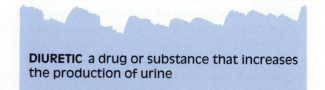

DIURETIC a drug or substance that increases the production of urine

hair of the dog that bit you" (from the old notion that the burnt hair of a dog is an antidote to its bite). This might help the person who is physically dependent, the same way giving heroin to a heroin addict will ease the withdrawal symptoms. The "hair of the dog" method might work by depressing the centers of the brain that interpret pain or by relieving a withdrawal response. Also consider the psychological factors involved in having a hangover; distraction or focusing attention on something else may ease the effects.

Another folk remedy is to take an analgesic compound like an aspirin-caffeine combination before drinking. Aspirin would help control headache; the caffeine may help counteract the depressant effect of the alcohol. These ingredients would have no effect on the actual sobering-up process. Products such as aspirin, caffeine, and Alka-Seltzer can irritate the stomach lining to the point where the person feels worse.

Long-Term Effects

Light or moderate drinking apparently does little permanent harm. (The exception is moderate drinking during pregnancy, in which case alcohol has little effect on the mother but can cause irreversible mental retardation in her child.) As we will see in the next section, when taken in large doses over long periods of time, alcohol can cause structural damage to several major organs. Summarized here are the following long-term effects of alcohol on various major organs of the body:

1. Prolonged heavy drinking can seriously damage nearly every organ and function of the body ("Centerpiece" 1993). One essential organ affected by alcohol is the heart, the myocardium. Laboratory investigations have shown that high concentrations of alcohol are directly toxic to the heart, and this effect can be fatal.
2. Heavy alcohol consumption also affects the kidneys and can cause liver damage (discussed further in the next section).
3. Heavy drinking over many years may result in serious mental disorders and permanent, irreversible damage to the brain and peripheral nervous system.
4. Heavy drinkers have lowered resistance to pneumonia and other infectious diseases.
5. Alcohol, especially when undiluted, irritates the gastrointestinal tract. Nausea, vomiting, and diarrhea are mild indications of trouble.

Effects of Alcohol on Organ Systems and Bodily Functions

As mentioned earlier, blood alcohol concentration depends on the size of the person, presence of food in the stomach, speed in drinking, amount of carbonation, and the ratio of muscle mass to body fat. Furthermore, we mentioned that alcohol has pervasive effects on the major organs and fluids of the body. The pervasive effects of alcohol on bodily organs are discussed in greater detail in the next section.

Brain and Nervous System

Every part of the brain and nervous system is affected and can be damaged by alcohol (Figure 7.3). "Initially, alcohol depresses subcortical inhibitions of the control centers of the cerebral cortex, resulting in disinhibition. In higher doses, alcohol depresses the cerebellum, resulting in slurred speech and staggering gait. In very high doses, alcohol can depress the respiratory centers of the medulla, resulting in death" (Levin 1990, 23). Furthermore, alcohol impairs the production and functioning of transmitters such as the dopamine and serotonin neurotransmitters, and neuromodulators such as the GABA and brain hormones. These neurochemical effects contribute to the fact that alcohol consumption can aggravate underlying psychiatric disorders such as depression and schizophrenia ("Centerpiece" 1993).

Liver

Among alcoholics, liver disorders are the most common causes of death (Hall 1985). How important is the liver? Royce (1989) calls it the body's chemical laboratory, where the following are manufactured: "bile, glycogen, albumin, globulin, prothombin and other substances for fighting in-

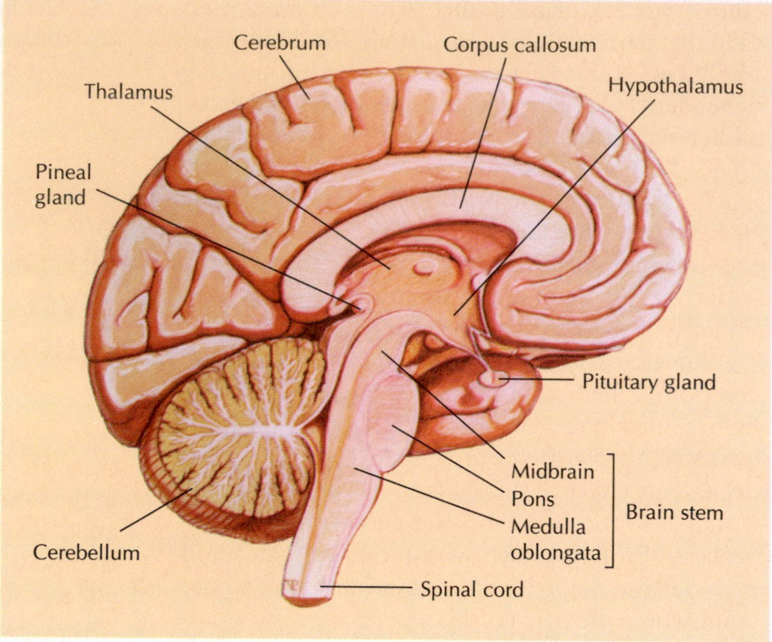

FIGURE 7.3 The principal control centers of the brain affected by alcohol consumption. Note also that all areas of the brain are interconnected.

fection, blood clotting (hence alcoholics show more bruises and bleeding), and general health. . . . The liver controls the levels of cholesterol, fatty acids, and triglycerides, which harm both liver and cardiovascular system" (Royce 1989, 63).

Among alcoholics, liver disorders are the most common causes of death (Hall 1985). There are three stages of alcohol-induced liver disease (see Figure 7.4). The first stage is known as *alcoholic fatty liver.* Essentially, liver cells increase the production of fat, which leads to a buildup of fat, resulting in an enlarged liver (Goldstein 1983). This direct toxic effect on liver tissue is known as **hepatotoxic effect.** This effect is reversible and can disappear if alcohol use is stopped. Several days of drinking five or six drinks of alcoholic beverages produce fatty liver in males. For females, as little as two drinks of hard liquor per day several days in a row can produce the same condition. After several days, if the drinker abstains from alcohol the liver returns to normal.

The second stage develops as the fat cells continue to multiply. Generally, irritation and swelling that result from continued alcohol intake causes **alcoholic hepatitis.**

At this stage, chronic inflammation sets in and this alone can be fatal. This second stage is also reversible if the intake of alcohol ceases.

Unlike stage 1 and 2, stage 3 is not reversible. Scars begin to form on the liver tissue during the third stage. These scars are fibrous, and they cause hardening of the liver as it shrinks and deteriorates. This condition of the liver is known as **cirrhosis,** where "the dead cells create acids that kill off more liver cells. Cirrhosis is the fifth leading cause of death among alcoholics and the third leading cause of death in males aged 25–65" (Royce 1989, 63) and affects approximately 15% of the alcoholic population.

Digestive System

The digestive system consists of structures involved in processing and digesting food and liquids, and includes the mouth, pharynx, esophagus, stomach, and small and large intestines. As alcohol travels through the digestive system, it irritates tissue and can even damage the tissue lining as it causes acid imbalances, inflammation, and acute gastric distress. Often the result is gastritis and heartburn. The more frequently consumption takes place, the greater the irritation; one out of three heavy drinkers suffers from chronic gastritis. Furthermore, the heavy drinker has double the probability of developing cancer of the mouth and other tis-

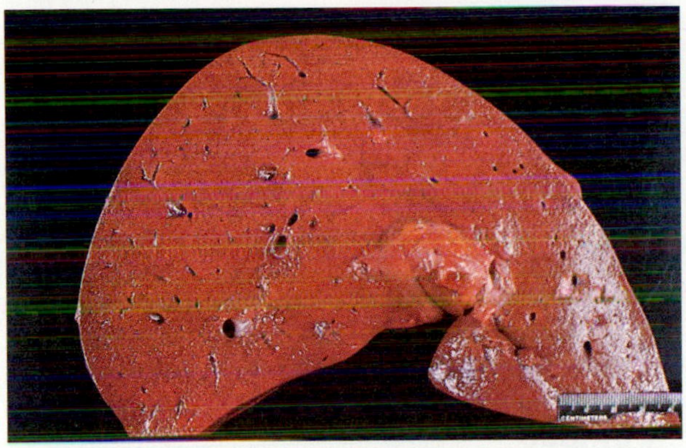

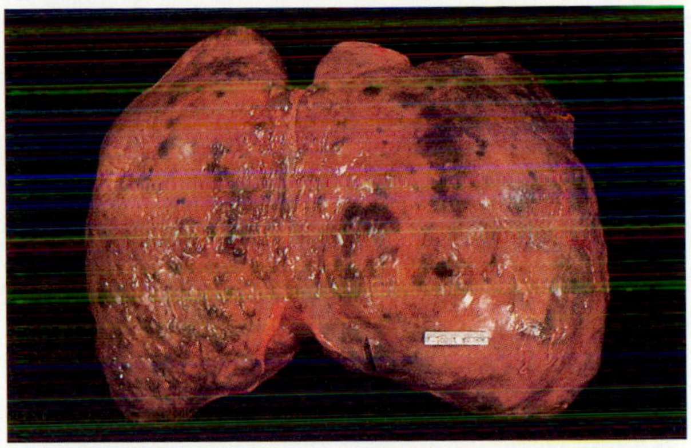

FIGURE 7.4 A normal liver as it would be found in a healthy human body. An abnormal liver that exhibits the effects of moderate to heavy alcohol consumption.

sues as alcohol passes these two organs on the way to the stomach.

Prolonged heavy use of alcohol may cause ulcers, hiatal hernia, and cancers in the digestive tract. The likelihood of cancers in the mouth, throat, and stomach dramatically increases (15 times) if the person is also a heavy smoker ("Centerpiece" 1993). The pancreas is another organ associated with the digestive system that can be damaged by heavy alcohol consumption. Alcohol can cause pancreatitis, pancreatic cirrhosis, and alcoholic diabetes ("Centerpiece" 1993).

Blood

Alcohol diminishes the effective functioning of the hematopoietic (blood-building) system. It decreases production of red blood cells, white cells, and platelets. Problems with clotting and immunity to infection are not uncommon among alcohol abusers. Often the result is lowered resistance to disease. Heavy drinking appears to affect the bone marrow, where various blood cells are formed. The suppression of the bone marrow contributes to alcoholic anemia, in which red blood cell production cannot keep pace with the need (Aldo-Benson 1988). Heavy drinkers are also likely to develop alcoholic bleeding disorders because they have too few platelets to form clots (Seixas 1980).

HEPATOTOXIC EFFECT when liver cells increase the production of fat, resulting in an enlarged liver

ALCOHOLIC HEPATITIS the second stage of alcohol-induced liver disease in which chronic inflammation occurs; reversible if alcoholic consumption ceases

CIRRHOSIS scarring of the liver and destruction of fibrous tissues; results from alcohol abuse. Once cirrhosis begins, it is irreversible.

Cardiovascular System

The effects of ethanol on the cardiovascular system have been extensively studied, but much is still unknown. Ethanol causes dilation of blood vessels, especially in the skin. This effect accounts for the flushing and sensation of warmth associated with alcohol consumption.

The long-term effects of alcohol on the cardiovascular system are dose dependent. Recent studies have demonstrated that regular light to moderate drinking (two drinks or less of wine a day) reduces heart diseases such as heart attacks, strokes, and high blood pressure. The type of alcoholic beverage consumed does not appear to be important as long as the quantity of alcohol consumed is moderate (1 to 2.5 ounces per day) (Margen 1992). Although the precise explanation for this coronary benefit is not known, it appears to be related to the effects of moderate alcohol doses in relieving stress and increasing the blood concentration of high-density lipoproteins (HDL). HDL is a molecular complex used to transport fat through the bloodstream, and its levels are negatively correlated with cardiovascular disease. In contrast, heavy drinking is a good way to *cause* heart disease.

Intense use of alcohol changes the composition of heart muscle by replacing it with fat and fiber, resulting in a heart muscle that becomes enlarged and flabby. Congestive heart failure from **alcoholic cardiomyopathy** often occurs when heart muscle is replaced by fat and fiber. Other results of alcohol abuse that affect the heart are irregular heartbeat or arrhythmia, high blood pressure, and strokes. A common example of damage is "holiday heart," so called because people drinking heavily over a weekend turn up in the emergency room with a dangerously irregular heartbeat. Chronic excessive use by people with arrhythmia causes congestive heart failure. Malnutrition and vitamin deficiencies associated with prolonged heavy drinking contribute to cardiac abnormalities (Ritchie 1980).

Sexual Organs

Although alcohol lowers social inhibition, its use interferes with sexual functioning. As Shakespeare said in *Macbeth,* alcohol "provokes desire, but it takes away the performance." Continued alcohol use causes prostatitis, which is an inflammation of the prostate gland. This condition directly interferes with the male's ability to maintain an adequate erection. Another frequent symptom of alcohol abuse is atrophy of the testicles, which results in lowered sperm count and diminished hormones in the blood.

Endocrines

Endocrine glands release hormones into the bloodstream. The hormones function as messengers that directly affect cell and tissue development. Alcohol abuse alters endocrine functions by influencing the production and release of hormones, and affects the hypothalamus, pituitary, and gonads. Because of alcohol abuse, there may be a reduction of testosterone (the male sex hormone), resulting in sexual impotence, breast enlargement, and loss of bodily hair in males. Females experience menstrual delays, ovarian abnormalities, and infertility.

ALCOHOLIC CARDIOMYOPATHY congestive heart failure due to the replacement of heart muscle with fat and fiber

FETAL ALCOHOL SYNDROME (FAS) a condition affecting children born to alcohol-consuming mothers that is characterized by facial deformities, growth deficiency, and mental retardation

Kidneys

Smaller than a fist, the kidneys weigh approximately 4 oz. and are the primary organs responsible for excretion. The kidneys' primary function is to strain the blood and remove both useless and/or used material after absorption. Consistent abuse of alcohol damages kidney functioning, resulting in improper (1) secretion of hormones, (2) production of vitamin D, and (3) regulation of the pH balance of the blood plasma. In addition to liver disease, alcoholics experience more urinary tract infections than do nondrinkers or moderate drinkers.

Mental Disorder and Damage to the Brain

Long-term heavy drinking can severely affect memory, judgment, and learning ability. Wernicke-Korsakoff's syndrome is a characteristic psychotic condition caused by alcohol use and the associated nutritional and vitamin deficiencies. Patients who are brain damaged (Royce 1989, 70) cannot remember recent events and compensate for their memory loss with confabulation (making up fictitious events that even the patient accepts as fact). Peripheral neuropathy (formerly called *neuritis*) initially begins with pain in the calf muscles and an inflammation of the nerves that causes burning and prickly sensations in the hands and feet and has the same origin. B-complex vitamins are often used to treat neuropathies and memory deficit, but the damage is not always reversible (Seixas 1980; Royce 1989).

The Fetus

In pregnant women, alcohol easily crosses the placenta and often damages the fetus in cases of moderate to excessive drinking. Fetal alcohol syndrome (discussed next) results in smaller babies and facial abnormalities. Spontaneous abortions may occur in women who abuse alcohol while pregnant.

Fetal Alcohol Syndrome A condition affecting children born to alcohol-consuming mothers, **fetal alcohol syndrome (FAS)** is characterized by facial deformities, growth deficiency, and mental retardation. Women who are alcoholics or who drink heavily during pregnancy have a higher rate of spontaneous abortion, suggesting that alcohol is toxic to the developing embryo. Infants born to alcoholic mothers have a high probability of being afflicted with fetal alcohol syndrome (FAS). These children have a characteristic pattern of facial deformities (see Figure 7.5), growth deficiency, joint and limb irregularities (Royce 1989), and mental retardation. The growth deficiency occurs in embryonic development, and the child usually does not catch up after birth. The mild to moderate mental retardation does not appear to improve with time, apparently because the growth impairment affects growth of the brain as well.

The severity of FAS appears to be dose–response related: the more the mother drinks, the more severe the fetal damage. A safe lower level of alcohol consumption has not been established for pregnant women ("Centerpiece" 1993). Birthweight decrements have been found at levels corresponding to about two drinks per day, on average. Clinical studies have established that alcohol clearly causes the syndrome; it is not related to the effects of smoking, maternal age, parity (number of children a woman has borne), social class, or poor nutrition (Streissguth et al. 1980; Streissguth and LaDue 1985; Royce 1989). Studies in experimental animals show that ethanol by itself can cause all the damage associated with FAS (Brown et al. 1979; Clarren et al. 1988; Miller 1988, 1987).

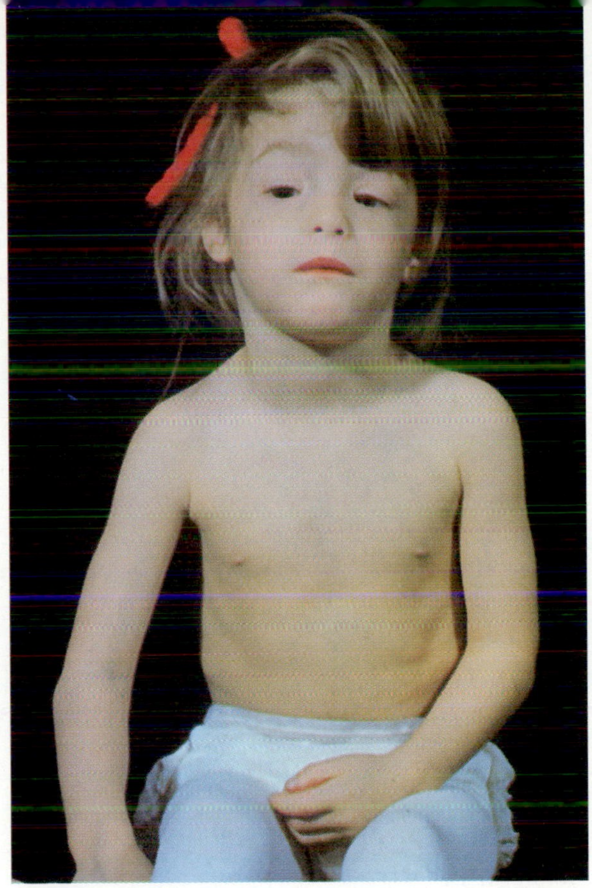

FIGURE 7.5 Fetal alcohol syndrome (FAS) is characterized by facial deformities, as well as growth deficiency and mental retardation.

Thus alcohol has the ability to damage most major organs of the body. The damage from alcohol can be direct or indirect. Direct damage involves the effect of repeated alcohol abuse on particular cells, organs, and tissues. Indirect damage results from alteration of the chemical environment in the body.

Review Questions

1. What evidence is there that alchohol is a drug like marijuana, cocaine, or heroin?
2. Explain how alcohol is made.
3. In the Western world, alcohol use has a long history. List and discuss some of these historical events.
4. Explain how alcohol affects the mouth, stomach, small intestine, brain, liver, and the bloodstream.
5. List at least five factors that affect the absorption rate of alcohol in the bloodstream.

6. List at least three short-term and three long-term effects of alcohol abuse.
7. Describe the symptoms and causes of a hangover.
8. What characterizes fetal alcohol syndrome?
9. In two sentences or less for each, how does alcohol abuse affect the normal functioning of brain and nervous system, liver, digestive system, blood, heart, sexual organs, endocrines, kidneys, and the fetus?

Key Terms

ethanol
social lubricant
fermentation
distillation
methyl alcohol
ethylene glycol
isopropyl alcohol
congeners
anesthetic
behavioral tolerance
absorption
distribution
elimination
polydrug use
disinhibition
alcoholic
diuretic
hepatotoxic effect
alcoholic hepatitis
cirrhosis
alcoholic cardiomyopathy
fetal alcohol syndrome (FAS)

Summary

1. Alcohol is a drug because it is a central nervous system depressant, and it affects both the mind and body functioning.
2. Three types of poisonous alcohols are methyl alcohol made from wood products; ethylene glycol, used as antifreeze; and isopropyl alcohol used as an antiseptic. The fourth type, ethanol, is the alcohol used for drinking purposes.
3. Absorption is the process in which the drug molecules reach the bloodstream, and occurs through the body's circulatory system. Distribution involves a drug moving through the bloodstream to the site of action. Elimination is the process of excreting the drug from the body.
4. The blood alcohol concentration (BAC) produced depends on the presence of food in the stomach, the rate of alcohol consumption, the concentration of alcohol, and the drinker's body composition.
5. Alcohol depresses CNS (central nervous system) activity at all doses. Low to moderate doses of alcohol interfere with motor activities, reflexes, and coordination. In moderate quantities, alcohol slightly increases heart rate; slightly dilates blood vessels in the arms, legs, and skin; and moderately lowers blood pressure. It stimulates appetite, increases production of gastric secretions, and at higher doses markedly stimulates urine output. The CNS depression incapacitates the individual, causing difficulty in walking, talking, and thinking.
6. Long-term heavy alcohol use directly causes serious damage to nearly every organ and function of the body.
7. Prolonged heavy drinking causes various types of muscle disease and tremors. Heavy alcohol consumption causes irregular heartbeat, affects the kidneys and commonly damages the liver. Heavy drinking over many years results in serious mental disorders and permanent, irreversible damage to the brain and peripheral nervous system. Memory, judgment, and learning ability can deteriorate severely.
8. Women who are alcoholics or who drink heavily during pregnancy have a higher rate of

spontaneous abortions. Infants born to drinking mothers have a high probability of being afflicted with fetal alcohol syndrome. These children have characteristic patterns of facial deformities, growth deficiency, joint and limb irregularities, and mental retardation.

9. Alcohol has pervasive effects on the major organs and fluids of the body. Every part of the brain and nervous system is affected and can be damaged by alcohol. Among alcoholics, liver disorders include alcoholic fatty liver, alcoholic hepatitis, and cirrhosis. Alcohol also irritates tissue and damages the digestive system. Heavy use of alcohol seriously affects the blood, heart, sexual organs, the endocrines, and kidneys, and as mentioned, damages the fetus.

References

Aldo-Benson, M. A. "Alcohol Directly Suppresses b Cell Response to Antigen." *Federation Proceedings* 2, no. 6 (1988): 9–12.

Brown, N. H., E. H. Goulding, and S. Fabro. "Ethanol Embryotoxicity: Direct Effects on Mammalian Embryos in Vitro." *Science* 206 (1979): 573–75.

Clarren, S. K., S. J. Astley, and D. M. Bowden. "Physical Anomalies and Developmental Delays in Nonhuman Primate Infants Exposed to Weekly Doses of Ethanol During Gestation." *Teratology* 37 (1988): 561–69.

"Centerpiece: Alcohol in Perspective." *Wellness Letter* 9 (February 1993): 4–6.

Doweiko, H. *Concepts of Chemical Dependency.* Pacific Grove, CA: Brooks/Cole, 1990.

Goldstein, D. B. *Pharmacology of Alcohol.* New York: Oxford University Press, 1983.

Hall, P., ed. *Alcoholic Liver Disease: Pathology, Epidemiology, and Clinical Aspects.* New York: Wiley, 1985.

Levin, J. D. *Alcoholism: A Bi-Psycho-Social Approach.* New York: Hemisphere, 1990.

Margen, S. "Ask the Expert." *Wellness Letter* 9 (1993): 8.

Miller, M. W. "Effect of Prenatal Exposure to Ethanol on the Development of Cerebral Cortex: I." *Alcoholism* 12 (1988): 440–49.

Miller, M. W. "Effect of Prenatal Exposure to Alcohol on the Distribution and Time of Origin of Corticospinal Neurons in the Rat." *Journal of Contemporary Neurology* 257 (1987): 372–82.

National Institute on Drug Abuse (NIDA). *NIDA Capsules.* Capsule 18. U.S. Department of Health and Human Services. Rockville, MD: NIDA, April 1988.

National Institute on Drug Abuse (NIDA). *Annual Emergency Room Data, 1990.* Statistical Series. DAWN, Series 1, No. (ADM) 10-A, DHHS Publication no. 91-1839. Washington, DC: U.S. Government Printing Office, 1991.

National Institute on Drug Abuse (NIDA). *Preliminary Estimates from the 1992 National Household Survey on Drug Abuse: Selected Excerpts.* Advance Report no. 3. Rockville, MD: NIDA, 1993.

Ritchie, J. M. "The Aliphatic alcohols." In *The Pharmacological Basis of Therapeutics,* 6th ed., edited by G. Gilman, L. S. Goodman, and A. Gilman. New York: Macmillan, 1980.

Royce, J. E. *Alcohol Problems and Alcoholism: A Comprehensive Survey.* New York: Free Press, 1989.

Samson, H., and R. Harris. "Neurobiology of Alcohol Abuse." *Trends in Pharmacological Sciences* 13 (1992): 206–11.

Schuckit, M. A. *Drug and Alcohol Abuse: A Clinical Guide to Diagnosis and Treatment,* 2d ed. New York: Plenum Press, 1984.

Seixas, F. A. "The Medical Complications of Alcoholism." In *Alcoholism: A Practical Treatment Guide,* edited by S. E. and H. S. Peyser Gitlow, 165–80. New York: Grune & Stratton, 1980.

Sellers, E., and R. Bendayan. "Pharmacokinetics of Psychotropic Drugs in *Selected Patient Populations." In Psychopharmacology: The Third Generation of Progress,* edited by H. Meltzer, 1397–1406. New York: Raven Press, 1987.

Streissguth, A. P., S. Landesman–Dwyer, J. C. Martin, and D. W. Smith. "Teratogenic Effects of Alcohol in Humans and Laboratory Animals." *Science* 209 (1980): 353–61.

Streissguth, A. P., and R. LaDue. "Psychological and Behavioral Effects in Children Prenatally Exposed to Alcohol." *Alcohol Health and Research World* 10, no. 1 (Fall 1985): 6–12.

White, Jason M. *Drug Dependence.* Englewood Cliffs, NJ: Prentice-Hall, 1991.

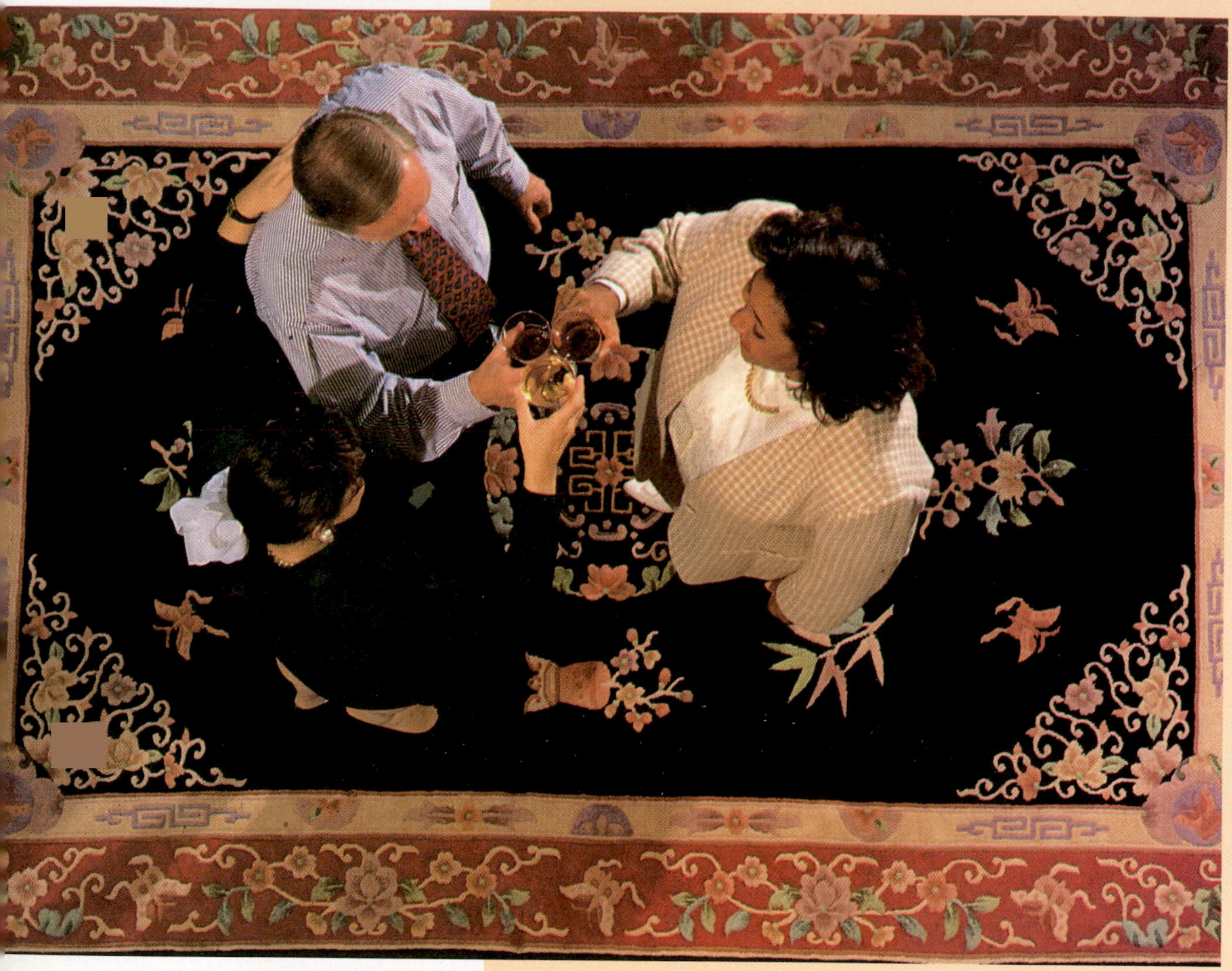

Chapter 8

DID YOU KNOW THAT . . .

- Alcohol kills over 100,000 people annually.
- Approximately 100 million Americans drink alcohol, and between 10 and 15 million are alcoholics.
- Problem drinking and alcoholism cost the United States well over $70 billion yearly.
- In 85% of homicides, either the attacker, the victim, or both had been drinking.
- In 50% of motor vehicle crashes, alcohol was involved.
- In the United States, alcohol consumption has dropped sharply since 1981.
- The higher the household income, the higher the percentage is of those who drink.
- Women are less likely to drink than men.
- In a recent National Institute on Drug Abuse (NIDA) study, 54% of eighth-graders, 72% of tenth-graders, and 77% of twelfth-graders reported drinking in the past year.
- African Americans have high rates of abstinence from alcohol and low rates of heavy drinking.
- Of all U.S. minority groups, Asian Americans have the highest rates of abstinence, the lowest rates of heavy drinking, and the lowest levels of drinking-related problems.
- Most people who consume alcohol do not develop into problem drinkers.
- Children of alcoholics are two to four times more likely to develop alcoholism.

Alcohol

A Behavioral Perspective

LEARNING OBJECTIVES

On completing this chapter, you will be able to

1. Discuss the ways in which ethanol use is costly for our society.
2. Discuss how beer, wines, rum, and whiskey relate to American history.
3. Discuss the main events of the temperance movement and the Prohibition era.
4. Define *set* and *setting*, and explain how these two processes affect alcohol consumption.
5. Name four different positions cultures may take regarding alcohol consumption. Give examples of cultures that exemplify each attitude toward drinking.
6. Cite four reasons why alcohol consumption has been decreasing since 1981.
7. List the major findings regarding alcohol consumption in America by social class and by religious, regional, gender, age, and youth groups.

continued

Healthy People **2000**

Reduce deaths caused by alcohol-related motor vehicle crashes to no more than 8.5 per 100,000 people.

Extend to 50 states legal blood alcohol concentration tolerance levels of 0.04% for motor vehicle drivers aged 21 and older and 0.00% for those younger than age 21.

LEARNING OBJECTIVES

8 Explain what social and psychological similarities exist among racial and ethnic minorities, gays, and the homeless in terms of their abuse of alcohol.
9 Define *alcoholism,* and cite the general characteristics of a typical alcoholic.
10 State the major causes of alcoholism according to the moral and medical models, psychological explanations, psychopathological theory, social learning and reinforcement theories, and sociological theories.
11 Define and explain *codependency* and *enabling.*
12 Describe children of alcoholics, and explain why these children are important to study.
13 Explain the differences between primary and secondary prevention.
14 Identify two stages of treatment for alcoholism, and name three helping agencies for treatment.

The Pervasive Costs of Alcohol Use

The term *alcohol* refers to a class of chemical agents that possess very diverse properties. In everyday usage, however, the word *alcohol* refers to the specific agent **ethanol** (ethyl alcohol, or grain alcohol) that belongs to this family of chemicals. Ethanol is the psychoactive ingredient found in so-called alcoholic beverages. Oddly enough, because of its availability and high degree of acceptance in U.S. society, ethanol is unique in that most individuals do not consider it a true drug but rather a **social substance.** As a result of this casual attitude toward ethanol, people are not as cautious about its consumption as they are about administering other equally potent or controlled drugs. The tragic consequences, which will be discussed at length throughout this chapter, are almost beyond comprehension. The misuse of ethanol and its impact on society far exceeds that of any other psychoactive substance, either legal or illegal.

ETHANOL the consumable type of alcohol that is the psychoactive ingredient in alcoholic beverages; often called *grain alcohol*

SOCIAL SUBSTANCE alcohol when it is not perceived as a drug

How Serious Is Alcohol Consumption?

Alcohol use continues to be one of the most used and abused drugs in our nation today (Moskowitz 1989, 54). Approximately 100 million Americans drink alcohol (Liska 1990, 218; Royce 1989, 20), and between 10 and 15 million are alcoholics (Doweiko 1990). Alcohol-related consequences affect not only drinkers themselves but also their spouses, children, friends, and employers, as well as strangers with whom they may come in contact.

There are 18 million problem drinkers in the United States and approximately 23,000 alcohol-related traffic deaths per year ("In These Times" 1989). In addition to traffic accidents, alcohol-involved injuries and deaths, serious medical consequences, and birth defects, alcohol abuse has been implicated in violence, crime, marital discord, suicide, and job loss.

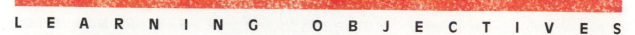

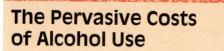

There are also serious economic consequences. Problem drinking and alcoholism cost the United States over $90 billion yearly (U.S. Department of Health and Human Services 1992): about 46% in

lost production, 29% in health and medical costs, 13% in motor vehicle accidents, 7% in violent crimes, 4% in social responses (public education on highway safety, role of alcohol abuse in decreased production, and so on), and 1% in fire losses.

Alcohol in America

Historical Considerations

Alcoholic beverages have played an important role in the history of the United States. The Pilgrims stopped at Plymouth Rock instead of going farther south because "[their] victuals were much spent, especially [their] beer." A decade later, other Puritans stocked their ship, the *Arabella,* with 10,000 gallons of wine, 42 tons of beer, and 14 tons of water (Lee 1963).

Although the early settlers were straightlaced, they did not frown on drinking in moderation (Royce 1989; Levin 1990). Homemade beers and wines were an important source of fluid and nutrition for early American farmers. Sanitation was unknown, and the family well was often contaminated by human and animal wastes. Cows' milk was known to transmit "milk sickness," a disease whose symptoms included weakness, vomiting, and constipation.

Although the alcoholic content of "home brew" must have helped to make the rugged nature of pioneer life more endurable, the alcohol was primarily a preservative for the beverage. Homemade beers and wines were not purified, as commercial products are today (Royce 1989). The nutritional and medicinal value of the yeast left over from the brewing process had been recognized by people around the world for centuries. Because American colonial beers and wines were not clarified but were consumed with the spent yeast, they supplied many of the vitamins and minerals needed for good nutrition (Brown 1978).

Rum, the alcoholic essence of fermented molasses, was probably invented by the first European settlers in the West Indies. The manufacturing of rum became New England's largest and most profitable industry in the so-called triangle trade. Yankee traders would sail with a cargo of rum to the west coast of Africa, where they bargained the "demon" for slaves. From there, they sailed to the West Indies, where they bartered the slaves for molasses. They took the molasses back to New England, where it was made into rum, thus completing the triangle. For many years, the New England distilleries flourished and the slave trade proved highly lucrative. This continued until 1807, when an act of Congress prohibited the importation of slaves. About this time, too, agricultural production of corn and rye made domestic whiskey cheaper (Roueché 1960).

Whiskey production in America was introduced by a post–Revolutionary War wave of Scottish and Irish settlers to whom the making of pot-still whiskey was a natural phase of farming. Almost every home had a still or fermentation crock to make beers, wines, or whiskeys. Whiskey first came into prominence as a backwoods substitute for rum in western Maryland and Virginia, southwestern Pennsylvania, and eastern Kentucky. Because it cost more to transport a barrel of flour made from the grain than the flour would have sold for in eastern markets, farmers converted grain into whiskey.

In 1794, many of these farmers became incensed when the new U.S. government levied a tax on liquor. Because they considered whiskey an economic necessity and used it as a medium of exchange, the farmers refused to pay the tax and tarred and feathered the revenue officers. President Washington, alarmed, summoned the militia of several states under the command of Alexander Hamilton and put down the rebellion. The consequences of this insurrection were significant: the federal government was in essence strengthened, and its authority regarding the right to make and enforce federal laws was established at the expense of the local farmers.

The period of heaviest drinking in America began during Jefferson's term of office (1800–1808). The nation was going through uneasy times, trying to stay out of the war between Napoleon and the British allies. There was an increase in the transient population, especially in the seaport cities, and the migration westward had begun. Heavy drinking had become a major form of recreation and a "social lubricant" at elections and public gatherings. Thus, the temperance movement began with the goal of *temperance* in the literal sense: "moderation." In the 1830s, at the peak of this early campaign, temperance leaders (many of whom drank beer and wine) recommended abstinence only from distilled spirits. Over the next decades, partly in connection with religious revivals, the meaning of *temperance* was gradually altered from "moderation" to "total abstinence." All alcoholic beverages were attacked as being unnecessary, harmful to health, and inherently poisonous. Over the course of the nineteenth century, the demand gradually arose for total prohibition (Austin 1978).

Almost every civilized country has passed prohibition laws, but few have worked for long. Attempts to control, restrict, or abolish alcohol have been made in the United States, but they have all met with abysmal failure. From 1907 to 1919, 34 states passed prohibition laws. Finally, in 1919, the Eighteenth Amendment to the Constitution was ratified in an attempt to stop the rapid spread of alcoholic addiction. As soon as such a widely used substance became illegal, criminal activity to satisfy the huge demand for alcohol flourished. Illegal routes were developed for purchasing liquor. Numerous not-so-secret **"speakeasies"** developed as illegal places where people could buy alcoholic beverages, and "bootlegging" was a widely accepted activity. In effect, then, such developments filled the vacuum for many drinkers during Prohibition.

During this time, doctors and druggists prescribed whiskey and other alcoholic patent medicines. By 1928, doctors made an estimated $40 million per year writing prescriptions for whiskey (Austin 1978). Patent medicines flourished, with alcoholic contents as high as 50%. Whisko, a "nonintoxicating stimulant," was 55 proof (or 27.5% alcohol). Another, Kaufman's Sulfur Bitters, was labeled "contains no alcohol" but was 40 proof (20% alcohol) and did not contain sulfur. There were dozens of others, many of which contained other types of drugs, such as opium.

Both Prohibitionists and critics of the law were shocked by the violent gang wars that broke out between rivals seeking to control the lucrative "black market" in liquor. More important, a general disregard for the law developed. Corruption among law enforcement agents was widespread. Organized crime was born and grew to be an enormous "business." In reaction to these developments, political support rallied against Prohibition, resulting in its repeal in 1933 by the Twenty-First Amendment.

Since then, alcoholic beverages have had a relatively secure place in the U.S. political and social scene, with varying degrees of regulation within states and local jurisdictions. Current projections for alcohol use and abuse show little change, even across selected age groups (see Figure 8.1). In short, alcohol use starts at an early age and remains heavily ingrained in U.S. culture. Although the percentage of light to moderate *drinkers* has been decreasing, the projections of *combined alcoholics and alcohol abusers* from 1985 and 1990 shows little change. In looking at the 1995 projections, there is some decrease in the 21–34 age group. In the 35–49 age group, some noteworthy increase is expected.

Cultural Considerations

Although the alcohol content of a drug such as an alcoholic beverage has an independent effect on the user, two additional factors contribute to the alcohol content, exerting independent effects. The first factor is called set and the second is setting (Zinberg 1984; Zinberg and Robertson 1972). **Set** is the individual's expectation of what a drug will do to his or her personality. **Setting** is both the physical and social environment where the drug is consumed.

Some psychologists contend that both set and setting can overshadow the pharmacological effects of most drugs. In fact, set and setting are even more influential in determining a drug user's experience when the less immediately addictive drugs, such as alcohol and marijuana, are used, in contrast to more potent addictive drugs, such as cocaine and heroin.

David Watts (1971), a sociologist, expands the setting to include culture. He specifically points to a culture's views and attitudes regarding the consumption of alcoholic beverages. David Pittman (1967), a sociologist who has long studied the effects of alcohol, refers to four different cultural viewpoints regarding alcohol consumption:

1. In the first group are what Pittman terms **abstinent cultures,** such as the Middle Eastern cultures and the country of India, where

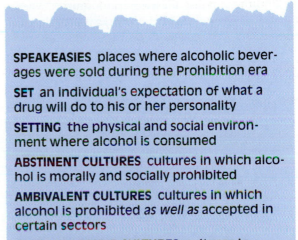

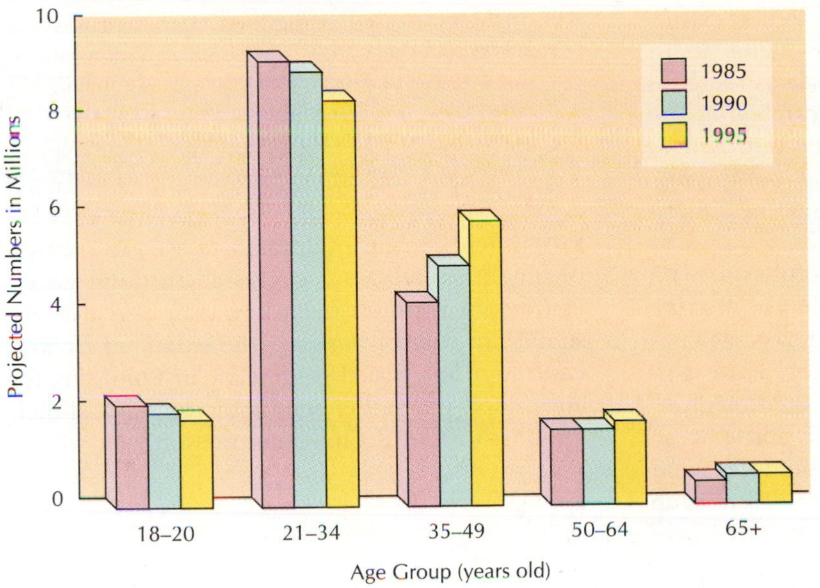

FIGURE 8.1 Projections of combined alcoholics and alcohol abusers, United States: resident, noninstitutionalized population, 1985–1995 *Source:* G. D. Williams et al., "Demographic Trends, Alcohol Abuse and Alcoholism, 1985–1995," *Alcohol Health and Research World* 11, no. 3 (1987):80–83.

alcohol is morally and socially prohibited, especially among more orthodox religious believers.

2. The second group consists of the **ambivalent cultures,** where in some regions or sectors of the culture alcohol is prohibited while, in contrast, other regions of the same culture approve its use. In the United States, for example, alcohol use is often socially and religiously prohibited in some religious communities of the Deep South while in other regions, such as Las Vegas, alcohol use is encouraged and normatively abused.
3. The third consists of **permissive cultures,** such as the Spanish and Italian. These two examples display more permissive attitudes toward the use of alcoholic beverages.
4. The last consists of **overpermissive cultures,** which use alcohol in excess, and where drinking is often viewed as an end in itself. Pittman cites as examples Camba society in eastern Bolivia, South America, and France. France and several other Scandinavian countries, such as Denmark and Finland (Pernanen 1989, 160), are examples of countries with the highest per capita rate of alcohol consumption throughout the world.

Attitudes Toward Drinking in the United States

Although cultures often maintain generalized (normative) attitudes regarding alcohol use and abuse, significant attitude differences also exist *within* cultures (Arkin and Funkhouser 1992; Inciardi 1992; Siegel 1989). As mentioned previ-

SPEAKEASIES places where alcoholic beverages were sold during the Prohibition era

SET an individual's expectation of what a drug will do to his or her personality

SETTING the physical and social environment where alcohol is consumed

ABSTINENT CULTURES cultures in which alcohol is morally and socially prohibited

AMBIVALENT CULTURES cultures in which alcohol is prohibited *as well as* accepted in certain sectors

OVERPERMISSIVE CULTURES cultures in which excessive use of alcohol is permitted

PERMISSIVE CULTURES cultures in which alcohol consumption is accepted ously, the United States is characterized as culturally ambivalent regarding alcohol use. This occurs because of dichotomies in the culture such as urban versus rural communities, and religious and ethnic differences. Other factors that contribute to diversity in attitudes include social upbringing, peer group dynamics, social class, income, education, and occupational differences.

What specific impact do such attitudes have on drinking? Attitudes are responsible for making alcohol consumption acceptable or unacceptable—or even relished as a form of behavior! For example, in one segment of impoverished African-American groups alcohol use and abuse is so common that it has become accepted behavior (Primm 1987). The following excerpt describes an accepted use of alcohol consumption.

> A party without liquor or a street rap without a bottle is often perceived as unimaginable. These attitudes about drinking are shaped as youth grow up seeing liquor stores in their communities next to schools, churches, and homes. Liquor stores and bootleg dealers frequently permeate the black residential community, where in traditionally white communities they are generally restricted to commercial or business zones. With liquor stores throughout the fabric of black residential life, black youth grow up seeing men drinking in the streets and relatives drinking at home. (Harper 1986)

Contrast this attitude with orthodox religious and fundamentalist lifestyle communities where the use of alcohol and other drugs is strictly prohibited:

> I was raised in a very religious, Seventh-Day Adventist family. My father was a pretty strong figure in our little church of 18 members. My mother stayed home most of the time, living in a way like an Old Testament kind of biblical life, so to speak. We were strict vegetarians, and all of us in the family had to be very involved with church life. The first time I ever saw alcohol outside of always hearing how corrupting it was to the mind and the body, was when I was 7. One day the father of a friend of mine—the only non-Adventist family friend I was allowed to play with—was drinking a beer in the kitchen when we walked in. I asked, "What's that?" The father's reply was "This is beer, dear John." I looked strangely at him and pretended to be amused at the father's answer. Actually, inside I remember being very surprised and scared at the same time for I was always told that people who drink alcohol were not doing what God wanted them to do in life. (Interview with an eighteen-year-old undergraduate second-year male university student, conducted by Peter Venturelli, on 21 May 1993.)

From these contrasting examples, we can see that communities of values expressed through group and family attitudes regarding drug use are very significant for determining the extent of alcohol consumption. (See also the Case in Point box for an example of another community group and their attitudes toward alcohol consumption.)

How Widespread Is Alcohol Use and Abuse?

Although estimates of consumption levels for the world's developed countries are somewhat variable, apparent per capita consumption of alcoholic beverages began to level off in most industrialized countries except the United States during the mid-1970s. And by the mid-1980s, many countries, including the United States, were experiencing declines over previous levels of consumption. Of the 25 countries surveyed between 1979 and 1989, nearly two-thirds experienced declines or stability in levels of per capita consumption. Only four of the nine countries where consumption increased had rates of increase greater than 1%. In contrast, consumption in some developing countries has continued to increase.

In the United States, alcohol consumption has dropped sharply since 1981, as is evident from data for the decade 1977 to 1987 shown in Figure 8.2. The decline in consumption of spirits led the dropoff, as shown in Figure 8.3. Beer consumption remained at the 1986 level of 1.34 gallons per capita, the lowest level of consumption since 1978 and 4% lower than the 1981 peak level of 1.39 gallons (see Figure 8.2). By 1987, for the first time in more than 10 years, wine consumption had also leveled off.

What explains the steady decline in alcohol

Case in Point

Cheap High Lures Youths to Malt Liquor "40s"

NEW YORK, April 15—The start of another "Fri-high-day" in the Bronx: With no questions asked and no proof of age demanded, a 19-year-old walks into a grocery store and buys a 40-ounce bottle of Olde English 800 malt liquor. Rejoining his friends on a stoop across the street, he lifts the fat bottle trumpet-like to his lips and gulps down the brew in loud, foamy swallows.

"It gets you nice," he says, passing the bottle to an eager friend.

"It gets you pumped up," adds the next boy. "I feel most comfortable when I'm drinking a 40."

Malt liquor—essentially beer brewed with sugar for an extra alcoholic kick—has long been popular with black and Hispanic drinkers. But in the outsize 40-ounce bottle, introduced in the late 1980's with aggressive marketing campaigns aimed at minority drinkers, it is fast becoming the intoxicant of choice for black and Hispanic youths in New York and other American cities.

Some teen-agers call malt liquor "liquid crack," in tribute to its potency. And to the dismay of drug counselors, social workers and ministers who see malt liquor as a dangerous drug in sheep's clothing, the 40-ounce bottles with brand names like King Cobra, Crazy Horse, Colt 45 and St. Ides have become an accessory to the youth-culture ensemble of baggy clothes, expensive work boots and street-hardened attitudes. "Tap the Bottle," a new song celebrating the consumption of 40-ounce malt liquor, has become a hit on the rap charts.

The essence of the 40 is its combination of size, power and price. At between $1.25 and $2.50, essentially the same as a quart bottle, and with an alcohol content of 5.6 to 8 percent, compared with 3.5 percent for regular beer, the 40-ounce malt liquor offers more punch for the money.

The brewing companies—which have long been criticized for marketing campaigns that target minority communities—argue that in selling and promoting the 40-ounce malt liquors, they are simply trying to maintain what has always been a crucial market. But to a chorus of critics, the creation and targeted marketing of the 40 is a cynical attempt to take advantage of poor youngsters in search of a cheap high. The results, they say, can be dangerous and occasionally disastrous, not least because of a misimpression that malt liquor is a relatively harmless pleasure.

"They are becoming alcoholics and don't even know it," said Eric Brent, a recovering cocaine addict who is the founder of Rescue, an anti-addiction program in the Hunts Point section of the Bronx. "Denial is such a monster in their lives."

The precise dimensions of the phenomenon are unknowable. But industry analysts say that in the last few years, malt liquor has become the fastest-growing segment of the beer market. And drug counselors and health officials say that while they know of no studies of malt-liquor consumption by young people in the inner city, they see signs of increasing underage drinking linked to the availability of the large bottles.

Seen as Alternative to Drugs

The popularity of the 40's comes as drug-treatment experts and the police are reporting modest drops in teen-age drug use. Some teen-agers in poor neighborhoods now see malt liquor as an alternative to drugs, according to Makani Thaemba, a public policy specialist for the Marin Institute for the Prevention of Alcohol and Other Drug Problems in San Rafael, Calif.

At the same time, some substance abuse authorities say they have been seeing growing numbers of young

(continued on next page)

Case in Point

Cheap High Lures Youths to Malt Liquor "40s" (continued)

people seeking treatment for twin addictions. Increasingly, one of the substances is alcohol, many say, and often that alcohol came by way of malt liquor sold in a 40-ounce bottle.

Some say, too, that they have noticed a growing association between drinking 40-ounce bottles of malt liquor and smoking marijuana. The combination, one teen-ager said, goes together like "cookies and milk."

The Bronx teen-ager who bought the Olde English 800 returned to the grocery store minutes later to purchase a 35-cent Philly Blunt cigar and, as street fad dictates, he hollowed it out and packed it with marijuana to smoke with the malt liquor.

Drug counselors said they are also concerned that habitually getting intoxicated on malt liquor at an early age may lead to the consumption of harder liquors and more dangerous substances.

Hoisting a 40 for Breakfast

Drinking a 40-ounce bottle of malt liquor for breakfast en-route to school is not unusual, said a Bronx teen-ager who said he used to do just that. Guzzling 40 ounces to intoxication, others added, is a major attraction at "hooky parties."

"It is just a thing we did," said Clifton W., a 16-year-old Bronx boy who is in treatment for substance abuse. "It just made me feel good."

Fakri A., a 17-year-old from the Bronx who is now in treatment, recalled that he was once so drunk after drinking six 40-ounce bottles of malt liquor that he staggered obliviously through a firefight between drug dealers. "I guess God was looking out for me that day," he mused.

Darryl McDaniels, a 28-year-old member of the rap group Run-DMC, recently told a rap magazine that he had been hospitalized for alcoholic pancreatitis, the result of years of drinking as many as eight 40-ounce bottles of malt liquor a day.

"That's an old man's disease," said Ms. Thaemba of the Marin Institute. "If we are not careful with this kind of push to heavy consumption patterns, which is new to us, we will see more of that."

"Pack a Lot of Punch"

The 40-ounce bottle was introduced beginning in the mid-80's as a "retailer and consumer convenience," according to Ron Richards, a spokesman for the Miller Brewing Company, maker of the Magnum brand of malt liquor. Store owners like them, he said, because they take up far less shelf space than six-packs.

And in the wake of their introduction, national malt liquor consumption has increased to 82.9 million 2.5-gallon cases in 1992 from 73.6 million in 1989, according to the Jobson Publishing Corporation's Beer Handbook, which predicts sales of 97.8 million cases this year.

The reason for such sales, market researchers say, is the promise of more alcohol for less money.

"If you measure your serving size by 40 ounces," said Peter Reid, editor of Modern Brewery Age, "it's going to pack a lot of punch."

In a comparative analysis, the Marin Institute found that 40 ounces of St. Ides, which at 8 percent alcohol is one of the most powerful malt liquors, has more alcohol than a six-pack of standard beer, and roughly the same amount as five 5-ounce glasses of wine or five 1.5-ounce glasses of mixed drinks.

Following Market Dictates

Brewery officials deny that their pursuit of a small but lucrative segment of the American liquor market is an effort to entice underage or irresponsible drinking, and they insist that they are not unduly targeting young minority drinkers. Noting that malt liquor sales have always been the highest among minority drinkers, they say they are simply following the dictates of maintaining a market they want to continue to serve.

"You obviously gear the advertising of any products to groups that tend to prefer them," said Randy Smith, a vice president of the G. Heileman Brewing Company of LaCrosse, Wis., the maker of Colt 45.

He and officials of other breweries say they regularly advertise against irresponsible and underage drinking. And they say they also sponsor a variety of service activities in minority neighborhoods, from concerts, to literacy programs, to scholarships.

"The industry is very sensitive and spends a lot of money to be responsible," said Frank Walters, director of research for M. Shanken Communications in New York, publishers of Impact and Market Watch, leading trade publications.

Two years ago, Heileman Brewing came under fire from black consumer groups and civil rights organizations after introducing Power Master, its most powerful malt liquor at 5.9 percent alcohol, and marketing it specifically to black drinkers. Regulators ordered it off the market, saying the word "power" on the label violated a law against using brand names to promote alcohol content.

Linking Success With Liquor

Heileman now faces criticism over an advertising campaign for Colt 45 that is aimed at a younger black consumer than before. Gone is the middle-aged black actor, Billy Dee Williams; instead, a polished, soft-spoken younger black man talks of commitment, giving back and success. As he does, he reaches for a can of Colt 45.

Linking black success with malt liquor is cynical and exploitative, critics of the ads say.

"All this speaks of a slick marketing campaign that has tremendous impact on African-Americans," said the Rev. Calvin O. Butts 3d of the Abyssinian Baptist Church in Harlem. Mr. Butts has led a campaign to stem the advertising of alcohol and tobacco products in poor neighborhoods.

"What they do is diabolical," Mr. Butts said of malt liquor makers' efforts. "They know exactly what they are doing."

Popular at Hooky Parties

Judy Corman, a spokeswoman for Phoenix House, a drug-rehabilitation organization, said she was surprised by the response when she asked a roomful of Manhattan teenagers recently if they had drunk 40-ounce malt liquor.

"You should have seen the hands go up," she said. "Nearly everyone raised their hands."

Jennifer O. was one of them.

The 16-year-old Bronx high school student said she seldom went to classes last year, preferring instead to attend hooky parties at friends' houses, in basements and on rooftops. "As long as there was music and people," recalled Jennifer, who is Puerto Rican.

"When I went to hooky parties, we used to have boxes and boxes and boxes of 40 ounces in the refrigerator, and we would go crazy," she said. She drank to impress her friends, she said, and her ability to drink two bottles of malt liquor back-to-back earned her the nickname, "Shorty Two Forties."

"The most I drank was three and a half bottles and I was drunk out of my mind," Jennifer said.

When asked if there was anything she regretted about her days of drunken malt liquor binges, she paused, and nodded.

"I lost my virginity," she said, "when I was drunk on 40's."

Source: Michel Marriott. "Cheap High Lures Youths to Malt Liquor '40s.'" *New York Times*, 6 April 1993:1, A12.

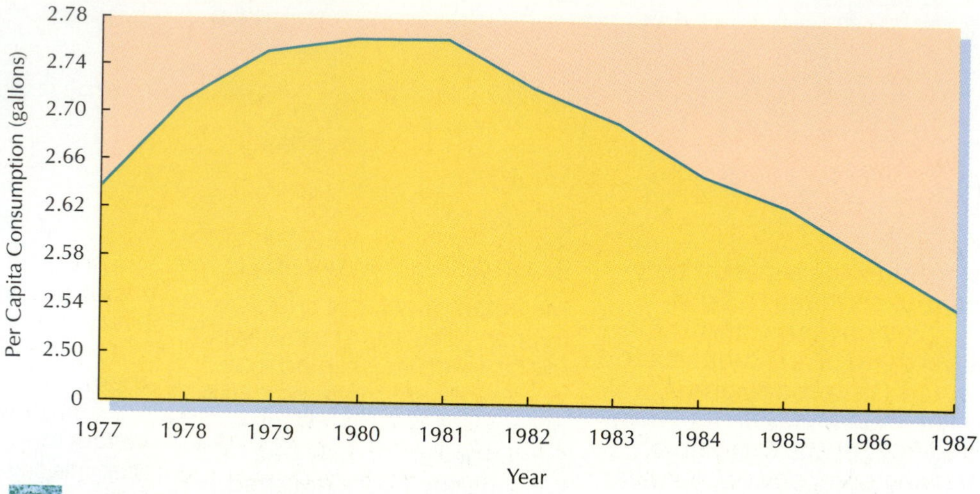

FIGURE 8.2 Apparent U.S. per capita consumption of pure alcohol: 1977–1987 *Source:* National Institute of Alcohol Abuse and Alcoholism. *Apparent Per Capita Alcohol Consumption: National, State and Regional Trends, 1977–1987*. Surveillance report no. 13. Washington, DC: U.S. Department of Health and Human Services, 1989.

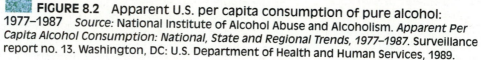

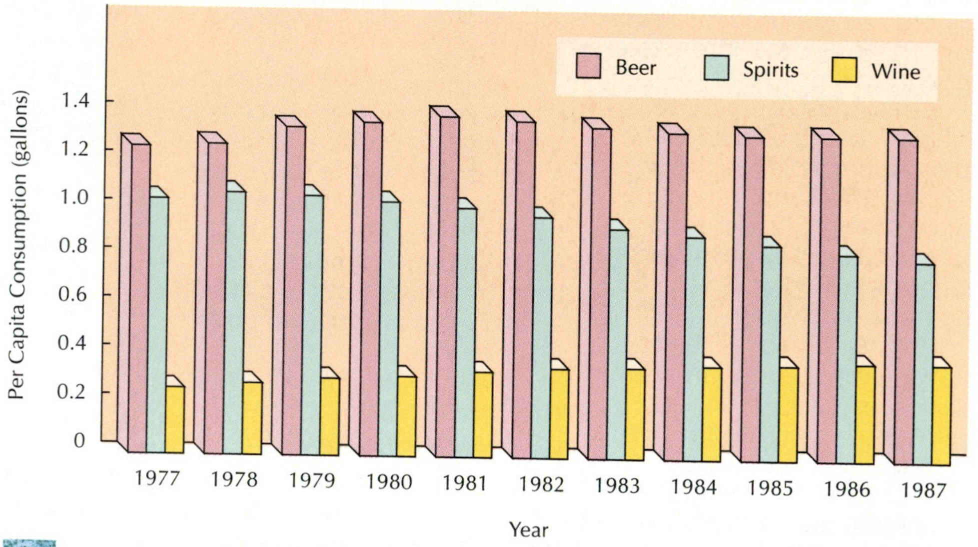

FIGURE 8.3 Apparent U.S. per capita consumption of beer, wine, and spirits: 1977–1987 *Source:* National Institute of Alcohol Abuse and Alcoholism. *Apparent Per Capita Alcohol Consumption: National, State and Regional Trends, 1977–1987*. Surveillance report no. 13. Washington, DC: U.S. Department of Health and Human Services, 1989.

Case in Point

Drinkers' Profiles

Which groups in America are most likely to say they drink, at least occasionally? Those under fifty, men, Catholics, those living on either coast, and those with higher levels of education and higher incomes.

Teetotalers are most likely to be women, older Americans, Protestants, less well-educated, to have lower incomes, and to live in the Midwest and the South.

There are fascinating differences by group in the type of alcoholic beverages Americans consume:

- Beer is very much a man's drink: two-thirds of men who have had a drink within the week prior to the survey said that they drink beer most often, compared to only 25 percent of women. Beer is also more likely to be the favorite of those without college educations, a young person's drink (dominant among those eighteen to twenty-nine), and most likely to be the favorite in the Midwest.
- Wine is the most common drink among women, and not nearly as common in the South and Midwest as on either coast. Wine is also more likely to be a favorite among college-educated Americans and those with the highest incomes.
- Hard liquor is clearly a drink of older Americans; it is the favorite of 45 percent of Americans aged fifty and older, but of only 8 percent of those eighteen to twenty-nine. Hard liquor is also more common in the South and East than in the Midwest and West.

Source: George Gallup, Jr., and Rank Newport. "Americans Now Drinking Less Alcohol." *Gallup Poll,* no. 303, January 1990.

consumption since 1981? Changing demographics may be a reason. For instance, the proportion of the population over age 60 continues to increase, and alcohol consumption in this age group is low. The 1980s and the 1990s were rather conservative decades, and the social acceptability of heavy drinking decreased steadily. Public awareness of the risks associated with alcohol use has increased. Although serious problems continue to exist in certain subgroups, the trend is that the mass population of drinkers have turned away from distilled spirits toward beverages with lower alcohol content. People have also become increasingly more health conscious. The general population is now preoccupied with maintaining a healthy diet and adequate physical fitness. Such attitudes militate against constant alcohol use and abuse.

Alcohol Use in U.S. Population Groups

Concern over patterns of abuse has led social researchers to focus on the common characteristics of various groups that seem most at risk (see the Case in Point box for more specific information). In this section, we identify and survey the distinctive problems of alcohol abuse experienced by several categories of people in America.

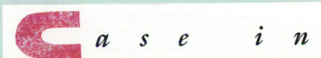

In the University of Michigan 1991 annual study titled *Monitoring the Future,* it was reported that among respondents ages 19–28, lifetime use of alcohol was 94%. Another recent Gallup poll found that 56% of Americans drank alcoholic beverages in 1989, while in 1988 it was 63% (Colasanto and Zeglarski 1989, 12). Including both licit and illicit drugs, alcohol continues to be the most widely used drug, followed by lifetime use of cigarettes at 74%, marijuana at 59%, and cocaine at 21%.

Although the widespread use of alcohol remains high, the total *amounts* and *frequency* of alcohol consumption have dropped. Regarding frequency, in 1990 52% of people who view themselves as drinkers had a drink within the week before being surveyed, compared to 67% the year before, in 1988 (Gallup and Newport 1990, 2).

There continue to be significant variations in drinking patterns among specific population groups. Gallup polls in 1989 and 1990 (Colasanto and Zeglarski 1989; Gallup and Newport 1990) show sharp differences in alcohol use among various groups.

Social Class Differences The higher the household income, the higher the percentage of those who drink. The percentage who drank involved 75% of household incomes $50,000 and over, 61% of households earning $30,000–$49,000, 50% of households earning $20,000–$29,999, and 46% of households under $20,000 (Colasanto and Zeglarski 1989, 14).

Alcohol Consumption Among Different Religions Concerning religious affiliation, the *Gallup Report* (1988, 24) found that 57% of the Protestants and 75% of the Catholics reported drinking. Interestingly, in response to the question "Do you drink?" 73% of the respondents indicated that they had no religious affiliation, and answered yes to this question (Gallup and Newport 1990, 4).

Alcohol Consumption Among Different Regions In the same *Gallup Report* (Gallup and Newport 1990, 4), the largest percentages were of drinkers on the East Coast (64%) and West Coast (62%). The South had the lowest percentage (50%), and the Midwest ranked second lowest (54%) in the percentage of drinkers.

Gender Differences In looking at the percentage who consider themselves drinkers, a 1994 Gallup Poll (McAneny 1994, 1) showed that 70% of the men and 61% of the women drank. This amounts to "seven in ten men and six in ten women [who] currently identify themselves as drinkers" (McAneny 1991, 1). (See also the Case in Point box for additional information.) The overall trend shows that the percentage of women drinking declined to 48% in 1989, but for the first time since 1985 women now exceed 60%. The percentage of women drinking is strongly affected by age. Younger women are more likely to drink, while women over 50 are less likely to drink and when they do they consume less (Gomberg and Lisansky 1989). Other findings show that generally, males continue to drink more than females and that not only is their percentage larger, but males consume more, drink more often, and their alcohol-related problems are greater.

As a group, alcohol-abusing women tend to drink alone or at home. High incidence of alcohol abuse is found in women who are unemployed and looking for work, while less alcohol abuse is likely to occur with women employed part time outside the home. Divorced or separated women, women who never marry, and those who are unmarried and living with a partner are more likely to use and abuse alcohol. Other high-risk groups are women in their twenties and early thirties and women with heavy-drinking husbands or partners. Wilsnack and others (1986) found that women who experience depression or reproductive problems also demonstrate heavier drinking behavior.

Looking at specific age groups, the following conclusions are drawn by the National Institute on Alcohol Abuse and Alcoholism (1990):

1. Women in the 21- to 34-year-old age group were least likely to report alcohol-related problems if they had stable marriages and were working full time. Thus, young mothers with full-time occupations reported less reliance on alcohol in comparison to childless women without full-time work.
2. In the 35- to 49-year-old age group, the heaviest drinkers were divorced or separated women without children in the home.
3. In the 50- to 64-year-old age group, the heaviest drinkers were women whose husbands or partners drank heavily.
4. Women 65 years and older comprised less than 10% of drinkers with drinking problems.

Interestingly, more alcohol consumption is also found in women who closely perform so-called masculine gender roles, such as female executives and women in traditional blue-collar occupations.

Case in Point

Survey Question: "I have a question about alcoholic beverages. Do you have occasion to use alcoholic beverages such as liquor, wine, or beer, or are you a total abstainer?"

PEPERCENTAGE WHO DRINK, BY GENDER—TREND

	Total	Men	Women		Total	Men	Women		Total	Men	Women
June 3–6, 1994	65%	70%	61%	1978	71	75	64	1951	59	70	46
1992	64	72	57	1977	71	77	65	1950	60	n.a.	n.a.
1990	64	64	51	1976	71	n.a.	n.a.	1949	58	66	49
1989	56	64	48	1974	68	77	61	1947	63	72	54
1988	63	72	55	1969	64	n.a.	n.a.	1946	67	n.a.	n.a.
1987	65	72	57	1966	65	70	61	1945	67	75	60
1985	67	72	62	1964	63	n.a.	n.a.	1939	58	70	45
1984	64	73	57	1960	62	n.a.	n.a.				
1983	65	71	58	1958	55	66	45				
1982	65	69	61	1957	58	67	50				
1981	70	75	66	1956	60	n.a.	n.a.				
1979	69	74	64	1952	60	68	53				

Source: Leslie McAney. "Alcohol in America: Number of Drinkers Holding Steady, But Drinking Less." Gallup Poll News Service 59 (17 June 1994):2.

Alcohol Use Among Different Age Populations Some correlation exists regarding age and the amount of alcohol consumed. In the same Gallup poll (Gallup and Newport 1990, 4), 61% of the respondents under age 30 drank, 64% between the ages of 30 and 49, and 47% age 50 and older reported drinking. It appears that after age 49 there is an appreciable drop in the percentage reporting drinking.

Alcohol Use Among the Youth In the 1993 National Institute on Drug Abuse (NIDA) study, it was found that 69% of eighth-graders, 53% of tenth-graders, and 37% of twelfth-graders reported drinking in the past year. Approximately "70% of eighth-graders say they have at least tried alcohol, 27% report having gotten drunk at least once, and 13% report having consumed five or more drinks in a row in just prior to the two weeks of the survey" (Johnston et al. 1993). Table 8.1 and the Here and Now box show these and other startling findings.

Although the results from another major survey, the 1988 National High School Senior Survey, showed that high school seniors categorized as "current drinkers" declined from 66 to 64% (NIAAA 1990, 26), the use of alcohol by teen-

Here and Now

Do Teenagers Have an Alcohol Problem?

Although nearly all age groups are consuming less alcohol, the following excerpts from a speech diminish our optimism:

- Junior and senior high school students drink 35% of all wine coolers sold in the United States (31 million gallons) and consume 1.1 billion cans of beer (102 million gallons) each year.
- Many teenagers who drink are using alcohol to handle stress and boredom and many of them drink alone, breaking the old stereotype of party drinking.
- Understanding labels is a big problem for this age group. Two out of three teenagers cannot distinguish alcoholic from nonalcoholic beverages because they appear similar on store shelves.
- Teenagers lack essential knowledge about alcohol. Very few are getting clear and reliable information about alcohol and its effects. [Millions of teenagers] . . . learn the facts from their peers; close to 2 million do not even know a law exists pertaining to illegal underage drinking.
- The federally mandated 21-year-old minimum drinking law is largely a myth; it is riddled with loopholes.
- Two-thirds of teens who drink, about 7 million kids, simply walk into a store and buy booze. . . .
- The health message is clear: "use of alcohol by young people can lead to serious health consequences—not to mention absenteeism, vandalism, date rape, random violence, and even death."

Source: Antonia C. Novello. "Alcohol and Kids: It's Time for Candor." *Christian Science Monitor* (26 June 1992):19.

agers remains alarmingly high. In fact, it was found that 8 million American teenagers (ages 13–19) use alcohol every week, and the amount of binge drinking has significantly increased.[1]

Alcohol Abuse Among Traditional and Nontraditional College Student Populations How much binge drinking occurs? In one study of traditional college students at 14 Massachusetts colleges (ages 18–23), more than one-half of men and one-third of women students were found to be binge drinkers (Wechsler and Isaac 1992). Another national study of 158,000 students at seventy-eight institutions nationwide found that "nationally, about 42% of the students" said they had binged at least once within the last two weeks, and nearly 19% said they had binged three or more times in that same period (Cage 1993, A30).

The researchers found that among college students, women drink less than men. Older, nontraditional college students (ages 24+) drank less than traditional-age students; and students at two-year institutions drank less than students at four-year institutions. In another study, 8% of 21-year-old men were reported to be drinking large quantities of alcohol, defined as 15 or more drinks per week (Jensen et al. 1992). On the bright side, however, there is little continuity in drinking behavior dur-

[1] Binge drinking is consuming five drinks in a row. This type of drinking involves heavy drinking during short periods of time, and it involves nearly "half a million teenagers [who] go on weekly binges" (Novello 1992, 19).

TABLE 8.1 Incidence of alcohol use: A comparison of responses from eighth-, tenth-, and twelfth-graders

	Reported Drinking	Binge Drinking[a]
Eighth-graders	69%	13%
Tenth-graders	55	23
Twelfth-graders	37	34

[a]Binge drinking is consuming five or more drinks in a row in rapid succession.

Source: National Institute on Drug Abuse. *National Survey Results on Drug Use from the Monitoring the Future Study, 1975–1992.* Vol. I: *Secondary School Students.* Rockville, MD: NIDA, 1993:137.

ing the transition years between adolescence and young adulthood. Drinking levels tend to decline substantially by age 30. Older adults display decreases in alcohol consumption patterns; there are more abstainers and fewer heavy drinkers in this age group than in the younger age groups. Generally, if we exclude cases of more serious stressful life experiences and older patients who have been hospitalized for non–alcohol-related causes, the prevalence of drinking-related problems is lower among older people.

Elderly Populations Most elderly people (aged 62+) who are diagnosed as alcoholics or alcohol abusers fall into two categories: (1) those who were previously addicted to alcohol, and (2) those who abuse alcohol because of stress from diminishing supportive resources (Jennison 1992). The same study finds that such supportive resources as spouse, family, friends, and church protect against the onset of loneliness. Other related stressful situations include neglect, ill health, severe depression, or side effects of medication. The latter group includes by far the largest number of elderly abusers.

However, when comparisons are made between younger people and people in their sixties and older, overall alcohol use is lower in older groups. The lower use of alcohol in the elderly population has been attributed to

1. Chronic health problems, combined with fear of alcohol interference with strong medication
2. Decreased income
3. Increased sensitivity and less tolerance for alcohol (resulting partly from the loss of body mass, leading to less body water content)
4. Changes in lifestyle resulting from retirement
5. The diminished capacity of drinking found in aging peer members

Racial Minorities and Ethnic Group Differences Four major racial and ethnic minority groups in the United States have been surveyed in terms of their percentages of nondrinkers (abstinence rates), heavy drinkers, and people subject to alcohol-related health problems. African Americans comprise 12% of the population in the United States, and they are the largest minority group in the total population. African Americans display high rates of abstention and low rates of heavy drinking, but they are at extremely high risk for health problems in which alcohol is a factor, such as liver cirrhosis, heart disease, and cancers of the esophagus, mouth, larynx, and tongue.

The next largest minority group is Hispanics, comprising 7% of the total population. Members of this group, particularly Mexican Americans, have high rates of both abstinence and heavy drinking and a higher prevalence of drinking-related problems than other racial and ethnic groups.

Asian Americans represent 2% of the total population. They have the highest rates of abstention, the lowest rates of heavy drinking, and the lowest levels of drinking-related problems.

Asian Americans have been found to have certain physiological responses to drug use (Chan 1986; Chi et al. 1988). Findings show that when Asians consume alcohol, they are prone to experience the "flushing response." This response is

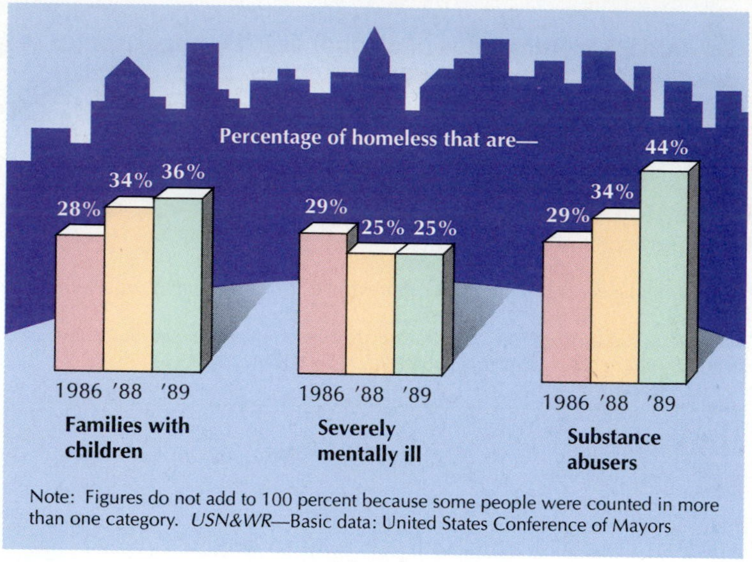

FIGURE 8.4 The changing homeless population: Alcoholics and drug abusers constitute an increasing portion of those who are homeless. *Source:* David S. Merrill. "The Changing Homeless Population." *U.S. News and World Report* (15 January 1990):27.

characterized by sudden reddening of the face and upper body, which follows consumption of light amounts of alcohol. For example, 47% of Japanese men and 43% of women were classified as flushers, compared with 33% of Japanese-American men and 38% of Japanese-American women (Parrish et al. 1990). Incidently, related low tolerance has also been found among American Indians, including Eskimos.

Native American groups—including American Indians and Alaskan Natives—are the smallest racial minority, comprising 1% of the total population. Native Americans vary widely in alcohol use but, as a whole, have very high mortality rates from causes that are most likely to be alcohol related: cirrhosis, unintentional injuries, homicide, and suicide. Native Americans are likely to feel stress from displacement and rejection from their homeland, as well as from high unemployment—all contributing factors to alcohol abuse. Many new alcohol rehabilitation programs for Native Americans have been started, and it is not unusual to find traditional tribal shamans assisting in these health and rehabilitation programs.

Among white Europeans, the heaviest drinking groups are the Irish, Italians, Jews, northern WASPs (white Anglo-Saxon Protestants), Slavs, Germans, and Scandinavians. More abstinence was found among Latins and southern WASPs (Cahalan and Room 1974; Greeley et al. 1980; U.S. Department of Health and Human Services 1987).

Alcohol Consumption Among Gay Populations Among homosexual men and women, who comprise approximately 6 to 10% of the population, alcohol and drug abuse is significant. How high is alcohol abuse among this group? "Approximately 23% of gay males and 13% of lesbian women reported that they use alcohol 'half the time' or more when coping with personal stress" (McKirnan and Peterson 1989, 559).

Research indicates that most of the excessive alcohol consumption is largely due to three primary factors: stress from having a different sexual orientation in a predominantly heterosexual society (arising from gay bashing or victimization from homophobia); from common discrimination, particularly in the form of verbal harassment and ostracism from mainstream heterosexual society; and "negative affectivity" or negative emotional states represented by "moderate depression, low self-esteem, alienation, and trait anxiety" (McKirnan and Peterson 1989; Watson and Clark 1984; Lewis and Jordan 1989).

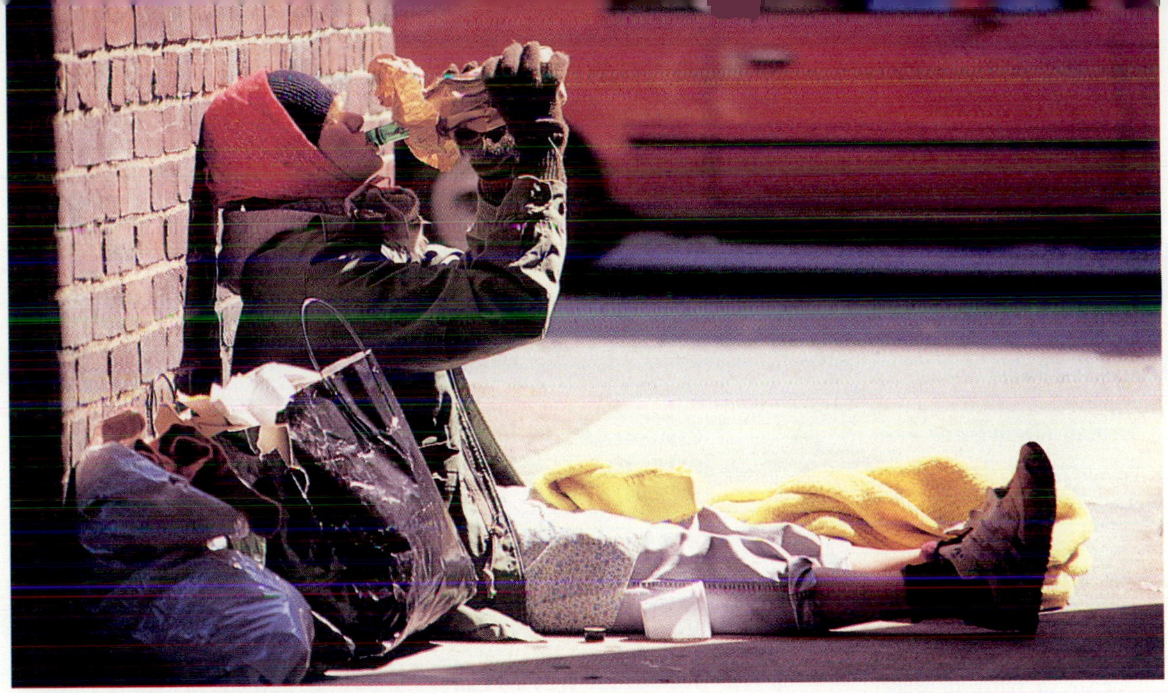

FIGURE 8.5 The more things change—While news reports focus on homeless families, alcoholism has been a growing problem in recent years.

In short, the excessive use of alcohol among this group is caused by the nonacceptance of homosexual behavior by the predominant heterosexual population. The discrimination and prejudice they experience contributes to use of alcohol and other licit and illicit drug use.

The Homeless Drug abusers and severely addicted alcoholics are the fastest-growing group among the homeless (Whitman et al. 1990). Figure 8.4 illustrates the increasing portion of homeless who are alcoholic and drug abusers.

It is estimated that 250,000 Americans are homeless on most nights, and as many as 3 million may experience some type of homelessness each year (Ropers and Bayer 1987). Alcohol abuse and alcohol dependence are serious problems among the homeless (see Figure 8.5). Prevalence estimates for current alcohol abuse and alcoholism range from 20 to 48% (Wright et al. 1987). Alcohol abuse among the homeless intensifies other major problems, such as health and psychiatric disorders. Alcohol is involved in one-third to one-half of all

Drinking and Driving

highway fatalities in the United States. Serious problem drinking has been implicated in almost half of these alcohol-related deaths; the other half involved young drinkers and social drinkers with high blood alcohol levels at the time of the accident. One-third of all traffic injuries are also related to alcohol (National Highway Traffic Safety Administration, or NHTSA 1988).

Such widespread destruction has prompted relatives and friends of victims of drunk drivers to form volunteer groups, which lobby for mandatory jail sentences and revocation of driving licenses for drivers convicted of driving while intoxicated. Such measures have proven to be successful deterrents to drunken driving in several European countries.

The leading cause of injury deaths in the United States is motor vehicle crashes (Baker et al. 1984). In the United States, 46,386 people die in

Self-Check

Attitudinal Test

Part 1: Alcohol Knowledge Test

In response to each statement, circle either T (true) or F (false).

T F 1. Mixing different kinds of drinks can increase the effect of alcohol.

T F 2. The average 4-oz. drink of wine is less intoxicating than the average 1-oz. drink of hard liquor.

T F 3. A can of beer is less intoxicating than an average drink of hard liquor.

T F 4. A cold shower can help sober up a person.

T F 5. A person can be drunk and not stagger or slur his or her speech.

T F 6. It is easy to tell if people are drunk even if you don't know them well.

T F 7. A person drinking on an empty stomach will get drunk faster.

T F 8. People's moods help determine how they are affected by alcohol.

T F 9. A person who is used to drinking can drink more.

T F 10. A person who weighs less can get drunk faster than a heavier person.

T F 11. Of every ten traffic deaths, up to five are caused by drinking drivers.

T F 12. The surest way to tell if the person is legally drunk is by the percent of alcohol in the blood.

T F 13. People who are drunk cannot compensate for it when they drive.

T F 14. In a fatal drunk-driving accident, the drunk is usually not the one killed.

T F 15. Drinking black coffee can help sober up a person.

T F 16. Alcoholic beverages are a stimulant.

Part 2: Alcohol Attitude Test

Directions: If you strongly agree with the following statements, write in 1. If you agree, but not strongly, write in 2. If you neither agree nor disagree, write in 3. If you disagree, but not strongly, write in 4. If you strongly disagree, write in 5.

Set 1

____ 1. If a person concentrates hard enough, he or she can overcome any effect that drinking may have on driving.

____ 2. If you drive home from a party late at night when most roads are deserted, there is not much danger in driving after drinking.

____ 3. It's all right for a person who has been drinking to drive, as long as he or she shows no signs of being drunk.

____ 4. If you're going to have an accident, you'll have one anyhow, regardless of drinking.

____ 5. A drink or two helps people drive better because it relaxes them.

____ Total score for questions 1 through 5

Set 2

____ 6. If I tried to stop someone from driving after drinking, the person would probably think I was butting in where I shouldn't.

____ 7. Even if I wanted to, I would probably not be able to stop some-

one from driving after drinking.

_____ 8. If people want to kill themselves, that's their business.

_____ 9. I wouldn't like someone to try to stop me from driving after drinking.

_____ 10. Usually, if you try to help someone else out of a dangerous situation, you risk getting yourself into one.

_____ Total score for questions 6 through 10

Set 3

_____ 11. My friends would not disapprove of me for driving after drinking.

_____ 12. Getting into trouble with my parents would not keep me from driving after drinking.

_____ 13. The thought that I might get into trouble with the police would not keep me from driving after drinking.

_____ 14. I am not scared by the thought that I might seriously injure myself or someone else by driving after drinking.

_____ 15. The fear of damaging the car would not keep me from driving after drinking.

_____ Total score for questions 11 through 15

Set 4

_____ 16. The 55-mph speed limit on the open roads spoils the pleasure of driving for most teenagers.

_____ 17. Many teenagers use driving to let off steam.

_____ 18. Being able to drive a car makes teenagers feel more confident in their relations with others their age.

_____ 19. An evening with friends is not much fun unless one of them has a car.

_____ 20. There is something about being behind the wheel of a car that makes one feel more adult.

_____ Total score for questions 16 through 20

Set 5

_____ 21. I usually do things that everybody else is doing.

_____ 22. What my friends think of me is the most important thing in my life.

_____ 23. I would ride in a friend's car even if that person had been drinking a lot.

_____ 24. Often I do things just so I won't feel left out of the group I'm with.

_____ 25. I often worry about what other people think about things I do.

_____ Total score for questions 21 through 25

Set 6

_____ 26. Adults try to stop teenagers from driving just to show their power.

_____ 27. I don't think it would help me to go to my parents for advice.

_____ 28. I feel I should have the right to drink if my parents do.

_____ 29. My parents have no real understanding of what I want out of life.

_____ 30. I wouldn't dare call my parents to come and take me home if either I or a friend I was with got drunk.

continued

Self-Check

Attitudinal Test *continued*

_____ Total score for questions 26 through 30

Scoring the Self-Test

Set 1 13–25 points: realistic in avoiding drinking-driving situations; 5–6 points: tends to make up excuses to combine drinking and driving.

Set 2 15–25 points: takes responsibility to keep others from driving when drunk; 5–9 points: wouldn't take steps to stop a drunk friend from driving.

Set 3 12–25 points: hesitates to drive after drinking; 5–7 points: is not deterred by the consequences of drinking and driving.

Set 4 19–25 points: perceives auto as means of transportation; 5–14 points: uses car to satisfy psychological needs, not just transportation.

Set 5 16–25 points: cares about what others think, but acts according to own beliefs and values; 5–10 points: goes along with the crowd.

Set 6 18–25 points: accepts adult and parental responsibility and concern for one's safety; 5–10 points: rejects parental concern or control.

Answers: (1) F, (2) F, (3) F, (4) F, (5) T, (6) F, (7) T, (8) T, (9) F, (10) T, (11) T, (12) T, (13) T, (14) F, (15) F, (16) F

Source: Courtesy of National Highway Traffic Safety Administration, National Center for Statistics and Analysis. From *Drug Driving Facts.* Washington, DC: NHTSA, 1988.

traffic accidents in a given year; approximately half of the deaths are alcohol related (NHTSA 1988). The National Highway Traffic Safety Administration (NHTSA) defines a *fatality* or *traffic crash* as alcohol involved or alcohol related when a participant (driver, pedestrian, or bicyclist) has a measured or estimated blood alcohol concentration (BAC) of 0.01% or above (NHTSA 1988; NIAAA 1990). In most states, the legal limit for intoxication is a BAC of 0.10% or greater.

Alcohol-related car accidents are particularly common among youth. Each year, 40% of all teenage deaths result from traffic accidents (NIAAA 1999), and another 40,000 youth are disfigured in accidents involving alcohol. Overall, approximately 24,000 people die annually in alcohol-related automobile crashes and about 500,000 others are physically seriously impaired. In 1987, motor vehicle crashes were the fifth leading cause of death in the United States, and half of these were alcohol related. It is estimated that members of our society have a 40% chance of becoming involved in an alcohol-related automobile accident and that two-thirds of all traffic fatalities involve alcohol-impaired drivers (NHTSA 1989).

Alcohol-related crashes are the leading cause of death for every age group between 6 and 30 years. Findings show that in 1991, more than 2,400 drivers between the ages of 15 (legal permit driving age) and 20 were involved in fatal crashes where the driver had been drinking. Single-vehicle fatal crashes where the driver was legally intoxicated on weekend nights approach 70% (Wagenaar 1994).

In an effort to address this high-risk group, NHTSA has devised a test that gauges the attitudes of teenagers toward drinking and driving. NHTSA wants to encourage young people to consider social-psychological factors associated with their urge to drink and drive or to ride with drink-

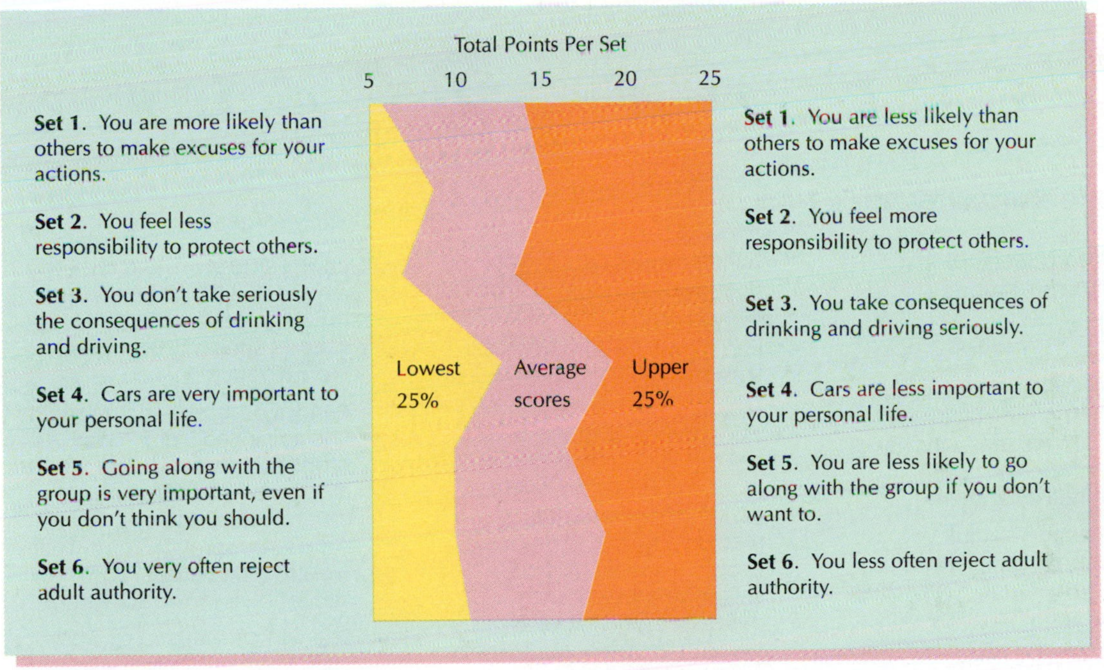

Total Points Per Set
5
10
15
20
25
Set 1. You are more likely than others to make excuses for your actions.
Set 2. You feel less responsibility to protect others.
Set 3. You don't take seriously the consequences of drinking and driving.
Set 4. Cars are very important to your personal life.
Set 5. Going along with the group is very important, even if you don't think you should.
Set 6. You very often reject adult authority.
Lowest 25%
Average scores
Upper 25%
Set 1. You are less likely than others to make excuses for your actions.
Set 2. You feel more responsibility to protect others.
Set 3. You take consequences of drinking and driving seriously.
Set 4. Cars are less important to your personal life.
Set 5. You are less likely to go along with the group if you don't want to.
Set 6. You less often reject adult authority.

FIGURE 8.6 Assessment of attitudes about drinking and driving
Source: Courtesy of National Highway Traffic Safety Administration, National Center for Statistics and Analysis. From *Drug Driving Facts*. Washington, DC: NHTSA, 1988.

ing friends. The two-part test lets respondents evaluate themselves and then compare their own knowledge, values, and beliefs about alcohol with an average profile compiled from responses of the students. Anyone can benefit from taking this test and plotting results against the profile for Pennsylvania teens in Figure 8.6.

Alcoholism Defined

Most people who consume alcohol do not develop into problem drinkers.[2] Thus, it is logical to assume that ethanol in alcohol is not the sole cause for developing an uncontrollable attachment to alcohol.

Alcoholics vary considerably. To many people, the stereotype of an alcoholic is the skid row or homeless derelict. In fact, this stereotype makes up less than 5% of America's problem drinkers. Most problem drinkers are employed, family-centered people, leading what may appear to be normal lives. Estimates vary, but it is believed that about three-fourths of problem drinkers are men and one-fourth are women. The proportion of women has risen in recent years, perhaps because they are increasingly willing to acknowledge the problem and seek treatment. Female problem drinkers may therefore now be more visible rather than numerous (see "Gender Differences" earlier in this chapter). "Alcoholism claims tens of thousands of lives each year (see the Case in Point box), ruins untold numbers of families and costs $117 billion a year in everything from medical bills to lost work days" (Desmond 1987). Approximately 7.3 million are alcohol abusers (NCADI 1991), and alcoholism is

[2] Problem drinkers are known as abusers of alcohol, and they are often alcoholics.

Case in Point

Profile of a Runaway Addiction

The following describes the drift into deeper stages of alcoholism:

Her skin is smooth and her face is pretty. Her blue eyes are clear and radiant. They weren't always that way. Randi is sixteen. She has been through hell with alcohol.

"Most teenagers think you can't become an alcoholic so young," said Randi. "They think you have to be drinking for thirty years and be forty years old, and that because you may not drink every day, you can't have a problem." Randi offers herself as proof of yet another misconception.

Randi's first drinking experience was at a family Christmas party when she was nine. Her alcoholic uncle kept feeding her rum and Cokes. He thought it was funny to see his little niece stumble around, lose control of herself, not be able to speak clearly.

Randi got drunk, passed out, blacked out, and got sick her very first time. She drank very infrequently after that, until age thirteen. Life at home had become unbearable. She had endured years of sexual and physical abuse by her stepfather. A cauldron of anger and guilt and helplessness had been building inside her, and it finally burst. "I just flew off the handle," she said. She was filled with hurt and despair. She discovered that alcohol was very good at numbing these feelings.

"I didn't think there was anything wrong with using alcohol this way," she said. "It made me forget anything going on, any problem, it just made me forget. It helped me escape my feelings. I was always very lonely and depressed, and I always thought drinking would make it better." The feelings would get soothed, temporarily. "But things never got better, only worse," she said.

Randi started hanging out with juniors and seniors—the "alcohol crowd," as she calls it. "To go out on a Friday night, there needed to be alcohol in the car or it just wasn't worth going out," she said.

She had always been a fine student, but by freshman year, Randi was absent 113 out of the 181 school days. "My grades went completely down the tubes. But, of course, I didn't have a problem. Not me." Randi laughed at her sarcasm.

More and more, drinking just seemed to be the thing to do. She drank not only to forget, but to have fun, to be cool. "I think I always saw the glamour involved with alcohol. The adults sitting around drinking a glass of wine or whatever. I put it together with the social scene." She could not imagine life without it.

Randi's progression was rapid. She advanced from Friday night parties to weekend-long alcohol binges. "I needed it so much toward the end, it was such a desperation for it, that I would drink before I went to school . . . if I went to school."

She was committed to a psychiatric hospital for a year because of several drunken suicide attempts. She lied about her drinking. She carved a hole in the floor of her room to hide bottles. Still, she had denial.

"I didn't want to blame my problems on my drinking," she said. "I was addicted to alcohol, but I just thought I was tired, or getting sick. I never really put my problems together with my drinking until later."

During the early stages of her drinking to excess, why do you think Randi did not realize she had a problem with alcohol?

Source: W. Coffey, *Straight Talk About Drinking: Teenagers Speak Out About Alcohol.* Markham, Ontario, Canada: Penguin Books Canada Limited, 1988:110-12. .

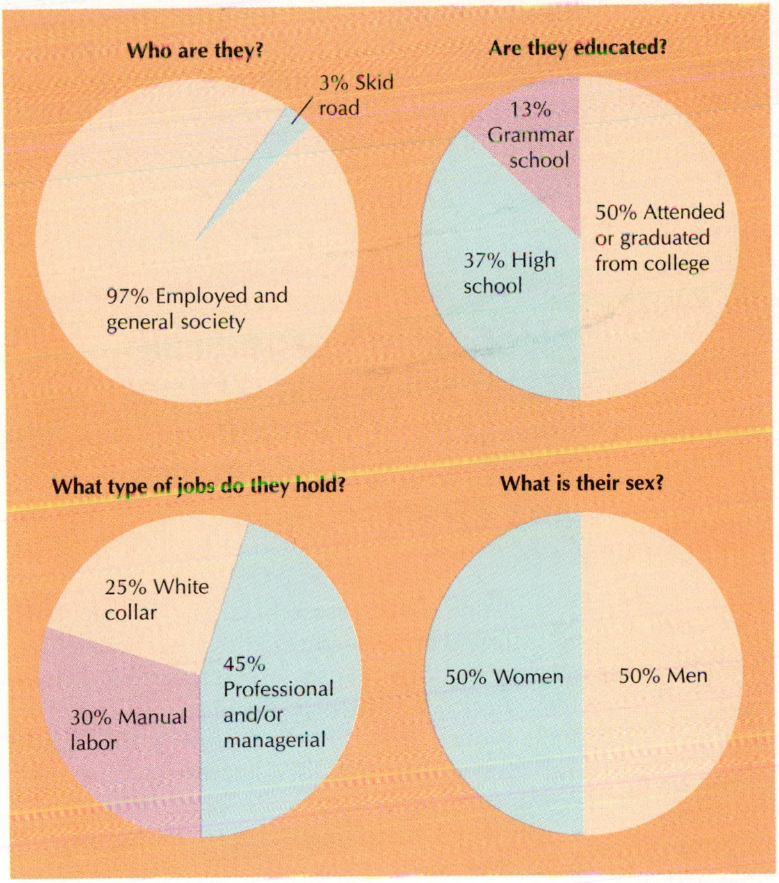

FIGURE 8.7 Who are alcoholics? *Source:* James E. Royce. *Alcohol Problems and Alcoholism*, rev. ed. New York: Free Press, 1989:5.

found in all age, ethnic, lifestyle, and social class groups (see Figure 8.7). Alcoholism is a worldwide affliction; it is particularly severe in France, Ireland, Poland, Scandinavia, and the former Soviet Union ("Alcoholism," no date).

Alcoholism is a state of physical and psychological addiction to the psychoactive substance ethanol. It was once viewed as a vice and dismissed as "sinful," but over the years, there has been a shift from this perspective to one that views alcoholism as a disease. The "sinfulness" perspective failed to focus on the fact that alcoholism is an addiction, an illness, and not the result of a lack of personal discipline and morality.

Attempts to expand the basic definition of alcoholism to include symptoms of the condition and psychological and sociological factors have been difficult; no one definition satisfies everyone. The World Health Organization defines the *alcohol dependence syndrome* as a state, psychic and usually also physical, resulting from taking alcohol and characterized by behavioral and other responses that always include a compulsion to take alcohol on a continuous or periodic basis to experience its psychic effects and sometimes to avoid the discomfort of its absence; tolerance may or may not be present (NIAAA 1980).

The following are two other widely accepted definitions of alcoholism:

> Alcoholism is a chronic behavioral disorder manifested by repeated drinking of alcoholic beverages in excess of the dietary and social uses of the community, and to an extent that interferes with the drinker's health or his social or economic functioning. (Keller 1958)

> Alcoholism is a chronic, primary, hereditary

> disease that progresses from an early, physiological susceptibility into an addiction characterized by tolerance changes, physiological dependence, and loss of control over drinking. Psychological symptoms are secondary to the physiological disease and not relevant to its onset. (Gold 1991, 99).

For many years, people with drinking problems were lumped together under the label *alcoholic,* and all were assumed to be suffering from the same illness. It has become evident that there are many kinds of drinking problems, many diverse types of people who have them, and many reasons why people begin and continue to drink to a harmful extent. The search for a single cause of alcoholism has shifted to interdisciplinary exploration of factors that might, singly or in combination, account for the development of problem drinking in various types of individuals.

There is no generally agreed-on universal model of how alcoholism starts; multiple circumstances are required to make a person become a problem drinker. A report from the NIAAA, "Facts About Alcohol and Alcoholism" (1980) and a report by the Cooperative Commission on the Study of Alcoholism (NIAAA 1980) suggests that an individual who displays the following characteristics is more likely to develop trouble with alcohol:

- Drinking in order to "cope with life"
- Often drinking to a state of intoxication, going to work inebriated, driving a car while intoxicated, drinking alone, and drinking early in the morning
- Responding to beverage alcohol in a certain way, perhaps physiologically determined, experiencing intense relief and relaxation
- Having certain personality characteristics, such as difficulty in dealing with others and difficulty in overcoming depression, frustration, and anxiety
- Being a member of a culture in which there is both pressure to drink and culturally induced guilt and confusion regarding what kinds of drinking behavior are appropriate

The importance of the different causal factors of alcoholism no doubt varies from one individual to another. Research into physiological, psychological, and sociological dimensions of this problem and integration of the findings in these and other areas have resulted in greater understanding of the conditions that precede, underlie, and maintain problem drinking.

Alcoholism: Large-Scale Major Models and Other Discipline-Oriented Explanations of Causes and Effects

Most distinguished researchers studying alcoholism believe that no single factor causes alcoholism and that multiple causes are responsible (Gold 1991; Peele et al. 1991; Pittman 1967; Royce 1989; Rudy 1986). Here we present two major large-scale models and discipline-oriented psychological (including "alcoholic personality type" theories) and sociological explanations for the causes of alcoholism.

Moral Model

This section outlines the two models that attempt to place in perspective why alcohol becomes abused. Two major models on the use and eventual abuse of alcohol are known as the **moral model** and the medical or disease model of alcohol addiction. Although some social scientists, psychologists, sociologists, and social workers distinguish between a moral model and free-will model (Schaler 1991), we combine both models under the moral model because at some points the assumptions of both models overlap and the differences are slight.

The view of alcohol abuse under the moral model basically says that excessive alcohol consumption reverts to a breakdown of individual social control. Abusers drink to excess because of personal choice (Nusbaumer 1994). The decision to abuse alcohol occurs because the moral enforcement against excessive use is either absent or has waned. In a sense, alcohol use is rewarded and is often supported by friends and associations (Akers 1992). To remedy this abuse, it is necessary to increase penalties and punishments so that alcohol abuse is no longer a rewarding choice. The types of punishments advocated are "fines, loss of certain privileges such as the revocation of drivers' licenses, mandatory alcohol or driving education [courses], or incarceration" (Nusbaumer 1994).

The therapy recommended under this model includes (1) promoting healthy choices; (2) increasing awareness of responsibility; (3) emphasizing value clarification; (4) supporting achievement of behavior goals; and (5) educating people with an emphasis on coping skills (Schaler 1991).

Medical Model

In contrast to the moral model, the **medical model** includes biological explanations for abusive alcohol consumption. Generally, this model views alcohol abuse as a disease that is innate and biologically determined in specific individuals. Thus the motivation to use and abuse alcohol results from an individual's constitutional and biological characteristics. This model assumes that alcohol abuse is uncontrollable and if the consumption is stopped or curtailed, the alcoholic is viewed as "recovering" but not "cured" of the disease. Other assumptions under this model are (1) excessive drinkers who become alcoholic are different from light to moderate drinkers, (2) alcoholics are compulsive drinkers, (3) the path to alcoholism is marked by distinct stages, and (4) addiction to alcohol is primarily a physical addiction (Little 1989).

The medical model is widely accepted and endorsed by such prestigious professional organizations as the American Medical Association, the American Health Association, the American Psychiatric Association, and the World Health Organization. The extent of agreement on the medical model was so strong that in 1970 the U.S. government succeeded in passing the Hughes Act establishing the National Institute of Alcohol Abuse and Alcoholism (NIAAA).

The medical model assumes that alcohol abusers have physiological differences based on a genetic source and that the conflict is between physiology and the attraction of the chemicals in the drugs where the response to alcohol use results from this interaction. Unlike the moral model, where the alcohol abuser loses rational control of his or her environment, the medical model maintains a mechanistic view in that alcohol abuse is believed to have a genetic basis. The alcohol abuser's conflict is between physiology and the attraction to the chemical properties in the drugs.

Research Using the Medical Model Much research on causation has been devoted to finding physiological factors—either in the alcoholic beverage itself or in the biological makeup of the alcoholic—that could account for alcoholic addiction.

A major difficulty with research into causes of alcoholism is that, although laboratory animals can be made dependent on alcohol and this process can be studied, there is no good model to study the spontaneous development of alcoholism as it occurs in humans. For example, if minute quantities of an alcohol solution are injected directly into rats' brains every two or three hours for several days, they will drink alcohol whenever it is offered to them. However, the drug must initially be forced on them in this or some other manner to make them dependent. Strains of mice have been bred that demonstrate a selective preference for alcohol, which they drink in large amounts. This preference is genetically determined; it is not affected even when the young mice are raised by females of a different strain or are exposed to various conditions of stress or isolation. However, the mice of these heavy-drinking strains also happen to be able to metabolize alcohol much more rapidly than mice of other strains. Thus, it is difficult to determine whether their increased alcohol intake is related to a particular taste for alcohol or to their ability to consume more alcohol without becoming intoxicated. As described earlier, under controlled conditions, both alcoholic and normal

MORAL MODEL view that excessive alcohol consumption results from a breakdown of individual social control

MEDICAL MODEL the view that alcohol abuse is a disease that is innate and biologically determined in specific individuals subjects have an increased rate of alcohol metabolism while consuming relatively large amounts (Lumeng and Li 1986). Therefore, the mouse data are probably irrelevant to the study of alcoholism.

Another interesting finding is that there is a 55% or higher concordance rate for alcoholism in identical twins, compared to a 28% rate for same-sex fraternal twins. In addition, studies using either the half-sibling method or adoption samples demonstrate a four times or higher increase in alcoholism for the children of alcoholics over those of nonalcoholics, even when the children had been separated from their natural parents shortly after birth and raised without knowledge of their parents' drinking problem. Children adopted through the same adoption agencies but without alcoholic biological parents showed low rates of alcoholism even if they were raised by an alcoholic parent figure or experienced a subsequent severe psychological trauma, such as parental death or divorce (Schuckit and Rayes 1979).

As discussed later, alcoholism occurs more frequently in adult children of alcoholics (ACOAs). Some researchers are confident that the specific gene that may be responsible for the development of alcoholism will be found (Bower 1991); other researchers believe that a "'drinking gene' does not exist" (Leerhsen and Namuth 1988). Despite the controversial gene theory of alcoholism, it remains true that children of alcoholic parents are four times more likely to develop a problem with alcohol even when these children are raised or adopted by nonalcoholic parents. Other findings "show that 50 to 80% of all alcoholics have had a close alcoholic relative" ("Alcoholism" no date).

To date, the extent to which genetic factors might contribute to alcoholism in the population remains unfounded. It is not as clear-cut as the genetic contribution to the development of diabetes, for example, although there are parallels. Perhaps future studies will either prove or disprove the role of genetics in the development of alcoholism.

Psychological Factors

What psychological factors cause or contribute to alcoholism? Evidence shows that alcoholics have psychological similarities that may contribute to the onset of alcoholism. The study of the relationship between psychological causes and alcoholism can be divided into two areas: family background and personality characteristics (Catanzaro 1967). Psychological explanations range from psychoanalytic to social learning and reinforcement to personality theories.

Psychoanalytic Theory The more Freudian psychoanalytic explanations consider that addiction to alcohol results from deep-seated anxieties that revolve around conflict (Levin 1990). Freud believed that all the later addictions to food, alcohol, or gambling, for example, are re-enactments of the original addiction to masturbation and that the use of an addiction is really self-punishment. In effect, alcoholism is a symbolic replacement of the first addiction, which is masturbation (Freud 1928). As far-fetched as this may appear, partly because of the brevity necessary in presenting Freud's reasoning on this matter, we do find that many alcoholics have serious inner conflicts and repressed feelings. Although some will disagree with Freud's emphasis on the importance or even relevance of "the first addition," this theory forces us to recognize the many inner psychological struggles that may be affecting the compulsive drinker. As we shall see later, feelings of anger, denial, and withdrawal re-emerge from the psychoanalytic perspective and are discussed in personality theories.

Psychopathological Theory The psychopathological theory of alcoholism focuses on antisocial behavior and depression and how such behavior affects the severity of dependence (Nathan 1990). The belief is that age, gender, and ethnicity affect developing antisocial behavior and depression; for example, younger drinkers tend to abuse alcohol, women combine alcohol abuse with depression, and blacks and Hispanics display patterns of abuse and antisocial behavior and depression. The terms *prealcoholic personality* and *alcoholic personality* have been used to define personality characteristics; however, there is little agreement on the identity of alcoholic personality traits or whether they may be the cause or the result of excessive drinking. Clinical psychologists and psychiatrists with a psychoanalytic perspective have described alcoholic drinkers who are in treatment as neurotic, maladjusted, unable to relate effectively to others, sexually and emotionally immature, isolated, dependent, unable to withstand frustration or tension, poorly integrated, and marked by deep feelings of sinfulness and unworthiness. Some therapists have suggested that alcoholism is a disastrous attempt at the self-cure of some inner conflict and that it might well be called "suicide by ounces." These observations are based on clinical impressions of alcoholics who are already in treatment because they were arrested, sick enough to be committed, rich enough to enter one clinic, or poor enough to enter another. No long-term studies have answered the question "What was the person like before he or she drank?" (Aronow 1980).

Social Learning and Reinforcement Theories

Social learning theory (Becker 1966; Sutherland 1947) emphasizes that alcohol use and later abuse result from early socialization experiences. Alcohol-drinking parents and/or significant others serve as role models who in effect teach children that drinking is okay.

Reinforcement theory (Akers 1985) explains alcohol use as resulting from some kind of positive "stroking," or benefit received from drinking. Peers and the mass media, including cinema and advertising in magazines and billboards, help reinforce the idea that consuming alcohol is expected and required during times of crisis, boredom, and celebration. By drinking, the individual may feel more accepted than if he or she abstained. Drinking may also bring attention from others that the drinker felt was lacking.

Alcoholic Types

Another personality type theory or system demarking the types of alcoholics is described by Jellinek (1960). The categories are

Alpha alcoholism. Mostly a psychological dependence on alcohol to bolster an inability to cope with life. The alpha type constantly needs alcohol and becomes irritable and anxious when it is not available.

Beta alcoholism. Mostly a social dependence on alcohol. Often this type is a heavy beer drinker who continues to meet social and economic obligations. Some nutritional deficiencies can occur, including organic damage such as gastritis and cirrhosis.

Gamma alcoholism. The most prevalent form of alcoholism. This type of alcoholic suffers from emotional and psychological impairment. Jellinek believed that this type of alcoholic suffered from a true disease and progressed from a psychological dependence to physical dependence. Loss of control over when alcohol is consumed, and how much, characterizes this latter phase of this type of alcoholism.

Delta alcoholics. Called the *maintenance* drinker (Royce 1989). The person loses control over drinking and cannot abstain for even a day or two. Many wine-drinking countries such as France and Italy contain delta-type alcoholics who sip wine throughout most of their waking hours. Being "tipsy" but never completely inebriated is typical of the delta alcoholic.

Epsilon alcoholic. This type of alcoholic is characterized as a binge drinker. The epsilon-type drinker drinks excessively for a certain period, then abstains completely from alcohol until the next binge period. The dependence on alcohol is both physical and psychological. Loss of control over the amount consumed is another characteristic of this type of alcoholic.

Zeta alcoholic. This type was added to Jellinek's types to typify the moderate drinker who becomes abusive and violent. Although this type is also referred to as a pathological drinker or "mad drunk," zeta types may not be drinkers addicted to alcohol.

SOCIAL LEARNING THEORY a theory that asserts that the use of alcohol results from early socialization experiences

REINFORCEMENT THEORY a theory that asserts that alcohol use results from positive "stroking," which leads to satisfying feelings

Other classifications include differentiating alcoholics by their reaction to the drug as quiet, sullen, friendly, or angry types. Finally, another method is to classify alcoholics according to drinking patterns: people with occupational, social, escape, and emotional disorders.

Social and Psychological Reactions to the Alcoholic Most often the typical alcoholic lives within a family environment. How does a spouse respond to a husband or wife that is alcoholic? Here we find that certain patterned stages emerge:

Stage 1. Denial or miminizing. Denial exists when the spouse of an alcoholic either denies or minimizes the extent of drinking by the alcoholic spouse. Although the nonaddicted spouse worries privately, he or she often makes excuses to neighbors, friends, and relatives that the drinking is normal.

Stage 2. Tension and isolation. This stage is characterized by social isolation. The nonaddicted spouse withdraws from socializing with the addicted spouse and reduces his or her visibility. Attempts are made to "hide the liquor" and empty the whiskey bottles. Tension mounts between the spouse and the addicted drinker.

Stage 3. Frustration and disorganization. At this stage, a sullen belief by the nonalcoholic spouse emerges that the drinking may be permanent. Past threats and attempts to rid the physical environment of alcohol have failed. The nonaddicted partner grows ever more distant from his or her alcoholic partner.

Stage 4. Reorganization and role shifts. Family life at this stage has become more difficult than ever before. The alcoholic spouse continues with binge drinking despite the concerns expressed by family members. There may not be any food in the house, verbal abuse and/or violence has occurred, and some nonalcoholic spouses may have abandoned the marriage. In other cases, the nonalcoholic spouse begins to assume the leadership role and the alcoholic becomes the subordinate partner. The nonaddicted spouse often hides money, and the alcoholic either sleeps on the couch or in a separate room. If children are present, the drinking partner is ignored and feels isolated. Some attempts are made to regain control of authority by the alcoholic, either through verbal or physical confrontations. Sometimes the nonaddicted partner of the marriage begins to plan for separation or divorce or contacts Al-Anon, an organized group of spouses seeking help for living with an alcoholic.

Stage 5. Separating or escaping. The nonalcoholic partner either separates or leaves the alcoholic spouse. The alcoholic can easily become very violent, threatening to kill his or her spouse and/or the children. The nonalcoholic spouse makes final plans for leaving. Often the nonalcoholic spouse leaves for a short time, and with each subsequent trial, the thought of permanent divorce or escape becomes easier to envision.

Stage 6. Life without the alcoholic. Although the alcoholic spouse continues to threaten, the nonalcoholic spouse reorganizes his or her life without the alcoholic spouse. The realization is that the alcoholic spouse is a sick person that cannot be rehabilitated. Other family members also begin to reorganize their lives without the alcoholic. The nonalcoholic spouse grows in her or his ability to be both the family mother and father.

Stage 7. Recovery and reorganization with the alcoholic. (This stage may or may not occur.) Here the alcoholic faces his or her problem and seeks out such outside help as AA (Alcoholics Anonymous) or other kinds of drug counseling and treatment. The recovery from alcohol addiction remains uncertain and the marriage bears many scars at this stage. Because of past drinking, the alcoholic confronts many strained and damaged relationships with family members. Furthermore, the marital partners have difficulty in problems that appear unresolvable in the absence of alcohol. Gradually, however, the drinking problems of the past either destroy the marriage or fade as the marriage readjusts itself in light of alcohol abstinence.

Destructive Support and Organizations for Victims of Alcoholics

Co-dependency and Enabling Generally co-dependency and enabling occur together. Co-dependency (some call this *coalcoholism*) refers to a relationship pattern, and enabling refers to a set of specific behaviors (Doweiko 1990). **Codependency** is defined as the behavior displayed by those nonaddicted family members (or codependents) who identify with the alcohol addict and cover up the excessive drinking behavior. Enablers are those close to the alcohol addict who deny or make excuses for enabling the excessive drinking. Often both codependency and enabling are done by the same person. An example is the husband who calmly conspires and phones his wife's place of employment and reports that his wife has a stomach flu when the addicted spouse is too drunk or hungover to even realize it's Monday morning. Such a husband is both codependent and an enabler. He lies for his wife's addiction and enables her not to face the irresponsible drinking behavior. In this example, the husband is responsible for perpetuating the spouse's addiction. Even quiet toleration of the alcoholic's addiction enables the drinker to continue.

Children of Alcoholics (COAs) and Adult Children of Alcoholics (ACOAs) It is estimated that there are 28.6 million COAs in the United States, and 6.6 million are under the age of 18 (National Clearinghouse for Drug and Alcohol Information, or NCADI 1992). The children of alcoholics are at a high risk of developing the same attachment to alcohol. Alcoholics are more likely than nonalcoholics to have an alcoholic father, mother, sibling, or other relative.

Within the last 10 years, both COAs and ACOAs have been studied extensively. Here are some findings concerning these two groups:

1. Children of alcoholics are two to four times more likely to develop alcoholism. In addition, both COAs and ACOAs are more likely to marry into families where alcoholism is prevalent.
2. Research studies show that approximately one-third of most alcoholics are from families where one parent was or is an alcoholic (NCADI 1992).
3. Both physiological and environmental factors appear to place COAs and ACOAs at a greater risk of becoming alcoholics.
4. COAs and ACOAs exhibit more symptoms of depression and anxiety than do children of nonalcoholics.
5. Small children of alcoholics exhibit an excessive amount of crying, bed wetting, and sleep problems, such as nightmares.
6. Teenagers display excessive perfectionism, hoarding, staying by themselves (loners), and excessive self-consciousness.
7. Finally, phobias develop, and difficulty with school performance is not uncommon.

Sociological Explanations

To what extent are the external factors responsible for excessive drinking? Sociologists take a much broader approach to the causes of alcoholism than do psychologists. Cultural values and attitudes, including ethnic differences, family drinking practices, peer influence, influence of mass media advertising of alcohol, and the degree to which people are bonded to major social institutions (for example, family, religion, economic, and political systems) all play a role.

Often sociologists pay particular attention to how drinking is viewed in a particular society. In our culture, for example, alcohol is seen as a social lubricant and drinkers are strongly affected by such cultural practices. In some cultural groups, like the Abipone Indians of Paraguay, drinking usually leads to violence, while in other cultures (the Yuruna Indians of South America) it leads to passiveness or (the Tarahumara of Mexico) to heightened sexual activity (MacAndrew and Edgerton 1969). MacAndrew and Edgerton refer to these

CODEPENDENCY a relationship pattern in which nonaddicted family members identify with the alcohol addict; coalcoholism

ENABLING denial or making up of excuses for the excessive drinking of an alcohol addict to whom someone is close vast cultural differences as **drunken comportment,** where it is not the frequency or the amount of alcohol consumed that affects how drinkers comport themselves, but instead the cultural values and norms that cause an independent outcome of drinking behavior.

Because people interpret reality in terms of their affiliation with the social groups with which they identify, the quality of social interaction with family, peers, and workmates affects our attitudes regarding alcohol use. Other sociological approaches look at the varying amounts of alcohol consumed by different societies and the resulting effects that consumption has on the drinkers. For example, Italians consume a large amount of wine but have moderate rates of alcoholism. The Irish, in contrast, consume large amounts of alcohol and have one of the highest rates of alcoholism (Little 1989, 194).

Still other sociological approaches look at family structures and their use of alcohol. For example, several studies have shown that families with children who do not experience significant alcohol problems are families that have the lowest incidence of alcoholism among the parents. The social psychological profile of these families emphasizes the following habits and attitudes:

1. The children are exposed to alcohol early in life, within a strong family or religious group.
2. The beverage is served in very diluted and small quantities. It is considered mainly as a food and is usually consumed with meals. Abstinence is socially acceptable. It is no more rude or ungracious to decline a drink than to decline a piece of bread.
3. Parents present a constant example of moderate drinking. Excessive drinking or intoxication is not socially acceptable. Such behavior is not considered stylish, comic, or tolerable.
4. No moral importance is attached to drinking; it is not viewed as proof of adulthood or virility.
5. Finally and perhaps most important, there is wide and usually complete agreement among members of the family on what might be called the "ground rules" of drinking (Aronow 1980; NIAAA 1990; Ullman 1958).

DRUNKEN COMPORTMENT cultural values and norms that cause an independent outcome of drinking behavior

PRIMARY PREVENTION prevention of alcohol consumption by means of techniques that are aimed at nonusers and early experimenters

SECONDARY PREVENTION prevention of alcohol consumption by means of techniques that are aimed at more experimental users

Prevention of Alcohol Abuse

Prevention of alcohol abuse differs from treatment in that it involves delaying or preventing alcohol consumption. Treatment entails withdrawing from alcohol consumption. Two major types of prevention are *primary* and *secondary prevention.* **Primary prevention** techniques are aimed at nonusers and early experimenters. **Secondary prevention** techniques are aimed at more experimental users. Often the goal is to prevent the early use of or increased involvement with alcohol and to avoid the health problems associated with alcohol abuse. Prevention efforts focused on the social conditions that foster alcohol abuse are usually undertaken by law enforcement officials, health professionals, educators, legislators, business leaders, and other concerned citizens. Such programs are based on prevention strategies closely tied to research.

Prevention programs and research concentrate on the following kinds of activities and areas of concern (NIAAA 1990, 210-33):

Basic Prevention Methods

1. Increase the price of alcoholic beverages (Babor 1985, 181). This has been found to curtail the amount of alcohol consumed, especially among the youngest age groups. The larger benefit is fewer driving-under-the-influence auto accidents.
2. Ban advertising and portrayals of alcohol consumption on television, in movies, and in

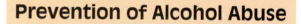

newspapers and magazines (Frankana et al. 1985).

Specific Social Environments

3. Research how the family influences attitudes toward drinking.
4. Prevent or discourage drinking during working hours. Focus on how the working environment promotes or can reduce alcohol consumption.
5. Analyze drinking establishments. Research shows that most cases of continued drinking while under the influence occur in licensed drinking establishments. Are there particular types of bars where heavy drinking occurs? Does the size of the drinking group influence how much is consumed?

Individual Characteristics

6. Analyze how age, gender, and ethnic differences affect consumption rates and the risk of becoming an alcoholic. Analyze personality traits in children and adults that are associated with the amount of alcohol consumed in later life.
7. Analyze accidents and trauma. How does the excessive use of alcohol lead to more accidents (such as fires, burns, and falls)?
8. Analyze how alcohol consumption contributes to violence, namely, family violence and marital stability.
9. Focus on adolescent risk factors and peer group formation. How does peer support of drinking lead to excessive individual use of alcohol? Analyze the relationship between smoking and drinking.

Applied Prevention

10. Increase the minimum drinking age. States that have increased the minimum drinking age from 18 to 21 also experience a reduction in fatal auto accidents.
11. Use planning and zoning ordinances to prevent the consumption and sale of alcoholic beverages in residential areas.
12. Toughen drinking-and-driving laws. Use a deterrent model, consisting of sobriety checkpoints on major highways, fines, license revocation, and imprisonment so as to prevent driving while intoxicated (DWI) or driving under the influence (DUI).
13. Develop more alcohol education programs, workshops, and videos, especially mandatory education for people convicted of DWI offenses.
14. Initiate server-training programs to educate people who are responsible for serving alcohol in private and public places.
15. Improve transportation services or alternatives, including designated driver programs and safe ride programs. In a designated driver program, one person in a group is selected to abstain from drinking and becomes responsible for driving the other members. Safe ride programs offer drinkers alternatives to driving themselves, providing free cab service or other means of transportation.

Programs to Change Individual Behaviors

16. Create mandatory drug education curriculums beginning in grade schools and high schools, and make prevention and treatment information readily available in boys' and girls' clubs, recreational centers, and public housing developments.

Treatment of Alcoholism

Alcoholism is a treatable illness from which about two-thirds of those affected can recover; that is, they can stop the compulsion to consume alcohol by their own efforts. Many of the misunderstandings about alcoholism make it difficult for alcoholics to seek and get the help they need. For instance, some people think of alcoholism as a form of moral weakness rather than an illness. This stigma causes problem drinkers and their families to hide the problem rather than face it and seek treatment. There is a widespread belief, even among physicians, that alcoholism is not treatable and that the alcoholic is unmanageable and unwilling to be helped. None of these assumptions is true.

About 70% of alcoholics are men and women who are married and living with their families, who hold jobs, and who are accepted and reasonably respected members of their communities. For those of this group who seek treatment, the outlook is optimistic.

One obstacle to treatment is that many individuals deny their alcoholism, even to themselves. They are not inclined to seek treatment until the pain, severity, and duration of their drinking problem become overwhelming or until a personal crisis forces assessment. As the circumstances in such a person's life fluctuate and become less painful, the motivation for recovery lessens; such an alcoholic may then discontinue treatment and relapse into a serious alcoholic condition.

In fact, it is quite possible for a person with a drinking problem to recover completely. This does not mean that he or she is cured; rather, it means that he or she can stop or control compulsive or uncontrolled drinking.

Rehabilitation Methods

Rehabilitation for alcohol abuse means a return to successful living without the need to have alcohol. The patient is rehabilitated when he or she has reestablished and can maintain a good family life, work record, and respectable position in the community. Relapses may occur, but they do not mean that the problem drinker or the treatment effort has failed.

Satisfactory rehabilitation of alcoholics can be expected in at least 60% of cases, according to the National Institute on Alcohol Abuse and Alcoholism (NIAAA). Some therapists report success in 70 to 80% of cases. The recovery rate depends on the personal characteristics of the patient, the competence of the therapist, the availability of treatment facilities, and the support of the family, employer, and community. Unfortunately, the prognosis is less optimistic for chronic alcoholics and patients with alcoholic psychoses, who are usually placed in psychiatric hospitals. Less than 10 to 12% of this segment of the alcoholic population achieves full recovery.

The type of therapy provided is less important than the patient's personal characteristics and environmental experiences. Motivation is the most important characteristic, followed by high socioeconomic status and social stability. Similar results are obtained regardless of whether treatment is provided in expensive inpatient settings or in less expensive outpatient and intermediate care settings. In outpatient therapy, the length of time the patient stays in treatment seems to have a positive effect on the outcome; this is a function of the patient's motivation. As with any other illness, the earlier treatment is begun, the better the prospects for improvement. Nonetheless, many alcoholics have been treated successfully after many years of excessive drinking.

Aspects of Treatment Methods

The treatment of alcoholism consists of getting the alcoholic safely through the withdrawal period, correcting the chronic health problems associated with alcoholism, and helping him or her to change long-term behavior so that destructive drinking patterns are not continued. The individual may begin treatment during a spell of temporary sobriety, during a severe hangover, or during acute intoxication. For many, it will be during the drying out or withdrawal stage.

Getting Through Withdrawal An alcoholic who is well nourished and in good physical condition can go through withdrawal with reasonable safety as an outpatient. However, an acutely ill alcoholic needs medically supervised care. A general hospital ward is best for preliminary treatment.

The alcohol withdrawal syndrome is quite similar to that described in Chapter 6 for barbiturates and other sedative hypnotics. Symptoms typically appear within 12 to 72 hours after total cessation of drinking but can appear whenever the blood alcohol level drops below a certain point. The alcoholic has severe muscle tremors, nausea, weakness, and anxiety. This condition is called the **delirium tremens (DTs),** or the "shakes." Grand mal seizures can occur but are less common than in barbiturate withdrawal, and there may be terrifying hallucinations.

The syndrome reaches peak intensity within 24 to 48 hours. About 5% of the alcoholics in hospitals and perhaps 20 to 25% who suffer the DTs without treatment die as a result. Phenobarbital,

DELIRIUM TREMENS (DTS) a condition that affects chronic abusers of alcohol during alcohol withdrawal; characterized by agitation, hallucinations, and involuntary body tremors chlordiazepoxide (Librium), and diazepam (Valium) are commonly used to prevent withdrawal symptoms. Controlled withdrawal may take from 10 to 21 days and cannot safely be hurried. Simultaneously, the alcoholic may need treatment for malnutrition and vitamin deficiencies (especially the B vitamins). Pneumonia is also a frequent complication (Jaffe 1980).

Once the alcoholic patient is over the acute stages of intoxication and withdrawal, CNS depressants may be continued for a few weeks, with care taken not to transfer dependence on alcohol to dependence on the depressants. Long-term treatment with sedatives (Librium, Valium) does not prevent a relapse of drinking or assist with behavioral adaptation. A prescription of disulfiram (Antabuse) may be offered to encourage patients to abstain from alcohol; it blocks metabolism of acetaldehyde, and drinking any alcohol will result in a pounding headache, flushing, nausea, and other unpleasant symptoms. The patient must decide about two days in advance to stop taking Antabuse before he or she can drink. Antabuse is an aid to other supportive treatments, not the sole method of therapy.

Psychological and Behavioral Therapies

After withdrawal symptoms are over, the person usually goes right back to drinking unless he or she can be persuaded to start other therapy to address the factors underlying the drinking problem. Most successful therapists say that pleading, exhortation, telling the patient how to live his or her life, and urging him or her to use more willpower are useless strategies and may even be destructive. They emphasize the need to create a warm, concerned relationship with the patient.

Psychotherapy is quite effective for some patients. For alcoholics, it is directed more to action, focusing on the patient's immediate life situation and drinking problem. Many therapists bring members of the patient's family into the therapy program; family support and understanding are often crucial to success. Sometimes a member of the family, perhaps more emotionally disturbed than the patient, may unconsciously support the alcoholic's drinking behavior.

A psychotherapeutic approach begins by getting the patient (and perhaps his or her family) to accept alcoholism as an illness, not as a moral problem or weakness. The patient must genuinely accept the idea that he or she needs help. Once these attitudes have been established, the therapist and patient try (1) to solve those problems that can be readily handled and (2) to find an approach that will enable the patient to live with those problems that cannot be solved.

Behavioral psychologists believe that drinking is learned behavior. Behavioral therapies try to reverse the reinforcement pattern so that abstinence or moderate drinking brings reward or avoids punishment. Techniques used include aversion therapies, assertiveness, relaxation, biofeedback (see Chapter 16), blood alcohol discrimination training, and controlled drinking. The current trend is to observe drinking patterns and develop techniques that will change them. Analysis of drinking behavior focuses on cues and stimuli, attitudes and thoughts, specific behaviors, and consequences of drinking. These factors are complex and highly individualized; careful assessment is required in order to change the attitudes and behaviors that lead a given patient to excessive drinking. No one treatment plan is suitable for everyone.

Sobering up means that the alcoholic must face a backlog of personal, family, financial, and social problems. Without help to work out these alcohol-related problems, the alcoholic will probably return to the same escape method as before: drinking. Moreover, effective treatment must be conducted on a consistent basis in order to deal with the root of the problem. Treatment should not constitute random sessions after occasional drinking episodes. Rather, treatment should be tailored to the individual's needs and rate of progress.

Helping Agencies for Alcohol Rehabilitation

It is important to remember that the alcoholic commonly has several social problems that must be successfully handled if the drinking is to stop. Many organizations and agencies, staffed largely by nonmedical personnel, aid countless thousands of alcoholics and help them re-establish better relations at home, at work, and in the community.

Alcoholics Anonymous (AA) is a loosely knit, voluntary fellowship of alcoholics whose sole purpose is to help themselves and one another get sober and stay sober. AA has been characterized first as a way back to life and then as a way of living.

In the AA approach, the alcoholic must admit that he or she lacks control over drinking behavior and that his or her life is unmanageable and intolerable. For some alcoholics, this realization may not come until they have lost everything and everyone. For a few, it may occur sooner, for instance, when they are arrested by police or are warned by their employers. At this point, "the individual must decide to turn over his life and his will to a power greater than his own." Much of the program has a nonsectarian, spiritual basis. Over 356,000 members belong to about 19,000 groups in the United States, and more than 200,000 members participate in 11,500 groups in Canada and other countries. Despite its scope, AA reaches only a small percentage of the approximately 10 million alcoholics and problem drinkers in the United States.

During the early years of AA, some members insisted that "only an alcoholic can understand an alcoholic." As a result, there was little cooperation between AA workers and physicians, clergy, and social workers. Through understanding of one another's roles, most AA members no longer hold this view and cooperate increasingly with professional therapists. Conversely, professionals strongly encourage membership in AA as part of the treatment programs in detoxification centers, general and psychiatric hospitals, clinics, and prisons.

However, many professionals emphasize that, as valuable and widely accessible as AA is, it should not be considered as a complete form of treatment for all alcoholics; instead, it should be viewed as a support to other forms of therapy. Some alcoholics simply do not fit the AA approach but can be helped by other treatment modalities. The AA model has been used for treatment of other drug addictions, such as heroin.

Al-Anon and Alateen were formed to help families cope with alcoholic members. Al-Anon is for spouses and other relatives of alcoholics; it does not matter whether the alcoholic is in AA or another rehabilitation program. Members learn that they are not alone in this predicament and benefit from the experiences of others. Alateen is a parallel organization for teenage children of alcoholic parents. (These organizations are listed in most phone directories.)

The National Council on Alcoholism (NCA) provides leadership in public education, advocacy of enlarged government involvement in prevention and treatment, and consultation services, particularly to industry. There are more than 200 member councils across the United States. At the community level, information and referral service and short-term pretreatment counseling are offered to problem drinkers and their families.

The Salvation Army and the Volunteers of America provide food, shelter, and rehabilitation services, often through halfway houses. Many religious groups have also developed programs and therapy groups to aid alcoholics and their families. Most clergy have training in counseling and some in psychotherapy; they provide a valuable service.

The U.S. Department of Transportation (DOT) has become involved in alcohol rehabilitation in an attempt to reduce the thousands of deaths and hundreds of thousands of serious accidents that occur on the highways each year because of drinking. The DOT has developed an information program to persuade people to prevent their friends from driving while drunk and a technical assistance program to help state and local governments develop systems for apprehending drunk drivers and bringing them for treatment.

The National Institute on Alcohol Abuse and Alcoholism provides federal policy guidance on alcohol-related problems. It also channels funds for research, training, prevention, and development of community-based services for treatment of alcoholics, a national information and education program, and other special projects.

The Veterans Administration (VA) hospitals conduct the largest alcoholism treatment and research program in the United States; over 100,000 alcoholic patients are treated yearly. Eligible alcoholic veterans are treated at no charge. Treatment for acute intoxication is available at any VA hospital in the country, and many offer comprehensive follow-up treatment and rehabilitation services.

Alcohol use and abuse is of concern to U.S. industry, as well. It is estimated that business, industry, and government employ about 5.8 million problem drinkers—up to 6% of the nation's labor force and perhaps 10% of its executives. Because the problem is substantial, the federal government and many industries have initiated programs to help employees whose job performance suffers due to their use of alcohol. Organized labor has also become involved. The unions have developed their own training programs and provide services for members in trouble with alcohol; some of these programs have been included in contract agreements. A good evaluation of job-based alcohol abuse treatment programs is presented in the *Handbook on Drug Abuse* (Trice 1979) (see also Roman 1988; Nathan and Skinstad 1987; Berg and Skutle 1986).

Job-based treatment programs have an average 70% success rate. Because the drinking problem is identified much earlier in alcoholic employees than in unemployed persons, treatment is begun before physical health has entirely deteriorated, before financial resources are totally gone, and while emotional support still exists in the family and community. Also, the threat of job loss motivates employees to accept treatment.

Review Questions

1. Why do you think alcohol remains as a legitimate drug despite the tremendous costs to our society?
2. Would a temperance movement and/or prohibition on alcohol be successful today? Why or why not? Give at least three reasons in support of your position.
3. Do you personally believe that set and setting can have a stronger effect on the alcohol user than the ethanol itself? In other words, do you think that nonalcoholic beer, for example, could possibly cause people to actually believe and act as if they were inebriated?
4. Of the four cultures cited by Pittman—namely abstinent, ambivalent cultures, permissive and overly permissive cultures—which type do you think would have the most alcoholics? Why?
5. Review the four reasons cited regarding the decrease of alcohol consumption since 1981. Which single reason do you believe is the most important for the decrease? Why?
6. Review the major findings regarding alcohol consumption among social class, religious, regional, gender, age, and youth groups. Describe two groups where the findings contradicted your commonsense expectations.
7. What theory discussed in Chapter 2 do you think best explains the reasons why racial and ethnic minorities, gays, and the homeless are prone to abuse so much alcohol?
8. From the views and theoretical explanations given for alcoholism in this chapter, which view or theoretical explanation best explains the causes of alcoholism? Why does the view or theory you selected provide more explanatory power than the others?
9. What specific factors do you think makes the children of alcoholics and adult children of alcoholics more likely to develop drinking problems?
10. Create an alcoholism prevention program targeted at grade-school children. What would you emphasize?
11. Create an alcoholism prevention program targeted at high school drug *users*. What would you emphasize differently, in contrast to a program aimed at grade-school children?
12. Visit an open session of either AA or Al-Anon. Report your observations to the class.
13. Visit an AA or Al-Anon chapter, collect their written information and analyze the brochures, pamphlets, and other written handouts you have gathered and report the findings to your class.

Key Terms

ethanol
social substance
set
setting
speakeasies
abstinent cultures
ambivalent cultures
permissive cultures
overpermissive cultures
moral model
medical model
social learning theory
reinforcement theory
codependency
enabling
drunken comportment
primary prevention
secondary prevention
delirium tremens (DTs)

Summary

1. Ethanol is the psychoactive ingredient found in alcoholic beverages. The ill effects of its misuse exceed those of any other legal or illicit drugs.
2. Alcohol use has occurred during most of our U.S. history.
3. In response to the heaviest drinking period in America during Jefferson's turn in office (1800–1808), the *temperance movement* occurred. The original goal of this movement was to promote moderate use of alcohol. Largely because it was unsuccessful, the temperance movement began advocating "total abstinence." Over the course of the nineteenth century, total prohibition was enacted into law. Shortly after Prohibition laws were enacted making alcohol use illegal, organized crime involved itself in producing and selling alcohol as an illicit drug.
4. Set and setting exert independent effects on the consumption of alcohol. Set is the drinkers' belief about what effect the drug will have on his or her personality. Setting consists of the physical and social environment where the drug is consumed. Set and setting are believed to greatly affect the drug user when less initially potent and addictive drugs such as alcohol and marijuana are used.
5. Cultures vary in the use of alcohol. Abstinent cultures strictly prohibit alcohol use. Ambivalent cultures have contradictory views on alcohol consumption. Permissive cultures promote alcohol consumption, and overpermissive cultures encourage alcohol use.
6. There has been a steady decline in alcohol consumption since 1981.
7. Groups in our society vary in their consumption of alcohol. The higher the household income the greater is the percentage who drink. Catholics drink more heavily than Protestants. People residing on the East and West Coasts drink more heavily than southerners and midwesterners. Women are less likely to drink than men, although the percentage of women drinking has been increasing in recent years. People over age 50 drink the least, while those under 30 through 49 drink the most. Although in the last few years the percentage of youth drinking alcohol has begun to decline, a disturbing percentage, well over 60% of all youth continue to drink alcohol.
8. Racial minorities and ethnic groups, gays, and the homeless are among the groups consuming a disproportionately high amount of alcohol.
9. There are several accepted definitions of alcoholism. Alcohol addiction involves both physical and psychological dependence on ethanol. Most definitions include chronic behavioral disorders, repeated drinking to the point of loss of control, health disorders, and difficulty functioning socially and economically.
10. The importance given to the causes of alcohol addiction is determined by the various perspectives on alcoholism. We have cited four major explanations: the moral model, the medical model, explanations based on psychological factors, and sociological explanations.
11. Codependency and enabling are often done by the same person. Codependency is the behavior displayed by those nonaddicted family members who identify with the alcohol addict. Enabling is the behavior of those close to the alcohol addict who deny or make excuses for excessive alcohol consumption. Both involve covering up the addiction.
12. Children of alcoholics (COAs) and adult children of alcoholics (ACOAs) are of particular interest in the study of alcoholism because research shows that these children and adults are two to four times more likely to develop alcoholism.
13. Prevention differs from treatment in that it involves delaying or preventing alcohol consumption. Treatment involves stopping the ongoing consumption of alcohol. Primary prevention techniques are aimed at nonusers and early experimenters. Secondary prevention techniques address experimenters or early users of alcohol.
14. Alcohol treatment is based on the view that alcoholism is a treatable illness from which two-thirds of those affected can recover. Treatment focuses on rehabilitative methods, getting past the DTs, and psychological behavioral therapies. Helping agencies include AA, Al-Anon, the VA, and industrial programs.

References

Akers, R. L. *Deviant Behavior: A Social Learning Approach,* 3d ed. Belmont: CA: Wadsworth, 1985.

Akers, R. L. *Drugs, Alcohol, and Society: Social Structure, Process, and Policy.* Belmont, CA: Wadsworth, 1992.

"Alcoholism." *Academic American Encyclopedia.* (Electronic data base on CARL system at the University of Colorado, Boulder). Grolier Electronic Publishing, no date.

Arkin, E. B., and J. E. Funkhouser, eds. *Communicating About Alcohol and Other Drugs: Strategies for Reaching Populations at Risk.* OSAP Prevention Monograph 5. Rockville, MD: Office of Substance Abuse Prevention, U.S. Department of Health and Human Services, 1992.

Aronow, L. *Alcoholism, Alcohol Abuse, and Related Problems: Opportunities for Research.* Washington, DC: National Academy Press, 1980.

Austin, G. A. *Perspectives on the History of Psychoactive Substance Use.* National Institute on Drug Abuse Research Issues 23. Washington, DC: U.S. Department of Health, Education, and Welfare, 1978.

Babor, T. F. "Alcohol, Economics and Ecological Fallacy: Toward an Integration of Experimental and Quasi-Experimental Research." In *Public Drinking and Public Policy,* edited by E. Single and T. Storm, 161–89. Proceedings of a Symposium on Observation Studies held at Banff, Alberta, 26–28 April 1984. Toronto: Addiction Research Foundation, 1985.

Baker, S. P., B. O'Neil, and R. Karpf. *Injury Fact Book.* Lexington, MA: Heath, 1984.

Becker, H. S. *Outsiders: Studies in the Sociology of Deviance.* New York: Free Press, 1966.

Berg, G., and A. Skutle. "Early Intervention with Problem Drinkers." In *Treating Addictive Behaviors: Processes of Change,* edited by W. R. Miller and N. Heather, 205–20. New York: Plenum, 1986.

Bower, B. "Gene in the Bottle" A Controversial Alcoholism Gene Gets a New Twist." *Science News* 140, (21 September 1991): 392–93.

Brazeau, R., and M. Sparrow. *International Survey: Alcoholic Beverage Taxation and Control Policies,* 6th ed. Ottawa: Brewers Association of Canada, 1986.

Brown, N. H., E. H. Goulding, and S. Fabro. "Ethanol Embryotoxicity: Direct Effects on Mammalian Embryos in Vitro." *Science* 206 (1979): 573–75.

Brown, S. C. "Beers and Wines of Old New England." *American Scientist* 66 (1978): 460–67.

Cage, M. C. "Alcohol Abuse by Students Is Found Most Severe on Campuses in Northeast." *Chronicle of Higher Education* (26 May 1993): A28, A30.

Cahalan, Don, and Robin Room. *Problem Drinking Among American Men.* New Brunswick, NJ: Rutgers Center for Alcohol Studies, 1974.

Catanzaro, R. J. "Psychiatric Aspects of Alcoholism." In *Alcoholism,* edited by D. J. Pittman. New York: Harper & Row, 1967.

Chan, A. W. K. "Racial Differences in Alcohol Sensitivity." *Alcohol and Alcoholism* 21 (1986): 93–104.

Chi, I., H. H. L. Kitano, and J. E. Lubben. "Male Chinese Drinking Behavior in Los Angeles." *Journal of Studies on Alcohol* 49 (1988): 21–25.

Coffey, W. *Straight Talk About Drinking: Teenagers Speak Out About Alcohol.* Markham, Ontario, Canada: Penguin, 1988.

Colasanto, D., and J. Zeglarski. "Alcoholic Beverages: Alcohol Consumption at Lowest Level in 30 Years." *Gallup Report,* 288 (September 1989).

Desmond, E. W. "Out in the Open: Changing Attitudes and New Research Give Fresh Hope to Alcoholics." *Time* (30 November 1987): 42–50.

Doweiko, H. E. *Concepts of Chemical Dependency.* Monterey, CA: Brooks/Cole, 1990.

Dryfoos, J. D. *Adolescents at Risk.* New York: Oxford University Press, 1991.

Frankana, M., M. Cohen, T. Danill, L. Ehrlich, N. Greenspun, and D. Kelman. "Alcohol Advertising, Consumption and Abuse." In *Recommendations of the Staff of the Federal Trade Commission: Omnibus Petition for Regulation of Unfair and Deceptive Alcoholic Beverage Marketing Practices,* edited by staff. Docket no. 290–346, Washington, DC: Federal Trade Commission, 1985.

Freud, Sigmund. "Dostoyevsky and Parricide." *The Standard Edition of the Complete Works of Sigmund Freud,* edited by J. Strachey, 340–386. London: Hogarth Press and Institute of Psychoanalysis, 1961.

Gallup, G., Jr., and F. Newport. "Americans Now Drinking Less Alcohol." *Gallup Poll Monthly* (December 1990).

Gallup Report, no. 276 (September 1988).

Gold, M. S. *The Good News About Drugs and Alcohol.* New York: Villard Books, 1991.

Gomberg, E., and S. Lisansky. "Historical and Political Perspective: Women and Drug Use." In *Drug Use and Misuse: A Reader,* edited by T. Heller, M. Gott, and C. Jeffery. New York: Wiley, 1989.

Greeley, Andrew M., W. C. McCreedy, and G. Theison. *Ethnic Drinking Subcultures.* New York: Praeger, 1980.

Harper, F. D. *The Black Family and Substance Abuse.* Detroit: Detroit Urban League, 1986.

Inciardi, J. A. *The War on Drugs II.* Mountain View, CA: Mayfield, 1992.

"In These Times." Chicago, IL: 18–24 October 1989.

Jaffe, J. H. "Drug Addiction and Drug Abuse." In *The Pharmacological Basis of Therapeutics,* 6th ed., edited by A. G. Gilman, L. S. Goodman, and A. Gilman, 494–534. New York: Macmillan, 1980.

Jellinek, E. M. *The Disease Concept of Alcoholism.* New Haven, CT: College and University Press, 1960.

Jennison, K. M. "The Impact of Stressful Life Events and Social Support on Drinking Among Older Adults: A General Population Survey." *International Journal of Aging and Human Development* (1992): 991–1023.

Jensen, M. A., T. L. Peterson, R. J. Murphy, and D. A. Emmerling. "Relationship of Health Behaviors to Alcohol and Cigarette Use by College Students." *Journal of College Students Development* 33 (1992): 170.

Johnston, L. D., P. O'Malley, and J. G. Bachman. "Smoking, Drinking, and Illicit Drug Use Among American Secondary School Students, College Students, and Young Adults, 1975–1991." In *Drugs, Society and Behavior 93/94,* edited by E. Goode. Guilford, CT: Dushkin, 1993.

Keller, M. "Alcoholism: Nature and Extent of the Problem." *Understanding Alcoholism, Annals American Academy Political and Social Science* 315 (1958): 1–11.

Kilbourne, J., Ed. "Advertising Addiction: The Alcohol Industry's Hard Sell." *Multinational Monitor* (Washington, DC) Vol. 10, no. 6 (June 1989): 13–16.

Lee, H. *How Dry We Were: Prohibition Revisited.* Englewood Cliffs, NJ: Prentice Hall, 1963.

Leerhsen, C., with T. Namuth. "Alcohol and the Family." *Newsweek,* (18 January 1988).

Levin, J. D. *Alcoholism: A Bio-psychosocial Approach.* New York: Hemisphere, 1990.

Lewis, G. R., and S. M. Jordan. "Treatment of the Gay or Lesbian Alcoholic." In *Alcoholism and Substance Abuse in Special Populations,* edited by G. W. Lawson and A. W. Lawson, 165–203. Gaithersburg, MD: Aspen, 1989.

Liska, K. *Drugs and the Human Body,* 3rd ed. New York: Macmillan, 1990.

Little, C. B. *Deviance and Control: Theory, Research, and Social Policy.* Itasca, IL: Peacock, 1989.

Lumeng, L., and Li, T.-K. "The Development of Metabolic Tolerance in the Alcohol-Preferring P Rats: Comparison on Forced and Free-Choice Drinking of Ethanol." *Pharmacological Biochemical Behavior* 25, no. 5 (1986): 1013–20.

MacAndrew, C., and R. B. Edgerton. *Drunken Comportment: A Social Explanation.* Chicago: Aldine, 1969.

McAneny, Leslie, "Alcoholism in America: Number of Drinkers Holding Steady but Drinking Less." *Gallup Poll News Service* 59 (17 June 1994): 1–4.

McKirnan, D. J., and P. L. Peterson. "Psychosocial and Cultural Factors in Alcohol and Drug Abuse: An Analysis of a Homosexual Community." *Addictive Behaviors* 14 (1989): 555–63.

Mathias, R. "Drug Use Among High School Seniors Continues 16-Year Decline." *NIDA Notes* 7, no. 3 (1992): 13.

Merrill, D. S. "The Changing Homeless Population." *U.S. News and World Report* (15 January 1990): 27.

Moskowitz, J. M. "The Primary Prevention of Alcohol Problems: A Critical Review of the Research Literature." *Journal of Studies on Alcohol* 50, no. 1 (1989): 54–88.

Nathan, P. E. "Integration of Biosocial and Psychosocial Research on Alcoholism." *Alcoholism: Clinical and Experimental Research* 14 (1990): 368–74.

Nathan, P. E., and A. H. Skinstad. "Outcomes of Treatment for Alcohol Problems: Current Methods, Problems, and Results." *Journal of Consulting Clinical Psychology,* 55 (1987): 332–40.

National Clearinghouse for Alcohol and Drug Information (NCADI). "The Fact is . . . Alcoholism Tends to Run in Families." Rockville, MD: NCADI, October 1991.

National Clearinghouse for Alcohol and Drug Information (NCADI). "The Fact is . . . Alcoholism Tends to Run in Families." OSAP Prevention Resource Guide. Rockville, MD: NCADI, 1992.

National Highway Traffic Safety Administration (NHTSA), National Center for Statistics and Analysis. *Drug Driving Facts.* Washington, DC: NHTSA, 1988.

National Highway Traffic Safety Administration (NHTSA), National Center for Statistics and Analysis. *Drug Driving Facts.* Washington, DC: NHTSA, 1989.

National Institute on Alcohol Abuse and Alcoholism (NIAAA). *Facts About Alcohol and Alcoholism.* Washington, DC: U.S. Government Printing Office, 1980.

National Institute on Alcohol Abuse and Alcoholism (NIAAA). *Apparent Per Capita Alcohol Consumption: National, State and Regional Trends, 1977–1987.* Surveillance report no. 13. Washington, DC: U.S. Government Printing Office, 1989.

National Institute on Alcohol Abuse and Alcoholism (NIAAA). "Seventh Special Report to the U.S. Congress on Alcohol and Health," 1990.

National Institute on Drug Abuse (NIDA). *National Survey Results on Drugs from the Monitoring the Future Study, 1975–1992. Vol. 1: Secondary School Students,* 137. Rockville, MD: NIDA, 1993.

Novello, A. C. "Alcohol and Kids: It's Time for Candor." *Christian Science Monitor* (26 June 1992): 19.

Nusbaumer, M. R. "Governmental Control of Deviant Drinking: The Manipulation of Morals and Medicine." *Drug Use in America: Social, Cultural and Political Perspectives,* edited by P. J. Venturelli, 13–22.

Boston: Jones and Bartlett, 1994.

Parrish, K., S. Higuchi, F. S. Stinson, et al. "Genetic or Cultural Determinants of Drinking: A Study of Embarrassment at Facial Flushing Among Japanese and Japanese-Americans." *Journal of Substance Abuse* 2 (1990): 439–47.

Peele, S., and A. Brodsky with M. Arnold. *The Truth About Addiction and Recovery.* New York: Simon & Schuster, 1991.

Pernanen, K. "Causal Inferences About the Role of Alcohol in Accidents, Poisonings and Violence." In *Drinking and Casualties: Accidents, Poisonings and Violence in an International Perspective,* edited by N. Giesbrecht, R. Gonzalez, M. Grant, E. Osterberb, R. Room, I. Rootman, and L. Towle. New York: Tavistock/Routledge, 1989.

Pittman, D. J., ed. *Alcoholism.* New York: Harper & Row, 1967.

Primm, B. J. "Drug Use: Special Implications for Black Americans." In *The State of Black America, 1987,* edited by J. Dewart, 145–66. New York: National Urban League, 1987.

Public Health Services. *Health United States 1989 and Prevention Profile.* Washington, DC: U.S. Department of Health and Human Services, 1990.

Public Health Services, U.S. Department of Health and Human Services. *Healthy People 2000, National Health Promotion and Disease Prevention Objectives, Full Report, with Commentary.* Boston: Jones and Bartlett, 1992.

Roman, P. M. "Growth and Transformation in Workplace Alcoholism Programming." In *Recent Developments in Alcoholism,* vol. 6, M. Galanter, ed., 131–58. New York: Plenum, 1988.

Ropers, R. H., and R. Bayer. "Homelessness as a Health Risk." *Alcohol Health Research World* 11, no. 3 (1987): 38–41.

Roueché, B. *The Neutral Spirit: A Portrait of Alcohol.* Boston: Little, Brown, 1960.

Royce, James E. *Alcohol Problems and Alcoholism,* rev. ed. New York: Free Press, 1989.

Rudy, D. R. *Becoming Alcoholic: Alcoholic Anonymous and the Reality of Alcoholism.* Carbondale: Southern Illinois University Press, 1986.

Schaler, J. A. "Drugs and Free Will." *Society* (September–October 1991): 42–49.

Schuckit, M. A., and V. Rayes. "Ethanol Ingestion: Differences in Blood Acetaldehyde Concentrations in Relatives of Alcoholics and Controls." *Science* 203 (1979): 54–55.

Siegel, R. K. *Intoxication: Life in the Pursuit of Artificial Paradise.* New York: Dutton, 1989.

Sutherland, Edwin H. *Principles of Criminology.* Philadelphia: Lippincott, 1947.

Trice, H. M. "Job-Based Alcohol and Drug Abuse Programs: Recent Program Developments and Research." In *Handbook on Drug Abuse,* edited by R. L. DuPont, A. Goldstein, and J. O. O'Donnell, 181–191. Washington, DC: National Institute on Drug Abuse, 1979.

Ullman, A. D. "Sociocultural Backgrounds of Alcoholism." In *Understanding Alcoholism, Annals American Academy Political and Social Science,* vol. 315, edited by S. D. Bacon, 48–54. 1958.

U.S. Department of Health and Human Services. *Facts About Alcohol and Alcoholism.* Rockville, MD: National Institute on Alcohol Abuse and Alcoholism, 1980.

U.S. Department of Health and Human Services. *Sixth Special Report to the U.S. Congress on Alcohol and Health from the Secretary of Health and Human Services.* Rockville, MD: National Institute on Alcohol Abuse and Alcoholism, 1987.

Wagenaar, A. C. "Protecting Our Future: Options for Preventing Alcohol-Impaired Driving Among Youth." In *Drug Use in America: Social, Cultural and Political Perspectives,* edited by P. J. Venturelli, 193–202. Boston: Jones and Bartlett, 1994.

Watson, D., and L. A. Clark. "Negative Affectivity: The Disposition to Experience Aversive Emotional States." *Psychological Bulletin* 96 (1984): 465–90.

Watts, D. W., Jr. *The Psychedelic Experience: A Sociological Study.* Beverly Hills, CA: Sage 1971.

Wechsler, H., and N. Isaac. "'Binge' Drinkers at Massachusetts Colleges." *Journal of the American Medical Association* 267 (1992): 2929–31.

Whitman, D., with D. Friedman and L. Thomas. "The Return of Skid Row: Why Alcoholics and Addicts Are Filling the Street Again." *U.S. News and World Report* (15 January 1990): 27–29.

Williams, G. D., F. S. Stinson, D. A. Parker, T. C. Harford, and V. Noble. "Demographic Trends, Alcohol Abuse and Alcoholism, 1985–1995." Epidemiologic Bulletin no. 15. *Alcohol Health and Research World* 11, no. 3 (1987): 80–83.

Wilsnack, S. C., R. W. Wilsnack, and A. D. Klassen. Epidemiological Research on Women's Drinking, 1978–1984." In *Women and Alcohol: Health-Related Issues.* Research Monograph no. 16. DHHS Pub. no. (ADM). Washington, DC: U.S. Government Printing Office, 1986.

Wright, J. D., J. W. Knight, E. Weber-Burdin, and J. Lam. "Ailments and Alcohol: Health Status Among the Drinking Homeless." *Alcohol Health and Research World* 11, no. 3 (1987): 22–27.

Zinberg, N. E. *Drug, Set, and Setting: The Basis for Controlled Intoxicant Use.* New Haven, CT: Yale University Press, 1984.

Zinberg, N. E., and J. A. Robertson. *Drugs and the Public.* New York: Simon & Schuster, 1972.

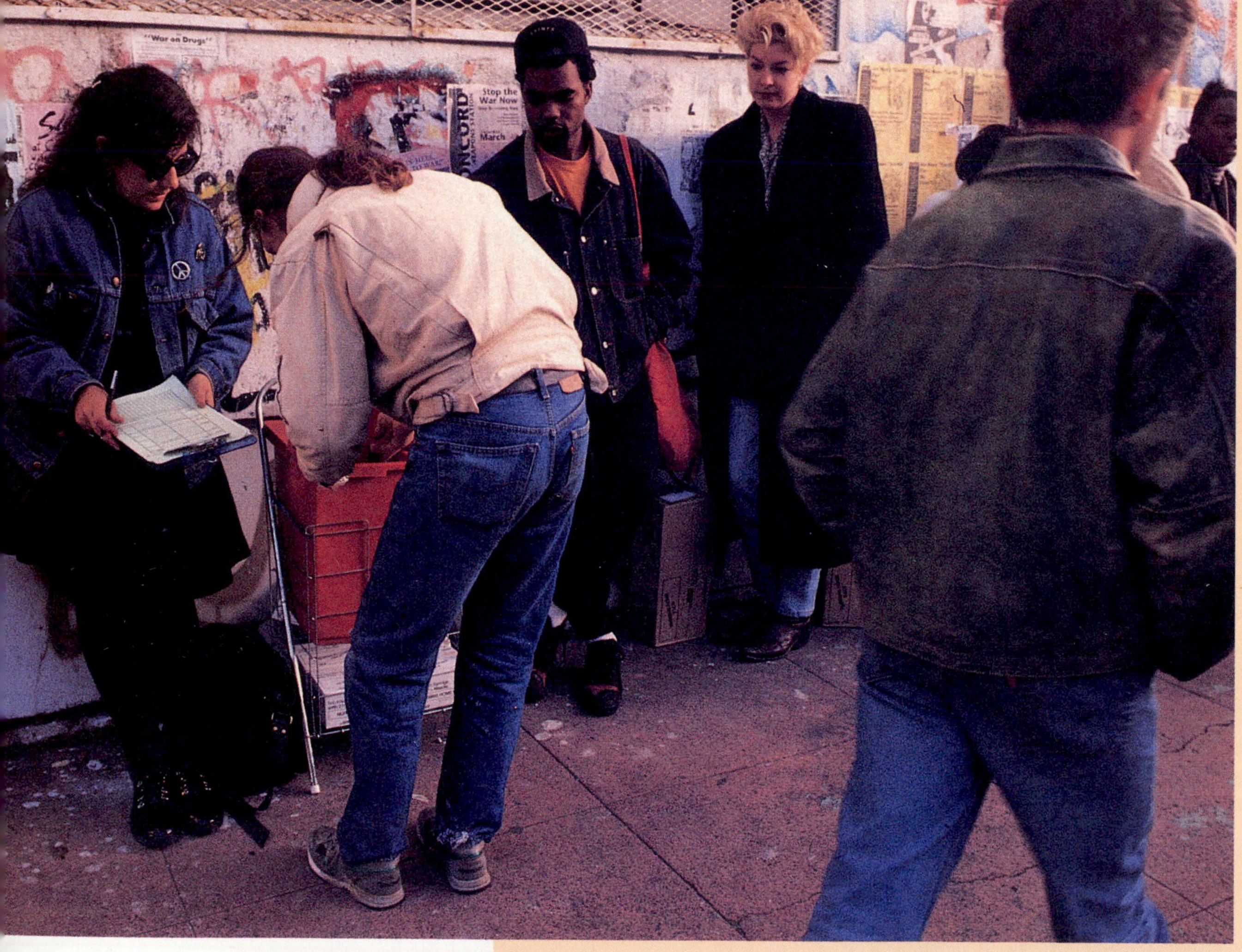

Chapter 9

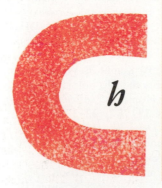

Narcotics (Opioids)

DID YOU KNOW THAT . . .

- The release of natural substances called *endorphins* can mimic the effects of narcotics such as heroin.
- By the end of the nineteenth century, almost 1 million Americans were addicted to opiates, primarily due to the use of patent medicines that contained opium products.
- Narcotics are the most potent analgesics available today.
- Extreme tolerance to the narcotics can develop with continual use, causing as much as a 35-fold increase in dosage to maintain the effects.
- Some people, called "chippers," can continue to use opioid narcotics daily without significantly altering their lifestyle and ability to function.
- Because heroin addicts often "mainline" the drug and share needles, almost one-half of these addicts have been exposed to the AIDS virus.
- One designer drug, made from the narcotic fentanyl, is 6,000 times more potent than heroin.
- Some heroin addicts have to be treated with the narcotic methadone for the rest of their lives.
- One contaminant of illegal narcotic manufacturing is called MPTP and can cause severe Parkinson's disease in a matter of days.

LEARNING OBJECTIVES

On completing this chapter, you will be able to

1. Describe the principal pharmacological effects of narcotics and their main therapeutic uses.
2. Identify the major side effects of the narcotics.
3. Identify the abuse patterns for heroin.
4. Outline the stages of heroin dependence.
5. Describe the association of AIDS with heroin abuse.
6. List the withdrawal symptoms that result from narcotic dependence, and discuss the significance of tolerance.
7. Describe the use of methadone and other long-acting narcotics in treating narcotic addiction.

(continued)

Healthy People 2000

Increase to at least 50% the estimated proportion of intravenous drug abusers not in treatment who use only uncontaminated drug paraphernalia.

Increase to at least 90% the proportion of cities with populations over 100,000 that have outreach programs to contact drug abusers (particularly intravenous drug abusers) to deliver HIV risk reduction messages.

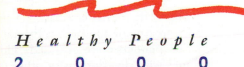

LEARNING OBJECTIVES

8 Identify the unique features of fentanyl that make it appealing to illicit drug dealers but dangerous to narcotic addicts.
9 Describe how "designer" drugs have been associated with the narcotics.
10 Distinguish among the narcotic agents fentanyl, morphine, codeine, pentazocine, and propoxyphene.

The term *narcotic* in general means CNS depressants that produce insensibility or stupor. However, the term has come to designate those drugs and substances with pharmacological properties related to opium and its drug derivatives. All opioid narcotics activate opioid receptors and have abuse potential. In addition, the narcotics are effective pain relievers **(analgesics)** and anticough medications, and are effective in the treatment of diarrhea.

In this chapter we introduce the opioid narcotics with a brief historical account. The pharmacological and therapeutic uses of these drugs are discussed, followed by a description of their side effects and problems with tolerance, withdrawal, and addiction. Narcotic abuse is presented in detail, with special emphasis on heroin. In addition, treatment approaches for narcotic addiction and dependence are included. This chapter concludes with descriptions of other commonly used opioid narcotics.

What Are Narcotics?

The word *narcotic* has been used to label many substances, from opium to marijuana to cocaine. The translation of the Greek word *narkoticos* is "benumbing or deadening." The term *narcotic* is sometimes used to refer to a central nervous system (CNS) depressant, producing insensibility or stupor, and at other times to refer to an addicting drug. Most people would not consider marijuana among the narcotics today, although for many years it was included in this category. Although pharmacologically cocaine is not a narcotic either, it is still legally so classified. Perhaps part of this confusion is due to the fact that cocaine, as a local anesthetic, can cause a numbing effect.

For purposes of the present discussion, the term *narcotic* will be used to refer to those naturally occurring substances derived from the opium poppy and their synthetic substitutes. These drugs are referred to as the **opioid** (or opiate) narcotics because of their association with opium and they have similar pharmacological features including abuse potential, pain-relieving effects (referred to as analgesics), cough suppression, and reduction in intestinal movement. Some of the most commonly used opioid narcotics are listed in Table 9.1.

ANALGESICS drugs that relieve pain without affecting consciousness

OPIOID relating to the drugs that are derived from opium

TABLE 9.1 Commonly used opioid narcotic drugs and products

Narcotic Drug	Common Product Name(s)	Most Common Use(s)
Heroin	Horse, smack, junk (street names)	Abuse
Morphine	(Several)	Analgesia
Methadone	Dolophine	Treat narcotic dependence
Meperidine	Demerol	Analgesia
Oxycodone	Percodan	Analgesia
Propoxyphene	Darvon	Analgesia
Codeine	(Several)	Analgesia, antitussive
Loperamide	Imodium A-D	Antidiarrheal
Diphenoxylate	Lomotil	Antidiarrheal
Opium tincture	Paregoric	Antidiarrheal

The History of Narcotics

The opium poppy, *Papaver somniferum*, from which opium and its narcotic derivatives are obtained, has been cultivated for millenia (see Figure 9.1). A 6,000-year-old Sumerian tablet has an ideograph for the poppy shown as "joy" plus "plant," suggesting that the addicting properties of this substance have been appreciated for many centuries. The Egyptians listed opium along with approximately 700 other medicinal compounds in the famous Ebers Papyrus (about 1500 B.C.).

The Greek god of sleep, Hypnos, and the Roman god of sleep, Somnus, were portrayed as

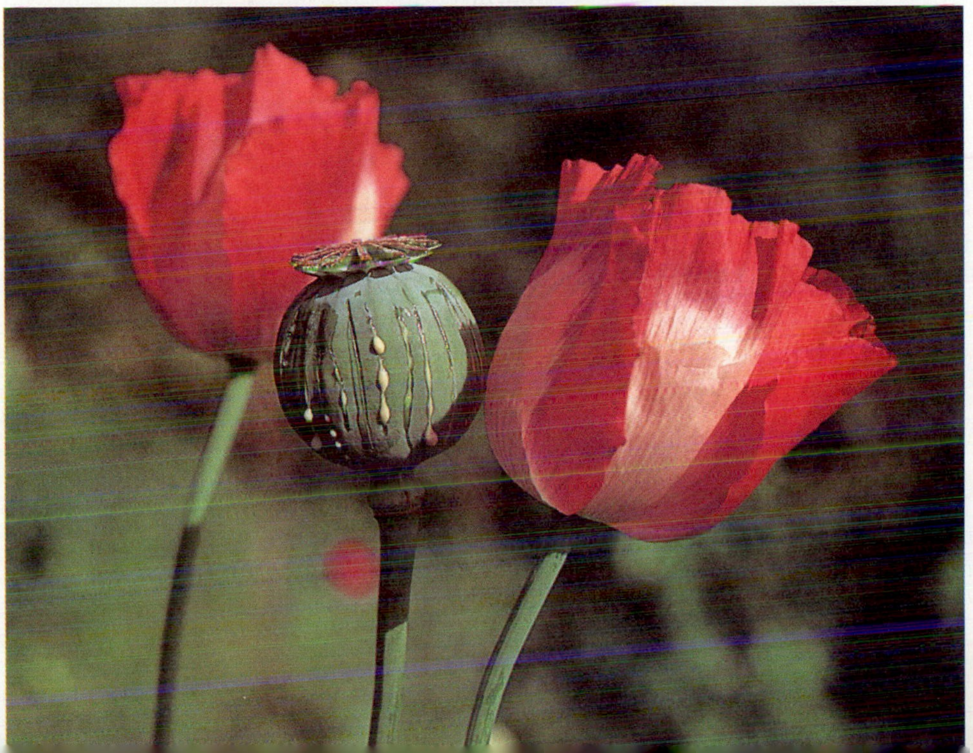

FIGURE 9.1
The opium poppy

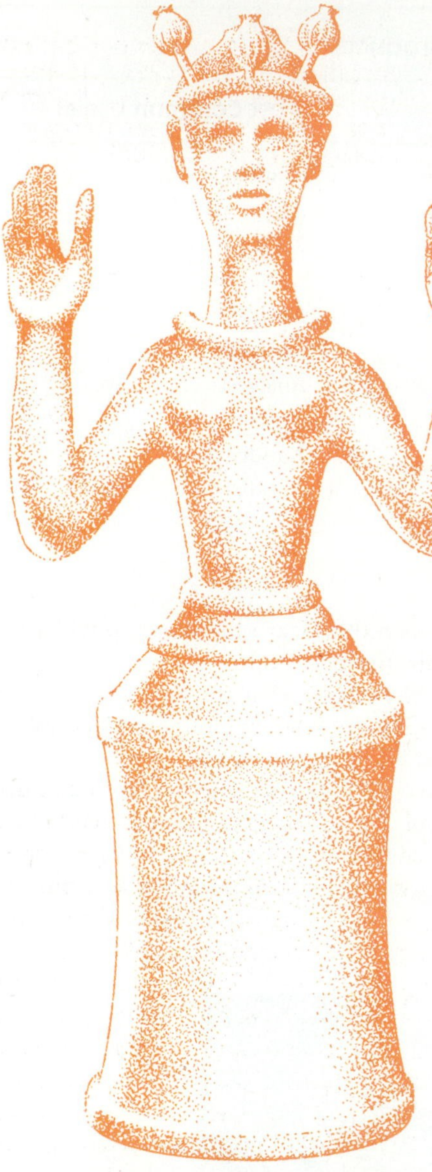

FIGURE 9.2 The Minoan goddess of sleep, wearing a headband of opium poppies

carrying containers of opium pods, and the Minoan goddess of sleep wore a crown of opium pods (see Figure 9.2). According to Greek mythology, the poppy was sacred to Demeter, the goddess of sowing and reaping, and to her daughter, Persephone.

During the so-called Dark Ages that followed the collapse of the Roman Empire, Arab traders actively engaged in traveling the overland caravan routes to China and to India, where they introduced opium. Eventually, both China and India grew their own poppies.

Opium in China

The opium poppy had a dramatic impact in China, causing widespread addiction. Initially, the seeds were used medically, as was opium later. However, by the late 1690s, opium was being smoked and used for diversion. The Chinese government, fearful of the weakening of national vitality by the potent opiate narcotic, outlawed the sale of opium in 1729. The penalty for disobedience was death by strangulation or decapitation.

Despite these laws and threats, the habit of opium smoking became so widespread that the Chinese government went a step further and forbade its importation from India, where most of the opium poppy was grown. The British East India Company (and later the British government in India) encouraged cultivation of opium. British companies were the principal shippers to the Chinese port of Canton, which was the only port open to Western merchants. During the next 120 years, a complex network of opium smuggling developed in China with the help of local merchants, who received substantial profits, and local officials, who pocketed bribes to ignore the smugglers. The amount of opium entering China rose from 200 chests in 1729 to 30,000 to 40,000 chests (weighing about 130 lbs. each) in 1838 (Austin 1978; Scott 1969).

Everyone involved in the opium trade, particularly the British, was profiting until the Chinese government ordered the strict enforcement of the edict against importation. Such actions by the Chinese caused conflict with the British government and helped trigger the Opium War of 1839 to 1842. Great Britain sent in an army, and by 1842, 10,000 British soldiers had won a victory over 350 million Chinese (see Figure 9.3).

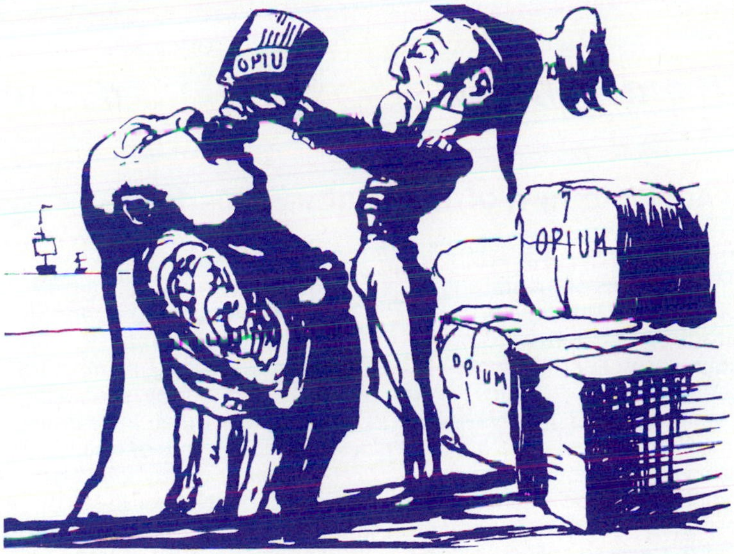

FIGURE 9.3 Famous cartoon, showing a British sailor shoving opium down the throat of a Chinese man, which dates back to the Opium War of 1839–1842.

Britain protested that the war was not over opium but rather over high import tariffs and corrupt Chinese courts. In reality, the British wanted to force China to open its ports to trade. Because of the war, the Treaty of Nanking was signed in 1842; five ports were opened to the British, the island of Hong Kong was ceded to them, and an indemnity of $6 million was imposed on China to cover the value of the destroyed opium and the cost of the war. In 1856, a second Opium War broke out. Peking was occupied by British and French troops, and China was compelled to make further concessions to Britain. The importation of opium continued to increase until 1908, when Britain and China made an agreement to limit the importation of opium from India (Austin 1978).

American Opium Use

Meanwhile, in 1803, a young German named Frederick Serturner extracted and purified the active ingredient in opium. It was 10 times more potent than opium itself and was named *morphine* after Morpheus, the Greek god of dreams. This discovery increased worldwide interest in opium, and by 1832, a number of different alkaloids had been isolated from the raw material. In 1832, the second compound was purified, *codeine,* named after the Greek word for "poppy capsule" (Maurer and Vogel 1967).

The opium problem was aggravated further in 1853, when Alexander Wood perfected the hypodermic syringe and introduced it in Europe and then America. Christopher Wren and others had worked with the idea of injecting drugs directly into the body by means of hollow quills and straws, but the approach was never successful or well received. Wood perfected the syringe technique with the intent of preventing an addiction to morphine by injecting the drug directly into the veins rather than by oral administration (Golding 1993). Unfortunately, just the opposite happened: Injection of morphine increased the potency and the chance of dependence (Maurer and Vogel 1967).

The hypodermic syringe was used extensively during the Civil War to administer morphine for treating pain, dysentery, and fatigue. A large percentage of the men who returned from the war were addicted to morphine. Opiate addiction became known as the "soldier's disease" or "army disease." Nevertheless, historical analysis shows that these returning soldiers did not necessarily contribute significantly to opiate addiction in the United States.

By 1900, an estimated 1 million Americans

Here and Now

The Life of a Functioning Opium Addict in Turn-of-the-Century America

The following account, published in 1907, tells of the typical life of a functioning opium addict:

> Some settle down to a certain dose and adhere to it for years; others devote their lives to the effort of absorbing all the opiate they can crowd into their systems. The life of the former runs on uneventfully. They live, perform a certain limited series of mental and physical evolutions, but their progress ceases, their career culminates. They gradually retire from the activities of the community and grow yearly more contracted in their operations and their sympathies. Ambition is dead, incentive has perished—they just live and no more. The man collects his little rents, sees to his little kitchen garden, eats a trifle, wears his old clothes and sits alone at home, reading a bit, meditating long, ruminating most of the time, producing nothing; a quiet, inoffensive, retiring hermit; of no use to himself or to anybody else, neither hated nor loved by any mortal man. Only the druggist knows the truth. (Sterne 1907)

were dependent on the opiates (Abel 1980). The effects of long-term opiate use on many of those who became addicted during this era are related by an addict in the Here and Now box. This drug problem was made worse because of (1) Chinese laborers, who brought with them to the United States opium to smoke (it was legal to smoke opium in the United States at that time); (2) the availability of purified morphine and the hypodermic syringe; and (3) the lack of controls on the large number of patent medicines that contained opium derivatives. Although opium smoking was not popular in the United States at the turn of the century, the use of morphine was. The widespread popularity of opiate-containing patent medicines and morphine was probably the main reason for the spread of and increase in opium addiction.

Until 1914, when the Harrison Narcotic Act was passed (regulating opium, coca leaves, and their products), the average opiate addict was a middle-aged, southern, white woman who functioned well and was adjusted to her role as a wife and mother. She bought opium or morphine legally by mail order from Sears, Roebuck or at the local store, used it orally, and caused very few problems. A number of physicians were addicted, as well. One of the best-known morphine addicts was William Holsted, a founder of Johns Hopkins Medical School. Holsted was a very productive surgeon and innovator, although secretly an addict for most of his career. He became dependent on morphine as a substitute for his cocaine dependence (Brecher 1972).

Looking for better medicines, chemists found that modification of the morphine molecule resulted in a more potent compound. In 1898, diacetylmorphine was placed on the market as a cough suppressant by Bayer. It was to be a "heroic" drug, without the addictive potential of morphine, thus the name *heroin* (see Figure 9.4).

Heroin was first used in the United States as a cough suppressant and to combat addiction to other substances. However, its inherent abuse potential was quickly discovered. When injected, heroin is more addictive than other narcotics because of its ability to enter the brain rapidly and cause a euphoric surge (DiChiara and North 1992). Heroin was banned from U.S. medicines in 1924, although it is still used legally as an analgesic in other countries.

The Vietnam War was an important landmark for heroin use in the United States. It has been estimated that as many as 40% of the U.S. soldiers serving in Southeast Asia at this time used heroin to combat the frustrations and stress associated with this unpopular military action. Although only 7% of the soldiers continued to use heroin after returning home, those who were addicted to this potent narcotic became a major component of the heroin-abusing population in this country (Golding 1993).

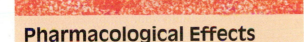

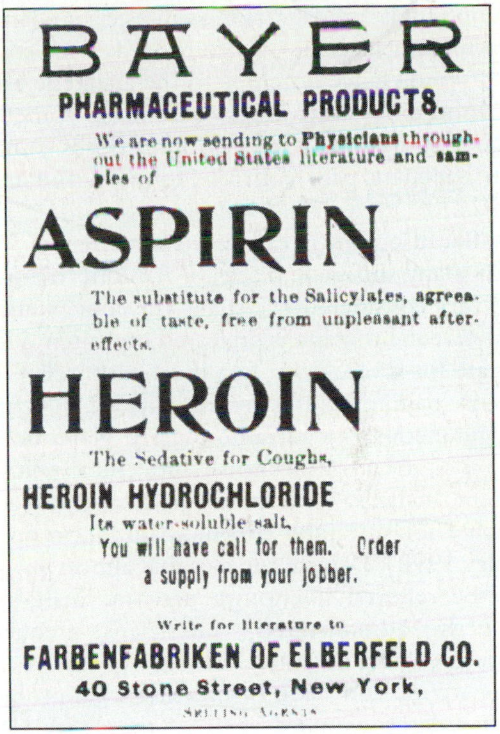

FIGURE 9.4 Bayer Pharmaceutical introduced two new products in the late 1800s: aspirin and heroin.

Pharmacological Effects

Even though opioid narcotics have a history of being abused, they continue to be important therapeutic agents.

Narcotic Analgesics

The most common clinical use of the opioid narcotics is as analgesics to relieve pain. These drugs are effective against most varieties of pain, including visceral (associated with internal organs of the body) and somatic (associated with skeletal muscles, bones, skin, and teeth) types (Johnson and Finley 1992). Used in sufficiently high doses, narcotics can even relieve the intense pain associated with some types of cancer (Nowak 1992).

The opioid narcotics relieve pain by activating the same group of receptors that are controlled by the endogenous substances called *endorphins.* As discussed in Chapter 5, the endorphins are peptides (small proteins) that are released in the brain, spinal cord, and from the adrenal glands in response to stress and painful experiences. When released, the endorphins serve as transmitters and stimulate receptors designated as an opioid type. Activation of opioid receptors by either the naturally released endorphins, or by administration of the narcotic analgesic drugs, blocks the transmission of pain through the spinal cord or brain stem and alters the perception of pain in the "pain center" of the brain. Because the narcotics work at all three levels of pain transmission, they are potent analgesics against almost all types of pain.

Interestingly, the endorphin system appears to be influenced also by psychological factors. It is possible that pain relief caused by administration of placebos or nonmedicinal manipulation such as acupuncture is due in part to the release of endorphins. This suggests that physiological, psychological, and pharmacological factors are intertwined in pain management, which makes it impossible to deal with one without considering the others.

Although the narcotics are very effective analgesics, they do cause some side effects that are particularly alarming; thus their clinical use usually is limited to the treatment of moderate-to-severe pain (Johnson and Finley 1992). Other drugs, such as the aspirin-type analgesics (see Chapter 14), are used for pain management when possible. Often the amount of narcotic required for pain relief can be reduced by combining a narcotic, such as codeine, with aspirin or acetaminophen (the active ingredient in Tylenol): such combinations reduce the chance of significant narcotic side effects (Johnson and Finley 1992).

Morphine is a particularly potent pain reliever

and often is used as the analgesic standard by which other narcotics are compared. With continual use, tolerance develops to the analgesic effects of morphine and other narcotics, sometimes requiring a dramatic escalation of doses to maintain adequate pain control (Johnson and Finley 1992).

Because pain is expressed in different forms with many different diseases, narcotic treatment can vary considerably. Usually the convenience of oral narcotic therapy is preferred but often is inadequate for severe pain. For short-term relief from intense pain, narcotics are effective when injected subcutaneously or intramuscularly. Narcotics can also be given intravenously for persistent and potent analgesia or administered by transdermal patches for sustained chronic pain (Johnson and Finley 1992). Despite the fact that almost any pain can be relieved if enough narcotic analgesic is properly administered, physicians frequently underprescribe narcotics. Because of fear of causing narcotic addiction or creating legal problems with federal agencies such as the DEA (Drug Enforcement Agency), it is estimated that less than 50% of the cancer patients in the United States receive enough narcotics for adequate pain relief (Nowak 1992). An important rule of narcotic use is that adequate pain relief should not be denied because of concern about the abuse potential of these drugs (Way and Way 1992). In fact, addiction to narcotics is rare in patients receiving these drugs for therapy unless they have a history of drug abuse or have an underlying psychiatric disorder (Pfefferbaum and Hagberg 1993).

Other Therapeutic Uses

Opioid narcotics are also used to treat conditions not related to pain. For example, these drugs suppress the coughing center of the brain so they are effective **antitussives.** Codeine, a natural opioid narcotic, is commonly included in cough medicine. In addition, opioid narcotics slow the movement of materials through the intestines, a property that can be used to relieve diarrhea. Paregoric contains an opioid narcotic substance and is commonly used to treat severe diarrhea.

When used carefully by the clinician, opioid narcotics are very effective therapeutic tools. Some precautions for avoiding unnecessary problems with these drugs include the following (Way and Way 1992):

1. Before beginning treatment, therapeutic goals should be clearly established.
2. Doses and duration of use should be limited as much as possible while permitting adequate therapeutic care.
3. If other, safer drugs (for example, nonnarcotic analgesics such as ibuprofen or aspirin) adequately treat the medical condition, narcotics usually should be avoided.

Mechanisms of Action

As mentioned, the opioid receptors are the site of action of the endorphin peptide transmitters and are found throughout the nervous system, intestines, and other internal organs. Because narcotic drugs such as morphine and heroin enhance the endorphin system by stimulating opioid receptors, these drugs have widespread influences throughout the body.

For example, the opioid receptors are present in high concentration within the limbic structures of the brain. Stimulation of these receptors by narcotics causes release of the transmitter, dopamine, in limbic brain regions. This effect contributes to the rewarding actions of these drugs and leads to dependence and abuse (Pothos et al. 1991).

Side Effects

The most common side effect of the opioid narcotics is constipation. Other side effects of these drugs include drowsiness, mental clouding, respiratory depression (suppressed breathing is usually the cause of death from overdose), nausea and vomiting, itching, inability to urinate, a drop in blood pressure, and constricted pupils. This array of seemingly unrelated side effects are due to widespread distribution of the opioid receptors throughout the body and their involvement in many physiological functions (Jaffe and Martin 1990). With continual use, tolerance develops to

ANTITUSSIVE drugs that block coughing

some of these undesirable narcotic responses (Johnson and Finley 1992).

Drugs that selectively antagonize the opioid receptors can block the effects of natural opioid systems in the body as well as reverse the effects of narcotic opiate drugs. When an opioid antagonist such as the drug naloxone is administered alone, it has little noticeable effect. The antiopioid actions of naloxone are most apparent when the antagonist is injected into someone who has taken a narcotic opioid drug. For example, naloxone will cause (1) a recurrence of pain in the patient using a narcotic for pain relief, (2) the restoration of consciousness and normal breathing in the addict who has overdosed on heroin, and (3) severe withdrawal effects in the opioid abuser who has become dependent on the narcotics.

TABLE 9.2 Common narcotics and their CSA schedules

Narcotic	Schedule[a]
Heroin	I
Morphine	II, III
Methadone	II
Fentanyl	II
Hydromorphone	II
Meperidine	II
Codeine	II, III, V
Pentazocine	IV
Propoxyphene	IV
Narcotics combined with NSAIDS	III

[a] According to Drug Enforcement Administration (DEA) classification, Controlled Substances Act (CSA).

Abuse, Tolerance, Dependence, and Withdrawal

All the opioid narcotic agents that activate opioid receptors have abuse potential and are classified as scheduled drugs (see Table 9.2). An estimated 2.5 million people in the United States abuse heroin or other narcotics (DiChiara and North 1992). The patterns of abuse are determined by the ability of these drugs to cause tolerance, dependence, and withdrawal effects.

The process of tolerance literally begins with the first dose of a narcotic, but does not become clinically evident until two to three weeks of frequent use (either therapeutic- or abuse-related). Tolerance occurs most rapidly with high doses given in short intervals. Doses can be increased as much as thirty-five times in order to regain the narcotic effect. Physical dependence invariably accompanies severe tolerance (Way and Way 1992). Psychological dependence can also develop with continual narcotic use, because these drugs can cause euphoria and relieve stress. Such psychological dependence leads to compulsive use (Way and Way 1992). Because all narcotics affect the same opioid systems in the body, developing tolerance to one narcotic drug means the person has tolerance to all the drugs in this group.

The development of psychological and physical dependence makes breaking the narcotic habit very difficult. Abstinence from narcotic use by a long-term addict can cause severe withdrawal effects such as exaggerated pain responses, agitation, anxiety, stomach cramps and vomiting, joint and muscle aches, runny nose, and an overall flu-like feeling. Although these withdrawal symptoms are not fatal, they are extremely aversive and encourage continuation of the narcotic habit (DiChiara and North 1992). Overall, the narcotics have similar actions; there are differences, however, in their potencies, severity of side effects, likelihood of being abused, and clinical usefulness.

Heroin Abuse

Heroin is currently classified as a Schedule I drug by the DEA. It is not approved for any clinical use in the United States and is the most widely abused illegal drug in European and Far Eastern countries. Heroin also was illicitly used more than any other drug of abuse in the United States (except for marijuana) until 15 years ago, when it was replaced by cocaine (DiChiara and North 1992).

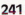

From 1970 through 1976, most of the heroin reaching the United States originated from the Golden Triangle region of Southeast Asia, which includes parts of Burma, Thailand, and Laos. During that period, the United States and other nations purchased much of the legal opium crop from Turkey in order to stop opium from being converted into heroin. From 1975 until 1980, the major heroin supply was from opium poppies grown in Mexico. The U.S. government furnished the Mexican government with helicopters, herbicide sprays, and financial assistance to destroy the poppy crop. Changes in political climates may well shift the source of supply back to the Golden Triangle, Turkey, or elsewhere in the future. The opium poppy can be cultivated commercially almost anywhere cheap labor is available during the brief harvesting season.

Heroin Combinations Pure heroin is a white powder. Other colors, such as brown Mexican heroin, result from unsatisfactory processing of morphine or from adulterants. Heroin is usually "cut" (diluted) with lactose (milk sugar) to give it bulk and thus increase profits. When heroin first enters the United States, it may be up to 95% pure, but by the time it is sold to users, its purity may be anywhere from 3 to 5%. However, occasionally the purity of street heroin unexpectedly rises. If addicts are unaware of these changes and do not adjust doses, such increases in purity can be extremely dangerous and occasionally fatal. Thus, in 1992 bags that contained 20–75% pure heroin were sold in Massachusetts and resulted in several fatal overdoses in the Boston area (Roche 1993).

Heroin has a bitter taste, so quite often it is "cut" with quinine, a bitter substance, to disguise the fact that the heroin content has been reduced. Quinine can be a deadly adulterant. Part of the "flash" from direct injection of heroin may be caused by quinine. It is an irritant, and it causes vascular damage, acute and potentially lethal disturbances in heartbeat, depressed respiration, coma, and death from respiratory arrest. Opiate poisoning causes acute pulmonary edema as well as respiratory depression. Heroin plus quinine has an unpredictable additive effect (Bourne 1976). To counteract the constipation caused by heroin, mannitol is often added for its laxative effect.

Another potentially lethal combination is when heroin is laced with the much more potent artificial narcotic fentanyl. This contaminated heroin is known on the streets as *Tango and Cash* or *Goodfellas* and can be extremely dangerous due to its unexpected potency. In February 1991, a batch of heroin cut with fentanyl sold for $10 a bag in a South Bronx neighborhood and killed 22 people, while sending more than 200 other users to area hospitals (Greenhouse 1992).

Heroin is also deliberately combined with other drugs when self-administered by addicts. Thus, according to the NIDA-sponsored Drug Abuse Warning Network (DAWN) survey of emergency rooms in the United States, 41% of the reported heroin abuse cases included other drugs of abuse in combination with this narcotic. Heroin was most frequently used with alcohol, but also frequently was combined with CNS stimulants, such as cocaine. It has been reported that street heroin addicts use cocaine to withdraw or detoxify themselves from heroin by gradually decreasing amounts of heroin while increasing amounts of cocaine. This drug combination is called "speedballing" (see the Case in Point box), and addicts claim the cocaine provides relief from the unpleasant withdrawal effects that accompany heroin abstinence in a dependent user. A possible explanation for this effect is that cocaine, like heroin, stimulates the natural endorphin systems of the brain (Kreek 1987).

Profile of Heroin Addicts Heroin addicts are always searching for the "dynamite bag" (the really potent one); however, if they do find an unusually potent batch of heroin, there is a good chance they will get more than they bargained for. Addicts are sometimes found dead with the needle still in the vein after injecting heroin. In such cases, as described earlier, the unsuspecting addict may have died in reaction to an unusually concentrated dose of this potent narcotic. Approximately 2,000-3,000 deaths occur annually in the United States from heroin overdoses (Drug Abuse Warning Network [DAWN] 1991). Death associated with heroin injection is usually due to concurrent use of alcohol or barbiturates and not the heroin alone.

It is typical for addicts to have a common place where they can stash supplies and equipment for their heroin encounters. These locations, called "shooting galleries," serve as gathering places for addicts. Shooting galleries can be set up in homes, but are usually located in less-established locations

Case in Point

A Firsthand Account of the Speedball

A speedball is a combination of the stimulant cocaine and the depressant heroin, which hits the system with two opposing drugs at the same time. The effect is described by Bobby Dalziel, a 37-year-old junkie in Los Angeles: "The initial effects is the rush of the coke, like you're taking off and then all of a sudden the dope comes up through your stomach and overtakes it to make you feel relaxed." Addicts frequently try to "make an angle" and become "cooker friends," bringing together dealers of heroin and cocaine so they can make the speedball mix (Bearak 1992). Why are drug combinations such as this particularly dangerous?

such as abandoned cars, cardboard lean-tos, and in weed-infested vacant lots. A $2 entrance charge often is required of the patrons. Conditions in shooting galleries are notoriously filthy, and these places are frequented by IV heroin users with blood-borne infections that can cause AIDS or hepatitis. Because of needle sharing and other unsanitary practices, shooting galleries have become a place where serious communicative diseases are spread to a wide range of people of different ages, races, sexes, and socioeconomic status (Bearak 1992). The heroin is typically prepared by adding several drops of water to the white powder in an improvised container (such as a metal bottle cap) and lightly shaken while heating over a small flame to dissolve the powder. The fluid is then drawn through a tiny wad of cotton to filter out the gross contaminants into an all-too-often used syringe ready for injection. A day's activities in the shooting gallery can cost from $50 to $200 (Bearak 1992).

Some addicts become fixated on the drug's paraphernalia (see Figure 9.5), especially the needle. They can get a psychological "high" from

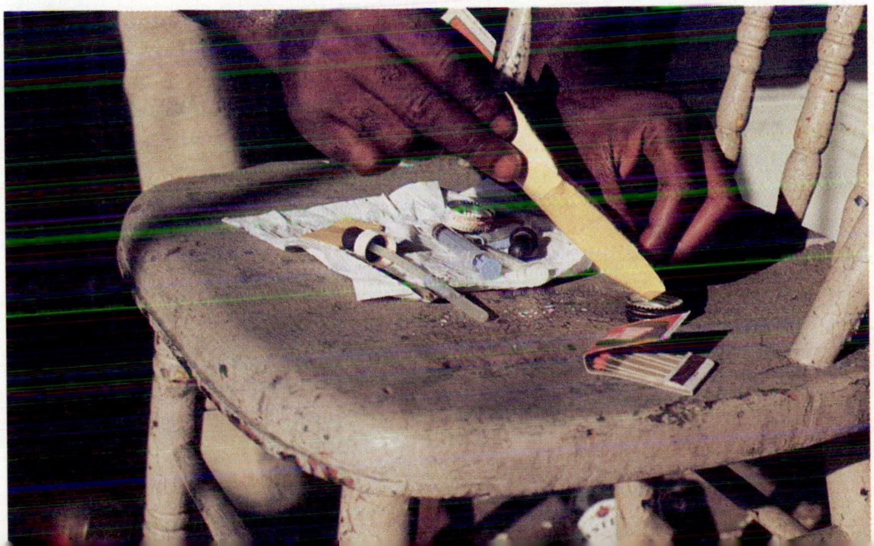

FIGURE 9.5 Heroin paraphernalia is usually simple and crude but effective: a spoon on which to dissolve the narcotic and a makeshift syringe with which to inject it.

TABLE 9.3 Prevalence of heroin and other opioid (in parentheses) abuse in high school seniors

Students	Annual Use			Lifetime Use		
	1989	1991	1992	1989	1991	1992
High School Seniors	0.6% (4.4%)	0.4% (3.5%)	0.6% (3.3%)	1.3% (8.3%)	0.9% (6.6%)	1.2% (6.1%)

Source: L. Johnston, "University of Michigan Annual National Survey of Secondary School Students." Lansing: University of Michigan News and Information Services, 9 April 1993.

playing with the needle and syringe. The injection process and syringe plunger action appear to have sexual overtones for them.

Heroin and Crime In 1971, the Select Committee on Crime in the United States released a report on methods used to combat the heroin crisis that arose in the 1950s and 1960s. This report was a turning point in setting up treatment programs for narcotic addicts. The report stated that drug arrests for heroin use had increased 700% since 1961, that there were as many as 4,000 deaths per year from heroin, and that the cost of heroin-related crimes was estimated to be over $3 billion a year. Other studies since that time have linked heroin addiction with crime (Hall et al. 1993).

Research shows most heroin users are poorly educated with minimal social integration. Because of these disadvantages, the typical heroin addict has a low level of employment, exists in unstable living conditions, and socializes with other illicit drug users (Hall et al. 1993). Clearly such undesirable living conditions encourage criminal activity; however, two other factors also likely contribute to the association between heroin use and crime. First, the use of heroin and its pharmacological effects encourage antisocial behavior that is crime-related. Depressants such as heroin diminish inhibition and cause people to engage in activities they normally would not. The effects of heroin and its withdrawal makes addicts self-centered, demanding, impulsive, and governed by their "need" for the drug: because heroin is expensive, the user is forced to resort to crime to support the drug habit. The second factor linking heroin and crime is that a similar personality is driven to both criminal behavior and heroin use. Often heroin addicts start heroin use about the same time they begin to become actively involved in criminal activity. In most cases the heroin user has been taking other illicit drugs, especially marijuana, years before beginning heroin (Hall et al. 1993). These findings suggest that for many heroin addicts the antisocial behavior caused the criminal behavior rather than resulting because of the heroin use. Thus, the more a drug such as heroin is perceived as being illegal, desirable, and addictive, the more likely it will be used by deviant criminal populations. Another factor is that, as heroin availability declines, its cost rises, increasing the likelihood that people dependent on this drug will resort to crime to support their habits (Hammersley et al. 1989).

Patterns of Heroin Abuse In the 1980s, U.S. attitudes toward narcotics changed when it became obvious that the problem was no longer confined to the inner city; narcotic use had infiltrated suburban areas and small towns. These new drug populations had more financial resources than people in the inner city and were usually able to obtain confidential medical surveillance. For these reasons, it has been and remains very difficult to determine the precise level of heroin use.

However, a study released in 1993 by the University of Michigan (Johnston 1993) found that, from 1989 to 1991, the annual use of heroin and other opioid narcotics had declined in high school

Here and Now

"Heroin Use Rises as Crack Wanes"

This headline in the *New York Times* (18 June 1991) reflects the trendy and whimsical nature of heroin abuse. This article reveals how heroin dealers made inroads into New York City's illicit drug market in 1990 and 1991. Because of the waning popularity of "crack," middle-level cocaine dealers have been switching to heroin and on many street corners have replaced "crack" dealers. The resulting increase in heroin use has been subtle and seen mostly in poor people living in inner-city sections. A director at the New York City Association for Drug Abuse and Prevention claimed that "people are pulling away from 'crack' because of what it does to you in terms of destruction, how it tears the body down. A lot of people are afraid of that. . . . If people know you're a crackhead they think you're stupid, you can't be trusted." Because the effects of heroin are viewed as gentler and less destructive, a shift in drug use patterns has been taking place and may be heralding the beginning of a new narcotic epidemic (Treaster 1991).

seniors (see Table 9.3). A 1991 report confirmed this decline in heroin use when it disclosed that total sales of heroin dropped from $15.5 billion in 1989 to $12.3 billion in 1990 (Meddis 1991).

This trend paralleled similar reductions seen with other drugs of abuse at the time and likely reflected a change in public attitudes about the recreational use of drugs in general.

However, since 1990 some disturbing trends have occurred. With the decline in the popularity of cocaine, there was evidence in the early 1990s that cocaine dealers switched to selling heroin (see Here and Now box). An apparent increase in heavy heroin use resulted in an increase in heroin-related emergencies and deaths in hospitals throughout the country ("Five-Year Trends," 1992; Swan 1992). Corresponding increases in heroin use and related emergencies occurred in such diverse populations as entertainers and celebrities (O'Dair 1992) and twelfth-graders (Johnston 1993). It is likely that because antidrug efforts during this time primarily were designed to stop cocaine abuse, they inadvertently encouraged some drug users to replace cocaine with heroin. Another reason for a switch to heroin dealing at this time was that this narcotic wholesaled for as much as $200,000 per kilogram in the United States, almost 13 times greater than the price for cocaine. This dramatic increase in value caused heroin to replace cocaine as the principal money crop from some Latin American countries (Dallas Morning News, 1992).

Stages of Dependence Initially, the effects of heroin are often unpleasant, especially after the first injection. It is not uncommon to experience nausea and vomiting or to feel sick after administration, but gradually, the euphoria overwhelms the aversive effects (Goldstein 1994). There are two major stages in the development of a psychological dependence on heroin or other opioid narcotics.

1. There is a rewarding stage, in which euphoria and positive effects occur to at least 50% of users. These positive feelings and sensations increase with continued administration and encourage use.
2. Eventually, the heroin or narcotic user must take the drug to avoid withdrawal symptoms

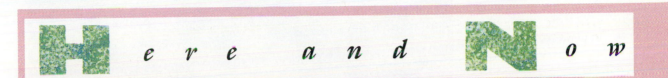

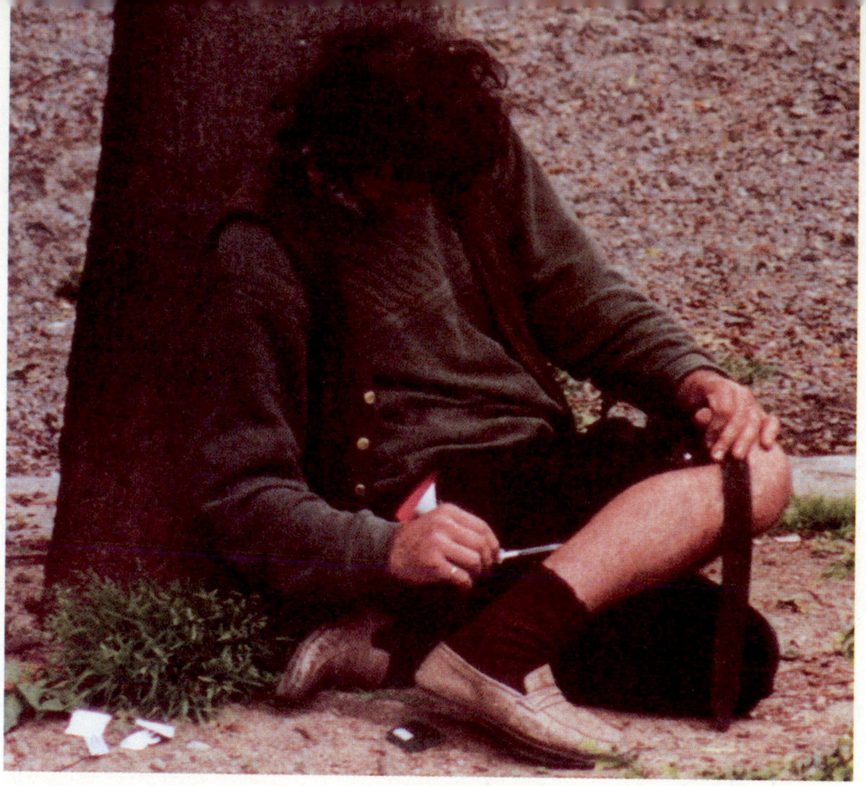

A heroin addict mainlining his drug.

that start about 6 to 12 hours after the last dose. At this stage, it is said that "the monkey is on his back." This is psychological dependence. If one grain of heroin (about 65 mg) is taken over a two-week period on a daily basis, the user becomes physically dependent on the drug.

Methods of Administration Many heroin users start by sniffing the powder or injecting it into a muscle (intramuscular) or under the skin ("skin popping"). Sometimes it is smoked, but most addicts consider this wasteful. In Vietnam, many of these who became addicted to heroin started out by smoking it with tobacco or marijuana or by sniffing it. The heroin available in Vietnam was nearly 95% pure.

Established heroin addicts usually **"mainline"** the drug (intravenous injection). The injection device can be made from an eyedropper bulb, part of a syringe, and a hypodermic needle (see Figure 9.5). "Mainlining" drugs causes the thin-walled veins to become scarred, and if it is done frequently, the veins will collapse. Once a vein is collapsed, it can no longer be used to introduce the drug into the blood. Addicts become expert in locating new veins to use: in the feet, the legs, the neck, even the temples (see photo). When addicts do not want "needle tracks" (scars) to show, they inject under the tongue or in the groin.

Heroin Addicts and AIDS As noted already, because needle sharing is a common occurrence in populations of heavy heroin users, the transmission of deadly communicable diseases such as acquired immune deficiency syndrome (AIDS) is a major problem (see Chapter 15). Approximately 40–50% of IV heroin users have been exposed to the AIDS virus (as demonstrated by viral-directed antibodies) (Brown et al. 1990).

Withdrawal Symptoms After the effects of the heroin wear off, the addict usually has four to six hours in which to find the next dose before severe withdrawal symptoms begin. A $10 bag (single "shot") of heroin only lasts 4–6 hours. It is enough to help addicts "get straight" or relieve the severe withdrawal symptoms called "dope sickness" but is not enough to give a desired "high"

"MAINLINING" intravenous injection of a drug of abuse

Here and Now

A Product of the Shooting Galleries

Early in 1993 George Vega tested positive for the human immunodeficiency virus (HIV). The news was expected because Vega was a heroin addict who had shared countless needles in shooting galleries. Resigned to his fate, Vega said, "I've seen lots of guys die already. They turned into skeletons and their teeth fell out and everything. I hope I die before I get that far. Maybe I'll be lucky and just die one night up in the gallery."

Source: B. Bearak. "Junkies Playing Roulette with Needles." *Salt Lake Tribune* (29 November 1992):A4.

(Bearak 1992). Withdrawal symptoms start with a runny nose, tears, and minor stomach cramps. The addict may feel as if he or she is coming down with a bad cold. Between 12 and 48 hours after the last dose, the addict loses all his or her appetite, vomits, has diarrhea and abdominal cramps, feels alternating chills and fever, and develops goose pimples all over (going "cold turkey"). Between two and four days later, the addict continues to experience some of the symptoms just described, as well as aching bones and muscles and powerful muscle spasms that cause violent kicking motions ("kicking the habit"). After four to five days, symptoms start to subside, and the person may get his or her appetite back (Way and Way 1992). However, attempts to move on in life will be challenging because compulsion to keep using the drug remains strong.

The severity of the withdrawal varies according to the purity and strength of the drug used and to the personality of the user. The symptoms of withdrawal from heroin, morphine, and methadone are summarized in Table 9.4. Withdrawal symptoms from opioids such as morphine, codeine, meperidine, and others are similar, although the time frame and intensity vary (Jaffe and Martin 1990).

TABLE 9.4 Symptoms of withdrawal from heroin, morphine, and methadone

Symptoms	Time in Hours		
	Heroin	Morphine	Methadone
Craving for drugs; anxiety	4	6	24–48
Yawning, perspiration, runny nose, tears	8	14	34–48
Pupil dilation, goose bumps, muscle twitches, aching bones and muscles, hot and cold flashes, loss of appetite	12	16	48–72
Increased intensity of preceding symptoms, insomnia, raised blood pressure, fever, faster pulse, nausea	18–24	24–36	72 plus
Increased intensity of preceding symptoms, curled-up position, vomiting, diarrhea, increased blood sugar, foot kicking ("kicking the habit")	26–36	36–48	

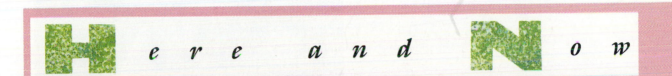

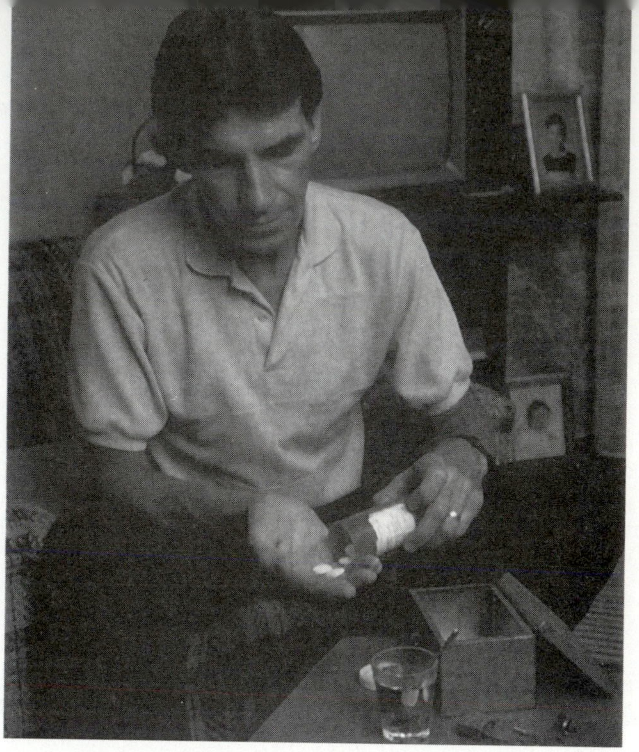

A heroin addict using methadone to treat narcotic dependence.

Treatment of Heroin and Other Narcotic Dependence

The ideal result of treatment for dependency on heroin or other narcotics is to help the addict live a normal, productive, and satisfying life without drugs. In reality, relatively few heroin users become absolutely "clean" from drug use; thus, therapeutic compromise is often necessary (Millstein 1992). In the real world, treatment of heroin dependency is considered successful if the addict (1) stops using heroin, (2) no longer associates with dealers or users of heroin, (3) avoids dangerous activities often associated with heroin use (such as needle sharing, injecting unknown drugs, frequenting shooting galleries, and so on), (4) improves employment status, (5) refrains from criminal activity, and (6) is able to enjoy normal family and social relationships (McLellan et al. 1993). For many heroin addicts, these goals can be achieved by substituting a long-lasting synthetic narcotic, such as methadone, in place of the short-acting heroin (see photo). The substitute narcotic is made available to heroin-dependent people from drug treatment centers under the direction of trained medical personnel. The dispensing of the substitute narcotic is tightly regulated by governmental agencies. The rationale for the substitution is that a long-acting drug, such as methadone, can conveniently be taken once a day to prevent the unpleasant withdrawal symptoms which occur within four hours after each heroin use (see Table 9.4). Although the substitute narcotic may also have abuse potential and be scheduled by the DEA (see Table 9.2), it is given to the addict in its oral form; thus its onset of action is too slow to cause a rush like heroin, so its abuse potential is substantially less.

Currently, methadone is approved by the FDA for "opiate maintenance therapy" in the treatment of heroin (or other narcotic) dependency (Swan 1993). Proper use of methadone has been shown to effectively decrease illicit use of narcotics and other undesirable behavior related to drug dependence (Strain et al. 1993). Another drug called LAAM (l-alpha-acetyl-methadol) recently has been clinically tested, and the FDA has approved it to treat narcotic addiction (*Facts and Comparisons Drug Newsletter* 1993; Goldstein 1995). LAAM is a very long-acting narcotic and is more convenient because it requires only three administrations per week to block heroin withdrawal symptoms ("LAAM" 1994). A third narcotic, buprenorphine, which is currently used as an analgesic, also is being tested in the treatment of narcotic dependence. Its minimal potential for dependence makes this drug a desirable substitute for heroin (Swan 1993). See Table 9.5 for comparison of these three drugs.

TABLE 9.5 Comparison of narcotic substitutes used in opiate maintenance therapy

Properties	Methadone	LAAM	Buprenophine
Administration	Oral	Oral	Oral or sublingual
Frequency of doses	Daily	Three times per week	Daily
Other uses	Analgesic	None	Analgesic
Physical dependence	Yes	Yes	Little
Causes positive subjective effects	Yes	Some	Yes
Abuse potential	Yes	Limited	Limited

Source: N. Swan. "Two NIDA-Tested Heroin Treatment Medications Move Toward FDA Approval." *NIDA Notes* (March–April 1993):45.

Unfortunately, many people, including professionals involved in drug abuse therapy, view heroin or narcotic addiction as a "failure of the will" and see methadone treatment as substituting one addiction for another (Goldstein 1994). So unrealistic treatment expectations are sometimes imposed on heroin addicts, resulting in high failure rates. For example, many methadone treatment programs may distribute inadequate methadone doses to maintain heroin or narcotic abstinence; or narcotic-dependent patients may be told their methadone will be terminated within six months regardless of their progress in the program (see Crosscurrents box). Such ill-advised policies often drive clients back to their heroin habits and demonstrate that many professionals who treat

CROSSCURRENTS

Addicts dependent on heroin are frequently treated by substituting a long-acting narcotic, such as methadone, for the short-acting heroin. There is controversy as to how methadone maintenance should be managed, as expressed in the following opposite views:

1. Methadone should only be used for a few months, to help the addict eliminate the heroin habit; then methadone must be withdrawn if treatment is to be successful.
2. Methadone should be used indefinitely if the addict is not willing to maintain a drug-free state. Continual use of methadone is much better than having the addict return to the heroin habit.

Choose a side, and support your position with arguments based on information in this text and other authoritative sources.

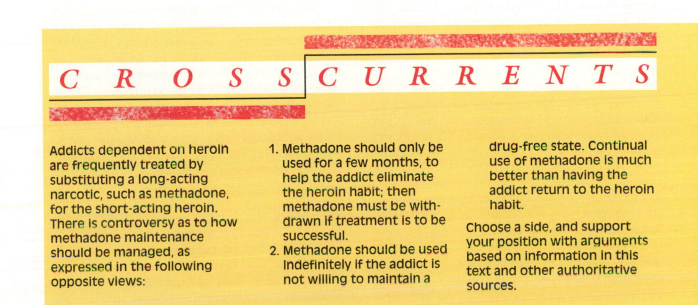

heroin and narcotic dependency do not understand that methadone is not a cure for heroin addiction, but is a means to achieve a healthier, more normal lifestyle (Millstein 1992).

It also is essential to understand that even proper use of methadone does not guarantee resolution of heroin or narcotic addiction. To maximize the possibility of successful treatment, the clients must also receive regular counseling sessions to help modify the drug-seeking behavior as well as receive on-site professional care, including job training, career development, education, general medical care and family counseling. The supplemental services dramatically improve the success rate of narcotic dependence treatment (McLellan et al. 1993).

Other Narcotics

A large number of narcotics are used for medical purposes. However, many are also distributed in the "streets": morphine, methadone, codeine, hydromorphone (Dilaudid), meperidine (Demerol), and other synthetics. A few of the most commonly abused opioids will be discussed briefly in the following sections. Except where noted, they are all Schedule II drugs.

Morphine

As noted earlier, morphine is the standard by which other narcotic agents are measured. It has been used to relieve pain from the time it was first isolated in 1803. Morphine has about half the analgesic potency of heroin but 12 times the potency of codeine.

Morphine is commonly used to relieve moderate to intense pain that cannot be controlled by less potent and less dangerous narcotics. Because of the potential for serious side effects, morphine is generally used in a hospital setting where emergency care can be rendered, if necessary. Most pain can be relieved by morphine if high enough doses are used (Johnson and Finley 1992); however, morphine works best against continuous dull pain.

The side effects that occur when using therapeutic doses of morphine include drowsiness, changes in mood, and inability to think straight. In addition, therapeutic doses depress respiratory activity; thus, morphine decreases the rate and depth of breathing as well as produces irregular breathing patterns. As with the other narcotics, morphine can cause an array of seemingly unrelated effects throughout the body, including nausea and vomiting, constipation, blurred vision, constricted pupils, and flushed skin.

The initial response to morphine is varied. In normal people who are not suffering pain, the first exposure can be unpleasant, with nausea and vomiting being the prominent reactions. However, continual use often leads to a euphoric response and encourages dependence. When injected subcutaneously, the effects of heroin and morphine are almost identical; this is because heroin is rapidly metabolized in the body into morphine. However, after intravenous administration, the onset of heroin's effects is more rapid and more intense than those of morphine because heroin is more lipid soluble and enters the brain faster. Because heroin is easier to manufacture and is more potent, it is more popular in illicit trade than morphine. Even so, morphine also has substantial abuse potential and is classified as a Schedule II substance (McEvoy 1993).

Tolerance to the effects of morphine can develop very quickly if the drug is used continuously. For example, an addict who is repeatedly administering the morphine to get a "kick" or maintain a "high" must constantly increase the dose. Such users can build up to incredible doses. One addict reported using 5 grams of morphine daily; the normal analgesic dose of morphine is 50 to 80 *milligrams* a day (Jaffe and Martin 1990). Such high doses are lethal in a person without tolerance to narcotics.

Methadone

Methadone was first synthesized in Germany in 1943, when natural opiate analgesics were not available because opium could not be obtained from the Far East during World War II. Methadone was first called *Dolophine,* after Adolph Hitler; one company still uses that trade name.

(On the "street," methadone pills are often called "dollies.") Today, methadone is often substituted for heroin in the treatment of narcotic-dependent people. It is an effective analgesic, equal to morphine if injected and more active if taken orally.

The physiological effects of methadone are the same as those of morphine and heroin. As a narcotic, methadone produces psychological dependence, tolerance, and then physical dependence if repeated doses are taken. Methadone is effective for about 24 to 36 hours; therefore, the addict must take methadone daily to avoid narcotic withdrawal. It is often considered as addictive as heroin if injected; consequently, because methadone is soluble in water, it is formulated with insoluble, inert ingredients to prevent it from being injected by narcotic addicts.

One of methadone's most useful properties is that of cross-tolerance with other narcotic drugs and a less intense withdrawal response. If it reaches a sufficiently high level in the blood, methadone blocks heroin euphoria. In addition, withdrawal symptoms of patients physically dependent on heroin or morphine and the postaddiction craving can be suppressed by oral administration of methadone. The effective dose for methadone maintenance is 50–100 mg per day to treat severe withdrawal symptoms (Millstein 1992).

The value of substituting methadone for heroin is its longer action. Because addicts no longer need the heroin to prevent withdrawal, they often can be persuaded to leave their undesirable associates, drug sources, and dangerous lifestyles. The potential side effects from methadone are the same as those from morphine and heroin, including constipation and sedation; yet if properly used, methadone is a safe drug. The only documented death directly related to methadone treatment occurred when a patient was using the drug as prescribed but untreated, severe constipation resulted.

When injecting methadone, some people feel the same kind of euphoria that can be obtained from heroin. Methadone addicts receiving maintenance treatment sometimes become euphoric if the dose is increased too rapidly. There are cases of people who injected crushed methadone pills and developed serious lung conditions from particles that lodged in the tissue, creating a condition somewhat like emphysema. The number of deaths from methadone overdose has been higher than those from heroin in some major cities like New York. Many of these deaths are in young children who get into methadone brought home by parents in maintenance programs or teenagers who try to shoot up with "street" methadone or methadone in combination with other drugs. Methadone overdoses can be reversed by the antagonist naloxone if the person is found in time.

Controlled Use of Methadone and Heroin

Some regular opiate users can keep jobs and are able to function quite normally. There are known cases of surgeons, lawyers, and other professionals who manage to perform while on opiates. Such narcotic users apparently are able to limit their use and do not become severely dependent.

Between one-third and one-half of those applying to methadone maintenance programs are turned away because they use heroin infrequently and are not considered to be truly dependent; they would likely become addicted to methadone during the course of treatment and be worse off. The estimated heroin-using population in the United States is between 3 and 4 million, of whom only 10% are addicted.

Very little is known about controlled users, or "chippers." They are extremely secretive, in contrast to the usual addicts found in treatment programs. No common personality type was found in one study of chippers; however, one similarity was that they are more afraid of being forced into abstinence than of losing control and becoming dependent on narcotics. This type of user regulates the circumstances and frequency of heroin use to prevent detection, addiction, and side effects. Typical examples of self-imposed rules are using the drug only on Friday and Saturday evenings, budgeting the amount of money spent on heroin, and being careful to sterilize injection equipment (Zinsberg 1979).

Fentanyl

Fentanyl (Sublimaze) is a very potent narcotic analgesic (200 times more potent than morphine) that is often administered intravenously for general anesthesia. It is also used in transdermal systems (patches on the skin) in the treatment of chronic pain (Duragesic). Fentanyl is not a natural opiate compound but is readily synthesized and can be modified into drugs that retain potent narcotic properties.

It is estimated that some 100 different active forms of fentanyl could be synthesized; up to now, about 10 derivatives have appeared on the "streets." They are considered to be "designer" drugs (see Chapter 4); because of their great potency and ease of production, they have sometimes been used to replace heroin on the "streets." Fentanyl-type drugs can appear in the same forms and colors as heroin, so there is nothing to alert users that they have been sold a heroin substitute (Henderson 1988). Due to their powerful effects, these drugs are especially dangerous, and incredibly small doses can cause fatal respiratory depression in an unsuspecting heroin user (Greenhouse 1992). (One "designer" fentanyl, 3-methyl fentanyl, is 6,000 times more potent than heroin.) More than 100 deaths in California have been caused by overdoses of fentanyl-related drugs. In spring 1991, four fentanyl-related deaths were identified in New York. Deaths from fentanyl overdoses have also occurred in other major U.S. metropolitan areas.

As yet, there is no reliable information regarding the extent of fentanyl abuse. (These drugs are sometimes very difficult to detect in the blood due to the small quantities used.) However, some authorities have speculated that fentanyl abuse has the potential to become a major drug problem in the United States (Henderson 1988).

Hydromorphone

Hydromorphone (Dilaudid) is prepared from morphine and used as an analgesic and cough suppressant. It is a stronger analgesic than heroin and is used to treat moderate to severe pain. Nausea, vomiting, constipation, and euphoria may be less marked with hydromorphone than with morphine (McEvoy 1993). On the "street," it is taken in tablet form or injected.

Meperidine

Meperidine (Demerol) is a synthetic drug that frequently is used as an analgesic for treatment of moderate pain; it can be taken in tablet form or injected. Meperidine is about one-tenth as powerful as morphine, and its use can lead to dependence. This drug has been given too freely by some physicians because tolerance develops, requiring larger doses to maintain its therapeutic action. With continual use, it causes physical dependence. Meperidine addicts may use large daily doses (3 to 4 g per day).

MPTP, a "Designer" Tragedy Attempts to synthesize illicit *designer* versions of meperidine by street chemists has proven to be tragic for some unsuspecting drug addicts. In 1976, a young drug addict with elementary laboratory skills attempted to make a meperidine-like drug by using short-cuts in the chemical synthesis. Three days after self-administering his untested drug product, the drug user developed a severe case of tremors and motor problems identical to Parkinson's disease, a neurological disorder generally occurring in the elderly. Even more surprising to attending neurologists was that this young drug addict improved dramatically after treatment with levodopa, a drug that is very effective in treating traditional Parkinson's disease. After 18 months of treatment, the despondent addict committed suicide. An autopsy revealed he had severe brain damage that was almost identical to that occurring in classical Parkinsonian patients (Davies et al. 1979). It was concluded that a by-product resulting from the sloppy synthesis of the meperidine-like designer narcotic was responsible for the irreversible brain damage.

This hypothesis was confirmed by a separate and independent event on the West Coast in 1981 when a cluster of relatively young heroin addicts (ages 22–42) in the San Francisco area also developed symptoms of Parkinson's disease. All these patients had consumed a new "synthetic heroin," obtained on the streets, that was produced by attempting to synthesize meperidine-like drugs (Langston et al. 1983). Common to both incidents was the presence of the compound MPTP, which was a contaminant resulting from the careless synthesis. MPTP is metabolized to a very reactive molecule in the brain that selectively destroys neurons containing the transmitter dopamine in the motor regions of the basal ganglia (see Chapter 5). Similar neuronal damage occurs in classical Parkinson's disease over the course of 50–70 years, whereas ingestion of MPTP dramatically accelerates the degeneration to a matter of hours (Goldstein 1995). As tragic as the MPTP incident was, it is heralded as an important scientific breakthrough: MPTP is now used by researchers as a tool to study why Parkinson's disease occurs and how to treat it effectively.

Codeine

Codeine is a naturally occurring constituent of opium and the most frequently prescribed of the narcotic analgesics. It is used principally to treat minor to moderate pain and as a cough suppressant. Maximum pain relief from codeine occurs with 30 to 50 mg. Usually, when prescribed for pain, codeine is combined with either a salicylate such as aspirin or with acetaminophen (Tylenol). Aspirin-like drugs and opioid narcotics interact in a synergistic fashion to give an analgesic equivalence greater than what can be achieved by aspirin or codeine alone.

Although not especially powerful, codeine may still be abused. Codeine-containing cough syrup is currently classified as a Schedule V drug. Because the abuse potential is considered minor, the FDA has ruled that codeine cough products can be sold without a prescription; however, the pharmacist is required to keep them behind the counter and must be asked in order to obtain codeine-containing cough medications. In spite of the FDA ruling, about 50% of the states have more restrictive regulations and require that codeine-containing cough products be available only by prescription.

Although codeine dependence is possible, it is not very common; most people that abuse codeine develop narcotic dependence previously with one of the more potent opioids. In general, large quantities of codeine are needed to satisfy a narcotic addiction; therefore, it is not commonly marketed on the "streets."

Pentazocine

Pentazocine (Talwin) was first developed in the 1960s in an effort to market an effective analgesic with low abuse potential. When taken orally, its analgesic effect is slightly greater than that of codeine. Its effects on respiration and sedation are similar to those of the other opioids, but it does not prevent withdrawal symptoms in a narcotic addict. In fact, pentazocine will precipitate withdrawal symptoms if given to a person on methadone maintenance who needs an analgesic (McEvoy 1993). Pentazocine is not commonly abused because its effects can be unpleasant, resulting in dysphoria. It is classified as a Schedule IV drug.

Propoxyphene

Propoxyphene (Darvon, Dolene) is structurally related to methadone, but it is a much weaker analgesic, about half as potent as codeine. Like codeine, propoxyphene is frequently given in combination with aspirin or acetaminophen. Although at one time an extremely popular analgesic, the use of propoxyphene has declined in the past few years as questions about its potency have been raised. Some research suggests this narcotic is no more effective in relieving pain than aspirin (McEvoy 1993). To a large extent, new, more effective nonnarcotic analgesics have replaced propoxyphene. In very high doses, it can cause delusions, hallucinations, and convulsions. Alone, propoxyphene causes little respiratory depression; however, when combined with alcohol or other CNS depressants, this drug can depress respiration.

Narcotic-Related Drugs

Dextromethorphan

Dextromethorphan is a synthetic used in cough remedies and can be purchased without prescription. Although its molecular structure is like codeine, this drug does not have analgesic action nor does it cause typical narcotic dependence. However, there have been recent, scattered reports across the country of high school students abusing cough medicines with dextromethorphan. It is claimed that high doses of this drug can cause mild hallucinations and stimulation, like PCP. Some abusers refer to the use of the antitussive product Robitussin as "roboing." As of 1993, the DEA had taken no steps to restrict the use of dextromethorphan.

Clonidine

Clonidine (Catapres) was discovered in the late 1970s. It is not a narcotic analgesic and has no direct effect on the opioid receptors; it stimulates receptors for noradrenaline, and its principal use is as an oral antihypertensive. Clonidine is mentioned here because it is the first nonaddictive, noneuphoriagenic prescription medication with demonstrated efficacy in relieving the effects of opiate withdrawal (such as vomiting and diarrhea). The dosing regimen is typically a 7- to 14-day inpatient treatment for opiate withdrawal. Length of treatment can be reduced to 7 days for withdrawal from heroin and short-acting opiates; the 14-day treatment is needed for the longer-acting methadone-type opiates. Because tolerance to clonidine may develop, opiates are discontinued abruptly at the start of treatment. In this way, the peak intensity of withdrawal will occur while clonidine is still maximally effective (McEvoy 1993).

One of the most important advantages of clonidine over other treatments for opiate withdrawal detoxification is that it shortens the time for withdrawal to 14 days compared to several weeks or months using standard procedures, such as methadone treatment. The potential disadvantage of taking clonidine is that it can cause serious side effects of its own, the most serious being significantly lowered blood pressure, which can cause fainting and blacking out (Washington et al. 1985). Overall, the lack of abuse potential makes clonidine particularly useful in treating narcotic dependence.

Naloxone

Naloxone is a relatively pure narcotic antagonist. This means the drug attaches to opiate receptors in the brain and throughout the body and does not activate it, but prevents narcotic drugs, such as heroin and morphine, from having an effect. By itself, naloxone does not cause much change, but it potently blocks or reverses the effects of all the narcotics. Because or its antagonistic properties, naloxone is a useful antidote in the treatment of narcotic overdoses; thus, administration of naloxone reverses life-threatening narcotic-induced effects on breathing and the cardiovascular system. However, if not used carefully, this antagonist will also block the analgesic action of the narcotics and initiate severe withdrawals in narcotic-dependent people (McEvoy 1993).

Review Questions

1. What effects of narcotics cause them to have abuse potential?
2. Why is the clinical use of heroin illegal in the United States while the use of morphine is not?
3. What are the principal clinical uses of the opioid narcotics?
4. What is the relationship between endorphin systems and the opioid narcotics?
5. Why has there recently been an increase in heroin abuse in the United States?
6. What are the principal withdrawal effects when heroin use is stopped in addicts?
7. How does "methadone maintenance" work for the treatment of narcotic dependence?
8. What are "shooting galleries," and why are they so important in the spread of AIDS?
9. What have been the consequences of "designer" narcotics?

Key Terms

analgesic
opioid
antitussive
"mainlining"

Summary

1. The term *narcotic* currently refers to naturally occurring substances derived from the opium poppy and their synthetic substitutes. These drugs are referred to as the opioid (or opiate) narcotics because of their association with opium. For the most part, the opioid narcotics possess abuse potential, but they also have important clinical value and are used to relieve all kinds of pain (they are analgesic), suppress coughing (they are antitussive), and stop diarrhea.
2. The principal side effects of the opioid narcotics, besides their abuse potential, include drowsiness, respiratory depression, nausea and vomiting, constipation, inability to urinate, and sometimes a drop in blood pressure. These side effects can be annoying or even life threatening, so caution is required when using these drugs.
3. Heroin is the most likely of the opioid narcotics to be severely abused; it is easily prepared from opium and has a rapid, intense effect. Heroin use is not limited to the inner-city ghettos but is found throughout the United States. From 1987 to 1991, the rate of narcotic use in the United States declined, although there is evidence that since 1991 heroin has been substituted for "crack" as the popularity of cocaine has diminished. The heroin addict usually "mainlines" the drug and often shoots up with other addicts in "shooting galleries." People dependent on narcotics such as heroin commonly engage in criminal activities to support their habits.
4. When narcotics such as heroin are first used by people not experiencing pain, the drugs can cause unpleasant, dysphoric sensations. However, euphoria gradually overcomes the aversive effects. The positive feelings increase with narcotic use, leading to psychological dependence. After psychological dependence, physical dependence occurs with frequent daily use, which reinforces the narcotic abuse. If the user stops taking the drug after physical dependence has occurred, severe withdrawal symptoms result.
5. Heroin addicts frequently administer their narcotic by IV routes using contaminated needles shared with other drug addicts. Due to such unsanitary dangerous practices, these individuals are at high risk to become infected with the AIDS virus or other pathogenic micro-organisms and to spread the infections to others.
6. Tolerance to narcotics can occur rapidly with intense use of these drugs. This tolerance can result in the use of incredibly large doses of narcotics that would be fatal to a nontolerant person. The withdrawal symptoms for narcotic dependency begin four to six hours after the last narcotic dose and become severe by 12 to 48 hours. The experience has been described as being like a bad case of the flu or a cold and includes a runny nose, stomach cramps, vomiting, diarrhea, chills and fever, and goose pimples. After four to five days, the symptoms begin to subside, but the urge to use the drug persists.
7. Methadone or LAAM are frequently used to help narcotic addicts stop using heroin or one of the other more addicting drugs. Oral methadone relieves the withdrawal symptoms that would result from discontinuing narcotics. Methadone can also cause psychological and physical dependence, but it is less addicting than heroin and easier to control; namely, when administered orally, methadone is a slower- and longer-acting drug. Because the effects of methadone last for 24 to 36 hours, it only needs to be administered once daily. Ultimately, the narcotic addict will be encouraged to stop using methadone; however, many addicts refuse and are maintained on methadone indefinitely. Two other long-acting narcotics, LAAM and buprenorphine, are also being used in narcotic maintenance programs.
8. Fentanyl is a very potent synthetic opioid narcotic. It is easily synthesized and can be converted into other fentanyl-like drugs that are as much as 3,000 to 6,000 times more potent than heroin itself. Detection and regulation of these fentanyl derivatives by law enforcement

agencies are very difficult. The fentanyl-type drugs are being used as heroin substitutes and have already killed many narcotic addicts, due to their unexpected potency.

9. Attempts to create designer narcotics has led to the synthesis of very potent fentanyl-like drugs responsible for a number of overdose deaths. In addition, attempts to synthesize a meperidine (Demerol) designer drug resulted in the inadvertent creation of MPTP: a very reactive compound that causes dramatic Parkinson's disease in the users.
10. Fentanyl and related drugs are the most potent of the opioid narcotics, making them useful clinical agents but also very dangerous. Morphine is still used for treatment of moderate to severe pain, usually in hospital settings. Codeine is the most commonly prescribed of the narcotic analgesics and is used to treat moderate pain and excessive coughing. Because of its low potency, codeine is not as likely to be abused as morphine or heroin; codeine is often combined with aspirin-like analgesics to give better pain relief. Pentazocine is a unique narcotic because it has both agonist and antagonist properties; it is less likely to be abused than most of the other narcotics and often causes dysphoria. Propoxyphene (Darvon) is the least potent of the commonly used narcotic analgesics. Its usefulness has been questioned, causing a decline in its popularity; because of its low potency, large doses are required by narcotic addicts to satisfy their dependency.

References

Abel, E. L. *Marijuana: The First Twelve Thousand Years.* New York: Plenum, 1980.

Austin, G. A. *Perspective on the History of Psychoactive Substance Use.* NIDA Research Issues no. 24. Washington, DC: U.S. Department of Health, Education, and Welfare, 1978.

Bearak, B. "Junkies Playing Roulette with Needles." *Salt Lake Tribune* (29 November 1992): A4.

Bourne, P. G., ed. *Acute Drug Emergencies: A Treatment Manual.* New York: Academic, 1976.

Brecher, E. M. *Licit and Illicit Drugs.* Boston: Little, Brown, 1972.

Dallas Morning News. "Deadly Heroin Trade Sprouting New Cash Crop in Columbia." *Salt Lake Tribune* 243 (16 February 1992): A28.

Davies, G., A. Williams, S. Markey, M. Ebert, E. Caine, C. Reickert, and I. Kopin. "Chronic Parkinsonism Secondary to Intravenous Injection of Meperidine Analogues." *Psychiatry Research* 1 (1979): 249–54.

DiChiara, G., and A. North. "Neurobiology of Opiate Abuse." *Trends in Pharmacological Sciences* 13 (May 1992): 185–93.

Drug Abuse Warning Network (DAWN). "Annual Medical Examiner Data, 1990." In *Data from the Drug Abuse Warning Network.* ADAMHA DHHS Publication no. 91–1880. Washington, DC: U.S. Department of Health and Human Services, 1991.

Facts and Comparisons Drug Newsletter. New Drugs 12 (September 1993): 65.

"Five-Year Trends: San Diego Cocaine Deaths Down, But Heroin Deaths Up." *Prevention Pipeline* 5 (July–August 1992): 93.

Golding, A. "Two Hundred Years of Drug Abuse." *Journal of the Royal Society of Medicine* 86 (May 1993): 282–86.

Goldstein, A. In *Addiction from Biology to Drug Policy,* 137–54. New York: Freeman, 1994.

Goldstein, F. "Pharmacological Aspects of Substance Abuse." In *Remington's Pharmaceutical Sciences,* 19th ed., edited by A. R. Genaro. Easton, PA: Mack, 1995.

Greenhouse, C. "NIDA Lays Plans for Quicker Response to Drug Crises." *NIDA Notes* 7 (January–February 1992): 20.

Hall, W., J. Bell, and J. Carless. "Crime and Drug Use Among Applicants for Methadone Maintenance." *Drug and Alcohol Dependence* 31 (1993): 123–29.

Hammersley, R., A. Forsyth, V. Morrison, and J. Davies. "The Relationship Between Crime and Opioid Use." *British Journal of Addiction* 84 (1989): 1029–43.

Henderson, G. "Designer Drugs: Past History and Future Prospects." *Journal of Forensic Sciences* 33 (1988): 569–75.

Jaffe, J., and M. Martin. "Opioid Analgesics and Antagonists." In *The Pharmacological Basis of Therapeutics,* 8th ed., edited by A. Gilman, T. Rall, A. Nies, and P. Taylor. New York: Pergamon, 1990.

Johnson, D., and R. Finley. "Pain Management." *American Druggist* (June 1992): 70–82.

Johnston, L. "University of Michigan Annual National Survey of Secondary School Students." Lansing: University of Michigan News and Information Services, 9 April 1993. Available from author at 412 Maynard Ave., Ann Arbor, MI.

Kreek, M. "Multiple Drug Abuse Patterns and Medical Consequences." In *Psychopharmacology: The Third Generation of Progress,* edited by Herbert Meltzer, 1597–1604. New York: Raven Press, 1987.

"LAAM—A Long-acting Methadone for Treatment of Heroin Addiction." *Medical Letter* 36 (10 June 1994): 52.

Langston, J., P. Ballard, J. Tetrud, and I. Irwin. "Chronic Parkinsonism in Humans due to a Product of Meperidine-Analogue Synthesis." *Science* 219 (1983): 979–80.

Maurer, D., and V. Vogel. *Narcotics and Narcotic Addiction,* 3d ed. Springfield, IL: Thomas, 1967.

McEvoy, G., ed. "Opiate Agonists." In *American Hospital Formulary Service Drug Information.* Bethesda, MD: American Society of Hospital Pharmacists, 1993.

McLellen, T., O. Arndt, D. Metzger, G. Woody, and C. O'Brian. "The Effects of Psychosocial Services in Substance Abuse Treatment." *JAMA* 269 (21 April 1993): 1953–59.

Meddis, S. "USA's Illegal Drug Bill: $40 Billion." *USA Today* (20 June 1991): 1A.

Millstein, R. "Methadone Revisited." *NIDA Notes* 7 (July–August 1992): 3–4.

Nowak, R. "Cops and Doctors: Drug Busts Hamper Pain Therapy." *Journal of NIH Research* 4 (May 1992): 27–29.

O'Dair, B. "X and Drugs and Rock and Roll." *Entertainment Weekly* 131 (14 August 1992): 8–9.

Pfefferbaum, B., and C. Hagberg. "Pharmacological Management of Pain in Children." *Journal of the American Academy of Child and Adolescent Psychiatry* 32 (1993): 235–42.

Pothos, E., P. Rada, G. Mark, and B. Hoebel. "Dopamine Microdialysis in the Nucleus Accumbens During Acute and Chronic Morphine, Naloxone-Precipitated Withdrawal and Clonidine Treatment." *Brain Research* 566 (1991): 348–50.

Roche, B. "High-Purity Drug Is Fatal Attraction." *Boston Globe* (14 July 1993): 21.

Scott, J. M. *The White Poppy: A History of Opium.* New York: Funk & Wagnalls, 1969.

Sterne, A. E. "A Life of Opium Addiction." *Journal of Inebriety* 29 (Autumn 1907): 203–09.

Strain, E., M. Stitzer, I. Liebson, and G. Bigelow. "Methadone and Treatment Outcome." *Drug and Alcohol Dependence* 33 (1993): 106–17.

Swan, N. "Heroin- and Cocaine-Related Visits to Hospital Emergency Rooms Continue to Increase Nationwide." *NIDA Notes* 7 (July–August 1992): 9–10.

Swan, N. "Two NIDA-Tested Heroin Treatment Medications Move Toward FDA Approval." *NIDA Notes* (March–April 1993): 45.

Swan, N. "Treatment Practitioners Learn About LAAM." *NIDA Notes* 9 (February–March 1994): 5.

Treaster, J. "Heroin Use Rises as Crack Wanes." *New York Times* (18 June 1991).

Washington, A. M., M. S. Gold, and A. C. Pottard. "Opiate and Cocaine Dependencies." *Drug Dependencies* 5 (1985): 46–47.

Way, W., and E. Way. "Opioid Analgesics and Antagonists." In *Basic and Clinical Pharmacology,* 5th ed., edited by B. Katzung, 420–36. Norwalk, CT: Appleton & Lange, 1992.

Zinsberg, N. E. "Nonaddictive Opiate Use." In *Handbook on Drug Abuse,* edited by R. L. Dupont, A. Goldstein, and J. O'Donnell. Washington, DC: National Institute on Drug Abuse, U.S. Department of Health, Education, and Welfare, 1979.

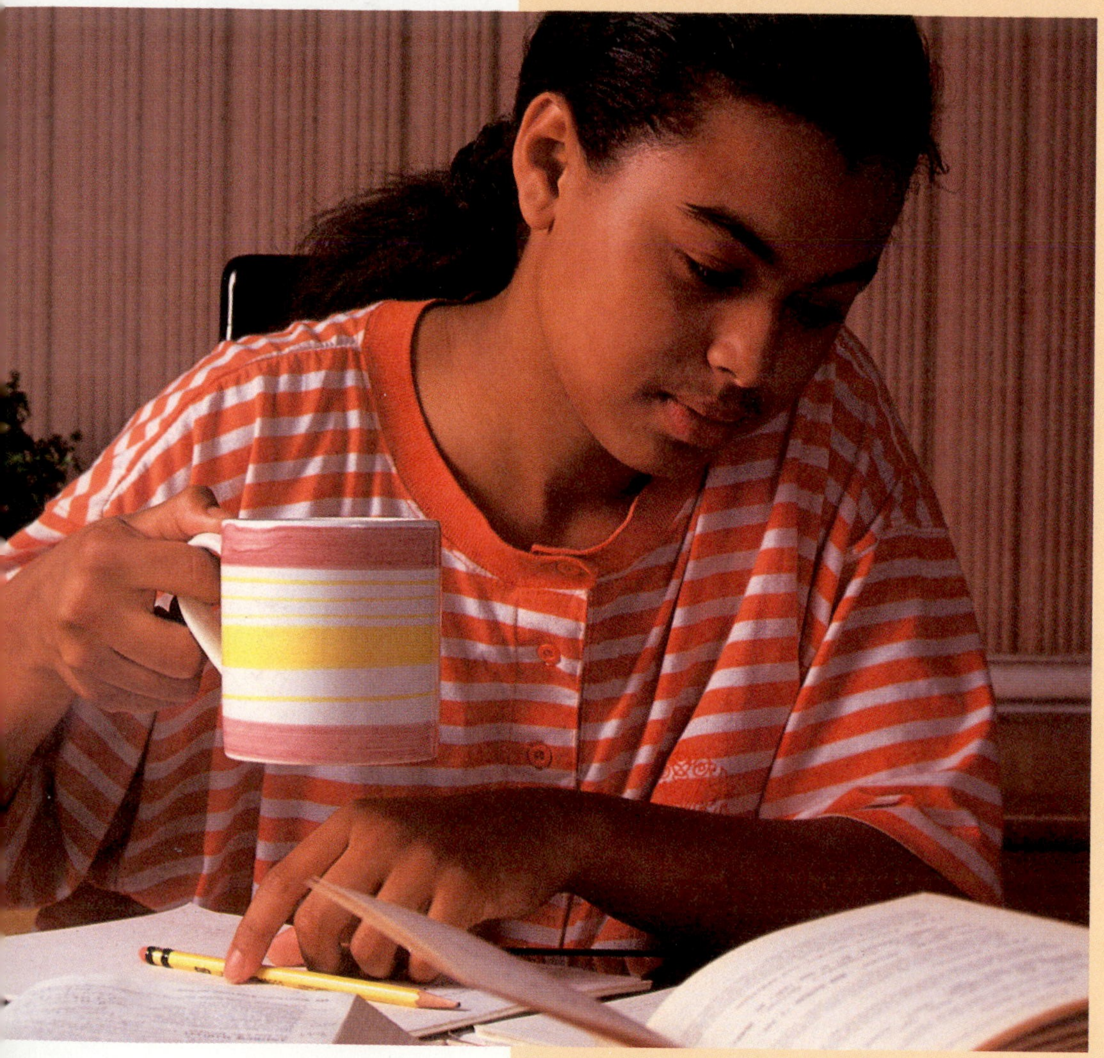

Chapter 10

Stimulants

Did You Know That . . .

- The first therapeutic use of amphetamines was in inhalers to treat nasal congestion.
- Ritalin is a type of amphetamine used to treat hyperactive (attention deficit disorder) children.
- The most common FDA-approved use of amphetamines is as a diet aid to treat obesity.
- "Ecstasy" is a "designer" drug that is chemically and pharmacologically related to amphetamines.
- The original Coca-Cola was a cocaine-containing tonic developed in the late 1800s.
- In the early 1980s, cocaine was viewed as a relatively harmless, glamorous substance by the media and some medical experts in this country.
- Smoking "freebased," or "crack," cocaine is more dangerous and more addicting than other forms of administration.
- Many people who abuse cocaine are attempting to self-medicate mood disorders, such as depression.
- Caffeine is the most frequently used stimulant in the world.
- OTC decongestant drugs usually contain mild CNS stimulants.

Learning Objectives

On completing this chapter, you will be able to

1. Explain how amphetamines work.
2. Identify the FDA-approved uses for the amphetamines.
3. Recognize the major side effects of amphetamines on brain and cardiovascular functions.
4. Identify the terms *"speed," "ice,"* and *"run"* as they relate to amphetamine use.
5. Explain what "designer" amphetamines are.
6. Identify the three cocaine eras.
7. Trace the changes in attitude toward cocaine abuse that occurred in the 1980s and explain why they occurred.
8. Compare the effects of cocaine to those of amphetamines.
9. Identify the four principal means of administering cocaine and their relative potencies.
10. Distinguish the properties of "crack" that make it unique from other cocaine forms.

continued

Healthy People 2000

Increase the proportion of high school seniors who perceive social disapproval associated with the heavy use of . . . and experimentation with cocaine.

Increase the proportion of high school seniors who associate risk of physical or psychological harm with the heavy use of . . . and experimentation with cocaine.

LEARNING OBJECTIVES

11 Identify the different stages of cocaine withdrawal.
12 Discuss the different approaches to treating cocaine dependence.
13 Identify and compare the major sources of the caffeinelike xanthine drugs.
14 List the principal physiological effects of caffeine.
15 Compare caffeine dependence and withdrawal to that associated with the major stimulants.

Stimulants are substances that act on the central nervous system (CNS). The user experiences pleasant effects initially, such as a sense of increased energy and a state of euphoria, or "high." But he or she may also feel restless and talkative and have trouble sleeping. High doses used over the long term can produce personality changes or even dangerous behavior. Many users self-medicate psychological conditions such as depression with stimulants. Because the initial effects of stimulants are so pleasant, these drugs are frequently abused, leading to dependence.

In this chapter, we examine the two principal classifications of stimulant drugs. Major stimulants, including amphetamines and cocaine, are addressed first, given their prominent role in current drug abuse problems in the United States. The chapter concludes with a review of minor stimulants, in particular caffeine. The stimulant properties of OTC sympathomimetics are also discussed.

(Because nicotine has unique stimulant properties, it is covered in Chapter 11, "Tobacco.")

Major Stimulants

All the major stimulants cause increased alertness, excitation, and euphoria; thus, these drugs are referred to as **"uppers."** The major stimulants are classified as either Schedule I ("designer" amphetamines) or Schedule II (amphetamine and cocaine) controlled substances because of their abuse potential. Toxic effects of the major stimulants account for almost half of all drug-related unexplained sudden deaths in the United States (Goldstein 1994). Although these drugs have properties in common, they also have unique features that distinguish them from each other. The similarities and differences of the major stimulants are discussed in the following sections.

Amphetamines

Amphetamines are potent CNS stimulants capable of causing dependence due to their euphorigenic properties and ability to eliminate fatigue. Despite their addicting effects, amphetamines can be legally prescribed by physicians. Consequently, amphetamine abuse occurs in people who acquire their drugs by both legitimate and illicit means.

The History of Amphetamines Amphetamine was first synthesized by the German pharmacologist L. Edeleano in 1887, but it was not until 1910 that this and several related compounds were tested in laboratory animals. Another 17 years passed before Gordon Alles, a researcher looking for a more potent substitute for ephedrine (used as a decongestant at the time), self-administered amphetamine and gave a firsthand account of its effects. Alles found that when inhaled or taken orally, amphetamine dramatically reduced fatigue, increased alertness, and caused a sense of confident euphoria (Grinspoon and Bakalar 1978).

Because of Alles's impressive findings, Benzedrine (amphetamine) inhalers became available in 1932 as a nonprescription medication in drugstores across America. The Benzedrine inhaler, marketed for nasal congestion, was widely abused and continued to be available over the counter until 1949. Because of a loophole in a law that was passed later, not until 1971 were all potent amphetamine-like compounds in nasal inhalers withdrawn from the market (Grinspoon and Bakalar 1978).

Because of the lack of restrictions during this early period, amphetamines were sold for a variety of different ailments. Advertisements for amphetamine inhalers made claims that they could be used to treat obesity, alcoholism, bed wetting, depression, schizophrenia, morphine and codeine addiction, nicotinism, heart block, head injuries, sea sickness, persistent hiccups, and caffeine mania. Today, most of these uses are no longer approved as legitimate therapeutics but would be considered forms of drug abuse.

World War II provided a setting in which both the legal and "black market" use of amphetamines flourished (Grinspoon and Bakalar 1978). The stimulating effects of amphetamines made them suitable for wide use in World War II to counteract fatigue. The Germans, Japanese, and British made extensive use of these drugs in the early 1940s. By the end of World War II, large quantities of amphetamines were readily available without prescription in seven different types of nasal inhalers. The inhalers were easily broken and the amphetamines removed and dissolved in coffee or alcohol for a stronger "kick." Not until 1947 was the extent of inhaler abuse finally documented in medical literature. Early reports cited abuse problems in the military, but it quickly became apparent that the problem was widespread.

In spite of warnings, the U.S. armed forces issued amphetamines on a regular basis during the Korean War. Korean veterans going back to college used amphetamine tablets to help cram for examinations, and other students quickly adopted the practice. Amphetamine use became widespread among truck drivers making long hauls; it is believed that among the earliest distribution systems for illicit amphetamines were truck stops along major U.S. highways. High achievers under continuous pressure in the fields of entertainment, business, and industry often relied on amphetamines to counteract fatigue. Homemakers used them for weight control and to combat boredom from unfulfilled lives. At the height of the U.S. epidemic in 1967, some 31 million prescriptions were written for **anorexiants** (diet pills) alone. About the same time, the Food and Drug Administration (FDA) estimated that more than 25 tons of legitimately manufactured amphetamine were diverted to illegal sales; at times, about 90% of the legal supply went into the illegal market.

In the late 1950s, some West Coast narcotic addicts used a combination of amphetamine and heroin to get an effect similar to that of heroin and cocaine. (Cocaine, for the most part, was unavailable at this time.) These addicts also used amphetamine alone when heroin could not be obtained. By the early 1960s, intravenous amphetamine was the first choice for a majority of drug users in West Coast cities. Individuals would get prescriptions for large amounts of methamphetamine for treatment of heroin addiction. The abuse of legally obtained methamphetamine became so prevalent that a number of physicians and pharmacists were prosecuted and convicted for encouraging this practice. And because of its abuse potential, injectable amphetamine was completely withdrawn from the market.

Although amphetamine abuse is typically thought of as an American phenomenon, the drug has been abused in many other industrial nations, as well. However, only Japan and Sweden have had large-scale epidemics of amphetamine abuse comparable to the experience in the United States in the 1960s.

Although a variety of related drugs and mixtures currently exist, the most common amphetamine substances are dextroamphetamine (Dexedrine), methamphetamine (Desoxyn), and amphetamine itself. Generally, if doses are adjusted, the psychological effects of these various drugs are similar, so they will be discussed as a group. Other drugs with similar pharmacological properties are phenmetrazine (Preludin), and methylphenidate (Ritalin). Common slang terms

"UPPERS" a slang term for CNS stimulants

ANOREXIANTS drugs that suppress the appetite for food

for the amphetamines include *speed, crystal, meth, bennies, dexies, uppers, pep pills, diet pills, jolly beans, copilots, hearts, footballs, white crosses,* and *ice.*

How Amphetamines Work Amphetamines are synthetic chemicals that are similar to natural neurotransmitters such as norepinephrine (noradrenaline), dopamine, and the stress hormone epinephrine (adrenaline). The amphetamines exert their pharmacological effect by increasing the activity of these catecholamine substances and serotonin (see Chapter 5), both in the brain and nerves associated with the sympathetic nervous system. Because amphetamines cause release of norepinephrine from sympathetic nerves, they are classified as *sympathomimetic* drugs. The amphetamines generally cause an arousal or activating response (also called the "fight-or-flight response") that is similar to the normal reaction to emergency situations or crises.

Amphetamines also cause alertness so that the individual becomes aroused, hypersensitive to stimuli, and feels "turned on." These effects occur even without external sensory input. This activation may be a very pleasant experience in itself, but a continual high level of activation may convert to anxiety, severe apprehension, or a feeling of panic.

Amphetamines have potent effects on dopamine in the reward (pleasure) center of the brain (see Chapter 5). This probably causes the "flash," or sudden feeling of intense pleasure that occurs when amphetamine is taken intravenously. Some users describe the sensation as a "whole-body orgasm," and many associate intravenous methamphetamine use with sexual feelings. Some report that use of amphetamines prolongs sexual activity, sometimes for hours. In contrast, others find that, while using amphetamines, they cannot reach orgasm under any circumstances. Although a minority of users actually report increased sexual activity while taking amphetamine, many users cite enhanced sexual pleasure as their principal reason for taking these stimulants (Jaffe and Martin 1990).

Amphetamines have two major actions on neurotransmission:

1. Amphetamines cause the release of the catecholamines and serotonin neurotransmitters from neurons.
2. Amphetamines block the enzyme that metabolizes these neurotransmitters (monoamine oxidase), thereby prolonging their effects.

What Amphetamines Can Do A curious condition commonly reported with heavy amphetamine use is **behavioral stereotypy,** or getting "hung up." This refers to a simple activity that is done repeatedly. An individual who is "hung up" will get caught in a repetitious thought or act for hours. For example, he or she may take objects apart, like radios or clocks, and carefully categorize all the parts, or sit in a tub and bathe all day, persistently sing a note, repeat a phrase of music, or repeatedly clean the same object. This phenomenon seems to be peculiar to potent stimulants such as the amphetamines and cocaine.

Behavioral stereotypy is said to occur in part because of the effects of amphetamines on dopamine in the brain. This neurotransmitter is associated with the complex controls for some of the body's motor functions. One theory is that, when dopamine activity is continually enhanced by amphetamine exposure, the associated neurons become sensitized so the effect of this transmitter becomes exaggerated and stereotypy occurs (Robinson 1991). Similar patterns of repetitive behavior also occur in psychotic conditions. This similarity suggests that the intense use of stimulants such as amphetamines or cocaine alters the brain in a manner like that which causes psychotic mental disorders (American Psychiatric Association, 1994).

Chronic use of high doses of amphetamines causes dramatic decreases in the brain content of the neurotransmitters dopamine and serotonin that persist for months, even after drug use is stopped (Jaffe 1990; Schmidt et al. 1985). These decreases have been shown to reflect the death of CNS neurons that release these transmitters. It is not clear why this neuronal damage occurs or how it affects behavior.

Approved Uses Until 1970, amphetamines had been prescribed for a large number of conditions, including depression, fatigue, and long-term weight reduction. In 1970, the FDA, acting on the recommendation of the National Academy of Sciences, restricted the legal use of amphetamines to three medical conditions: (1) narcolepsy, (2) hyperkinetic (attention deficit disorder) behavior, and (3) short-term weight reduction programs (Goldstein 1995).

Narcolepsy. Amphetamine treatment of **narcolepsy** is not widespread because this is a relatively rare disorder. The term *narcolepsy* comes from the Greek words for "numbness" and "seizure." A person who has narcolepsy falls asleep as frequently as 50 times a day if he or she stays in one position very long. Taking low doses of amphetamines helps keep narcoleptic people alert.

Hyperkinetic Behavior. This common behavioral problem in children and adolescents involves an abnormally high level of physical activity **(hyperkinesis)** and an inability to focus attention. About 4 out of every 100 grade-school children and 40% of schoolchildren referred to mental health clinics because of behavioral disturbances are hyperactive. Boys are much more likely to be diagnosed as hyperactive than girls. Such children have short concentration spans, are aggressive, lack clear direction, and are hard to anticipate. Their aggressive, talkative, restless, and impulsive behavior disrupts the classroom and often home life as well. Such behavior problems usually impede learning.

The drug commonly used to treat hyperkinetic (attention deficit disorder) children is the amphetamine-related methylphenidate or Ritalin. It is a mild stimulant of the central nervous system that counteracts physical and mental fatigue while having only slight effects on blood pressure and respiration. Its stimulant potency is intermediate between that of amphetamine and caffeine. Methylphenidate and amphetamine are about equally effective in treating hyperkinesis, but methylphenidate is thought to interfere with growth less than amphetamine (Weiner 1980) and to have less abuse potential. Stimulants have a paradoxical calming effect on children with hyperkinesis; the reason for this is unknown.

Similar attention deficit problems also appear in some adults. It is not clear if the mechanisms for the problem are the same in both children and adults, but Ritalin appears to be equally effective in the treatment of both populations.

Weight Reduction. By far the most common legal use of amphetamines is for the treatment of obesity. According to accepted medical and health standards, 24 to 45% of American adults are overweight (Appelt 1990). Amphetamines and chemically similar compounds are used as anorexiants to help such people control appetite. Amphetamines are thought to act by affecting the appetite center in the hypothalamus of the brain and decrease food intake. The FDA has approved short-term use of amphetamines for weight loss programs.

Unless the dose is continuously increased, the appetite-suppressing action of this drug, together with the pleasant stimulating effects, usually wear off after about two to four weeks of treatment. At high doses, the anorexic effect returns, but an even greater tolerance will result. Because of this buildup of tolerance, the FDA has issued a warning about the danger of long-term use of amphetamines.

Many experts feel that the euphoric effect of amphetamines is the primary motivation for their continued use in weight reduction programs. It is possible that many obese people have a need for gratification that can be satisfied by an amphetamine-like drug. If the drug is taken away, these individuals return to food to satisfy their need and sometimes experience "rebound," causing them to gain back more weight than they lost. Because of the particularly fragile psychological state of many obese patients and the potentially severe side effects of amphetamines, support for these drugs as diet aids is diminishing. Most clinicians who work with weight loss programs prefer to use nonmedicinal approaches, such as behavioral modification, counseling techniques, and support group therapy.

Side Effects of Therapeutic Doses The two principal side effects of therapeutic doses of amphetamines include (1) abuse potential, which has already been discussed at length, and (2) cardio-

BEHAVIORAL STEREOTYPY meaningless repetition of a single activity

HYPERKINESIS excessive movement

NARCOLEPSY a condition causing spontaneous and uncontrolled sleeping episodes vascular toxicities. As early as 1935, reports in medical journals suggested that Benzedrine might cause serious cardiovascular problems (Grinspoon and Bakalar 1978). Many of these effects are due to the amphetamine-induced release of epinephrine from the adrenal glands and norepinephrine from the nerves associated with the sympathetic nervous system. The effects include increased heart rate, elevated blood pressure, and damage to vessels, especially small veins and arteries (Max 1991). In users with a history of heart attack, coronary arrhythmia, or hypertension, amphetamine toxicity can be severe or even fatal.

Current Misuse Because amphetamine drugs can be readily synthesized in makeshift laboratories for illicit sales, accurate figures on the amount of illegal drugs manufactured and sold are not available. However, estimates run from 10 to 25% of the amount on the legal market. Surveys suggest that there was a decline in the abuse of amphetamines in the late 1980s and early 1990s in parallel with the trend in cocaine abuse (Johnston 1993). However, in 1993 the declines were replaced by an alarming rise in the number of adolescents that abused amphetamines compared to 1992 (approximately 10%). It is not clear if this increase was merely an aberration or the beginning of a pattern of escalating amphetamine abuse (Johnston 1994).

Since the late 1970s, U.S. medical associations have asked all physicians to be more careful in the use of prescribed amphetamines. In fact, presently, use is recommended only for narcolepsy and some cases of hyperactivity in children. In spite of FDA approval, most medical associations do not recommend the use of amphetamines for weight loss. Probably less than 1% of all prescriptions now written are for amphetamines, in contrast to 8% in 1970.

Amphetamine abusers commonly administer a dose of 10 to 30 mg. Besides the positive effects of this dose—the "high"—it can also cause hyperactive, nervous, or jittery feelings that encourage the use of a depressant such as benzodiazepine, barbiturate, or alcohol to relieve the discomfort of being "wired" (Jaffe 1990).

A potent and commonly abused form of amphetamine is **"speed,"** an illegal methamphetamine available as a white crystalline powder for injection. The profit for the speed manufacturer is substantial enough to make illicit production financially attractive. Methamphetamine is relatively easy to synthesize even by individuals without expertise in chemistry. Such people, referred to as "cookers," produce methamphetamine batches by using cookbook-style recipes (often obtained while in jail). At least two predominant methods for making methamphetamine are used in the United States and result in highly variable products from clandestine laboratory to laboratory (Irvine and Chin 1991). Due to the ease of production and the availability of chemicals used to prepare methamphetamine, there continues to be a constant supply of this drug.

Today, so-called meth or speed labs are frequently raided by law enforcement agencies across the country as local drug entrepreneurs try to get in on the profits. In fact, the number increased from 88 seizures in 1981 to 652 in 1989. Since 1987 over 80% of all clandestine laboratories seized have been involved in the manufacturing of methamphetamine (Irvine and Chin 1991).

Patterns of High-Dose Use. Amphetamines can be taken orally, intravenously, or by smoking. The intensity and duration of effects vary according to the mode of administration. The "speed freak" uses chronic, high doses of amphetamines intravenously. Another approach to administering amphetamines is smoking **"ice,"** which can cause effects as potent, but perhaps more prolonged and erratic, than intravenous doses (Fitzpatrick 1992). The cycle or pattern of use often starts with several days of repeated administrations, usually of "speed," gradually increasing in amount and frequency. This pattern of intense stimulant use is called a **"run."** Some users inject up to several thousand milligrams in a single day (Goldstein 1995). Initially, the user may feel energetic, talkative, enthusiastic, happy, confident, and powerful and may initiate and complete highly ambitious tasks. He or she will be unable to sleep and will usually eat very little. His or her pupils will be dilated, mouth dry, and body temperature elevated **(hyperpyrexia).**

After the first day or so, unpleasant symptoms become prominent as the dosage is increased. Symptoms commonly reported at this stage are teeth grinding, disorganized patterns of thought and behavior, stereotypy, irritability, self-conscious-

TABLE 10.1 Summary of the effects of amphetamine on the body and mind

	Body	Mind
Low Dose	Increased heartbeat	Decreased fatigue
↓	Increased blood pressure	Increased confidence
	Decreased appetite	Increased feeling of alertness
	Increased breathing rate	Restlessness, talkativeness
	Inability to sleep	Increased irritability
	Sweating	Fearfulness, apprehension
	Dry mouth	Distrust of people
	Muscle twitching	Behavioral stereotypy
	Convulsions	Hallucinations
	Fever	Psychosis
	Chest pain	
	Irregular heartbeat	
High Dose	Death due to overdose	

ness, suspiciousness, and fear. Hallucinations and delusions can occur that are similar to a paranoid psychosis and indistinguishable from schizophrenia (American Psychiatric Association 1994). The person is likely to show aggressive and antisocial behavior for no apparent reason. Severe chest pains, abdominal discomfort that mimics appendicitis, and fainting from overdosage are sometimes reported. "Cocaine bugs" is one bizarre effect of high doses of potent stimulants such as amphetamines: The user experiences strange feelings, like insects crawling under the skin. The range of physical and mental symptoms from low to high doses is summarized in Table 10.1.

SPEED an injectable methamphetamine used by drug addicts

"ICE" a smokable form of methamphetamine

"RUN" intense use of a stimulant, consisting of multiple administrations over a period of days

HYPERPYREXIA elevated body temperature

Toward the end of the run, which usually lasts from three to five days, the adverse symptoms dominate. When the drug is discontinued because the supply is exhausted or the symptoms become too unpleasant, prolonged sleep follows, sometimes lasting several days. On awakening, the person is lethargic, hungry, and often severely depressed. The amphetamine user may overcome these effects with another smoke of ice or injection of speed, initiating a new cycle. Barbiturates, benzodiazepines, and opiate narcotics are sometimes used to ease the "crash" or to terminate an unpleasant run (see Chapter 6).

Continued use of massive doses of amphetamine often leads to considerable weight loss, sores in the skin, nonhealing ulcers, liver disease, hypertensive disorders, cerebral hemorrhage (stroke), heart attack, kidney damage, and seizures (Hall and Hando 1993). Experiments in which rhesus monkeys received chronic intravenous injections of methamphetamine resulted in direct injury to the small arteries and veins, causing them to rupture and produce severe brain damage. Oral methamphetamine given to monkeys and rats can result in cerebral vascular changes and kidney damage as serious as that caused by intravenous methamphetamine (Rumbaugh 1977). For some of these effects, it is impossible to tell whether they are caused by the drug, poor eating habits, or other factors associated with the lifestyle of people who inject methamphetamine.

Speed freaks are generally unpopular with the rest of the drug-taking community, especially "acid-heads" (addicts who use LSD), because of the aggressive, unpredictable behavior associated with use of potent stimulants. In general, drug abusers who take high doses of these agents, such as amphetamines or cocaine, are more likely to be involved in violent crimes than those who abuse other drugs (Miller and Kozel 1991). Consequently, these individuals may live together in "flash houses" totally occupied by chronic amphetamine or stimulant addicts. Heavy users are generally unable to hold steady jobs because of their drug habits and often have a parasitic relationship with the rest of the illicit drug-using community.

Although claims have been made that amphetamines do not cause physical dependence, it is almost certain that the depression (sometimes suicidal), lethargy, and abnormal sleep patterns occurring after high chronic doses are part of withdrawal (Goldstein 1995). This type of rebound effect is opposite to those of drugs that are CNS depressants (see Chapter 6). Withdrawal from depressants causes severe and toxic overstimulation, even to the point of convulsions.

Amphetamine Combinations. Amphetamines are frequently used in conjunction with a variety of other drugs, such as barbiturates, benzodiazepines, alcohol, and heroin (Hall and Hando 1993). Amphetamines intensify, prolong, or otherwise alter the effects of LSD, and the two drugs are sometimes combined. The majority of speed users have also had experience with a variety of psychedelic and other drugs. In addition, people dependent on opiate narcotics frequently use amphetamines or cocaine. (The combinations are called **"speedballs."**)

"Designer" Amphetamines. Underground chemists have been synthesizing drugs that mimic the psychoactive effects of amphetamines. Although the production of such drugs has diminished recently, occasional outbreaks continue (Greenhouse 1992). These substances have become known as **designer drugs** (see Chapter 3).

Designer amphetamines sometimes differ from the parent compound by a single element. These "synthetic spinoffs" pose a significant abuse problem because often several different designer amphetamines can be made from the parent compound and retain the abuse potential of the original substance.

For many years the production and distribution of designer amphetamines were not illegal, even though they were synthesized from controlled substances. However, in the mid-1980s the DEA actively pursued policies to curb their production and sale. Consequently, many designer amphetamines are currently outlawed under the Substance Analogue Enforcement Act (1986), which makes illegal any substance that is similar in structure or psychological effect to any substance already scheduled, if it is manufactured, possessed, or sold with the intention it will be consumed by humans (Beck 1990).

The principal types of designer amphetamines are

1. Derivatives from amphetamine and methamphetamine that retain the CNS stimulatory effects such as 4-methylaminorex (U4EUH) and ICE.
2. Derivatives from amphetamine and methamphetamine that have prominent hallucinogenic effects besides their CNS stimulatory action, such as MDMA (Ecstasy).

Because the basic amphetamine molecule can be easily synthesized and readily modified, new amphetamine-like drugs continue to appear on the streets. Although these designer amphetamines are thought of as new drugs when they first appear, in fact, most were originally synthesized from the 1940s to the 1960s by pharmaceutical companies trying to find new decongestant and anorexiant drugs to compete with the other amphetamines. Some of these compounds were found to be too toxic to be marketed but have been rediscovered by "street chemists" and are being sold to unsus-

"SPEEDBALL" a combination of amphetamine or cocaine with an opioid narcotic, often heroin

TABLE 10.2 "Designer" amphetamines

Amphetamine Derivative	Properties
Methylenedioxy**methamphetamine** (MDMA, "Ecstasy")	Stimulant and hallucinogen
Methylenedioxy**amphetamine** (MDA)	More powerful stimulant and less powerful hallucinogen than MDMA
4-Ethoxy-2, 5-dimethoxy**amphetamine**	Effects like MDA (stimulant and hallucinogen)
4-Methylaminorex	CNS stimulant like amphetamine
3-, 4-Methylenedioxy-N, N-dimethyl**amphetamine**	Mild MDMA
N, N-Dimethyl**amphetamine**	One-fifth potency of amphetamine
4-Thiomethyl-2, 5-dimethoxy**amphetamine**	Hallucinogen
Para-methoxymeth**amphetamine**	Weak stimulant

Source: F. Sapienza, H. McClain, M. Klein, and J. Tolliver. "New Controlled Analogues of Interest to DEA." Abstract, Annual Meeting of the Committee on Problems of Drug Dependence. Washington, DC: Drug Control Section, Drug Enforcement Administration, 1989.

pecting victims trying to experience a new sensation. See Table 10.2 for a list of these designer amphetamines.

The Here and Now box on page 268 presents an excerpt from San Francisco street literature promoting a designer amphetamine called "U4Euh." This drug was developed in the early 1960s as an appetite suppressant but was never marketed because it was found to cause serious damage to the lungs as well as seizures. Despite the known danger from this drug, it was sold illegally from 1987 to 1990 on the streets of several states, causing a number of deaths (Hanson et al. 1992).

Other designer drugs of abuse that are chemically related to amphetamine include DOM (STP), methcathinone (called "Cat" or "Bathtub Speed"), MDA, and MDMA (or methylenedioxymethamphetamine, called "Ecstasy," "X," "E," "XTC," or "Adam"). All these drugs are currently classified as Schedule I agents.

MDMA (Ecstasy) Of the designer amphetamines, MDMA continues to be the most popular. It had widespread popularity in the United States throughout the 1980s, and its use peaked in 1987 despite its classification as a Schedule I drug in 1985 by the DEA. At the height of its use, 39% of the undergraduates at Stanford University reported to have used MDMA at least once (Randall 1992a). In the late 1980s and early 1990s use of MDMA declined in this country, but about this time it was "reformulated": this reformulation was not in a pharmacological sense but in a cultural context. The "rave" scene in England provided a new showcase for MDMA or Ecstasy (Randall 1992a)—see Here and Now box on page 269. Partygoers attired in "Cat in the Hat" hats and psychedelic jumpsuits paid $20 to dance all night to heavy electronically generated sound mixed with computer-generated video and laser light shows.

For another $20, an Ecstasy tablet could be purchased for the sensory enhancement caused by the drug (Randall 1992b). The British "rave" counterculture and its generous use of Ecstasy was exported to the United States in the early 1990s with its high-tech music and video trappings encouraged by low-tech laboratories that illegally manufactured the drug in this country. Some have compared the "rave" culture of the 1990s and their use of MDMA to the acid-test parties of the 1960s and their use of LSD and amphetamines (Randall 1992a).

The patent for MDMA was first issued in 1914 to E. Merck in Darmstadt, Germany, as an appetite

Here and Now

"Street" Advertisement for an Illicit "Designer" Amphetamine

The following is an excerpt from 1986 San Francisco "street" literature on the amphetamine "designer" drug called "U4Euh" (officially, 4-methylaminorex):

> U4Euh is an "experimental substance which undoubtedly will never be approved by the Food and Drug Gestapo for human use. . . . U4Euh HCl is available in extremely limited quantities to qualified individuals. (Due to unpredictably greater duration of the free-base, the freebase is not presently being offered.) Appreciate it, enjoy it, use it, do NOT abuse it. THOSE WHO ABUSE IT, DON'T ABUSE IT FOR LONG. Let's try to keep THIS one from being outlawed.*
>
> . . . Here are some comments: "One of the best things that happened to me this year. . . . At the end of a three-month national book tour, I feel like the first day of the tour." . . . "Fun . . . a unique stimulation." . . . "Like a cross between coke and speed but milder than speed." . . . "Gave me a feeling of irresponsibility." . . . This is the dawning of the age of U4Euh!

*They were unsuccessful—"U4Euh" was classified Schedule I in 1989.

suppressant. No pharmaceutical company has ever manufactured MDMA for public marketing, and the FDA has never approved it for therapy (Beck 1990). MDMA was first found by the DEA on the streets in 1972 in a drug sample bought in Chicago (Beck 1990). The DEA earnestly began gathering data on MDMA abuse a decade later, which led to its classification as a Schedule I substance in 1985 despite the very vocal opposition by a number of psychiatrists who had been using MDMA since the late 1970s to facilitate communication, acceptance, and fear reduction in their patients (Beck 1990). MDMA and related designer amphetamines are somewhat unique from other amphetamines in that, besides causing excitation, they have prominent hallucinogenic effects, as well (see Chapter 12). These drugs have been characterized as combining the properties of amphetamine and LSD. The psychedelic effects of MDMA are likely caused by release of the neurotransmitter serotonin. After using hallucinogenic amphetamines, the mind is often flooded with a variety of irrelevant and incoherent thoughts and exaggerated sensory experiences and is more receptive to suggestion.

MDMA is often viewed as a "smooth amphetamine" and does not appear to cause the severe depression, or "crash" often associated with frequent high dosing of the more traditional amphetamines. Most users tend to be predominantly positive when describing their initial MDMA experiences (Taylor 1994). They claim the drug causes a dramatic drop in defense mechanisms or fear responses, while feeling an increased empathy for others. Combined with its stimulant effects, this often increases intimate communication and association with others (Beck 1990; Goldstein 1995).

However, many users do experience adverse effects, such as loss of appetite, grinding of teeth, muscle aches and stiffness, sweating, and a rapid heartbeat. In addition, fatigue can be experienced for hours or even days after use (Randall 1992a). Despite these side effects, there are few reports of severe toxicity or death in the United States from

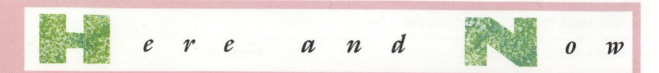

Here and Now

Here We Go Again

Some experts are making comparisons between LSD-laced "acid parties" of a quarter-century ago and MDMA-laced "rave parties" of the early 1990s. The scene appeared to have gone full circle when in 1992 several Los Angeles "raves" were hosted by the son of Timothy Leary. Dr. Timothy Leary was a former Harvard psychology professor who was an enthusiastic advocate of the use of LSD in the 1960s. He made several appearances at his son's "raves," referring to them as "high-tech acid test." Dr. Leary's son was only one of thousands of young adults who have again "tuned in" to the hallucinogenic scene.

Source: T. Randall. "'Rave' Scene. Ecstasy Use, Leap Atlantic." *JAMA* 268 (1992):1506.

using MDMA (Taylor 1994): in contrast, at least 15 young people in England were killed in the early 1990s because of this designer amphetamine. In every case a recreational dose of this drug had been taken by the victim at a "rave" where crowds were packed together and dancing vigorously (Randall 1992a). In these fatal cases, the victims collapsed unconscious while dancing and started to convulse. The combination of rapidly rising body temperature (up to 110°F), racing pulse, and plummeting blood pressure resulted in death from 2 to 60 hours after hospital admission. The lethality of MDMA under these conditions appears to be related to its ability to elevate body temperature and cause dehydration: thus, mixed with the crowded, hot environment of a "rave" and extreme physical exertion while dancing, the drug causes a deadly episode of hyperthermia (Taylor 1994). Authorities are very concerned that as raves become popular in the United States, use of MDMA may lead to similar fatal consequences in this country.

Methylphenidate: A Special Amphetamine

Methylphenidate (Ritalin) is related to the amphetamines but is a relatively mild central nervous system stimulant that has been used to alleviate depression. Research now casts doubt on its effectiveness for treating depression, but it is effective in treatment of narcolepsy. As explained previously, methylphenidate has also been found to aid in calming children suffering from attention deficit disorder and is currently the drug of choice for this purpose. The potency of methylphenidate lies between that of caffeine and amphetamine. It is not used much on the street because, compared to other amphetamines, it has less abuse potential. Even so, methylphenidate has been classified as a Schedule II drug, like the other prescribed amphetamines.

Cocaine

Over the last 10 to 15 years, cocaine abuse has become one of the greatest drug concerns in U.S. society. In the so-called war against drugs, cocaine eradication is considered to be a top priority. The tremendous attention recently directed at cocaine reflects the fact that from 1978 to 1987 the United States experienced the largest cocaine epidemic in history. Antisocial and criminal activities related to the effects of this potent stimulant have become highly visible and widely publicized (Grinspoon 1993).

As recently as the early 1980s, cocaine use was not believed to cause dependency because it did not cause gross withdrawal effects, as do alcohol and narcotics (Goldstein 1994). In fact, a 1982 article in *Scientific American* stated that cocaine was "no more habit forming than potato chips" (Van Dyck and Byck 1982). This has clearly been proven false: cocaine is so highly addictive that it is readily self-administered not only by humans but by laboratory animals as well (Fischman and Foltin 1992). Studies suggest that 30 to 40 million Americans have tried cocaine sometime during their life (Brown et al. 1992).

There is no better substance than cocaine to illustrate the "love–hate" relationship that people can have with drugs. Many lessons can be learned by understanding the impact of cocaine and the social struggles that have ensued as people have tried to determine their proper relationship with this substance.

The History of Cocaine Use Cocaine has been used as a stimulant for thousands of years. Its history can be classified into three eras, based on geographical, social, and therapeutic considerations. Studying each era will help us understand current attitudes about cocaine.

The First Cocaine Era. The first cocaine era was characterized by an almost harmonious use of this stimulant by South American Indians living in the regions of the Andean Mountains. One record dates cocaine use back to about 2500 B.C. in Peru, where coca leaves and even a chewed quid (wad) of coca were found near gravesites. Natives of Peru, Bolivia, and Colombia have long chewed the leaves of the *Erythroxylon coca* shrub, found in the high altitudes of the Andean Mountains. Leaves of this coca plant contain up to 1% of the alkaloid stimulant cocaine.

It is believed that the stimulant properties of cocaine played a major role in the advancement of this isolated civilization, providing its people the energy and motivation to realize dramatic social and architectural achievements while being able to endure tremendous hardships in barren, inhospitable environments. This hypothesis is supported by artifacts including monolithic idols (500 B.C. to A.D. 200) with distended cheeks of coca chewers and ancient bells cast in the shape of human faces, showing prominent bulges in the cheeks (Aldrich and Barker 1976). These and many other Indian artifacts underscore the religious reverence with which coca was held by these people until the time of the Spanish Conquistadors (Golding 1993).

The first written description of coca chewing in the New World was by explorer Amerigo Vespucci in 1499:

> They were very brutish in appearance and behavior, and their cheeks bulged with the leaves of a certain green herb which they chewed like cattle, so that they could hardly speak. Each had around his neck two dried gourds, one full of that herb in their mouth, the other filled with a white flour like powdered chalk. . . . [This was lime, which was mixed with the coca to enhance its effects.] When I asked . . . why they carried these leaves in their mouth, which they did not eat, . . . they replied it prevents them from feeling hungry, and gives them great vigor and strength. (Aldrich and Barker 1976, 3)

When the Spanish conqueror Francisco Pizarro invaded Peru in the sixteenth century, he found coca to be the center of the Incan social and religious systems. According to legend, the coca plant was divine. The Incan word *coca* simply meant "the tree," and this plant was viewed as the source of power for the expanding Incan empire.

It is ironic that there are no indications that these early South American civilizations had any significant social problems with cocaine, considering the difficulty it has caused contemporary civilizations. The ancient Indians appeared to be able to live harmoniously with this drug and even take advantage of its unique pharmacological properties to advance their societies. There are three possible explanations for their positive experiences with coca:

1. The Andean Indians maintained control of the use of cocaine. For the Incas, coca could only be used by the conquering aristocracy, chiefs, royalty, and other designated honorables (Aldrich and Barker 1976).
2. These Indians used the unpurified form of

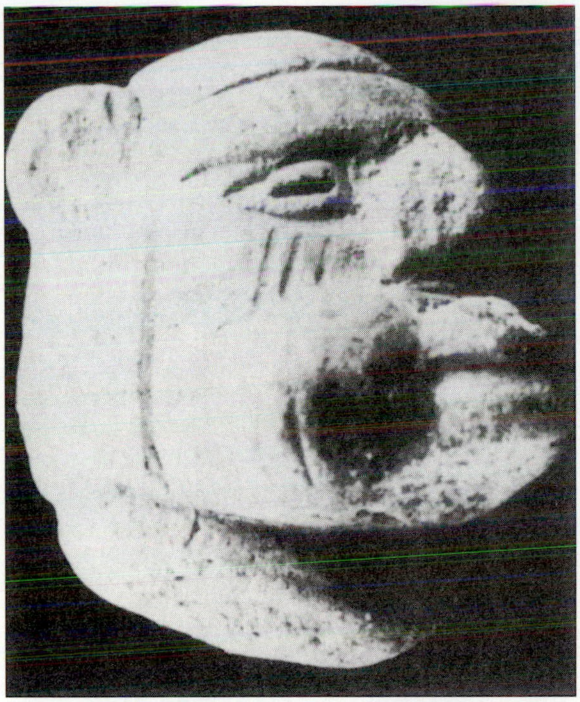

This sculpture from ancient Colombian civilization (ca. A.D. 1300) represents the head of a coca chewer.

cocaine in the coca plant, while later civilizations purified the drug and thus dramatically increased its potency and the likelihood of abuse.

3. Chewing the coca leaf was a slow, sustained form of administering the drug; therefore, the effect was much less potent than snorting, intravenous injection, or smoking—techniques most often used today.

The Spanish conquerors forbade the use of coca at first because they did not understand its significance to the Indians. It was outlawed and declared to be a form of satanic idolatry. However, in the mid-1500s, Spanish commercialism took precedence when the conquistadores learned that coca helped their Indian laborers to endure and work harder; coca was then used to pay the slaves. Taxes were also paid in coca leaves as were tithes to the Catholic Church (Aldrich and Barker 1976).

The Second Cocaine Era. A second major cocaine era began in the nineteenth century. During this period, scientific techniques were used to elucidate the pharmacology of cocaine and identify its dangerous effects. It was also during this era that the threat of cocaine to society—both its members and institutions—was first recognized (DiChiara 1993).

Reports from highly regarded naturalists of the virtues of coca leaves stirred the imagination of Europeans. In 1859, Paolo Mantegazza, an eminent Italian physician, wrote the following account after chewing an ounce of fresh coca leaves: "Borne on the wings of two coca leaves, I flew about in the spaces of 77,438 worlds, each one more splendid than the others. . . . I prefer a life of ten years with coca to one of a hundred thousand without it" (Gay et al. 1973). At about this time, scientists in North America and Europe began experimenting with a purified, white, powdered extract made from the coca plant.

In the last half of the nineteenth century, Corsican chemist Angelo Mariani removed the active ingredients from the coca leaf and identified cocaine. This purified cocaine was added into cough drops and into a special Bordeaux wine called *Vin Mariani*. The Pope gave Mariani a

The "refreshing" element in Vin Mariani was coca extract.

medal in appreciation for the fine work he had done. The cocaine extract was publicized as a magical drug that would free the body from fatigue, lift the spirits, and cause a sense of well-being, and the cocaine-laced wine became widely endorsed throughout the civilized world. Included in a long list of luminaries who advocated this product for an array of ailments were the Czar and Czarist of Russia; the Prince and Princess of Wales; the Kings of Sweden, Norway, and Cambodia; commanders of the French and English armies; President McKinley of the United States; H. G. Wells; August Bartholdi (sculptor of the Statue of Liberty); and some 8,000 physicians.

The astounding success of this wine attracted imitators, all making outlandish claims. One of these cocaine tonics was a nonalcoholic beverage named Coca-Cola, which was made from African kola nuts and advertised as the "intellectual beverage and temperance drink" and contained 4–12 mg per bottle of the stimulant (DiChiara 1993). By 1906 Coca-Cola no longer contained detectable amounts of cocaine, but caffeine had been substituted in its place.

In 1884, the esteemed Sigmund Freud published his findings on cocaine in a report called "Uber Coca." Freud recommended this "magical drug" for an assortment of medical problems, including depression, hysteria, nervous exhaustion, digestive disorders, hypochondria, "all diseases which involve degenerations of tissue," and drug addiction.

In response to a request by Freud, a young Viennese physician, Karl Koller, studied the ability of cocaine to cause numbing effects. He discovered that it was an effective local anesthetic that could be applied to the surface of the eye and permit painless minor surgery to be conducted. This

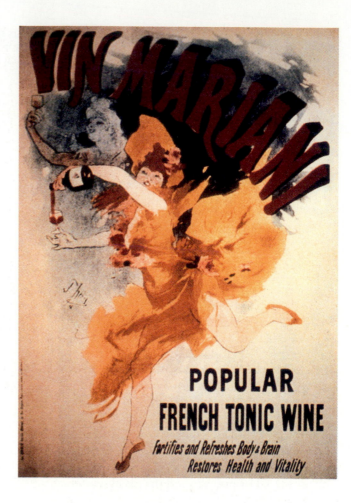

discovery of the first local anesthetic had tremendous worldwide impact. Orders for the new local anesthetic, cocaine, overwhelmed pharmaceutical companies.

Soon after the initial jubilation over the virtues of cocaine came the sober realization that, with its benefits, cocaine also had severe disadvantages. As more people used more cocaine, particularly in tonics and patent medicines, the CNS side effects and abuse liability became painfully evident. By the turn of the century, cocaine was being processed from the coca plant and purified routinely by drug companies. In its purified form, people began to snort or inject the popular powder, which increased both the effects and the dangers. The controversy over cocaine exploded before the American public in newspapers and magazines.

In the early 1900s, anticocaine sentiment arose that resembled the racist attitudes of the Spanish conquistadores several hundred years earlier. At this time, black laborers in the South began using cocaine to help them endure heavy labor and long working days. Plantation owners encouraged such use by issuing cocaine rations to their black laborers to help increase their productivity. As cocaine use spread north, into black, urban slums, white lawmakers became frightened of cocaine-driven blacks and pushed to outlaw the use of this stimulant. As medical and police reports of cocaine abuse and toxicities escalated, public opinion demanded that cocaine be banned. In 1914, the Harrison Act incorrectly classified both cocaine and coca as narcotic substances (cocaine is a stimulant) and outlawed their uncontrolled use.

Although prohibited in patent and nonprescription medicines, prescribed medicinal use of cocaine continued into the 1920s. Medicinal texts included descriptions of therapeutic uses for cocaine to treat fatigue, vomiting, seasickness, melancholia, and gastritis. However, prescriptions also included lengthy warnings about excessive cocaine use, "the most insidious of all drug habits" (Aldrich and Barker 1976).

Little of medical or social significance occurred for the next few decades. The medicinal use of cocaine was replaced mostly by the amphetamines during World War II because cocaine could not be supplied from South America. (Cocaine is not easily synthesized, so even today, the supply of cocaine, both legal and illegal, continues to come from the Andean countries of South America.) During this period, cocaine continued to be employed for its local anesthetic action, was available on the "black market," and was used recreationally by musicians, entertainers, and the wealthy. Because of the lack of availability, the cost of cocaine was prohibitive for most would-be consumers. Cocaine abuse problems were of minor concern until the 1980s.

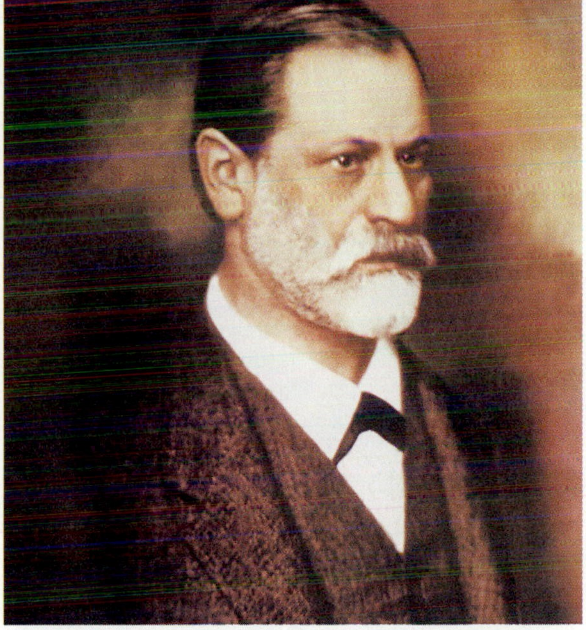

Sigmund Freud was an early advocate of cocaine, which he referred to as a "cure-all."

The Third Cocaine Era. With the 1980s came the third major era of cocaine use. This era started much like the second in that the public and even the medical community were naive and misinformed about the drug. Cocaine was viewed as a glamorous substance and portrayed by the media as the drug of celebrities. Its use by prominent actors, athletes, musicians, and other fast-paced elite was common knowledge. By 1982, over 20 million Americans had tried cocaine in one form or another, compared to only 5 million in 1974 (Green 1985).

The following is an example of a report from a

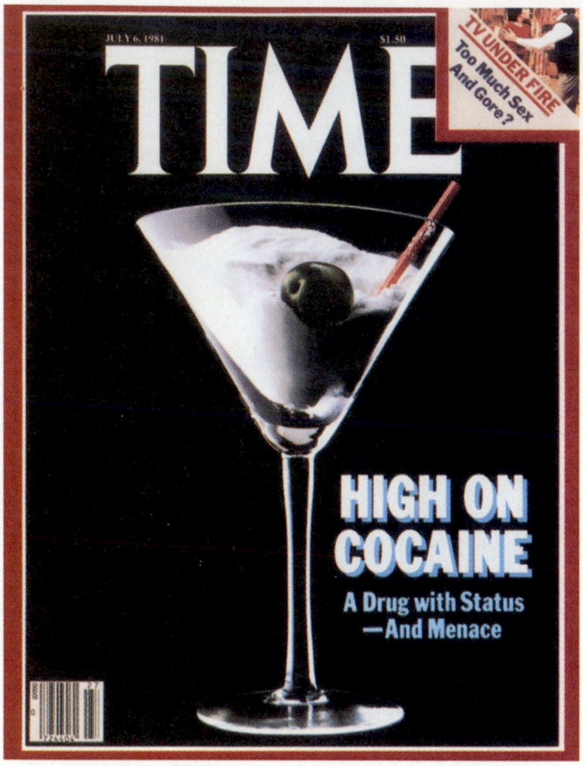

In the early 1980s, cocaine was a glamorous drug used by glamorous people. This cover of *Time* magazine (6 July 1981) depicts the public's cavalier attitude about cocaine use during that time.

Los Angeles television station in the early 1980s, which was typical of the misleading information being released to the public:

> Cocaine may actually be no more harmful to your health than smoking cigarettes or drinking alcohol; at least that's according to a six-year study of cocaine use. It concludes that the drug is relatively safe and, if not taken in large amounts, it is not addictive. The study appears in the new issue of *Scientific American*. (Byck 1987)

With such visibility, an association with prestige and glamour, and what amounted to an indirect endorsement by medical experts, the stage was set for another epidemic of cocaine use. Initially, the high cost of this imported substance limited access. However, with increased demand came increased supply, and prices tumbled from an unaffordable $100 a "fix" to an affordable $10. The epidemic began.

By the mid-1980s, cocaine permeated all elements of society. No group of people or part of the country was immune from its effects. Many tragic stories were told of athletes, entertainers, corporate executives, politicians, fathers and mothers, high school students, and even children using and abusing cocaine. It was no longer the drug of the laborer or even the rich and famous. It was everybody's drug and everybody's problem (Golding 1993).

Cocaine Production Because cocaine is derived from the coca plant, which is imported from the Andean countries, America's problems with this drug have had a profound effect on several South American countries. With the dramatic rise in U.S. cocaine demand in the early 1980s, coca production in South America increased just as dramatically. The coca crop is by far the most profitable agricultural venture in some of these countries. In addition, this crop is easily cultivated, easily maintained (the coca plant is a perennial and remains productive for decades), and can be harvested several times a year (on average, two to four). The coca harvest has brought many jobs and some prosperity to these struggling economies. According to *National Geographic,* coca exports bring between $0.5 and $1 billion to Bolivia annually. In U.S. terms, this is a relatively small amount, but for a poor country such as Bolivia, this money can be the difference between life and death for many impoverished families (Boucher 1991).

In 1988, 2,500 hectares (there are 2.47 acres in a hectare) of coca were eliminated in Bolivia in response to U.S. pressures, but 6,800 hectares of new coca took their place. In spite of U.S. efforts, coca production increased by 25% in Peru in 1989. The profits, combined with the traditional view held by the people in Latin American countries that coca is a desirable substance, have made it difficult to persuade farmers to change crops just to satisfy the demanding gringos.

In conjunction with local governments (and likely after a few bribes, possibly in the form of foreign aid), the United States has attempted to destroy coca crops directly by burning, cutting, spraying herbicides, and even the introduction of coca-eating caterpillars (Boucher 1991).

Obviously, attempts like these to eliminate the livelihood of coca farmers does not improve the image of the United States in foreign lands. Such strategies have turned many peasants against the United States and their own governments, as well. One result has been public support for political opponents, such as members of ruthless cocaine cartels and leftist guerrillas.

Cocaine Processing Cocaine is one of several active ingredients from the leaves of *Erythroxylon coca* (its primary source). The leaves are harvested two or three times a year and used to produce coca paste, which contains up to 80% cocaine. The paste is processed in clandestine labs to form a pure, white hydrochloride salt powder. Often purified cocaine is **adulterated** (or "cut") before it is sold on the "streets" with substances such as powdered sugar, talc, arsenic, lidocaine, strychnine, and methamphetamine. Adverse responses to administering street cocaine are sometimes caused by the additives, not the cocaine itself. The resultant purity of the cut material ranges from 10 to 60%. This technique of diluting the cocaine is intended to make the drug go farther and increase the profit margin for the "pusher" (Farrar and Kearns 1989).

Cocaine is often sold in the form of little pellets, called "rocks," or as flakes or powder. If it is in pellet form, it must be crushed before used. Such exotic names as Peruvian rock and Bolivian flake are bandied about to convince the buyer that the "stash" is high grade. Other street names used for cocaine include *blow, snow, flake, leaf, C, coke, toot, white lady, girl, cadillac, nose candy, gold dust,* and *stardust.*

Current Attitudes and Patterns of Abuse Given contemporary medical advances, we have greater understanding of the effects of cocaine and the toxicities and dependence it produces. The reasons for abusing cocaine are better understood, as well. For example, it is clear that as many as 30% of chronic cocaine users are self-medicating psychiatric disorders such as depression, attention deficit disorders, or anxiety (Grinspoon 1993). Such knowledge helps in identifying and administering effective treatment. The hope is that society will never again be fooled into thinking that cocaine abuse is glamorous or an acceptable form of entertainment.

Attempts are being made to use this understanding (some recently acquired, some merely relearned) to educate people about the true nature of cocaine. Such education was likely responsible for trends of declining cocaine use observed from 1987 to 1991 (see Figure 10.1). Decreases occurred in virtually every age group evaluated during this period. Surveys during this time revealed that, in general, cocaine use became less acceptable; these changes in attitude almost certainly contributed to the dramatic reduction in use (Johnston 1993). However, in 1992 and 1993, the declining trend in cocaine abuse appeared to stop (Johnston 1994). Although it is not clear why the declines ceased, some experts have speculated that attitudes about cocaine use are again changing and eventually may lead to a new era of cocaine problems (Johnston 1994).

It is important to note that in general even while cocaine use was declining dramatically over the past decade, there still existed a population of hard-core stimulant users who continued to self-administer large quantities of cocaine that often led to severe toxicity requiring emergency care. For example, from 1989 to 1991, the percentage of U.S. high school students who used any form of cocaine within 30 days of the survey fell by half, from 2.8% to 1.4% (*NIDA Notes* 1992, 19). In contrast, cocaine-related visits to hospital emergency rooms nationwide during this same time period were reduced by a slight 5% (*NIDA Notes* 1992, 9). These findings suggest that those cocaine users who are severely dependent and most likely require emergency treatment from toxicity resist the trends of declining usage and continue to self-administer large quantities of this drug.

Cocaine Administration Cocaine can be administered orally, inhaled into the nasal passages, injected intravenously, or smoked. The form of administration is important in determining the

ADULTERATED contaminating substances are mixed in to dilute the drugs

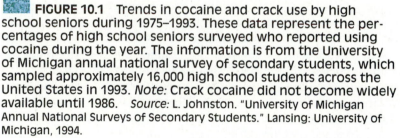

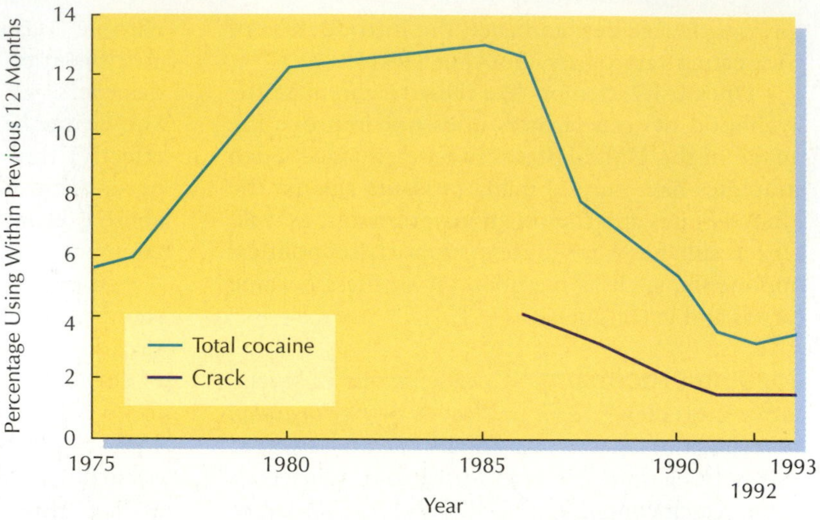

FIGURE 10.1 Trends in cocaine and crack use by high school seniors during 1975–1993. These data represent the percentages of high school seniors surveyed who reported using cocaine during the year. The information is from the University of Michigan annual national survey of secondary students, which sampled approximately 16,000 high school students across the United States in 1993. *Note:* Crack cocaine did not become widely available until 1986. *Source:* L. Johnston. "University of Michigan Annual National Surveys of Secondary Students." Lansing: University of Michigan, 1994.

intensity of cocaine's effects, its abuse liability, and the likelihood of toxicity.

Oral administration of cocaine produces the least potent effects; most of the drug is destroyed in the gut or liver before it reaches the brain. The result is a slower onset of action with a milder, more sustained stimulation. This form is least likely to cause health problems and dependence (Grinspoon 1993). South American Indians still take cocaine orally to increase their strength and for relief from fatigue. Administration is usually done by prolonged chewing of the coca leaf resulting in the consumption of about 20–400 mg of the drug (DiChiara 1993). Oral use of cocaine is not common in the United States.

"Snorting" involves inhaling cocaine hydrochloride powder into the nostrils, where deposits form on the lining of the nasal chambers and approximately 100 mg of the drug passes through the mucosal tissues into the bloodstream (DiChiara 1993). Substantial CNS stimulation occurs in several minutes, persists for 30 to 40 minutes, and then subsides. The effects occur faster and are shorter lasting and more intense than those achieved with oral administration, as more of the drug gets into the brain more quickly. Because concentrations of cocaine in the body are higher after snorting than after oral ingestion, the side effects are more severe. One of the most common consequences of snorting cocaine is rebound depression, or "crash," which is of little consequence after oral consumption. As a general rule, the intensity of the depression correlates with the intensity of the euphoria (Goldstein 1995).

According to studies by the National Institute on Drug Abuse, about 10 to 15% of those who try intranasal (snorting) cocaine go on to heavier forms of dosing, such as intravenous (IV) administrations. Intravenous administration of cocaine is a relatively recent phenomenon because the hypo-

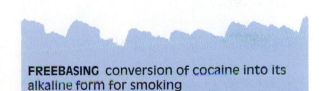

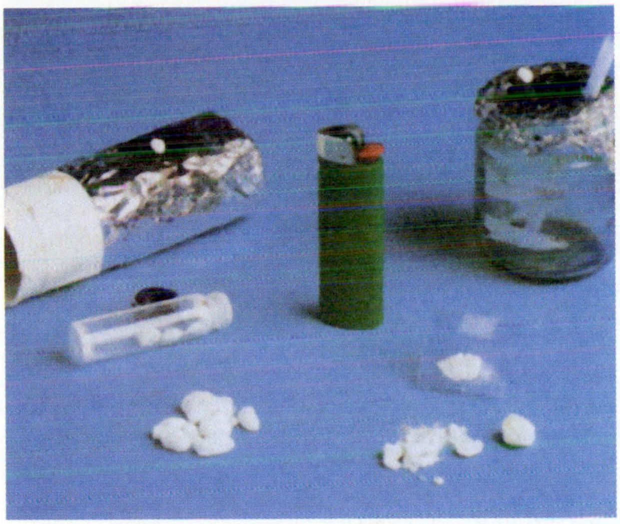

FIGURE 10.2 "Freebasing" paraphernalia. A water pipe is often used to smoke freebased cocaine, or "crack." Cocaine administered by smoking is very potent and fast acting; the effect lasts for 10 to 15 minutes, after which depression occurs. This is the most addicting form of cocaine.

dermic needle was not widely available until the late 1800s. This form of administration has contributed to many of the cocaine problems that appeared at the turn of the century. IV administration allows large amounts of cocaine to be introduced very rapidly into the body and causes severe side effects and dependence. Within seconds after injection, cocaine users experience an incredible state of euphoria. The "high" is intense but short lived; within 15 to 20 minutes, the user experiences dysphoria and is heading for a "crash." In order to prevent these unpleasant rebound effects, cocaine is readministered every 10 to 30 minutes. Readministration continues as long as there is drug available.

This binge activity resembles that which occurs with the methamphetamine "run." When the cocaine supply is exhausted, the binge is over (Goldstein 1994). Several days of abstinence may separate bingeing episodes; the average cocaine addict binges once to several times a week, with each binge lasting 4 to 24 hours. Cocaine addicts claim that all thoughts turn toward cocaine during binges; everything else loses significance. This pattern of intense use is how some people blow all of their money on cocaine.

Freebasing is a method of reducing impurities in cocaine and preparing the drug for smoking. It produces a type of cocaine that is more powerful than normal cocaine hydrochloride. One way to "freebase" is to treat the cocaine hydrochloride with a liquid base such as sodium carbonate or ammonium hydroxide. The cocaine dissolves, along with many of the impurities commonly found in it (such as amphetamines, lidocaine, sugars, and others). A solvent, such as petroleum or ethyl ether, is added to the liquid to extract the cocaine. The solvent containing the cocaine floats to the top and is drawn off with an eyedropper; it is placed in an evaporation dish to dry, and crystallized cocaine residue is then crushed into a fine powder, which can be smoked in a special glass pipe (see Figure 10.2).

The effects of smoked cocaine are as intense or greater than those achieved through intravenous administration. The onset is very rapid, the euphoria is dramatic, the depression is severe, the side effects are dangerous, and the chances of dependence are high (Grinspoon 1993). The reason for these intense reactions to inhaling cocaine into the lungs is that the drug passes rapidly through the lining of the lungs into the many blood vessels present; it is then carried almost directly to the brain.

Freebasing became popular in the United States in the 1980s due to the fear of diseases such

FREEBASING conversion of cocaine into its alkaline form for smoking as AIDS and hepatitis that are transmitted by sharing contaminated hypodermic needles. But freebasing involves other dangers. Because the volatile solvents required for freebasing are very explosive, careless people have been seriously burned or killed during processing (Siegel 1985). "Street" synonyms used for freebased cocaine include *baseball, bumping, white tornado, world series,* and *snow toke.*

"Crack" Between 1985 and 1986, a special type of freebased cocaine known as **"crack"** or "rock" appeared on the streets (Goldstein 1994). By 1988, approximately 7% of the young adult population had tried crack; however, as of 1992 the use of crack had fallen substantially to 1.5% and remained unchanged in 1993 (see Figure 10.1). This cocaine product is inexpensive and can be smoked without the dangerous explosive solvents mentioned earlier in the discussion of freebasing. Crack is made by taking powdered cocaine hydrochloride and adding sodium bicarbonate (baking soda) and water. The paste that forms removes impurities as well as the hydrochloride from the cocaine. The substance is then dried into hard pieces called *rocks,* which may be as high as 90% pure cocaine. Other slang terms for "crack" include *base, black rock, gravel, Roxanne,* and *space basing.*

Like freebased cocaine, crack is usually smoked in a glass water pipe (see Figure 10.2). When the fumes are absorbed into the lungs, they act rapidly, reaching the brain within 8 to 10 seconds. An intense "rush" or "high" results, and later a powerful state of depression, or "crash," occurs. The high may last only 3 to 5 minutes, and the depression may persist from 10 to 40 minutes or longer in some cases. As soon as crack is smoked, the nervous system is greatly stimulated by the release of dopamine, which seems to be involved in the rush. Cocaine prevents resupply of this neurotransmitter, which may trigger the crash.

Because of the abrupt and intense release of dopamine, smoked crack is viewed as a drug with tremendous potential for addiction (Grinspoon 1993) and is considered by users to be more enjoyable than cocaine administered intravenously (Fischman and Foltin 1992). In fact, some people with serious cardiovascular disease continue their use of crack despite knowledge of the serious risk for heart attacks and strokes (Fischman and Foltin 1992). Crack marketing and use are often associated with criminal activity (see Here and Now Box). In some of the larger metropolitan areas, such as New York and Los Angeles, more than 50% of the cocaine-related arrests have involved crack (Central Ohio Lung Association 1986).

In general, crack use is more common among the African and Hispanic populations than among white Americans. However, the difference in prevalence does not appear to be racially related, but rather due to socioeconomic circumstances (Lillie-Blanton et al. 1993). Of special concern is the use of crack among women during pregnancy. Children born under these circumstances have been referred to as "crack babies" and estimated to include as many as 900,000 infants from 1989–1992 (Knight-Ridder News Service 1992). Even though the effects of crack on fetal development are not fully understood, many clinicians and researchers have predicted that the "crack babies" will be an enormous social burden. However, other experts have expressed concern that the impact of cocaine on the fetus is grossly overstated and behavioral problems seen in these children are more a consequence of social environment than direct pharmacological effects (Mathias 1992; Grinspoon 1993). Clearly, more studies are required in order to determine the full impact of using this drug during pregnancy.

It is not coincidental that the popularity of crack use paralleled the AIDS epidemic in the mid-1980s. Because crack administration does not require injection, theoretically the risk of contracting the HIV virus from contaminated needles is avoided. Even so, there is still a very high incidence of HIV infection in crack users. This is due in part to the fact that most of the crack smokers also use cocaine intravenously and 30–40% of the IV users are HIV positive (Des Jarlais 1992)—see Chapter 15. Another reason for the high incidence of HIV infections (as well as other venereal diseases such as syphilis and gonorrhea) among crack

"CRACK" already processed and inexpensive "freebased" cocaine, ready for smoking

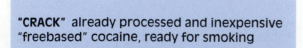

Here and Now

Crack Makes Riots of 1990s Deadlier

The list of casualties from the 1992 Los Angeles riots suggest that urban upheavals in the 1990s are likely to be more violent and far deadlier than those in the 1960s. The use of crack cocaine is of a particular concern in explosive social environments. The combination of sophisticated, rapid-fire weapons (often purchased with profits from cocaine dealing) combined with the fanatical, paranoid delusional thinking that is caused by crack use can change social unrest into urban warfare. The lack of sophisticated guns and the routine use of the depressant heroin made the riots of the 1960s more manageable and less devastating.

Source: Tribune Wire Services. "Arms, Drugs Make '90s Riots Deadlier." *Salt Lake Tribune* 244 (12 May 1992):A-1.

users is the dangerous sexual behavior in which these people participate. Crack is commonly used as payment for sex, not to mention that while under the influence of crack the users are much less inclined to be cautious about their sexual activities (Des Jarlais 1992).

Major Effects of Cocaine Cocaine has profound effects on several vital systems in the body. With the assistance of modern technology, the mechanisms whereby cocaine alters body functions are better understood today. Such knowledge will hopefully lead to better treatment of cocaine dependence.

Most of the pharmacological effects of cocaine use stem from enhanced activity of the catecholamine (dopamine, noradrenaline, adrenaline) and serotonin transmitters. It is believed that the principal action of the drug is to block the reuptake of these substances following their release from neurons. The consequence of such action is to prolong the activity of these transmitter substances at their receptors and substantially increase their effects. The summation of cocaine's effects on these four transmitters causes CNS stimulation (Woolverton and Johnston 1992). The increase of noradrenaline activity following cocaine administration increases the effects of the sympathetic nervous system and alters cardiovascular activity (see discussion later).

Central Nervous System. Because cocaine has stimulant properties, it has antidepressant effects, as well. In fact, some users self-administer cocaine to relieve severe depression (Case in Point box) or the negative symptoms of schizophrenia (Seibyl et al.

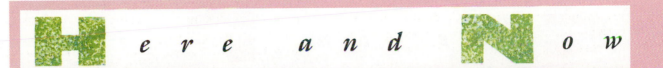

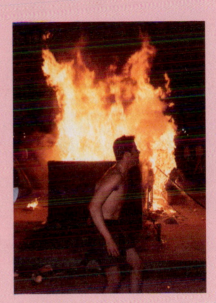

Case in Point

The following are examples of how cocaine is sometimes self-administered to relieve depression.

1. A 39-year-old man began using intravenous cocaine immediately after a divorce. Due to severe reactive depression, he was using up to 8 grams of cocaine (30 to 40 injections) daily. He said, "I never did street drugs in my life until six months ago. . . . I would never have started if I wasn't so lonely."
2. A 30-year-old male had been using cocaine for approximately 10 years, injecting himself with about 0.5 grams once a month. Clinical evaluation revealed a history of chronic depression that he had been self-medicating with cocaine.

Both patients were effectively treated for cocaine dependency by successful treatment of their underlying depression with traditional antidepressant medication, such as Prozac. Should these cocaine addicts be treated differently from addicts who use the drug for recreational purposes?

Source: L. Pagliaro, L. Jaglalsingh, and A. Pagliaro. "Cocaine Use and Depression." *Canadian Medical Association Journal* 147 (1992):1636.

1992), but in general its short-term action and abuse liability make cocaine unsatisfactory for the treatment of depression disorders. The effects of stimulation appear to increase both physical and mental performance while masking fatigue. High doses of cocaine cause euphoria (based on the form of administration) and enhance the sense of strength, energy, and performance. Because of these positive effects, cocaine has intense reinforcing properties, which encourage continual use and dependence (Woolverton and Johnston 1992).

The feeling of exhilaration and confidence caused by cocaine can easily transform into irritable restlessness and confused hyperactivity (Grinspoon 1993). In addition, high chronic doses alter personality, frequently causing psychotic behavior that resembles paranoid schizophrenia (American Psychiatric Association 1994). In some urban hospitals as many as 38% of the patients admitted for psychiatric reasons abuse cocaine (Galanter et al. 1992). In addition, cocaine use heightens the risk of suicide (Ehrman 1992), major trauma, and violent crimes (Brookoff et al. 1993). In many ways, the CNS effects of cocaine are like those of amphetamines although perhaps with a more rapid onset, a more intense high (this may be due partially to the manner in which the drugs are administered), and a shorter duration of action (Goldstein 1995).

Besides dependence, other notable CNS toxicities that can be caused by cocaine use include headaches, temporary loss of consciousness, seizures, and death (Benowitz 1992). Some of these effects may be due to the increased body temperature caused by this drug (Grinspoon 1993).

Cardiovascular System. Cocaine can cause pronounced changes in the cardiovascular system by enhancing the sympathetic nervous system, increasing the levels of adrenaline, and causing vasoconstriction (Grinspoon 1993). The initial effects of cocaine are to increase the heart rate and elevate blood pressure. At the same time that the heart is being stimulated and working harder, the vasoconstriction effects deprive the cardiac muscle of needed blood (Keegan 1991). Such a combination can cause severe heart arrhythmia (an irregular contraction pattern) or heart attack. This can happen to even the young user; a fatal cardiac response to cocaine has been reported in patients as young as 19 years of age (Weiss 1986). Other degenerative processes have also been described in the hearts and blood vessels of chronic cocaine users (Keegan 1991). In addition, the vasoconstrictive action of this sympathomimetic can cause damage to other tissues, prompting a stroke, lung damage in those who smoke cocaine, destruction of nasal cartilage in those who snort the drug, and damage to the gastrointestinal tract (Goldstein 1995).

Local Anesthetic Effect. Cocaine was the first local anesthetic used routinely in modern-day medicine. There is speculation that the ancient Andes Indians of South America used cocaine-filled saliva from chewing coca leaves as a local anesthetic for surgical procedures (Aldrich and Barker 1976). However, this assumption is contested by others (Byck 1987). Even so, cocaine is still a preferred local anesthetic for minor pharyngeal (back part of the mouth and upper throat area) surgery due to its good vasoconstriction (reduces bleeding) and topical, local numbing effects. Although relatively safe when applied topically, significant amounts of cocaine can enter the bloodstream and, in sensitive people, cause CNS stimulation, toxic psychosis, or even on rare occasions, death.

Cocaine Withdrawal There has been considerable debate as to whether cocaine withdrawal actually happens and if so, what it involves. With the most recent cocaine epidemic and the high incidence of intense, chronic use, it has become apparent that nervous systems do become tolerant to cocaine and that, during abstinence, withdrawal symptoms occur (Goldstein 1995). In fact, because of CNS dependence, the use of cocaine is less likely to be stopped voluntarily than is the use of other illicit drugs (Schwartz et al. 1991). Certainly, if the withdrawal experience is adverse enough, a user will be encouraged to resume the cocaine habit.

The intensity of cocaine withdrawal is proportional to the duration and intensity of use. However, the physical withdrawal symptoms are relatively minor compared to those caused by long-term use of CNS depressants and by themselves are not considered to be life threatening (Woolverton and Johnston 1992). Short-term withdrawal symptoms include depression (chronic cocaine users are 60 times more likely to commit suicide than others), sleep abnormalities, craving for the drug, agitation, and anhedonia (inability to experience pleasure). The long-term withdrawal effects include a return to normal pleasures, accompanied by mood swings and occasional craving triggered by cues in the surroundings (Grinspoon 1993).

Of particular importance to treatment of the chronic cocaine users is that abstinence after bingeing appears to follow three unique stages, each of which must be dealt with in a different manner if relapse is to be prevented. These phases are classified as phase 1, or "crash" (occurs 9 hours to 4 days after drug use is stopped), phase 2, or withdrawal (1 to 10 weeks), and finally, phase 3, or extinction (indefinite). The basic features of these phases are outlined in Table 10.3 (Gawin 1992).

Treatment of Cocaine Dependence Cocaine dependency is classified as a psychiatric disorder by the American Psychiatric Association (1994). Treatment of cocaine dependence has improved as experience working with these patients has increased. Even so, success rates vary for different programs. From 30–90% of the patients who persist in outpatient treatment programs are considered to be "successfully treated" (Gawin 1991). The problem with such assessments is that they do not take into account patients who drop out of programs. Also, there are no clear-cut criteria for qualifying success. For example, is success considered to be abstaining from cocaine for one year, two years, five years, or forever?

No one treatment technique has been found to be significantly superior to others or universally effective (Grinspoon 1993); consequently, there is substantial disagreement as to what is the best strategy for treating cocaine dependency. Most treatments are directed at relieving craving (Kleber 1992). Major differences in treatment approaches include (1) whether outpatient or inpatient status is appropriate, (2) which drugs and what dosages should be used to treat patients during the various

TABLE 10.3 Cocaine abstinence phases

	Phase		
	1—"Crash"	2—Withdrawal	3—Extinction
Time Occurs After Last Binge	24–48 hours	1–10 weeks	Indefinite
Features	*Initial* Agitation, depression, anorexia, suicidal thoughts	*Initial* Mood swings, sleep returns, some craving, little anxiety	Normal pleasure, mood swings, occasional craving, cues trigger craving
	Middle Fatigue, no craving, insomnia	*Middle and Late* Anhedonia, anxiety, intense craving, obsessed with drug seeking	
	Late Extreme fatigue, no craving, exhaustion		

Source: Adapted from F. Gawin and H. Kleber. "Evolving Conceptualizations of Cocaine Dependence. *Yale Journal of Biology and Medicine* 61 (1988):123–36.

stages of abstinence, and (3) what length of time the patient should be isolated from cocaine-accessible environments. It is important to treat each individual patient according to his or her needs. Some factors that need to be considered when formulating a therapeutic approach include the following:

- Why did the patient begin using cocaine, and why has dependency occurred?
- What is the severity of abuse?
- How has the cocaine been administered?
- What is the psychiatric status of the patient; are there underlying or coexisting mental disorders, such as depression or attention deficit disorder?
- What other drugs are being abused with the cocaine?
- What is the patient's motivation for eliminating cocaine dependence?
- What sort of support system (family, friends, co-workers, and so on) will sustain the patient in the abstinence effort?

Outpatient Versus Inpatient Approaches. The decision as to whether to treat a patient dependent on cocaine as an outpatient or inpatient depends on a number of issues. For example, inpatient techniques allow greater control than outpatient; thus, the environment can be better regulated, the training of the patient can be more closely supervised, and his or her responses to treatment can be more closely monitored. In contrast, the advantages of the outpatient approach are that supportive family and friends are better able to encourage the patient, the surroundings are more comfortable and natural, potential problems that might occur when the patient returns to a normal lifestyle are more likely to be identified, and treatment is less expensive.

Cocaine-dependent patients should be matched to the most appropriate strategy based on their personalities and the conditions of their addiction. For instance, a cocaine addict who lives in the ghettos, comes from a home with other drug-dependent family members, and has little support probably would do better in the tightly

TABLE 10.4 Medications used in treatment of cocaine abstinence at various phases

Phase	Drug	Drug Group (Rationale)
1. Crash	Benzodiazepines	Depressants (relieve anxiety)
	Haloperidol	Antipsychotic (relieve psychosis)
2. Withdrawal	Bromocryptine, L-dopa	Dopamine agonist (relieve craving)
3. Extinction	Desipramine, imipramine	Antidepressant (relieve depression and craving)

Source: Based on T. Kosten. "Pharmacotherapeutic Interventions for Cocaine Abuse Matching Patients to Treatments." *Journal of Nervous and Mental Disease* 177 (1989):379–90.

controlled inpatient environment. However, a highly motivated cocaine addict who comes from a supportive home and a neighborhood that is relatively free of drug problems would probably do better on an outpatient basis.

Therapeutic Drug Treatment. Several drugs have been used to treat cocaine abstinence. Table 10.4 lists those that have been used in each of the three principal phases of cocaine abstinence (Kosten 1989). Besides relieving acute problems of anxiety, agitation, and psychosis, drugs can also diminish cocaine craving; this is done by giving drugs such as bromocryptine or L-dopa that stimulate the dopamine transmitter system. As mentioned, the pleasant aspects of cocaine likely relate to its ability to increase the activity of dopamine in the limbic system. When cocaine is no longer available, the dopamine system becomes less active, causing depression and anhedonia, which results in tremendous craving for cocaine. The intent of bromocryptine or L-dopa is to stimulate dopamine activity and relieve the cravings. Although this approach often works initially, it is temporary. In the third phase of cocaine abstinence, antidepressants such as desipramine are effective for many cocaine-dependent patients in relieving the subtle mood problems and occasional cravings.

The beneficial effects of these drugs can persist for months but are not fully understood and not well studied. There is some debate over their use. Drugs are, at best, only adjuncts in the treatment of cocaine dependence; they are never long-term solutions by themselves (Carrol 1994). Successful treatment of cocaine abuse requires intensive counseling; strong support systems from family, friends, and co-workers; and a highly motivated patient. However, it is important to realize that there is never a complete "cure" from cocaine dependence: ex-addicts cannot return to cocaine and control its use (Kleber 1992).

Recovery from Cocaine Dependence. Although there are numerous therapeutic approaches to treating cocaine addiction, successful recovery is not likely unless the individual is substantially benefited by giving up the drug. Research has shown that treatment is most likely to succeed in patients who are middle class, employed, and married; for example, 85% of the addicted medical professionals recover from cocaine addiction. These people can usually be convinced that they have too much to lose in their personal and professional lives by continuing their cocaine habit. In contrast, a severely dependent crack addict who has no job, family, home, or hope for the future isn't likely to be persuaded that abstinence from cocaine would be advantageous, so therapy usually is not successful (Grinspoon 1993).

Polydrug Use by Cocaine Abusers. Treatment of most cocaine abusers is complicated by the fact that they are polydrug (multiple drug) users. It is unusual to find a person who only abuses cocaine. Greater than 50% of those dependent on cocaine are also dependent on alcohol (McCance-Katz et al.

1993). In general, the more severe the alcoholism the greater the severity of the cocaine dependence. For most cases, the alcoholism develops after the cocaine abuse pattern (Carroll et al. 1993) because the alcohol is used to relieve some of the unpleasant cocaine effects, such as anxiety, insomnia, and mood disturbances (Sands and Ciraulo 1992). This drug combination is a particularly dangerous one for several reasons:

1. The presence of both cocaine and alcohol (ethanol) in the liver results in the formation of a unique chemical product called *cocaethylene,* which is formed from the reaction of ethanol with a cocaine metabolite. Cocaethylene is often found in high levels in the blood of victims of fatal drug overdoses and appears to enhance the euphoria as well as the cardiovascular toxicity of cocaine (Carroll et al. 1993).
2. Both cocaine and alcohol can damage the liver, thus their toxic effects on the liver are summed when the drugs are used in combination (Sands and Ciraulo 1992).
3. The likelihood of damaging a fetus is enhanced when both drugs are used together during pregnancy (Sands and Ciraulo 1992).
4. Cardiovascular stress is substantially enhanced in the presence of both drugs; thus, people with underlying coronary artery disease are 18 times more likely to suffer sudden death from cardiovascular factors when using this combination (Sands and Ciraulo 1992).

As with amphetamines, cocaine abusers also frequently coadminister narcotics, such as heroin (Kosten 1989). Cocaine users often take other depressants, such as benzodiazepines, or marijuana (Sands and Ciraulo 1992) to help reduce the severity of the crash after their cocaine binge. Codependence on cocaine and a CNS depressant can complicate treatment but must be considered.

Cocaine and Pregnancy One of the consequences of widespread cocaine abuse is that literally thousands of babies are born each year in the United States having been exposed to cocaine in the womb. Cocaine use during pregnancy is highest in poor, inner-city regions and estimates range from 3 to 50% according to the metropolitan area (Mayes 1992). It is likely that in the United States $0.5 to 1 billion dollars are spent annually for maternal care of cocaine-using women during their pregnancies (Tanne 1991). The majority of these **cocaine babies** are abandoned by their mothers and left to the welfare system for care.

It is not clear exactly what types of effects cocaine has directly on the developing fetus. It is known that cocaine use during pregnancy can cause vasoconstriction of placental vessels, thus interfering with oxygen and nutrient exchange between mother and child, or contraction of the uterine muscles, resulting in trauma or premature birth. Current data also suggest that infants exposed to cocaine during pregnancy are more likely to suffer a small head (microencephaly), premature delivery, and reduced birthweight (Coles et al. 1992). Some controversial early studies suggested that cocaine use during pregnancy can also cause permanent malformation of the brain, strokes, SIDS (sudden infant death syndrome), permanent learning deficits, and behavioral disorders. However, these studies have been criticized because (1) the pregnant populations examined were not well defined and properly matched, (2) use of other drugs (such as alcohol) with cocaine during pregnancy was often ignored, and (3) the effects of poor nutrition, bad living conditions, and a traumatic lifestyle were not considered when analyzing the results. Due to these problems, much of the earlier work examining prenatal effects of cocaine is flawed and the conclusions are questionable (Richardson and Day 1991; Grinspoon 1993). Unfortunately, because of the dubious findings of these studies the popular press has predicted a devastating long-term outcome for the "cocaine babies" without reliable scientific proof. Consequently, these children are often difficult to place in adopting families and due to the social rejection, the predictions of behavioral and social problems may come true, but not because of prenatal exposure to cocaine (Mathias 1992).

COCAINE BABIES children exposed to cocaine while in the womb

TABLE 10.5 Caffeine content of beverages and chocolate

Beverage	Caffeine Content (mg)/cup	Amount
Brewed coffee	90–125	5 oz.
Instant coffee	14–93	5 oz.
Decaffeinated coffee	1–6	5 oz.
Tea	30–70	5 oz.
Cocoa	5	5 oz.
Coca-Cola	45	12 oz.
Pepsi-Cola	30	12 oz.
Chocolate bar	22	1 oz.

Minor Stimulants

Minor stimulants enjoy widespread use in the United States because of the mild lift in mood caused by their consumption. The most popular of these routinely consumed agents are methylxanthines (commonly called *xanthines*), such as caffeine, which are consumed in beverages made from plants and herbs. Other minor stimulants are contained in OTC medications, such as cold and hay fever products; these will be mentioned briefly in this chapter but discussed at greater length in Chapter 14. Because of their frequent use, some dependence on these drugs can occur; however, serious dysfunction due to dependence is infrequent. Consequently, abuse of xanthines such as caffeine is not viewed as a major health problem (Heishman and Henningfield 1992).

Caffeinelike Drugs (xanthines)

Caffeine is the world's most frequently used stimulant and perhaps its most popular drug (Heishman and Henningfield 1992). Beverages and foods containing caffeine are consumed by almost all adults and children living in the United States today (see Table 10.5). In this country, the average daily intake of caffeine is 4 mg/kg (280 mg per 70-kg man or the equivalent of approximately 3 cups of coffee) with 3% of the population consuming 600 mg or more per day (Heishman and Henningfield 1992). The most common sources of caffeine include coffee beans, tea plants, kola nuts, maté leaves, guaraná paste, and yoco bark.

Although the consumption of caffeine-containing drinks can be found throughout history, the active stimulant caffeine was discovered by German and French scientists in the early 1820s. Caffeine was described as a substance with alkaloid (basic) properties that was extracted from green coffee beans and referred to as *kaffebase* by Ferdinand Runge in 1820 (Gilbert 1984). In the course of the next 40 to 60 years, caffeine was identified in several other genera of plants, which were used as sources for common beverages. These included tea leaves (originally the drug was called *thein*); guaraná paste (originally the drug was called *guaranin*); Paraguay tea, or maté; and kola nuts. Certainly, the popularity of these beverages over the centuries attests to the fact that most consumers find the stimulant effects of this drug desirable.

The Chemical Nature of Caffeine Caffeine belongs to a group of drugs that have similar chemical structures and are known as the xanthines. Besides caffeine, other xanthines are theobromine (means "divine leaf"), discovered in cacao beans (used to make chocolate) in 1842, and theophylline (means "divine food"), isolated from tea leaves in 1888. These three agents have unique pharmacological properties (which are discussed later), with caffeine being the most potent CNS stimulant.

Beverages Containing Caffeine In order to understand the unique role that caffeine plays in U.S. society, it is useful to gain perspective on its most common sources: unfermented beverages.

Coffee. Coffee is derived from the beans of several species of *coffea* plants. The *coffea arabica* plant grows as a shrub or small tree and is 4 to 6 meters high when growing wild. Coffee beans are primarily cultivated in South America and East Africa and constitute the major cash crop for exportation in several underdeveloped countries.

The name *coffee* was likely derived from the Arabian word *kahwa;* some argue it was named after the Ethiopian province *Kaffa,* the suggested site of origin for the coffee tree. From Ethiopia, the coffee tree was carried to Arabia and cultivated (Kihlman 1977).

Coffee became an important element in Arabian civilization and is mentioned in writings dating back to A.D. 900. In fact, in Mecca, coffee drinking was so popular that people spent more time in coffeehouses than in mosques, and the use of coffee was outlawed for a short period of time. However, illicit coffeehouses sprang up immediately, and the coffee prohibition was repealed.

Coffee probably reached Europe through Turkey and was likely used initially as a medicine. By the middle of the seventeenth century, there were coffeehouses in England and in France—places to relax and talk, to learn the news, to make business deals, and perhaps to hatch political plots. These coffeehouses turned into the famous "penny universities" of the early eighteenth century, where for a penny a cup, you could listen to some of the great literary and political figures of the day.

Coffee was originally consumed in the Americas by English colonists, although tea was initially preferred. Tea was replaced by coffee following the Revolutionary War. Because tea had become a symbol of English repression, the switch to coffee was more a political statement than a change in taste. The popularity of coffee grew as U.S. boundaries moved west. In fact, daily coffee use continued to increase until it peaked in 1986, when annual coffee consumption averaged 10 pounds per person. Although concerns about the side effects associated with caffeine use have since caused some decline in coffee use, it still plays a major role in the lifestyles of most Americans (Sawynok and Yaksh 1993).

Tea. Tea is made from the *Camellia sinensis* plant, which is native to China and parts of India, Burma, Thailand, Laos, and Vietnam. As mentioned, tea contains two xanthines: caffeine and theophylline. As with coffee, the earliest use of tea is not known.

Although apocryphal versions of the origin of tea credit Emperor Shen Nung in 2737 B.C., the first reliable account of the use of tea is from an early Chinese manuscript written around A.D. 350. This record describes tea as a medicinal plant, supposedly good for tumors, abscesses, bladder trouble, and many other ailments. The popular use of tea slowly grew. The Dutch brought the first tea to Europe in 1610, where it was accepted rather slowly; however, with time, it was adopted by the British as a favorite beverage and an integral part of their daily activities. In fact, one of the major elements of the English economy became the tea trade. From about 1760, the British promoted the sale of tea through a strong advertising program, and profits grew. Tea revenues made it possible to colonize India and also helped to bring on the Opium Wars in the 1800s, which benefited British colonialism (see Chapter 9). Because so many people in England drank tea, the tax revenues from alcoholic beverages dropped, so in order to compensate, a special tax was charged on tea.

The British were constantly at odds with the Dutch as they attempted to monopolize the tea trade. Even so, the Dutch introduced the first tea into America at New Amsterdam in about 1650. Later, the British gained exclusive rights to sell tea to the American colonies. Because of the high taxes levied by the British government on tea being shipped to America, tea became a symbol of resistance to British rule.

Soft Drinks. The second most common source of caffeine is soft drinks. In general, the caffeine content per 12-ounce serving ranges from 30 to 60 mg (see Table 10.6). Soft drinks account for most of the caffeine consumed by U.S. children

TABLE 10.6 Caffeine content in 12-ounce servings of soft drinks

Brand	Caffeine Content (mg)
Colas	
Coca-Cola	45
Diet Coke	45
Shasta Cola	44
Pepsi Cola	38
Diet Pepsi	36
RC Cola	36
Diet Rite Cola	36
Canada Dry Diet Cola	1.2
Others	
Sugar Free Mr. Pibb	60
Mountain Dew	54
Tab	47
Mr. Pibb	41
Dr. Pepper	40

and teenagers, and for many people, a can of cola has replaced the usual cup of coffee (90–125 mg per cup).

Social Consequences of Consuming Caffeine-Based Beverages. It is impossible to accurately assess the social impact of consuming beverages containing caffeine, but certainly the subtle (and sometimes not so subtle) stimulant effects of the caffeine present in these drinks has had some social influences. These beverages have been integrated into social customs and ceremonies and recognized as traditional drinks.

Today, for many people, drinks containing caffeine are consumed with ritualistic devotion the first thing in the morning, following every meal, and at frequent interludes throughout the day known as "coffee breaks" or "tea times." The immense popularity of these products is certainly a consequence of the stimulant actions of caffeine. Both the dependence on the "jump-start" effect of caffeine as well as the avoidance of unpleasant withdrawal consequences in the frequent user assure the continual popularity of these products.

Other Natural Caffeine Sources Although coffee and tea are two of the most common sources of natural caffeine in the United States, other caffeine-containing beverages and food are popular in different parts of the world (see Table 10.7).

Guaraná is thought to have the highest caffeine content of the natural xanthine-containing beverages (see Table 10.7). With a caffeine content of 2 to 6%, guaraná causes significant stimulation. This beverage is used mostly in the Amazon Valley of Brazil and is the chief beverage of the Brazilian state of Mato Grosso. Pasta guaraná is sold in the form of hard, reddish-brown sticks or

TABLE 10.7 Caffeine content of common herbs

Beverage (herb)	Form	Caffeine Content
Coffee *(Coffea arabica)*	Beans	0.8%–2.4%
Tea *(Camellia sinensis)*	Leaves	3%–4%
Cola drinks *(Cola nitida)*	Seeds	1.5%–3.5%
Guaraná *(Paullnia cupana)*	Beans	2%–6%
Maté *(Ilex paraguayenas)*	Leaves	1.1%–1.9%

Source: Based on R. Gilbert. "Caffeine Consumption." In *The Methylxanthine Beverages and Foods: Chemistry, Consumption, and Health Effects.* New York: Liss, 1984.

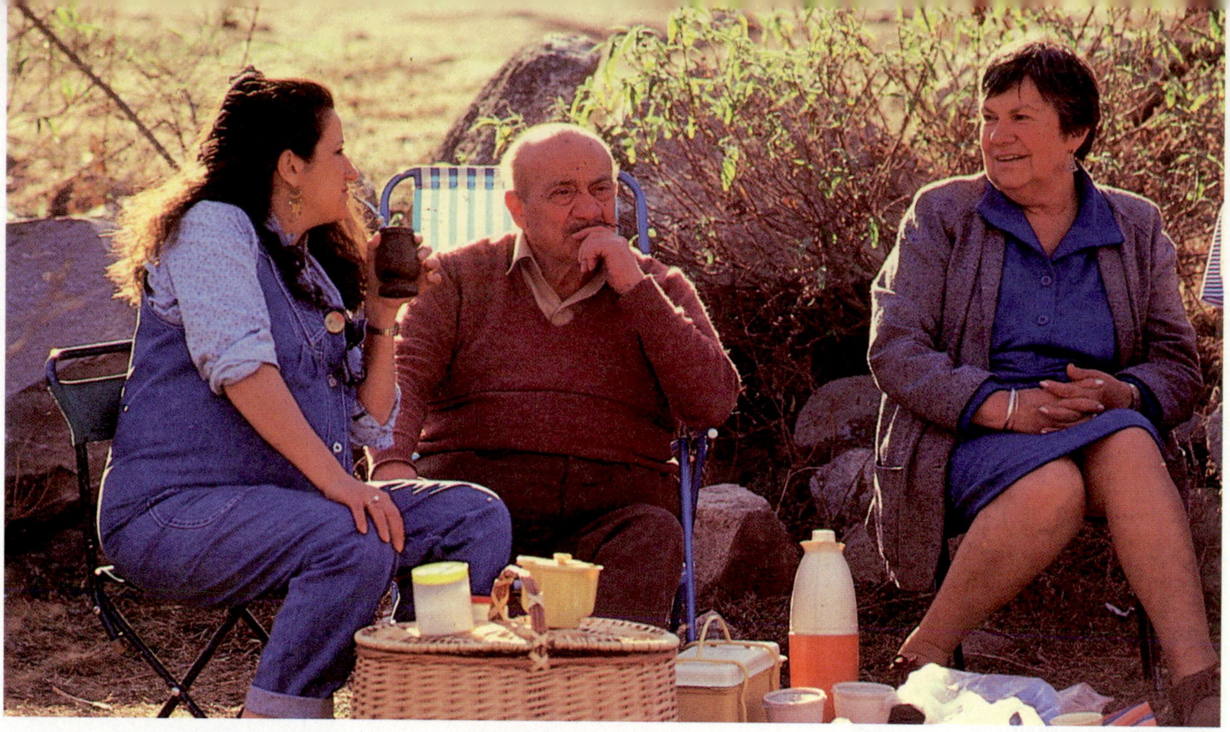

Maté is consumed by many people in South America.

bars or sometimes molded into the shapes of Brazilian fruits and animals. To prepare the beverage, the pasta is powdered, combined with hot water, and then sweetened, much like cocoa.

Maté is also known as Paraguay tea and contains 1 to 2% caffeine. When Spanish invaders conquered the Incas, they learned about the use of a beverage prepared from the maté plant. The Spaniards began using maté and believed it "gave a physical sensation and a moral value to life," which relieved fatigue and apprehension. Today, large quantities of maté are cultivated and consumed by some 20 million people, principally in Argentina, southern Brazil, and Paraguay.

Kola nuts are not generally used in beverages but are most often chewed in solid form. Although carbonated soft drinks marketed as colas are flavored with kola extract, kola accounts for only a minor portion of the caffeine content of these drinks (only a few milligrams). Most of the caffeine in cola drinks is synthetic and added to give the beverage additional "kick." The FDA allows up to 20 mg of caffeine per 100 ml of carbonated cola drink. Several species of kola nuts are edible (or chewable) and are cultivated in West Africa, the West Indies, and South America (Kihlman 1977).

Chocolate Although chocolate contains small amounts of caffeine (see Table 10.5), the principal stimulant in chocolate is the alkaloid theobromine, named after the cocoa tree, *Theobroma cacao*. (*Theobroma* is an Aztec word meaning "fruit of the gods.") The Aztecs thought very highly of the fruit and seed pods from the cacao tree, and they used the beans as a medium of exchange in bartering. The Mayan Indians adopted the food and made a warm drink from the beans that they called *chocolatl* (meaning "warm drink"). The original chocolate drink was a very thick concoction that had to be eaten with a spoon. It was unsweetened because the Mayans apparently did not know about sugar cane.

Hernando Cortés, the conqueror of Mexico, took some chocolate cakes back to Spain with him in 1528, but the method of preparing them was kept a secret for nearly 100 years. It was not until

CROSSCURRENTS

Caffeine: Addiction Versus Therapy

Caffeine is the most widely consumed CNS stimulant in the United States. Recently, caffeine has also been found to be an effective analgesic in the relief of some pains. Because of its abuse potential, there is controversy whether the FDA should approve caffeine as an OTC analgesic ingredient. The following statements represent two opposite views.

1. There are already millions of adults and children who are dependent on caffeine and consume it daily. If the FDA authorizes OTC marketing of caffeine as an analgesic, it will give therapeutic legitimacy to this addicting drug and result in even more use and greater problems of addiction.
2. Caffeine is no more addicting than OTC cough medicines and causes relatively few social problems. This drug is already combined with aspirin in several well-known OTC analgesic products. Consequently, official FDA approval of caffeine as an OTC analgesic will have no significant impact on its use patterns.

Select one of these positions, and defend it based on information in this text and other authoritative references.

1828 that the Dutch worked out a process to remove much of the fat from the kernels to make a chocolate powder. This was the forerunner of the cocoa we know today. The cocoa fat, or *cocoa butter* as it is called, was later mixed with sugar and pressed into bars. In 1847, the first chocolate bars appeared on the market. By 1876, the Swiss had developed milk chocolate, which is so popular in today's confectionaries.

OTC Drugs Containing Caffeine Although the consumption of beverages is by far the most common source of xanthines, a number of popular OTC products contain significant quantities of caffeine. For example, many OTC analgesic products contain approximately 30 mg caffeine per tablet (Anacin, Excedrin). Higher doses of 100 mg to 200 mg per tablet are included in stay-awake (No-Doz, Caffedrine) and "picker-upper" (Vivarin) products (PDR 1994). The addition of caffeine to these OTC medications is highly controversial and has been criticized by clinicians who are unconvinced of caffeine's benefits. Some critics believe that the presence of caffeine in these OTC medicines is nothing more than a psychological gimmick to entice customers because of the mild euphoric effects this stimulant provides.

Despite these criticisms, there is accumulating evidence that caffeine has some analgesic (pain-relieving) properties of its own (Sawynok and Yaksh 1993). Recent studies suggest that 130 mg, but not 65 mg, of caffeine is superior to a placebo in relieving nonmigraine headaches. In addition, the presence of caffeine has been shown to enhance aspirin-mediated relief from surgical pain (such as tooth extraction). Based on such findings, more clinicians are recommending the use of caffeine in the management of some types of headaches and minor to moderate pains (Sawynok and Yaksh 1993) (see Crosscurrents box).

Physiological Effects of the Xanthines

The xanthines significantly influence several important body functions. Although the effects of these drugs are generally viewed as minor and short term (Goldstein 1994), when used in high doses or by people who have severe medical problems, these drugs can be dangerous. The following sections summarize the responses of the major systems to xanthines.

CNS Effects. Of the common xanthines, caffeine has the most potent effect on the central nervous system, followed by theophylline; theobromine has relatively little influence. Although the CNS responses of users can vary considerably, in general, 100 to 200 mg of caffeine enhance a sense of alertness, cause arousal, and diminish the sense of fatigue (Heishman and Hennington 1992). Caffeine is often used to block drowsiness and facilitate mental activity, such as when cramming for exams into the early hours of the morning. In addition, caffeine stimulates the formation of thoughts but does not improve learning ability. The effects of caffeine are most pronounced in unstimulated, drowsy consumers (Goldstein 1994). The CNS effects of caffeine also diminish the sense of boredom (Nehlig et al. 1992). Thus, people engaged in dull, repetitive tasks, such as assembly-line work, or nonstimulating and laborious exercises, such as listening to a boring professor, often consume caffeine beverages to help compensate for the tedium. Most certainly, xanthine drinks are popular because they cause these effects on brain activity.

Adverse CNS effects usually occur with doses greater than 300 mg per day. Some of these include insomnia, an increase in tension, anxiety, and initiation of muscle twitches. Doses over 500 mg/kg of body weight often are dysphoric (unpleasant) and can cause panic sensations, chills, nausea, and clumsiness. Extremely high doses of caffeine, from 5 to 10 grams, frequently result in seizures, respiratory failure, and death (Heishman and Henningfield 1992).

Cardiovascular and Respiratory Effects. Drugs that stimulate the brain usually stimulate the cardiovascular system. The response of the heart and blood vessels to xanthines is dependent on dose and previous experience with these mild stimulants. Tolerance to the cardiovascular effects occurs with frequent use (Heishman and Hennington 1992). With low doses (100 mg to 200 mg), heart activity can either increase, decrease, or do nothing; at higher doses (over 500 mg), the rate of contraction of the heart increases. Xanthines usually cause minor vasodilation in most of the body. In contrast, the cerebral blood vessels are vasoconstricted by the action of caffeine. In fact, cerebral vasoconstriction likely accounts for this drug's effectiveness in relieving some minor vascular headaches caused by vasodilation of the cerebral vessels.

Of the xanthines, theophylline has the greatest effect on the respiratory system, causing air passages to open and facilitate breathing. Because of this effect, tea has often been recommended to relieve breathing difficulties, and theophylline is frequently used to treat asthma-related respiratory problems.

Other Effects. The methylxanthines have noteworthy albeit mild effects on other systems in the body. They cause a minor increase in the secretion of digestive juices in the stomach, which can be significant to individuals suffering from stomach ailments such as ulcers. These drugs also increase urine formation (as any heavy tea drinker undoubtedly knows). In addition, consuming high doses of caffeine increases the metabolism of the body; the significance of this effect on body functions is not known.

Caffeine Intoxication Consuming occasional low doses of the xanthines (equivalent of two to three cups of coffee per day) is relatively safe for most users (Heishman and Hennington 1992; Margen 1994). However, frequent use of high doses causes psychological as well as physical prob-

CAFFEINISM symptoms caused by taking high chronic doses of caffeine lems called **caffeinism.** This condition is found in about 10% of the adults who consume coffee (Heishman and Hennington 1992).

The CNS components of caffeine intoxication are recognized as a "Psychoactive Substance-Induced Psychiatric Disorder" in *DSM-IV* (American Psychiatric Association 1994) criteria established by the American Psychiatric Association. The essential features of this disorder are restlessness, nervousness, excitement, insomnia, flushed face, diuresis, muscle twitching, rambling thoughts and speech, and stomach complaints. These symptoms can occur in some people following a dose as low as 250 mg per day. Caffeine doses in excess of 1 g per day may cause muscle twitching, rambling thoughts and speech, heart arrhythmias, and motor agitation. With higher doses, ringing in the ears and flashes of light can occur.

Some researchers suggest consumption of large quantities of caffeine is associated with cancers of the bladder, ovaries, colon, and kidneys. These claims have not been reliably substantiated (Margen 1994).

One problem with many such studies is that they actually assess the effect of coffee consumption on cancers rather than caffeine itself. Because coffee contains so many different chemicals, it is impossible to determine specifically the effect of caffeine in such research (Bennett 1986). Other reports claim that caffeine promotes cyst formation in female breasts. Although these conclusions also have been challenged, many clinicians advise patients with mammillary cysts to avoid caffeine (Margen 1994). Finally, there are reports that very high doses of caffeine given to pregnant laboratory animals can cause stillbirths or offspring with low birthweights or limb deformities. Recent studies found that moderate consumption of caffeine (less than 300 mg per day) did not significantly affect human fetal development (Mills 1993); however, intake of more than 300 mg/day during pregnancy has been associated with an increase in spontaneous fetal loss (*Facts and Comparisons Drug Newsletter 1994*). Mothers are usually advised to avoid or at least reduce caffeine use during pregnancy (Bennett 1986; Margen 1994).

Based on the information available, there is no strong evidence that moderate use of caffeine leads to disease (Margen 1994). There are, however, implications that people with existing severe medical problems—such as psychiatric disorders (such as severe anxiety, panic attacks, and schizophrenia), cardiovascular disease, and possibly breast cysts—are at greater risk when consuming caffeine. Realistically, other elements—such as alcohol and fat consumption and smoking—are much more likely to cause serious health problems (Bennett 1986).

TABLE 10.8 Caffeine withdrawal syndrome

Symptom	Duration
Headache	Several days to 1 week
Decreased alertness	2 days
Decreased vigor	2 days
Fatigue and lethargy	2 days
Nervousness	2 days

Source: Based on S. Holtzman. "Caffeine as a Model Drug of Abuse." *Trends in Pharmacological Sciences* 11 (1990):355–56.

Caffeine Dependence Caffeine causes limited dependence, which is relatively minor compared to that of the potent stimulants; thus, the abuse potential of caffeine is also much less and dependence is less likely to interfere with normal daily routines (Heishman and Henningfield 1992). However, caffeine is so readily available and socially accepted (almost expected) that the high quantity of consumption has produced many modestly dependent users (Holtzman 1990). The degree of physical dependence on caffeine is highly variable but related to dose and is also considerably less than that with the major stimulants. However, a recent study reported that caffeine doses as low as 100 mg/day can cause significant withdrawal effects, such as headaches, fatigue, mood changes, muscle pain, flulike symptoms, and nausea in some people (Holtzman 1990). With typical caffeine withdrawal, these effects can persist for several days (see Table 10.8). Although these withdrawal symptoms are unpleasant, they usually are not severe enough to prevent most people from giving

TABLE 10.9 Common OTC sympathomimetics

Drug	OTC Product (form)
Phenylpropanolamine	Decongestant, diet aid (oral)
Ephedrine	Decongestant (oral, nasal spray or drops)
Levodesoxyephedrine	Decongestant (nasal inhalant)
Naphazoline	Decongestant (nasal spray or drops)
Oxymetazoline	Decongestant (nasal spray or drops)
Phenylephrine	Decongestant (oral, nasal spray or drops, eye drops)
Psuedoephedrine	Decongestant (oral)
Tetrahydozoline	Decongestant (eye drops)
Xylometazoline	Decongestant (nasal spray or drops)

Source: Based on B. Bryant and T. Lombardi. "Cold and Allergy Products." In *Handbook of Nonprescription Drugs,* 10th ed., edited by T. Covington. Washington, DC: American Pharmaceutical Association, 1993.

up their coffee or cola drinks, if desired. However, it is noteworthy that two-thirds of those patients who are treated for caffeinism relapse into their caffeine-consuming habits (Heishman and Henningfield 1992).

Variability in Responses Caffeine is eventually absorbed entirely from the gastrointestinal tract after oral consumption. In most users 90% of the drug reaches the bloodstream within 20 minutes and is distributed into the brain and throughout the body very quickly (Sawynok and Yaksh 1993). However, the rate of absorption of caffeine from the stomach and intestines differs from person to person as much as sixfold. Such wide variation in the rate at which caffeine enters the blood from the stomach likely accounts for much of the variability in responses to this drug (Nehlig et al. 1992).

OTC Sympathomimetics

Although often overlooked, the sympathomimetic decongestant drugs included in OTC products such as cold, allergy, and diet aid medications have stimulant properties like those of caffeine (Bryant and Lombardi 1993; Appelt 1993). For most people, the CNS impact of these drugs is minor, but for those people who are very sensitive to these drugs, they can cause jitters and interfere with sleep. For such individuals, OTC products containing the sympathomimetics should be avoided prior to bedtime.

The common OTC sympathomimetics are shown in Table 10.9 and include ephedrine and phenylpropanolamine. In the past, these two OTC agents were packaged to look like amphetamines (called "look-alike drugs") and legally sold on the "streets," usually to children or high school age adolescents. Although much less potent than amphetamines, even these minor stimulants can be abused and have caused several deaths. Attempts to regulate look-alike drugs resulted in passage of the federal and state Imitation Controlled Substances Acts. These statutes prohibit the packaging of OTC sympathomimetics to appear like amphetamines.

These laws have not resolved the problem. Other products called "act-alikes" have been created. Although the packaging of the act-alikes does not resemble that of amphetamine capsules, these minor stimulants are promoted on the streets as "harmless speed" and "OTC uppers." It is likely that use of such products will lead to the abuse of more potent stimulants (Brown 1991).

Review Questions

1. Should the FDA continue to approve amphetamines for the treatment of obesity? Why?
2. How are methamphetamine and Ecstasy similar, and how do they differ?
3. What are the dangers of designer drugs in general, and of designer amphetamines in particular?
4. What have past experiences taught us about cocaine? Do you think we have finally learned our lesson concerning this drug?
5. Why does the method of cocaine administration make a difference in how a user is affected by this drug? Use examples to substantiate your conclusions.
6. Why do people use cocaine, and what are the major toxicities caused by use of high doses of this stimulant?
7. How is cocaine dependence treated? What are the rationales for the treatments?
8. How does caffeine compare to cocaine and amphetamine as a CNS stimulant?
9. Because of caffeine's potential for abuse, do you think the FDA should control it more tightly? Defend your answer.
10. Do you believe dependence on caffeine can lead to dependence on more potent CNS stimulants? Why?

Key Terms

"uppers"
anorexiants
behavioral stereotypy
narcolepsy
hyperkinesis
"speed"
"ice"
"run"
hyperpyrexia
"speedball"
designer drugs
adulterated
"freebasing"
"crack"
cocaine babies
caffeinism

Summary

1. Amphetamines were originally developed as decongestants and used in nasal inhalers. These potent stimulants enhance the activity of dopamine, norepinephrine, epinephrine, and serotonin.
2. Some amphetamines have been approved by the FDA (a) as diet aids to treat obesity, (b) to treat narcolepsy, and (c) to treat hyperkinetic problems (attention deficit disorder) in children.
3. In therapeutic doses, amphetamines can cause agitation, anxiety, and panic due to their effects on the brain; in addition, they can cause an irregular heartbeat, increased blood pressure, and heart attack or stroke. Intense, high-dose abuse of amphetamines can cause severe psychotic behavior, stereotypy, and seizures as well as the severe cardiovascular side effects just mentioned.
4. *"Speed"* refers to the use of intravenous methamphetamine. *"Ice"* is smoked methamphetamine. A *"run"* is a pattern of intense, multiple dosing over a period of days that can cause serious neurological, psychiatric, and cardiovascular consequences.
5. "Designer" amphetamines are chemical modifications of original amphetamines. In spite of the chemical changes, designer amphetamines, such as "Ecstasy," retain abuse potential and are often marketed "on the streets" under exotic and alluring names.
6. Cocaine was used by societies as early as 2500 B.C. The first cocaine era was characterized by harmonious use of the coca plant by ancient South American Indians living in the regions of the Andean Mountains. The second period began in the 1800s and was characterized by unrestricted use of this drug in Europe and the United States. The final era began around

1980. Use of cocaine became widespread, and the devastating effects of its uncontrolled use were abundant. "War" was declared against this drug, and its mechanism of action was identified.

7. In the late 1970s and early 1980s, cocaine was commonly viewed by the U.S. public as a relatively safe drug with glamorous connotations. Medical experts did little to change this public opinion. By the mid-1980s, it was apparent that cocaine was a very addicting drug with dangerous side effects. About this time, governmental and social agencies declared "war" on cocaine and tried to prevent distribution, discourage use, and educate people about its potential dangers. By 1988, use patterns had reversed and cocaine abuse was declining. However, hard core use changed little.
8. The CNS and cardiovascular effects of both amphetamines and cocaine are similar. However, cocaine's effects tend to occur more rapidly, be more intense, and wear off more quickly than those of amphetamines.
9. The intensity of the cocaine effect and the likelihood of dependence occurring are directly related to the means of administration. Going from least to most intense effect, the modes of cocaine administration include chewing, "snorting," injecting, and smoking (or "freebasing").
10. "Crack" is cocaine that has been converted into its "freebase" form and is intended for smoking. Because inhaled cocaine rapidly enters the bloodstream and gets into the brain, crack has potent CNS effects, causes an intense "high," and is very addicting.
11. Cocaine withdrawal goes through three main stages: (a) the "crash," the initial abstinence phase consisting of depression, agitation, suicidal thoughts, and fatigue; (b) withdrawal, including mood swings, craving, anhedonia, and obsession with drug seeking; and (c) extinction, when normal pleasure returns, cues trigger craving and mood swings.
12. Treatment of cocaine dependence is highly individualistic and has variable success. The principal strategies include both inpatient and outpatient programs. Drug therapy often is used to relieve short-term cocaine craving and to alleviate mood problems and long-term craving. Psychological counseling and support therapy are essential components of treatment throughout.
13. Caffeine is the most frequently consumed stimulant in the world. It is classified as a xanthine (methylxanthine) and is found in a number of beverages, such as coffee, tea, guaraná, maté, and some soft drinks. It is also included in some OTC medicines such as analgesics and "stay-awake" products.
14. The principal physiological effects of caffeine include minor to moderate CNS stimulation. These effects are most pronounced in users who are tired and drowsy; in such people, performance of mental and physical tasks can be improved. Caffeine causes minor stimulation of cardiovascular activity, kidney function (it is a diuretic), and gastric secretion.
15. Dependence on caffeine can occur in people who regularly consume large doses. Withdrawal can cause headaches, agitation, and tremors. Although unpleasant, withdrawal from caffeine dependence is much less severe than that from amphetamine and cocaine dependence.

References

Aldrich, M., and R. Barker. *Cocaine: Chemical, Biological, Social and Treatment Aspects,* edited by S. J. Mule. Cleveland, OH: CRC, 1976.

American Psychiatric Association. "Substance-Related Disorders." In *Diagnostic and Statistical Manual,* 4th ed. [*DSM-IV*], A. Francis, chairperson, 175–272. Washington, DC: American Psychiatric Association, 1994.

Appelt, G. "Weight Control Products." In *Handbook of Nonprescription Drugs,* 10th ed., edited by T. Covington, 339–49. Washington, DC: American Pharmaceutical Association, 1993.

Beck, J. "The Public Health Implications of MDMA Use." In *Ecstacy,* edited by S. Peroutka, 77–103. Norwell, MA: Kluwar, 1990.

Bennett, W., ed. "Coffee: Grounds for Concern." *Harvard Medical School Health Letter* 11 (October 1986): 1–4.

Benowitz, N. "How Toxic Is Cocaine?" In *1992 Cocaine: Scientific and Social Dimensions,* edited by Ciba, 125–48. Ciba Foundation Symposium 166. New York: Wiley 1992.

Boucher, D. "Cocaine and the Coca Plant." *BioScience* 41 (1991): 72–76.

Brookoff, D., E. Campbell, and L. Shaw. "The Underreporting of Cocaine-Related Trauma." *American Journal of Public Health* 83 (1993): 369–71.

Brown, E., J. Prager, H. Lee, and R. Ramsey. "CNS Complications of Cocaine Abuse: Prevalence, Pathophysiology, and Neuroradiology. *American Journal of Radiology* 159 (July 1992): 137–47.

Brown, M. *Guide to Fight Substance Abuse.* Nashville, TN: International Broadcast Services, 1991.

Bryant, B., and T. Lombardi. "Cold and Allergy Products." In *Handbook of Nonprescription Drugs,* 10th ed., edited by T. Covington. Washington, DC: American Pharmaceutical Association, 1993.

Byck, R. "Cocaine Use and Research: Three Histories." In *Cocaine: Chemical and Behavioral Aspects.* London: Oxford University Press, 1987.

Carroll, K., B. Rounsaville, and K. Bryant. "Alcoholism in Treatment-Seeking Cocaine Abusers: Clinical and Prognostic Significance." *Journal in Studies of Alcohol* 54 (1993): 199–208.

Carroll, K., B. Rounsaville, L. Gordon, C. Nich, P. Jatlow, R. Bisighini, and F. Gawin. "Psychotherapy and Pharmacotherapy for Ambulatory Cocaine Abusers." *Archives of General Psychiatry* 51 (1994): 177–87.

Central Ohio Lung Association. *Crack—The Facts.* Columbus, OH: Central Ohio Lung Association, 1986.

Coles, C., K. Platzman, I. Smith, M. James, and A. Falek. "Effects of Cocaine and Alcohol Use in Pregnancy on Neonatal Growth and Neurobehavioral Status." *Neurotoxicology and Teratology* 14 (1992): 23–33.

Des Jarlais. "AIDS and HIV Infections in Cocaine Users." In *Cocaine: Scientific and Social Dimensions,* edited by Ciba, 181–95. Ciba Foundations Symposium 166. New York: Wiley, 1992.

DiChiara, G. "Cocaine: Scientific and Social Dimensions. *Trends in Neurological Sciences* 16 (1993): 39.

Ehrman, J. "Cocaine Heightens Risk for Suicides." *ADAMHA News* 18 (May–June 1992): 17.

Facts and Comparisons Drug Newsletter. "Fetal Loss Associated with Caffeine." 13 (March 1994): 22.

Farrar, H., and G. Kearns. "Cocaine: Clinical Pharmacology and Toxicology." *Journal of Pediatrics* 115 (1989): 665–75.

Fischman, M., and R. Foltin. "Self-Administration of Cocaine by Humans: A Laboratory Perspective." In *Cocaine: Scientific and Social Dimensions,* edited by Ciba, 165–80. New York: Wiley, 1992.

Galanter, M., S. Egelko, G. DeLeon, C. Rohrs, and H. Franco. "Crack/Cocaine Abusers in the General Hospital: Assessment and Initiation of Care. *American Journal of Psychiatry* 149 (1992): 810–15.

Gawin, F. "Cocaine Addiction: Psychology and Neurophysiology." *Science* 251 (1991): 1580–86.

Gawin, F., and H. Kleber. "Evolving Conceptualizations of Cocaine Dependence." *Yale Journal of Biology and Medicine* 61 (1988): 123–36.

Gay, C. R., C. Sheppar, D. Inaba, and J. Newmeyer. "Cocaine in Perspective: 'Gift from the Sun God' to 'The Rich Man's Drug.'" *Drug Forum* 2 (1973): 409.

Gilbert, R. "Caffeine Consumption." In *The Methylxanthine Beverages and Foods: Chemistry, Consumption, and Health Effects.* New York: Liss, 1984.

Golding, A. "Two Hundred Years of Drug Abuse." *Journal of the Royal Society of Medicine* 86 (May 1993): 282–86.

Goldstein, A., In *Addiction from Biology to Drug Abuse,* 179–89. New York: Freeman 1994.

Goldstein, F. "Pharmacological Aspects of Substance Abuse." In *Remington's Pharmaceutical Sciences,* 19th ed., edited by A. R. Genaro. Easton, PA: Mack, 1995.

Green, E. "Cocaine, Glamorous Status Symbol of the 'Jet Set,' Is Fast Becoming Many Students' Drug of Choice." *Chronicle of Higher Education,* 13 (November 1985): 1, 34.

Greenhouse, C. "Designer Drugs at a Glance." *NIDA Notes* 7 (January–February 1992): 20–22.

Grinspoon, L. "Update on Cocaine." Parts 1 & 2. *Harvard Mental Health Letter* 10 (August–September 1993): 1–4.

Grinspoon, L., and J. Bakalar. "The Amphetamines: Medical Use and Health Hazards." In *Amphetamines Use, Misuse and Abuse,* edited by D. Smith. Boston, MA: Hall, 1978.

Hall, W., and J. Hando. "Illicit Amphetamine Use Is a Public Health Problem in Australia." *Medical Journal of Australia* 159 (1993): 643–44.

Hanson, G. R., C. F. Bunker, M. Johnson, L. Bush, and J. Gibb. "Response of Monoaminergic and Neuropeptide Systems to 4-methylaminorex: A New Stimulant of Abuse." *European Journal of Pharmacology* 218 (1992): 287–93.

Heishman, S., and J. Henningfield. "Stimulus Functions of Caffeine in Humans: Relation to Dependence

Potential." *Neuroscience and Biobehavior Review* 16 (1992): 273–87.

Holtzman, S. "Caffeine as a Model Drug of Abuse." *Trends in Pharmacological Sciences* 11 (1990): 355–56.

Irvine, G., and L. Chin. "The Environmental Impact and Adverse Health Effects of the Clandestine Manufacture of Methamphetamine." In *Methamphetamine Abuse: Epidemiologic Issues and Implications,* 33–42. NIDA Research Monograph Series 15. Washington, DC: U.S. Government Printing Office 1991.

Jaffe, J. "Drug Addiction and Drug Abuse." In *The Pharmacologic Basis of Therapeutics,* 8th ed., edited by A. Gilman, T. Rall, A. Nies, and P. Taylor, 522–73. New York: Pergamon, 1990.

Jaffe, J., and M. Martin. "Opioid Analgesics and Antagonists." In *The Pharmacological Basis of Therapeutics,* 8th ed., edited by A. Gilman, T. Rall, A. Nies, and P. Taylor. New York: Pergamon, 1990.

Johnston, L. "University of Michigan Annual National Surveys of Secondary Students." Lansing: University of Michigan, 1993. Available from author at 412 Maynard, Ann Arbor, MI.

Johnston, L. "University of Michigan Annual National Surveys of Secondary Students." Lansing: University of Michigan, 1994. Available from author at 412 Maynard Ave., Ann Arbor, MI.

Keegan, A. "Scientists Get to the Heart of Cocaine's Toxic Effects on the Cardiovascular Systems." *NIDA Notes* 6 (Summer–Fall 1991): 21–23.

Kihlman, B. *Caffeine and Chromosomes.* Amsterdam: Elsevier, 1977.

Kleber, H. "Treatment of Cocaine Abuse: Pharmacotherapy." In *Cocaine Scientific and Social Dimensions,* edited by Ciba, 195–206. Ciba Foundation Symposium 166. New York: Wiley, 1992.

Knight-Ridder News Service. "Experts Call War on Drugs a $32 Billion Stalemate." *Salt Lake Tribune* 244 (21 September 1992): A-2.

Kosten, T. "Pharmacotherapeutic Interventions for Cocaine Abuse Matching Patients to Treatments." *Journal of Nervous and Mental Disease* 177 (1989): 379–90.

Lillie-Blanton, M., J. Anthony, and C. Schuster. "Probing the Meaning of Racial/Ethnic Group Comparisons in Crack Cocaine Smoking." *JAMA* 269 (1993): 993–97.

Margen, S. "Caffeine: Grounds for Concern." *U.C. Berkeley Wellness Letter* 10 (March 1994): 4.

Mathias, R. "'Crack Babies' Not a Lost Generation, Researchers Say." *NIDA Notes* 7 (January–February 1992): 16.

Max, B. "This and That: The Ethnopharmacology of Simple Phenethylamines and the Questions of Cocaine and the Human Heart." *Trends in Pharmacological Sciences* 12 (1991): 329–33.

Mayes, L., R. Granger, M. Bornstein, and B. Zucker. "The Problem of Prenatal Cocaine Exposure." *JAMA* 15 (1992): 406–08.

McCance-Katz, E., L. Price, C. McDougle, T. Kosten, J. Black, and P. Jatlow. "Concurrent Cocaine-Ethanol Ingestion in Humans: Pharmacology, Physiology, Behavior, and the Role of Cocaethylene." *Psychopharmacology* 111 (1993): 39–46.

Miller, M., and N. Kozel. "Introduction and Overview." In *Methamphetamine Abuse: Epidemiologic Issues and Implications,* 1–5. NIDA Research Monograph Series 115. Washington, DC: U.S. Government Printing Office, 1991.

Mills, J., et al. "Moderate Caffeine Use and the Risk of Spontaneous Abortion and Intrauterine Growth Retardation." *JAMA* 269 (1993): 593–602.

Nehlig, A., J. Daval, and G. Debry. "Caffeine and the Central Nervous System: Mechanisms of Action, Biochemical, Metabolic and Psychostimulant Effects." *Brain Research Review* 17 (1992): 139–70.

Pagliaro, L., L. Jaglalsingh, and A. Pagliaro. "Cocaine Use and Depression." *Canadian Medical Association Journal* 147 (1992): 1636.

Randall, T. "Ecstasy-Fueled 'Rave' Parties Become Dances of Death for English Youths." *JAMA* 268 (1992a): 1505–06.

Randall, T. "'Rave' Scene, Ecstasy Use, Leap Atlantic." *JAMA* 268 (1992b): 1506.

Richardson, G., and N. Day. "Maternal and Neonatal Effects of Moderate Cocaine Use During Pregnancy." *Neurotoxicity and Teratology* 13 (1991): 455–60.

Robinson, T. "The Neurobiology of Amphetamine Psychosis: Evidence from Studies with an Animal Model." In *Biological Basis of Schizophrenic Disorders,* edited by Tsuneyuki Nakazawa, 185–201. Japan Scientific Societies Press, 1991.

Rumbaugh, C. L. "Small Vessel Cerebral Vascular Changes Following Chronic Amphetamine Intoxication." In *Cocaine and Other Stimulants,* edited by E. H. Ellinwood, Jr., and M. M. Kilbey. New York: Plenum, 1977.

Sands, B., and D. Ciraulo. "Cocaine Drug–Drug Interactions." *Journal of Clinical Psychopharmacology* 12 (1992): 49–55.

Sapienza, F., H. McClain, M. Klein, and J. Tolliver. "New Controlled Substance Analogues of Interest to DEA." Abstract, Annual Meeting of the Committee on Problems of Drug Dependence. Washington, DC: Drug Control Section, Drug Enforcement Administration, 1989.

Sato, M. "A Lasting Vulnerability to Psychosis in Patients with Previous Methamphetamine Psychosis." *The Neurobiology of Drug and Alcohol Addiction.*

Annals of the New York Academy of Sciences 654 (28 June 1992): 160–70.

Sawynok, J. and T. Yaksh. "Caffeine as an Analgesic Adjuvant: A Review of Pharmacology and Mechanisms of Action." *Pharmacological Reviews* 45 (1993): 43–85.

Schmidt, C., J. Ritter, P. Sonsalla, G. R. Hanson, and J. W. Gibb. "Role of Dopamine in the Neurotoxic Effects of Methamphetamine." *Journal of Pharmacology and Experimental Therapeutics* 233 (1985): 539–44.

Schwartz, R., M. Lyenberg, and N. Hoffman. "Crack Use by American Middle-Class Adolescent Polydrug Users." *Journal of Pediatrics* 118 (1991): 150–55.

Seibyl, J., L. Brenner, J. Drystal, R. Johnson, and D. Charney. "Mazindol and Cocaine Addiction in Schizophrenia." *Biological Psychiatry* 31 (1992): 1172–83.

Siegel, R. K. "Treatment of Cocaine Abuse." *Journal of Psychoactive Drugs* 17 (1985): 52.

Tanne, J. "Jail for Pregnant Cocaine Users in U.S." *British Medical Journal* 303 (1991): 873.

Taylor, J. "All-New MDMA FAQ." Internet (computer networking service), Usenet News, sci.med.pharmacy (27 May 1994).

Van Dyck, C., and R. Byck. "Cocaine." *Scientific American* 246 (1982): 128–41.

Weiner, N. "Norepinephrine, Epinephrine, and the Sympathomimetic Amines." In *Pharmacological Basis of Therapeutics,* 6th ed., edited by A. G. Gilman, L. S. Goodman, and A. Gilman. New York: Macmillan, 1980.

Weiss, R. "Recurrent Myocardial Infarction Caused by Cocaine Abuse." *American Heart Journal* 111 (1986): 793.

Woolverton, W., and K. Johnston. "Neurobiology of Cocaine Abuse." *Trends in Pharmacological Sciences* 13 (1992): 193–200.

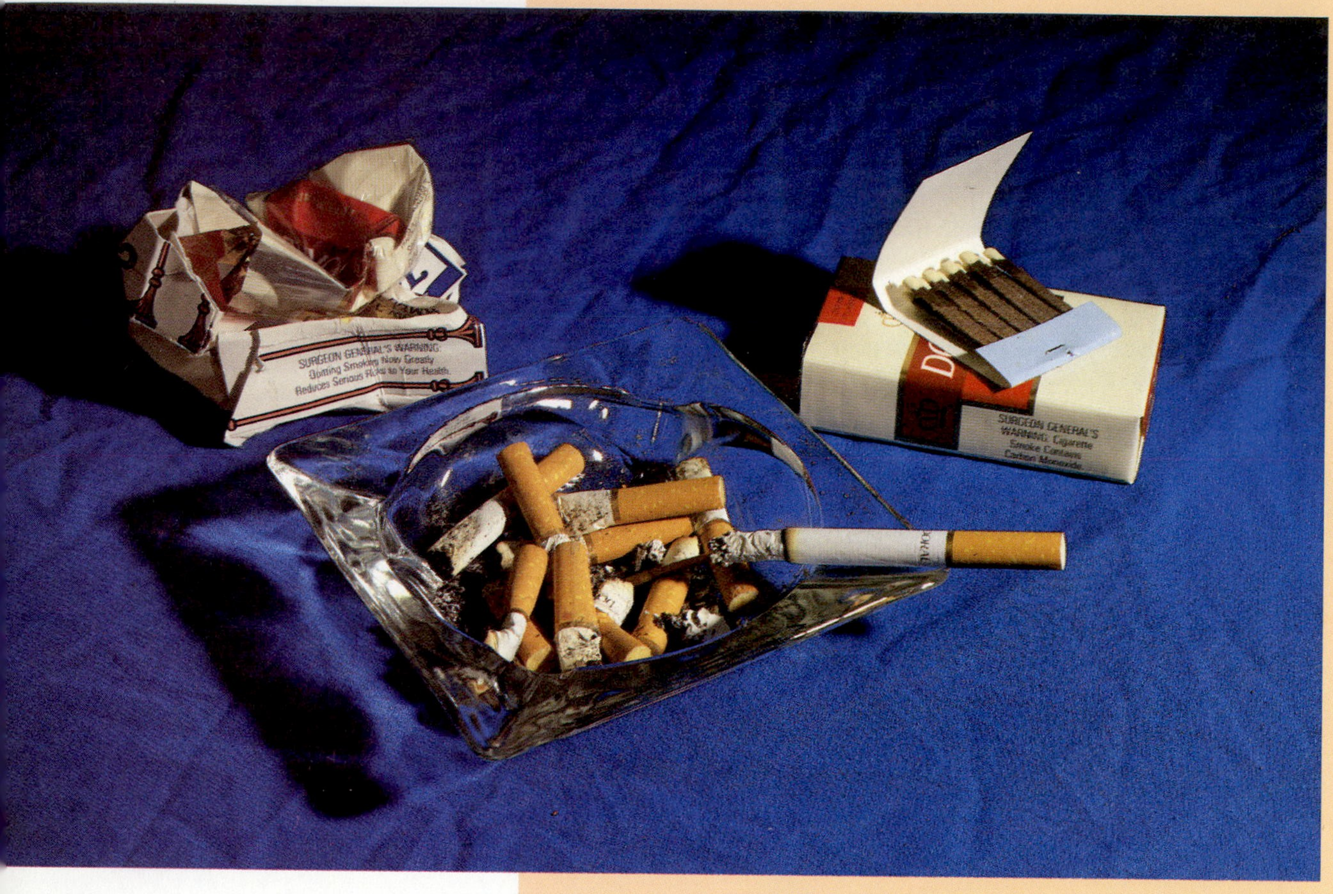
SURGEON GENERAL'S WARNING:
Quitting Smoking Now Greatly
Reduces Serious Risks to Your Health.
SURGEON GENERAL'S
WARNING: Cigarette
Smoke Contains
Carbon Monoxide

Chapter 11

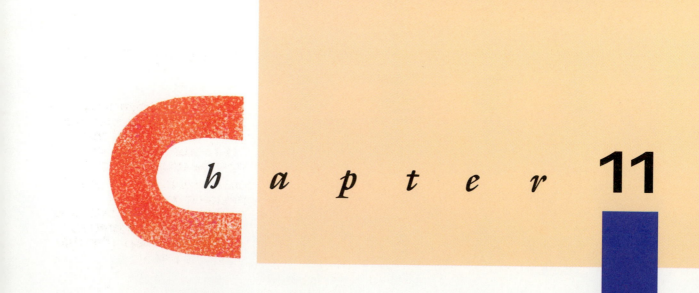

Tobacco

Did You Know That . . .

- Seventy-five percent of the U.S. population has used cigarettes, and nearly one-third currently use cigarettes.
- Chewing and snuffing were the most common ways of using tobacco in the United States especially before the turn of the century.
- Tar and nicotine levels in cigarettes have dropped considerably over the last 40 years.
- The cost of making cigarettes (not counting the tobacco) is about three cents a pack.
- Before the 1960s, tobacco was perceived as lacking any negative consequences.
- The risk of premature death is 70% higher for cigarette smokers than nonsmokers.
- Nicotine has been used as a lethal insecticide.
- Tobacco is the sixth largest cash crop in the United States.
- In 1988, the former U.S. Surgeon General publicly proclaimed that nicotine was as addictive as cocaine and heroin (Tolchin 1988).
- Over 4,000 substances have been identified in tobacco smoke, including several carcinogens.
- In the 1600s Turkey, Russia, and China all imposed the death penalty for smoking.
- Cigarette smoking has declined in the United States but risen in Third World countries.
- Daily cigarette smokers, as opposed to nonsmokers, are 10 times more likely to engage in the use of controlled substances, such as marijuana and cocaine.
- Uninhaled smoke from a lit cigarette has higher concentrations of carbon monoxide, nicotine, and ammonia than inhaled (mainstream) smoke.
- The American Cancer Society estimates that, on average, 90% of lung cancer deaths are caused by smoking.
- Health damage from smoking is estimated to cost Americans over $27 billion a year in medical care, absenteeism, decreased work productivity, and accidents.
- The cartoon figure "Joe Camel" used to advocate cigarette smoking is especially appealing to children and teens.

Learning Objectives

On completing this chapter, you will be able to

1. Assess how addictive nicotine is.
2. Discuss the value of tobacco as a cash crop in the United States.
3. Explain how the quality of leaf tobacco has changed since the mid-1950s.
4. Report what the latest findings show regarding cigarette consumption in the United States.
5. Report what national health surveys reveal about tobacco use with regard to gender, education, and race and ethnicity.
6. Describe the relationship between "gateway" drugs and the use of licit and illicit drugs.
7. Define the following: *smokeless tobacco products, sidestream smoke, and secondhand smoke.*
8. Explain the effect of nicotine on the nervous system.
9. Report what research shows about health issues and the tar and nicotine contents of cigarettes.

(continued)

Healthy People 2000

Reduce the initiation of cigarette smoking by children and youth so that no more than 15% have become regular cigarette smokers by age 20.

Increase to at least 50% the proportion of cigarette smokers aged 18 and older who stopped smoking cigarettes for at least one day during the preceding year.

LEARNING OBJECTIVES

10 Describe the two opposing groups that have come into existence as a result of the negative publicity regarding cigarette smoking.

11 List the three main types of behavioral treatments for the cessation of smoking.

Tobacco Use: Scope of the Problem

Cigarette smoking is the major, most preventable cause of disease and premature death in the United States. In surveys of such legitimate drugs as alcohol, nicotine, and caffeine, the number one killer drug continues to be cigarettes. They are responsible for approximately 1,096 deaths every day and 400,000 annually, while alcohol kills approximately 100,000 annually (Kilbourne 1989; U.S. Department of Health and Human Services [USDHHS] 1989). Another series of statistics show that 115,000 die of coronary heart disease, 27,000 from stroke, 136,000 from cancer, 60,000 from chronic pulmonary disease and other causes (USDHHS 1989). Furthermore, 150,000 yearly cases of bronchitis and pneumonia result in young children whose parents are smokers (*CBS Evening News* 1994). For every five deaths in the United States, at least one is caused by tobacco use (Office of Smoking and Health 1989).

Current Use of Tobacco

Of the U.S. population age 12 and over, 71% has used cigarettes, and 29% currently use them (National Institute on Drug Abuse [NIDA] 1991b; Substance Abuse and Mental Health Services Administration [SAMHSA] 1993). Current use[1] of cigarettes and smokeless tobacco combined among youth ages 12–17 is approximately 12%. Among young adults ages 18–25 and adults ages 26–34, the figure is 38%. Finally, among older adults ages 38 and older, the percentage is 29% (SAMHSA 1993).

The History of Tobacco Use

Indigenous to the United States, tobacco was one of the New World's contributions to the rest of humanity. The word *tobacco* may have come from *tabacco*, which was a two-pronged tube used by the natives of Central America to take snuff. Columbus reported receiving tobacco leaves from the natives of San Salvador in 1492. However, the natives had been smoking the leaves for many centuries before Columbus arrived. Practically all the natives from Paraguay to Quebec used tobacco. The Mayas regarded tobacco smoke as divine incense that would bring rain in the dry season. The oldest known representation of a smoker is a stone carving from a Mayan temple, showing a priest puffing on a ceremonial pipe. The Aztecs used tobacco in folk medicine and religious ritual.

Indeed, Native Americans used tobacco in every manner known: smoked as cigars and cigarettes (wrapped in corn husks) and in pipes; as a syrup to be swallowed or applied to the gums; chewed and snuffed; and administered rectally as a ceremonial enema (Schultes 1978; Tobacco Institute 1982).

[1] Current use is defined as having smoked in the past month, when the survey was administered.

Popularity in the Western World

Tobacco reached Europe and was at first merely a curiosity, but its use spread rapidly. Europeans had no name for the process of inhaling smoke, so they called this "drinking" smoke. Perhaps the first European to inhale tobacco smoke was Rodrig de Jerez, a member of Columbus's crew. He had seen people smoking in Cuba and brought the habit to Portugal. When he smoked in Portugal, his friends, seeing smoke coming from his mouth, believed he was possessed by the devil! He was placed in jail for several years (Heimann 1960).

In 1559, the French ambassador to Portugal, Jean Nicot, grew interested in this novel plant and sent one as a gift to Catherine de Medici, Queen of France. The plant was named ***Nicotiana tabacum*** after him.

The next several hundred years saw a remarkable increase in the use of tobacco. Portuguese sailors smoked it and left tobacco seeds scattered around the world. Over the next 150 years, the Portuguese introduced tobacco to trade with India, Brazil, Japan, China, Arabia, and Africa. Many large tobacco plantations around the world were started by the Portuguese at this time.

An early Christian religious leader, Bishop Bartolome de las Casas (1474–1566), reported that Spanish settlers in Hispaniola (Haiti) smoked rolled tobacco leaves in cigar form like the natives. When the bishop asked about this disgusting habit, the settlers replied that they found it impossible to give up.

As the use of tobacco spread, so did the controversy about whether it was bad or good. Tobacco use was the first major drug controversy of global dimensions. As a medicine, tobacco was at first almost universally accepted. Nicholas Monardes, in his description of New World plants (dated 1574), recommended tobacco as an infallible cure for 36 different maladies. It was described as a holy, healing herb, a special remedy sent by God to humans.

Opponents of tobacco use disputed its medical value. They pointed out that tobacco was used in the magic and religion of Native Americans. (Monardes had also described ritual use by native priests.) Tobacco was attacked as an evil plant, an invention of the devil. King James I of England was fanatically opposed to smoking. In an attempt to limit tobacco use, he raised the import tax on tobacco and also sold the right to collect the tax (Austin 1978).

Nevertheless, tobacco use increased. By 1614, the number of tobacco shops in London had mushroomed to over 7,000, and demand for tobacco usually outstripped supply. Tobacco was literally worth its weight in silver, so to conserve, it was smoked in pipes with very small bowls. Use of tobacco grew in other areas of the world as well.

In 1642, Pope Urban VIII issued a formal decree forbidding the use of tobacco in church under penalty of immediate excommunication. Priests and worshippers had been staining church floors with tobacco juice. One priest in Naples sneezed so hard after taking snuff that he vomited on the altar in full sight of the congregation. Pope Innocent X issued another edict against tobacco use in 1650, but the clergy and the laity continued to take snuff and smoke. Finally, in 1725, Pope Benedict XIII, himself a smoker and "snufftaker," annulled all previous edicts against tobacco (Austin 1978).

In the 1600s, Turkey, Russia, and China all imposed the death penalty for smoking. Sultan Murad the Cruel executed many of his subjects caught smoking. The Romanov tsars publicly tortured smokers and exiled them to Siberia. The Chinese decapitated anyone caught dealing in tobacco with the "outer barbarians." Yet smoking continued to grow to epidemic proportions. Despite their opposition to anything foreign, the Chinese became the heaviest smokers in Asia, thus facilitating the later spread of opium smoking. Thus, no nation whose population has learned to use tobacco products has been successful in outlawing use or getting people to stop.

Snuffing first became fashionable in France during the reign of Louis XIII and spread throughout European aristocracy. Snuffing was regarded as daintier and more elegant than constantly exhaling smoke. King Louis XIV, however,

NICOTIANA TABACUM the primary tobacco plant species cultivated in North America detested all forms of tobacco and would not permit its use in his presence. (He would have banned it, but he needed the tax revenue tobacco brought in.) His sister-in-law, Charlotte of Orleans, was one of the few at court who agreed with him. As she wrote to her sister, "It is better to take no snuff at all than a little; for it is certain that he who takes a little will soon take much, and that is why they call it 'the enchanted herb,' for those who take it are so taken by it that they cannot go without it." Napoleon is said to have used seven pounds of snuff per month (Corti 1931).

Tobacco Use in America

Tobacco played a significant role in the successful colonization of the United States (Langton 1991, 21). In 1610, John Rolfe was sent to Virginia to set up a tobacco industry. At first, the tobacco planted in Virginia was a native species, *Nicotiana rustica,* that was harsh and did not sell well. But in 1612 Rolfe managed to obtain some seeds of the Spanish tobacco species *Nicotiana tabacum,* and by 1613 the success of the tobacco industry and the Virginia colony was ensured.

The history of tobacco smoking in the United States is rich in terms of the tremendous number of laws, rules, regulations, and customs that have arisen out of the habit of smoking. Many states have had laws prohibiting the use of tobacco by young people as well as women of any age. In the 1860s, for instance, it was illegal in Florida for anyone under the age of 21 to smoke cigarettes. A 20-year-old caught smoking could be taken to court and compelled to reveal his source (the cigarette "pusher"). In Pennsylvania, as in South Carolina, any child not informing on his or her cigarette supplier was a criminal.

Up to the turn of the century, chewing and snuffing were the most common ways of using tobacco in the United States. In 1897, half of all tobacco was prepared for chewing. Law required that spittoons be placed in all public buildings until 1945 ("Cigars" 1988).

Cigars became popular in the United States in the early 1800s. Cigar manufacturers fought the introduction of cigarettes for many years. They spread rumors that cigarettes contained opium, were made with tobacco from discarded cigar butts and with paper made by Chinese lepers, and so on. By about 1920, cigarette consumption started to exceed that of cigars. The introduction of the cigarette-rolling machine in 1883 spurred cigarette consumption because they became cheaper than cigars. By 1885, a billion cigarettes a year were being produced. Americans consumed over 815 billion cigarettes in 1988, or about 5,000 per person age 18 or older. More recent estimates show that "[i]n 1991, an estimated 89.8 million (49.8 percent) adults in the United States at one time were smokers, and 46.3 million (25.7 percent) were current smokers. Approximately 43.5 million persons (48.5 percent of all smokers) . . . were former smokers during 1991" ("Cigarette Smoking Among Adults" 1993, 230). Although a higher percentage of men are smokers than women, 34 versus 28% (Fiore et al. 1989), men (39%) are more likely to quit smoking than women (30%). Furthermore, as educational levels increase, men are increasingly more likely to quit smoking than are women.

Tobacco Production Tobacco farming is the sixth largest legal cash crop in the United States, ranking behind corn, soybeans, hay, wheat, and cotton (Foster et al. 1989, 121). North Carolina and Kentucky are the two leading growers of tobacco.

While there are over 60 species of plants, *Nicotiana tabacum* is the primary species of tobacco cultivated in the United States. The mature leaves are 1 foot to 2.5 feet long. The nicotine content is from 0.3 to 7%, depending on the variety, leaf position on the stalk (the higher the position, the more nicotine), and growing conditions. The flavor of tobacco comes from *nicotianin,* also called *tobacco camphor* (U.S. Surgeon General 1979).

After harvesting and drying, the tobacco leaves are shredded, blown clean of foreign matter and stems, remoisturized with glycerine or other chemical agents, and packed in huge wooden barrels called *hogsheads.* These barrels are placed in storehouses for one to two years to age, during which time the tobacco gets darker and loses moisture, nicotine, and other volatile substances. When aging has been completed, moisture is again added and the tobacco is blended with other varieties.

There are many types of tobacco, with varying characteristics of harshness, mildness, and flavor. *Bright,* also called *flue-cured* or *Virginia,* is the most common type used in cigarettes. (Flue-cured tobacco is heated in curing sheds to speed the drying process.) Developed just before the Civil War, this technique made tobacco smoke more readily inhalable.

The amount of leaf tobacco in a cigarette has gone down about 25% since 1956. There are two reasons for this, not considering the introduction of filtertip cigarettes. (If a filtertip is the same size as a plain cigarette, it has about one-third less tobacco.) The first reason is the use of reconstituted sheets of tobacco. Parts of the tobacco leaves and stems that were discarded in earlier years are now ground up; combined with many other ingredients to control factors such as moisture, flavor, and color; and then rolled out as a flat, homogenized sheet of reconstituted tobacco. This sheet is shredded and mixed with regular leaf tobacco, thus reducing production costs. Nearly one-quarter of the tobacco in a cigarette comes from tobacco scraps made into reconstituted sheets.

A second technological advance further reduces the amount of tobacco needed. This process, called *puffing*, is based on freeze-drying the tobacco and then blowing air or an inert gas, such as carbon dioxide, into it. The gas expands, or puffs up, the plant cells so they take up more space, are lighter, and can absorb additives better.

Tobacco additives are not controlled by the Food and Drug Administration (FDA) or any other government agency. Additives may include extracts of tobacco, as well as nontobacco flavors such as licorice, cocoa, fruit, spices, and floral compositions. (Licorice was first use in tobacco as a preservative around 1830 and became appreciated as a sweetener.) Synthetic flavoring compounds also may be used.

In the 1870s, a "cigarette girl" could roll about four cigarettes per minute by hand. When James Duke leased and improved the first cigarette-rolling machine in 1883, he could make about 200 cigarettes per minute. This was the last link in the chain of development leading to the modern American blended cigarette. Today's machines make over 3,600 uniform cigarettes per minute.

Tar and nicotine levels in cigarettes have dropped considerably over the last 40 years (Palfai and Jankiewicz 1991). Most cigarettes today are low-tar and low-nicotine types. The filtertip, in which the filter is made of cellulose or charcoal, has also become common; over 90% of all cigarettes sold currently in the United States are filtertips (Stellman and Garfinkel 1986; *Tobacco Industry Profile* 1988). The filter does help remove some of the substances in smoke, but most, such as carbon monoxide, pass through into the mouth and lungs. Over 4,000 substances have been identified in burning tobacco and paper. Many are known carcinogens, whereas the health consequences of many more have not been adequately analyzed.

The cost of making cigarettes (not counting the tobacco) is about three cents a pack. Total cost varies with the manufacturer but usually is not more than five to seven cents a pack. The total amount spent by the American consumer is about $25 billion a year for all tobacco products, with over 90% of that for cigarettes. In 1986, the tax revenue on all cigarettes to the U.S. government was about $4 billion, with over $1.5 billion more in state taxes.

Government Regulation In the early 1960s, attitudes toward tobacco use began to change in the United States. Prior to this time, tobacco was perceived as being devoid of any negative consequences. After years of study and hundreds of research reports about the effects of smoking, the Advisory Committee to the U.S. Surgeon General reported in 1964 that "cigarette smoking is causally related to lung cancer in men; the magnitude of the effects of cigarette smoking far outweighs all other factors." Congress passed legislation in 1965, setting up the National Clearinghouse for Smoking and Health. This organization has the responsibility of monitoring, compiling, and reviewing the world's medical literature on the health consequences of smoking.

Reports were published in 1967, 1968, and 1969. The statistical evidence presented in 1969 made it difficult for Congress to avoid warning the public that smoking was dangerous to their health. Since 1 November 1970, all cigarette packages and cartons have had to carry this label: "Warning: The Surgeon General Has Determined That Cigarette Smoking Is Dangerous to Your Health." In 1984, Congress enacted legislation requiring cigarette advertisements and packages to post four distinct warnings (see Figure 11.1), which are to be rotated every three months (see also Here and Now box).

SURGEON GENERAL'S WARNING: Quitting Smoking Now Greatly Reduces Serious Risks to Your Health.

SURGEON GENERAL'S WARNING: Smoking Causes Lung Cancer, Heart Disease, Emphysema, and May Complicate Pregnancy.

SURGEON GENERAL'S WARNING: Smoking by Pregnant Women May Result in Fetal Injury, Premature Birth, and Low Birth Weight.

SURGEON GENERAL'S WARNING: Cigarette Smoke Contains Carbon Monoxide.

FIGURE 11.1 Warnings on cigarette labels. Four warnings must be rotated on cigarette packages. The messages are based on the reports of the U.S. Surgeon General on *The Health Consequences of Smoking* (1985) and went into effect on 12 October 1985.

Further pressure on Congress prompted passage of laws that prohibited advertising tobacco on radio and television after January 2, 1971. The intent was to limit the media's ability to make smoking seem glamorous and sophisticated. The loss in revenue to radio and television was enormous.

The 1979 publication *Smoking and Health: A Report of the Surgeon General* gave up-to-date information on research about the effects of tobacco on cardiovascular disease, bronchopulmonary disease, cancer, peptic ulcer, and pregnancy. It also emphasized the increase in smoking by women and girls over the past 15 years. The 1981 U.S. Surgeon General's report, *The Changing Cigarette*, gave further information, and the 1985 report, *The Health Consequences of Smoking*, gave research findings showing the relationship of smoking, cancer, and chronic lung disease in the workplace. See Figure 11.1.

Pharmacology of Nicotine

In 1828, nicotine was separated from tobacco. Nicotine is a colorless, highly volatile liquid alkaloid. It has no therapeutic application or action, and it is considered a volatile and powerful poison. Usually administered through inhalation, "Tobacco smoke is an aerosol, a colloid system consisting of a liquid dispersed in a gaseous medium, as in a fog or disinfectant spray (Palfai and Jankiewicz 1991, 348). In smoking, tobacco enters the lungs as a water-soluble liquid contained in the watery portion of the mucous membranes. Another popular method of incorporating nicotine is through chewing where nicotine is extracted from chewing or absorbing finely ground tobacco leaves in the mouth.

Tobacco chewing involves the absorption of nicotine through the mucous lining of the mouth; **snuff dipping** is another method of administration, which involves placing a pinch of tobacco between the gums and the check.

The amount of tobacco absorbed varies according to (1) number and intensity of puffs, (2) the length of the cigarette smoked, (3) volume of smoke inhaled, and (4) the number of cigarettes smoked throughout the day.

Where Is the Reward in Smoking? Nicotine produces an intense effect on the central nervous system, and inhalation of tobacco smoke as well as mouth absorption of smokeless tobacco is akin to an intravenous injection of nicotine. "Cigarette tobacco contains between 1.5 and 3 percent nicotine, with each cigarette containing between

TOBACCO CHEWING the absorption of nicotine through the mucous lining of the mouth

SNUFF DIPPING placing a pinch of tobacco between the gums and the cheek

Here and Now

Cigarette Advertising

The cigarette companies spent nearly $2.4 billion in 1986 to promote the sale of their products. Almost $1 billion was for advertising, $630 million went to retailers in promotional allowances, and the remainder was spent for a myriad of promotional enterprises—premiums, testimonials, public entertainment, direct mail promotions, and street corner and mail order sampling. The companies sponsor or support many sporting events, such as tennis tournaments, auto races, and basketball games. One company publishes a magazine that it distributes free to 11 million addressees.

The cigarette companies were the largest advertisers on television and radio until 1971, when Congress banned such advertising, and they are now among the leaders in magazine and national newspaper advertising. They are first in outdoor and transit advertising.

CIGARETTE ADVERTISING AND PROMOTION, 1986 (MILLIONS OF DOLLARS)

Advertising		
Newspapers	$120	
Magazines	340	
Outdoor	301	
Transit	35	
Point of sale	136	
Total		$932
Promotional allowances to retailers		630
Other:		
Sampling	99	
Premiums and other items	210	
Public entertainment	71	
All others	440	
Total		$820
Total		2,382

Federal Trade Commission

Source: U.S. Department of Health and Human Services. *Smoking, Tobacco and Health: A Fact Book.* DHHS Publication no. (CDC) 87-8397. Washington, DC: U.S. Department of Health and Human Services, 1989:27.

29 to 30 milligrams of the drug (Fort 1969, 154–155). (In 1980 an average cigarette contained less than 1 mg of nicotine.) Although tolerance to nicotine does build up rapidly, the fatal dose for adults is 60 milligrams and a cigar contains between 15 and 40 milligrams of nicotine (Fort 1969, 155). Death from overdose occurs from a paralysis of the respiratory muscles. Other findings include the following: "Nicotine distributes quickly and widely, concentrating in the brain at up to five times the blood level, also the sympathetic ganglia, adrenal medulla, parotid glands, stomach, thyroid, pancreas, and kidneys" (Palfai and Jankiewicz 1991, 349—see the diagram of the body human on page 145, Chapter 5).

The smoker who inhales gets about 90% of the nicotine in his or her bloodstream, compared to 20 to 50% from smoke taken into the mouth and then exhaled (Volle and Koelle 1975). The blood carries nicotine to the heart, which distributes the substance rapidly throughout the body. Nicotine from inhaled tobacco smoke reaches the brain in seven seconds—twice as fast as from intravenous administration in the arm.

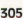

Physiological Effects

In large doses, nicotine is highly toxic. It has been used as an insecticide, and at higher concentration levels, it has the same effects as a poison. The symptoms of nicotine poisoning are sweating, vomiting, mental confusion, diminished pulse rate, and breathing difficulty. Respiratory failure from the paralysis of muscles usually causes death to occur.

Nicotine is believed to be the substance in tobacco that causes dependence, based on how it is metabolized and the effects it produces. Regular users commonly smoke about 20 to 30 cigarettes per day, or one every 30 to 40 minutes.

Nicotine is a curious drug because it first stimulates and then depresses the nervous system. The stimulus effect is due to release of norepinephrine and the fact that nicotine mimics the action of acetylcholine. Nicotine thus stimulates cholinergic receptors (nicotinic type) first but is not removed from the receptors very rapidly; the next effect is depression, caused by blocked nerve activity. Nicotine increases the respiration rate at low dose levels because it stimulates the receptors in the carotid artery (in the neck) that monitor the brain's need for oxygen. Nicotine stimulates the cardiovascular system by releasing epinephrine, causing increases in coronary blood flow, heart rate, and blood pressure. The effect is to increase the oxygen requirements of the heart muscle but not the oxygen supply. This may trigger heart attacks in susceptible people (Armitrage et al. 1985).

Nicotine causes an initial stimulation of salivary and bronchial secretions, followed by inhibition. The excess saliva associated with smoking is caused by the irritating smoke, not the nicotine (Taylor 1980; Benowitz 1988).

Nicotine and perhaps other substances in tobacco smoke tend to inhibit hunger contractions in the stomach for up to one hour. At the same time, it causes a slight increase in blood sugar and deadens the taste buds. These factors may be responsible for decreased feelings of hunger by many smokers. Smokers have often reported that they gain weight after they stop smoking and that their appetite increases. In addition, when someone who smokes one or more packs a day quits, there may be a decrease in heart rate (two to three beats per minute) and up to a 10% decrease in basal metabolic rate. The body is being stressed less, so it converts more food into fat.

Nicotine and other products in smoke, such as carbon monoxide, produce still other effects. Up to 10% of all the hemoglobin in smokers may be in the carboxyhemoglobin form. This form of hemoglobin cannot carry oxygen, so up to 10% of the smoker's blood is effectively out of circulation as far as normal oxygen–carbon dioxide exchange is concerned. This situation could easily cause a smoker to become out of breath from exertion. It is a factor in heart attacks and in the lower birthweight and survival rate of infants born to women who smoke during pregnancy (see also later in this chapter).

Mortality Rates

Although over the past 25 years there has been a steady decline in cigarette consumption (Office on Smoking and Health 1989), the risk of premature death is significantly higher (about 70%) for cigarette smokers than nonsmokers. According to the U.S. Surgeon General, estimates of premature deaths associated with cigarette smoking range from 320,000 to 400,000 per year, including 115,000 deaths from heart disease, 106,000 from lung cancer, 32,000 from other forms of cancer, 57,000 from chronic lung disease, 28,000 from stroke, and abut 52,000 from other conditions.

A 35-year-old male who smokes two packs a day has a life expectancy that is 8.1 years shorter than his nonsmoking counterpart (U.S. Surgeon General 1985; Callahan 1987). The death rate increases with the amount smoked: A two-pack-a-day smoker has a mortality rate twice as high as a nonsmoker. Overall mortality rates are greater for those who smoke longer; death rates are directly proportional. Thus, the longer you smoke, the higher the mortality rate.

Various cigarettes have different tar and nicotine contents; this means that the effects they produce and thus the mortality rate vary, as well. Smokers of low-tar and -nicotine cigarettes have a mortality ratio 50% greater than that of nonsmokers but 15 to 20% less than that of cigarette smokers as a group (U.S. Surgeon General 1981; DeAngelis 1989).

Overall mortality ratios decline the longer ex-smokers abstain from smoking. People who stop smoking before age 50 reduce their risk of dying over the next 15 years by 50%. The mortality rate for ex-smokers is related to the *number* of cigarettes they used to smoke per day and the *age* at which they started to smoke. The mortality rate for cigar smokers is somewhat higher than that for nonsmokers and is related to the number of cigars smoked daily. The mortality rate for pipe smokers is slightly greater than that for nonsmokers.

Chronic Illness

Not only do cigarette smokers tend to die at an earlier age than nonsmokers, but they also have a higher probability of contracting certain diseases (Schuckit 1984; American Cancer Society 1990). Following the U.S. Surgeon General's report in 1964, the National Center for Health Statistics began collecting information on smoking. These findings have been helpful in assessing the relationships between tobacco use and illnesses, disability, and other health indicators. Among other things, the center found that men and women currently smoking cigarettes have more chronic health problems than people who never smoked. What's more, there is a dose–response relationship between the number of cigarettes smoked per day and particular illnesses. For instance, men who smoke two packs of cigarettes a day have a four times higher rate of chronic bronchitis and/or **emphysema** than do nonsmokers. The rate for women smoking two or more packs a day is nearly ten times higher.

Other indicators of sickness studied were workdays lost, days spent in bed because of illness, and days of limited activity resulting from chronic disease. Male smokers had a 33% excess and female smokers a 45% excess of workdays lost compared to nonsmokers. Male former smokers had a 41% excess and female former smokers a 43% excess of workdays lost. The 1974 survey calculated that more than 81 million workdays are lost in the United States every year by smokers compared to nonsmokers. This is a tremendous financial and productivity loss for the nation.

Data on disability and illness show continued high risk among former smokers. The most likely reason for this is that smokers quit because of a smoking-related illness that has already severely damaged the cardiovascular system or lungs.

Cardiovascular Disease There is now overwhelming proof that cigarette smoking increases the risk of cardiovascular disease (Callahan 1987; Fiore et al. 1989). Data collected from the United States, the United Kingdom, Canada, and other countries show that smoking is a major risk factor for heart attack. The probability of heart attack is related to the amount smoked, which has a synergistic relationship to other risk factors, such as obesity.

Smoking cigarettes is a major risk factor for arteriosclerotic disease and for death from arteriosclerotic aneurysm of the aorta (Palfai and Jankiewicz 1991). (An *aneurysm* is a weakened area in a blood vessel that forms a blood-filled sac and may rupture.) Smokers have a higher incidence of atherosclerosis of the coronary arteries that supply blood to the heart (the arteries become blocked with fat deposits), and the effect is dose related. Both the carbon monoxide and the nicotine in cigarette smoke can precipitate angina attacks (painful spasms in the chest when the heart muscle does not get the blood supply it needs).

Smokers of low-tar and low-nicotine cigarettes have less risk of coronary heart disease, but their risk is still greater than that of nonsmokers. The risk goes down if the person quits; after about 10 years, the risk of coronary disease in ex-smokers approaches that of nonsmokers. Women who smoke and use oral contraceptives have a significantly higher risk of death or disability from stroke, heart attack, and other cardiovascular diseases than nonsmokers both on and off "the pill."

Cancer Currently, lung cancer is the leading cause of cancer death in the United States, claiming 125,000 victims a year (American Cancer Society 1990). There were an estimated 560,000 deaths from all types of cancer in 1988, of which 135,600 were from lung cancer. Lung cancer is the most common type in men and in women. There has been a dramatic increase in lung cancer in

EMPHYSEMA a common type of lung disease

women: fourfold in 25 years. Lung cancer mortality rates for women are increasing more rapidly than for men. Women who smoke die sooner, just as male smokers do; there is a direct relationship between smoking and lung cancer in both genders.

Approximately 85% of lung cancer cases in men and 75% in women are caused by cigarette smoking. Less than 10% of nonsmokers get lung cancer. What's more, 85% to 90% of all deaths from lung cancer are smoking related (Callahan 1987).

The risk of lung cancer increases with

- Amount smoked, as measured by the number of cigarettes smoked per day
- Duration of smoking
- Age at which the person started smoking
- Degree of inhalation
- Tar and nicotine content of the cigarettes

Use of filter cigarettes and of lower tar and nicotine cigarettes decreases the lung cancer mortality rate, but it is still significantly higher than that for nonsmokers. If a smoker quits, the lung cancer mortality rate goes down but will not approach the nonsmoker rate until 10 years of abstinence.

Pipe and cigar smokers are more likely to contract lung cancer than nonsmokers but less so than habitual cigarette smokers. Common types of cancers among cigar and pipe smokers include cancers of the mouth, larynx, and esophagus.

Exposure to certain air pollutants in the environment or in industry—especially the asbestos, uranium, nickel, and chemical industries—acts synergistically with cigarette smoking to increase lung cancer mortality rates far above what would be the rate for each separately.

Cancer of the larynx is significantly higher in smokers compared to nonsmokers and is related to the amount smoked. A compounding effect has also been shown to exist between smoking and alcohol consumption and between exposure to asbestos and smoking, increasing the likelihood of getting cancer of the larynx. The risk of laryngeal cancer goes down if the person stops smoking but like lung cancer, this form of cancer does not reach the level for nonsmokers for nearly 10 years.

There is also a causal relationship between smoking and cancers of the oral cavity, esophagus, urinary bladder, pancreas, and kidneys.

Bronchopulmonary Disease Cigarette smoking is the most important cause of bronchopulmonary disease, which includes a host of lung ailments. Cigarette smokers have higher death rates from pulmonary emphysema and chronic bronchitis and more frequently have impaired pulmonary function and other symptoms of pulmonary disease than nonsmokers (U.S. Surgeon General 1979; Callahan 1987; Cook et al. 1990).

Respiratory infections are more prevalent and more severe among cigarette smokers, particularly heavy smokers, than among nonsmokers. The risk of developing or dying from bronchopulmonary disease among pipe or cigar smokers is higher than that for nonsmokers but less than for cigarette smokers. Ex-smokers have lower death rates from bronchopulmonary disease than do continuing smokers.

The cause of lung damage may be impaired immune system activity in lung tissue, genetic factors, and deficiencies in certain substances in the tissues. It is known that people with a low amount of an enzyme called *alpha-1-antitrypsin* are more likely to develop emphysema. Smoking is especially dangerous for such people.

As mentioned, smokers are more prone to develop bronchopulmonary disease in the presence of air pollutants, such as sulfur oxides and asbestos, than are nonsmokers. Coal dust, cotton dust, and chlorine have additive effects with cigarette smoking in damaging the lungs. Likewise, exposure to fumes and dust—especially talc and carbon black in the rubber industry and uranium and gold dust in the mining industry—act synergistically with cigarette smoking in the development of bronchopulmonary disease.

It is now understood how cigarette smoking can cause one of the most common lung diseases, emphysema. Cigarette smoking produces inflammation of the lung tissue as well as an increase in the protein elastase in the tissue. Elastin, a structural material in the lungs, is broken down by elastase enzyme. In the long run, the lung tissue is damaged extensively, causing emphysema (U.S. Surgeon General 1984).

Effects on the Fetus

Cigarette smoking during pregnancy has a significantly harmful effect on the development of the fetus, the survival of the newborn infant, and the continued development of the child. Adverse effects on pregnancy range from increase risk for spontaneous abortion, impaired fetal growth, stillbirth, premature birth, and neonatal death. Babies born to mothers who smoke have a lower average body weight and length and have a smaller head circumference. The amount a woman smokes will impact the size of the child she bears. If a smoking woman gives it up for the entire duration of the pregnancy, her child will probably be of normal size and strength.

The below-average weight of babies born to smokers is caused by carbon monoxide and nicotine (Cook et al. 1990). Carbon monoxide reduces the oxygen-carrying capacity of the fetus's blood, just as it does the mother's. Fetal growth is retarded because the tissue is starved for oxygen. Inhaled nicotine enters the mother's blood from her lungs and rapidly constricts the blood flow to the placenta, reducing available oxygen and nutrients until the effect of the nicotine has worn off. In addition, nicotine crosses the blood–placenta barrier to the fetal bloodstream. It has the same effects on the fetus's nervous system and blood circulation as on the mother's. However, the fetus cannot metabolize nicotine efficiently, so the effects last longer for the child than for the mother.

One known carcinogen in tobacco smoke, *benzo(a)pyrene,* crosses the placenta and enters the fetal blood. Experiments with pregnant mice exposed to benzo(a)pyrene showed that their offspring had a markedly higher incidence of cancer. The impact of smoking during pregnancy on the incidence of cancer in infants is not known.

Infants born to mothers who smoke have a reduced probability of survival. They are more likely to die from **sudden infant death syndrome (SIDS)** and other causes related to their retarded growth. Long-term effects may be observed in physical growth, mental development, and behavioral characteristics of those babies who survive the first four weeks of life. And it appears that children of mothers who smoke do not catch up with children of nonsmoking mothers in various stages of development, at least up to age 11. Smoking during pregnancy may also be a cause of hyperkinesis in children.

If the father smokes even when the mother does not, the fetus may be affected through **secondhand smoke** or through damage to the sperm. There is a much higher mortality rate for newborn infants whose fathers smoke more than 10 cigarettes per day. Babies fathered by heavy smokers have twice the expected incidence of severe birth defects.

Clove Cigarettes

Indonesian clove cigarettes were first used in the 1980s by young Americans. Figures show that in 1980, 12 million cigarettes were sold and by 1984, sales increased to 150 million. Currently the popularity of clove cigarettes has begun to diminish. Because of their aroma, which masks the negative physical effects of nicotine, adolescents assume that these cigarettes are safer than common cigarettes. The truth, however, is that these clove cigarettes contain well over 60% tobacco and possess a greater amount of tar, nicotine, and carbon monoxide than regular cigarettes sold in the United States ("Beware Those Spicy Cigarettes" 1985). Some users have also reported excessive wheezing, fluid retention in the lungs, and bloody phlegm.

Taking Tobacco Without Smoking

Although it is customary to associate the effects of tobacco use with smoking, there are in fact millions of nonsmokers who experience some tobacco effects, voluntarily or involuntarily, through **smokeless tobacco** products and exposure to secondhand smoke.

SUDDEN INFANT DEATH SYNDROME (SIDS) unexpected and unexplainable death that occurs while infants are sleeping

SECONDHAND SMOKE the smoke from burning tobacco that pollutes the air and is breathed by smokers and nonsmokers alike

SMOKELESS TOBACCO two types exist: chewing and snuff tobacco. This type of tobacco consists of tobacco leaves that are shredded and twisted into strands.

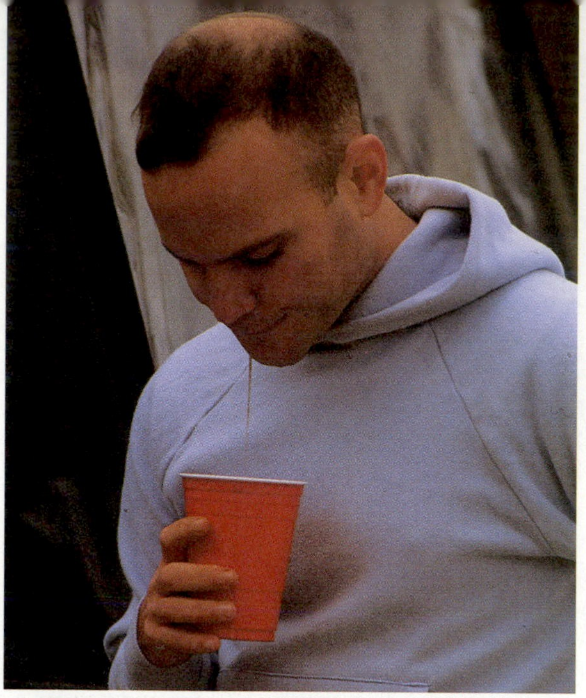

Despite the well-known health hazards of tobacco products, athletes, such as this baseball player, often use smokeless tobacco.

Smokeless Tobacco

Two types of tobacco products are classified as smokeless tobacco: chewing tobacco and snuff. Both consist of tobacco leaves that are shredded and twisted into strands and then either chewed or placed in the cheek between the lower lip and gum.

Interestingly, smokeless tobacco was used in the United States *before* cigarettes became popular. "In 1991, an estimated 5.3 million (2.9%) of U.S. adults were current users of smokeless tobacco, including 4.8 million (5.6%) men and 533,000 (0.6%) women" (USDHHS and Centers for Disease Control [CDC] 1993, 1). The use of smokeless tobacco declined until the early 1980s, when both chewing tobacco and snuff re-emerged. The increase in use is partly due to more effective and persistent advertising campaigns, depicting famous athletes using such products. However, the perceived linkage between health hazards and the use of smokeless tobacco remains understated (CDC 1989).

Who is more likely to use and/or abuse smokeless tobacco, and what is the percentage of users in various categories? In a survey reported in *Morbidity and Mortality Weekly Report* (USDHHS and CDC 1993) of a sample of total population ranging in ages from 18 to 75, 4% had currently used snuff or chewing tobacco at least 20 times and were using it at the time of the survey. Whites are more likely to use this product than African Americans (3 to approximately 2%) and American Indians and Alaskan Natives reported approximately 5% use. Non-Hispanics were more likely to use this drug than Hispanics 3 to 0.9%. Less educated people (less than 12 years of education) were more likely to use this drug than the more educated, approximately 5% in comparison to college graduates at 1%. Residents classified as rural reported 6% use while urban dwellers reported 2% use. Finally, survey respondents below the poverty level were more likely to use this drug, 4% in comparison to 3% of the respondents classified as above the poverty level (USDHHS and CDC 1993).

Accelerated use is found in young males. In some areas of the country, between 25 and 35% of adolescent males use products such as Beech Nut or Red Man (both loose-leaf tobaccos) or Copenhagen or Skoal (canned, moist snuff). The U.S. Centers for Disease Control found that in Alaska 17% of 5-year-old girls and 10% of 5-year-old boys use smokeless tobacco (Wolfe 1987). Currently, 14 American states allow the sale of smokeless tobacco to minors.

How safe are smokeless tobacco products in comparison to cigarettes? A study conducted by the University of Southern California found that taking one pinch of snuff has effects equivalent to those of smoking three or four cigarettes. The likelihood of getting oral cancer increases significantly for anyone who uses smokeless tobacco daily for 3.5 years of more (Perry 1990, 20–23) (see also Here and Now box). Other evidence has shown that continued use of smokeless products can cause cancer of the pharynx and esophagus, as well. The incidence of developing these cancers is related to the duration of use and the type of product used because "long-term snuff users have a 50% greater risk of developing oral cancer than nonusers" ("Smokeless Tobacco" 1990). Other less serious effects of using smokeless tobacco include severe inflammation of gum tissue, tooth decay, and receding gums and tooth loss ("Smokeless Tobacco" 1990).

Here and Now

Think Twice About "Chewing"

Dear Readers:
What follows is an edited version of an article by Susan Miller Degnan of the Miami Herald. It was sent to me by an 84-year-old fan in Harlingen, Texas, who urged me to "keep up the good work." I hope you will be as moved by it as I was. Here it is:

"There may never have been a quieter time in the 117-year history of the Philadelphia Phillies than when Rick Bender, a longtime sandlot ballplayer, walked into their clubhouse in early March with the U.S. surgeon general.

"Bender's face—what was left of it—jolted the Phillies so much that when they took the field that day, not a single cheek was filled with tobacco.

"'Put it this way,' said Bender, 31, a beekeeper in Montana, 'I have a face you will never forget.'

"Half a jaw. Partial tongue. Cavernous neck. Three remaining teeth. And scars he can't help but cut when he shaves the few hairs that still grow after radiation treatments. It took four operations to halt the mouth cancer doctors attributed to Bender's daily use of two cans of finely ground tobacco snuff, also known as dip, which he packed between his lower lip and gum.

"'He scared me out of the chimney,' said pitcher Terry Mulholland, who dipped for 17 years. 'I thought, "I'm 30 years old. It's time to grow up."'

"If major league baseball had its way, it would sever the growth at its roots. Smoking, dipping and chewing tobacco neither promote physical health nor portray a wholesome image for young people who idolize athletes.

"Mulholland quit dipping, but his teammates couldn't last. By the ninth inning, cheeks were bulging.

"Smokeless tobacco has been linked to baseball since the game's rules were roughed out in 1845. It was as easy to spit on the baseball field as on the corn field. Still is. A 1988 study funded by the National Cancer Institute found that 40 percent of pro players dip or chew, a figure that dwarfs use in other sports.

"Dipping half a tin of snuff daily is like inhaling 30 to 40 cigarettes. The nicotine is so addictive that it has been compared to heroin.

"Along with alcohol and cigars, Babe Ruth chewed vigorously and dipped. He even snorted snuff and was advised to stop because of impacted nasal passages. Ruth continued to do it all and died of throat cancer in 1948. He was 53.

"'A tobacco ban in baseball?' Pirates manager Jim Leyland responded with a cigar dangling from his mouth. 'It's ridiculous, a total invasion of privacy. We have a lot of other things we should be paying attention to rather than telling some poor SOB he can't put chew in his mouth.'"

And now this is Ann talking: I hope every baseball player who uses smokeless tobacco will take this seriously. Youngsters look up to you and think everything you do is cool. Do you want to be responsible for some kid ending up like Rick Bender? Please think about it.

Source: Susan Miller Degnan, Miami *Herald*, 9 October 1993: LIVING Section.

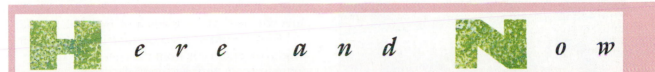

Major brands of chewing tobacco display prominent health warnings.

Since the mid-1980s, sales of chewing tobacco have declined, primarily because of negative publicity, price hikes, and legislation. Recent laws require that rotating warning labels be placed on smokeless products, as they are on cigarettes. What's more, smokeless tobacco can no longer be advertised on television and radio.

Secondhand and "Sidestream" Smoke

Studies of smoking and its effects have given increased attention to what is termed *secondhand smoke*—the smoke from burning tobacco that pollutes the air and is breathed in by smokers and nonsmokers alike. **"Sidestream" smoke**—that which comes directly from the lighted tip of a cigarette between puffs—is especially dangerous.

"Sidestream" smoke has much higher concentrations of some irritating and hazardous substances—such as carbon monoxide, nicotine, and ammonia—than inhaled ("mainstream") smoke. A recent national evening news telecast reported that secondhand smoke kills 50,000 nonsmokers yearly (*CBS Evening News* 1994). If several people smoke in an enclosed area, the carbon monoxide (CO) level may exceed the safe limit recommended by the Environmental Protection Agency (EPA). Nine parts CO per million (ppm) parts air is the regulatory limit, but this can easily be exceeded. Under conditions of heavy smoking and poor ventilation, concentrations of CO as high as 50 ppm can occur from sidestream smoke. CO is a gas and is not removed by most standard air filtration systems. It can only be diluted by increasing ventilation with fresh air containing low levels of CO. Formation of CO can be reduced by increasing the amount of oxygen available during the burning of the tobacco. This can be done by using perforated cigarette paper and perforated filtertips. Regular and small cigars produce more CO than cigarettes because the tobacco leaf wrapper reduces the amount of oxygen available at the burning zone. The levels of CO created by smokers may cause nonsmokers with coronary disease to have angina attacks.

Nicotine from sidestream smoke has a tendency to settle out of the air. The body absorbs small amounts from heavily polluted air, which are probably not hazardous.

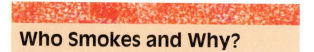

"SIDESTREAM" SMOKE smoke released into the air directly from the lighted tip of a cigarette

Who Smokes and Why?

Given what we know today about the effects of smoking, it's hard to understand why people smoke. Lifetime users are understandably addicted; quitting is hard. But why would anyone start smoking?

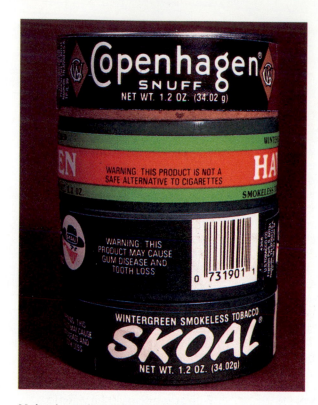

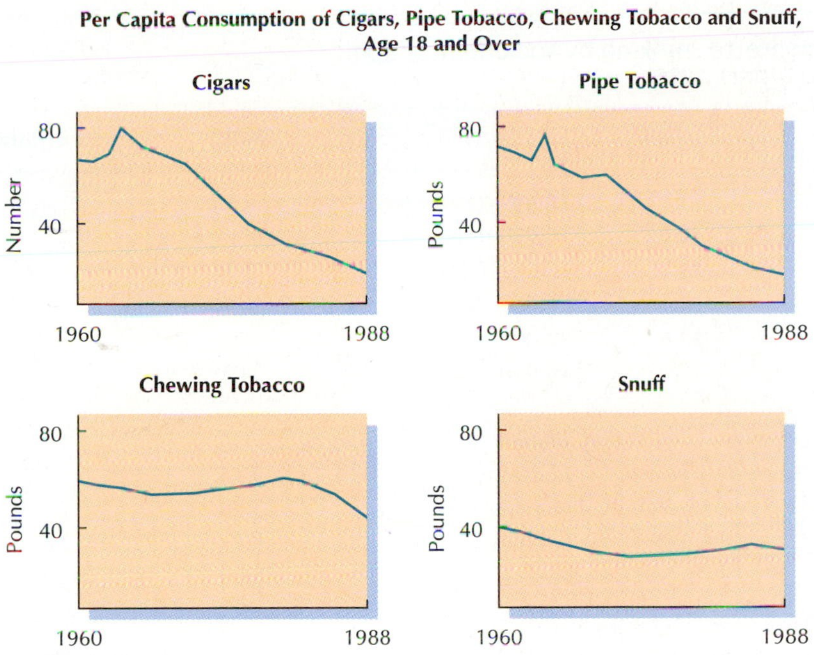

FIGURE 11.2 Per capita consumption of cigars, pipe tobacco, chewing tobacco and snuff, age 18 and over

The use of pipes, cigars, and smokeless tobacco has been declining for many years, except for one product, moist snuff. Sales of this product increased during the early 1980s.

Tobacco in any form is addictive and presents health risks. Those who smoke pipes and cigars are at greater risk of cancers of the oral cavity, larynx, pharynx, and esophagus and have higher death rates than nonsmokers, although not nearly as high as those of cigarette smokers. Smokeless tobacco is a cause of mouth cancer, other oral diseases, and other adverse health effects.

Young people who use smokeless tobacco often move on to cigarette smoking. In 1986, Congress became concerned that the use of smokeless tobacco was increasing among young people. It enacted legislation that bans its advertising on radio and television and requires health warnings on packages and in advertising. The warnings are "This product may cause mouth cancer," "This product may cause gum disease and tooth loss," and "This product is not a safe alternative to cigarettes."

Source: U.S. Department of Health and Human Services and Centers for Disease Control. *Smoking, Tobacco and Health: A Fact Book.* DHHS Publication no. (CDC) 87-8397. Washington, DC: USDHHS, October 1989:18.

Characteristics of Smokers

Recent surveys show that there has been a steady decline in tobacco use in the United States. Figure 11.2 illustrates a marked decline in the use of cigars, chewing tobacco, and smoking tobacco (used largely in pipes). Snuff consumption, on the other hand, increased in the early 1980s, after years of gradual decline. Reasons for this increase likely include the following: (1) snuff can be used anywhere, even in "no smoking" areas; (2) there has been an increase in outdoor advertising of the product; and (3) the fear associated with tobacco consumption has weakened somewhat in recent years (Foster et al. 1989, 124). In part, this is because the constant advertised messages and medical reports warning of the harmful effects of nicotine use may have saturated the environment of current smokers to the point of denying the harmful effects of tobacco use and/or abuse. As shown in Figure 11.2, however, the use of snuff has dropped off slightly in the last few years.

A long-term study on cigarette smoking found

TABLE 11.1 Prevalence of cigarette smoking by sociodemographic characteristics (17 years and older), 1986

	Male	Female		Male	Female
Marital status			***Household Income***		
Never married	25.5%	20.6%	10,000 or less	35.5	25.9
Currently married	29.5	24.1	10,001–20,000	31.8	25.6
Widowed	27.1	16.1	20,001–30,000	34.9	28.1
Separated or divorced	41.8	38.6	30,001–40,000	30.0	25.1
			40,000+	24.1	20.0
Education			***Region***		
11 or fewer years	38.0	27.8	Midwest	32.3	21.7
12 years	33.2	25.9	Northeast	28.0	24.0
13–15 years	25.4	22.9	Southeast	30.4	26.1
16+ years	18.0	13.5	West	26.7	22.7

Teenagers and Smoking

Teenagers appear to be turning away from cigarettes. In the years between 1976 and 1981, the percentage of high school seniors who smoke every day declined from 29% to 20%; since then, a small decline has occurred. Young men are doing much better than young women, and there are now more girls who smoke than boys.

Children take up smoking in three stages. The first is experimental; 70% of children experiment with smoking during the course of their childhood, 40% while they are still in grade school. The second, and more dangerous stage, is occasional use, on weekends, at parties, on dates. The final stage is when the young person becomes a confirmed, regular smoker. By the time the age of 20 is reached, the process is usually completed. About a third of the young men and young women at this age have become smokers and two-thirds have escaped.

Source: U.S. Department of Health and Human Services and Centers for Disease Control. *Smoking, Tobacco and Health: A Fact Book.* DHHS Publication no. (CDC) 87-8397. Washington, DC: USDHHS, October 1989:6.

that from 1944 to 1987 the percentage of U.S. adults (18 years and older) who smoke dropped nearly 10%. Furthermore, the latest findings show the following:[2]

1. Men smoke more than women. Twenty-four million men smoke, representing 32% of the total population, while 22.2 million women currently smoke cigarettes, representing 27% of the total population.
2. The highest percentage of smokers (37%) is between the ages of 35 and 44, and the second highest percentage of smokers (35%) is between the ages of 25 and 34.3. Smoking is highest among American Indians–Alaskan Natives and blacks, and Asian Pacific Islanders report the lowest.
3. Smoking is highest among American Indians–Alaskan Natives.
4. In comparing whites with African Americans, more African Americans smoke cigarettes (34% to 29%). Although the smoking rate for African Americans is higher than for white smokers, black smokers smoke fewer cigarettes per day. Also, in comparing these two races, African-American smokers suffer from a

[2] Numbers 1–4 are summarized from USDHHS and CDC 1993.

higher incidence of smoking-related illnesses than white smokers.

5. Smoking decreased with increasing educational levels. High school dropouts were most likely to smoke (36%), while college graduates were least likely to smoke (16%). (Also see Table 11.1 for additional sociodemographic findings.)
6. Overall findings show that the number of smokers in 1991 was virtually the same in 1990 (CDC 1990).

Other findings regarding the question "Have you, yourself, smoked any cigarettes in the past week?" is shown in Table 11.2. With the exceptions of certain years, cigarette smoking has been steadily declining from 40% in 1974 and 31% in 1986, to 27% in 1989 and 1990. National health surveys have also found that gender, education, and race and ethnicity strongly affect who is most likely to smoke. But researchers believe that educational achievement levels are better predictors of who is likely to smoke than gender (Pierce et al. 1989).

TABLE 11.2 Answers to the question: *"Have you smoked any cigarettes in the past week?"*

	Yes	No
1991 October–November	28%	72%
1990	27	73
1989	27	73
1988	32	68
1987	30	70
1986	31	69
1985	35	65
1983	38	62
1981	35	65
1978	36	64
1977	38	62
1974	40	60
1972	43	57
1971	42	58
1969	40	60
1957	42	58
1954	45	55
1949	44	56
1944	41	59

Source: Larry Hugick and Jennifer Leonard. "Despite Increasing Hostility, One in Four Americans Still Smokes." *Gallup Poll* 56, no. 29 (1 December 1991):4.

Youth and Smoking

Figure 11.3 shows that when comparing twelfth-graders (high school seniors) in their use of major licit and illicit drugs, tobacco use ranks highest (88%) lifetime prevalence and approximately 28% daily use (see also Table 11.1, "Teenagers and Smoking"). Other findings regarding cigarette smoking and youth are

1. By late adolescence, sizable proportions of young people still are establishing regular cigarette habits.
2. Of high school students who dropped out between the ages of 16 and 17, 55% reported smoking cigarettes as compared to 17% of students who smoke cigarettes but did not quit school (NIDA 1991a, 23).
3. The daily cigarette smoking rate for seniors did drop considerably between 1977 and 1981 (29 to 20%). However, it has dropped very little during the intervening 11 years (by another 3.1%, to 17.2%). Nearly a third of the seniors still do not feel there is a great risk associated with smoking.
4. Of serious concern, only 51% of eighth-grade students and 59% of tenth-grade students think that one-pack-a-day-smokers run a great risk of harm from smoking. In sum, our current health messages are not reaching U.S. youngsters.

Reasons for Smoking

About 30% of Americans continue to smoke, even though they are aware of its many potentially detrimental effects. Nearly 25% smoke over a pack a day.

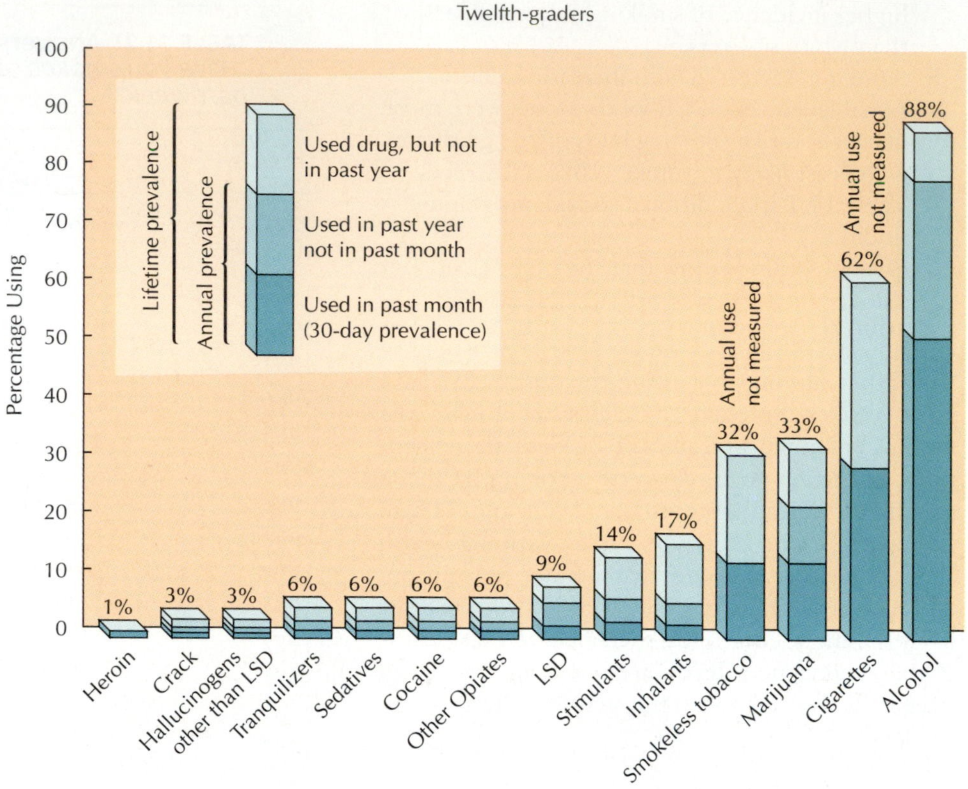

FIGURE 11.3 Prevalence and recency of use: various types of drugs for eighth-, tenth-, and twelfth-graders, 1992 *Source:* Lloyd D. Johnston, Patrick M. O'Malley, and Jerald G. Bachman. *National Survey Results from the Monitoring the Future Study, 1975–1992.* Vol. 1: *Secondary School Students.* Rockville, MD: National Institute on Drug Abuse, 1993:36.

If you were to ask tobacco users why they smoke, their answers would be quite similar:

1. It's relaxing.
2. It decreases the unpleasant effects of tension, anxiety, and anger.
3. It satisfies the craving.
4. It's a habit.
5. I do it for the stimulation, increased energy, and arousal.
6. I like manipulating objects/have become satisfying habits (the cigarette, pipe, and so on).

In addition,

7. Female high school students (34%) smoke to lose weight (Rovner 1991).
8. Nicotine functions as a mild tranquilizer moderating anxious or aggressive moods (Krough 1992).
9. Parents and/or siblings smoke (Rovner 1991).

A high level of dependence on tobacco should be expected, for a number of reasons:

1. The habit can be rapidly and frequently reinforced by inhaling tobacco smoke (about 10 reinforcements per cigarette, or 200 with one pack).

2. The rapid metabolism and clearance of nicotine allows frequent and repeated use, which is encouraged by the rapid onset of withdrawal symptoms.
3. Smoking has complex pharmacological effects, both central and peripheral, that may satisfy a variety of the smoker's needs.
4. Some groups offer psychological and social rewards for use, especially the peer groups of young people.
5. Smoking patterns can be generalized; that is, the smoker becomes conditioned to continue smoking with other activities. For example, some smokers feel the need to smoke after a meal, when driving, and so on.
6. Smoking is reinforced by both pharmacological effects and ritual.
7. There is no marked performance impairment; in fact, smoking enhances performance in some cases. (Nicotine produces a state of alertness, prevents deterioration of reaction time, and improves learning.)

These reasons may explain not only why people continue to smoke, but also why it is hard for them to stop. Smokers appear to regulate their intake of nicotine. The smoker with a low-nicotine cigarette is likely to smoke more and inhale more deeply. There appear to be specific nicotinic receptors in the brain that respond to nicotine. Consider that the average one-pack-a-day smoker is estimated to self-administer 70,000 pulses (one pulse per inhalation) of nicotine in a year. This surpasses by far the rate of any other known form of substance abuse. A habit that is reinforced as frequently and easily as smoking is very hard to break (Krasnegor 1979).

An incident that happened at Synanon, a treatment program for heroin addicts, illustrates how strong the smoking habit is. According to Synanon policy, addicts cannot use any drugs while being rehabilitated. In 1970, Synanon decided to ban cigarettes because of cost and because they seemed to serve as a crutch for people getting off other drugs. About 100 people left and chose possible readdiction to hard drugs rather than stay at Synanon without cigarettes. Residents of Synanon noted that the withdrawal symptoms for tobacco lasted much longer than those for other drugs, and they believed it was easier to quit heroin than cigarettes!

How to Stop Smoking

After having reached an epidemic peak in 1963—when per capita cigarette consumption among young adults, adults, and senior citizens aged 18 years and older was 4,345 cigarettes (USDHHS 1989, 2), per capita—cigarette smoking has been steadily decreasing, to 3,121 cigarettes in 1988. Today per capita number of cigarettes consumed is the lowest in 32 years. Although cigarette use steadily declines, "over 50 million adults still smoke, and each year one million teenagers take up smoking" (USDHHS 1989, 2).

In 1985, approximately 48.5 million Americans smoked cigarettes (Pierce et al. 1989, 63). The health damage has been estimated to cost the nation $37 billion a year in medical care, absenteeism, decreased work productivity, and accidents. As stated previously, smoking is the single most preventable environmental factor contributing to illness, disability, and death in the United States (Cook et al. 1990).

Withdrawal and Readdiction

When habitual smokers stop smoking, they may experience a variety of unpleasant withdrawal effects: craving for tobacco, irritability, restlessness, sleep disturbances, gastrointestinal disturbances, anxiety, and impairment of concentration, judgment, and psychomotor performance. The intensity of withdrawal effects may be mild, moderate, or severe and are not necessarily correlated to the amount the person smoked. (See the Case in Point box as an example of how difficult it is to permanently quit smoking.) The onset of these symptoms may occur within hours or days after quitting and may persist from a few days to several months. Frustration over these symptoms leads many people to start smoking again (Pomerleau 1979; Cook et al. 1990).

Even after the ex-smoker has overcome withdrawal symptoms during the first few weeks, he or she is still at risk. Various internal and external stimuli may serve as triggers for craving or withdrawal symptoms. Stressful situations—such as an

Case in Point

Profile of a Smoker

The following narrative, based on an interview with a 53-year-old man, illustrates some of the dilemmas faced by an older generation of smokers.

I guess I started smoking even before it was considered a drug! I was about 10, and we would steal cigarettes from our parents and smoke them in the back yard or away from our homes. At that age, we thought we were doing something against adults, and it felt fun to do something naughty. When we started, we didn't even know how to inhale.

Off and on until I was 17 or 18, I smoked occasionally, whenever my friends offered me a cigarette. I would follow the crowd. At 17 or so, I was buying cigarettes and carrying them around. I recall the menthols—Newport, Kool, Salem—also other nonmenthol cigarettes.

No health hazards were publicized when I was a kid, as this was before the Surgeon General issued his famous finding that smoking is hazardous to your health. I remember that it was more common to find adults smoking than not smoking. Movies and television programs were filled with smokers. Smoking was as normal as wearing clothes! Over the years, I really got used to smoking. I tried quitting four times, and sometimes I stopped for over two years. I switched to a pipe, then cigars, then cigarettes again. I think I tried smoking everything available in order to avoid any possible health hazards.

My health is fine, but I still worry whether I will ever develop cancer from smoking. I may have the beginnings of cancer right now and not even know it. I guess what you don't know, you don't worry about—until it's too late. Now I smoke about a pack of cigarettes per day, and just recently, I've been thinking about quitting again. I remember that, when I would go through weeks without smoking, I would slowly begin to feel better. No big change—just small things that add up to simply feeling better. I can usually breathe more clearly, my sinuses are not congested, and I don't have to look for out-of-the-way places to smoke so that people will not disapprove.

That's another thing: Today, society is against smoking. I never thought this would happen. I know several regular smokers who have to hide in their bedrooms or backrooms and offices with the doors shut in order to smoke a cigarette. This reminds me of the days when I used to smoke pot. Because it was illegal, we had to hide our smoking a joint. First spitting in public places became a violation of law when I was about 10 years old. Now, it won't be long before smoking cigarettes will be against the law.

Quitting is very hard once you're addicted to nicotine. In a London subway, I once saw a sign that said, "Addiction to nicotine is worse than addiction to heroin." At the time I first read this sign, I thought it was a complete exaggeration. But now, eight years later, I am convinced it's true.

Whenever I quit smoking, I go through weeks of anguish and craving for just one more cigarette. Yeah, quitting is really tough, especially during the first few days. The desire to smoke is very strong at first. But then slowly, ever so so slowly, the craving begins to fade. After three months, the worst is over. Yet, even after a year, you can suddenly think of how great it would be to have just one cigarette.

Whenever I go back to smoking after having stopped for several months, I would always convince myself that I could easily stop again and that my health would be fine if I only had one to three cigarettes per day. Now that I think back, I realize that I am probably a life-addicted person. I'm a lifer! Don't let anyone kid you: Nicotine is really a "hard-core" drug, and it's horribly addictive.

In this profile, can you find direct evidence proving the addictive qualities of tobacco?

Source: Interview conducted by Peter Venturelli, May 18, 1991.

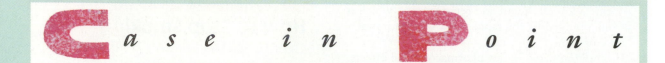

argument with a spouse, being with friends who smoke, and various types of social events—may cause a response similar to withdrawal. This sets the stage for readdiction.

Behavioral Treatments

The behavioral modification approach has proven successful in helping people to quit smoking. In most, fewer than half of the smokers quit, and of those who do, only 25 to 30% are still not smoking 9 to 18 months later. The long-term abstinence rate is about 13% (Pomerleau 1979). Most smokers who successfully quit first make five attempts (CDC, 1989). The three main types of behavioral treatment involve (1) punishment and aversive therapy, (2) stimulus control, and (3) substitute smoking procedures. Aversive conditioning techniques use cigarettes themselves to break the behavior pattern of smoking by making it so intense that it becomes unpleasant. A method called *rapid smoking* illustrates one successful use of aversive conditioning. The procedure is to have the person smoke cigarettes at a rapid rate, inhaling smoke about six seconds after each exhalation, until he or she cannot bear any more. Sessions are repeated daily until the person no longer desires to smoke. Follow-up sessions are held if the desire returns. The rapid smoking method essentially involves acute self-poisoning at a rate the person finds physiologically uncomfortable, compared to maintenance self-poisoning at the usual rate of smoking. This technique can be dangerously stressful for a person who has cardiovascular problems or reduced bronchopulmonary function.

Use of stimulus control is another approach to modification of smoking behavior. It is based on the assumption that smoking is associated with or controlled by environmental cues and that these cues contribute to the persistence of the habit. Programmed restriction of the stimuli that trigger smoking theoretically leads to a gradual elimination of smoking behavior. The person might be asked to keep a daily record of the circumstances in which he or she smokes each cigarette, which increases his or her awareness of smoking. Designated daily quotas can then be assigned as targets for reduction.

Generally, stimulus control by itself is not very effective. Better results are obtained when stimulus control procedures are combined with reward methods (for example, deposited money is reimbursed for reaching a goal) and other techniques. Multiple-method approaches give results about equal to those of the rapid smoking method, with 61% of the participants quitting smoking after eight sessions of treatment and 32% remaining nonsmokers after a year. Over longer periods of time, there is about a 50% return to addiction after treatment (Pomerleau 1979).

The American Cancer Society has developed a list of alternative activities the new ex-smoker might try as aids to get through the withdrawal period. When the craving for a cigarette arises, the smoker may substitute these behaviors:

Sip a glass of water.
Nibble on fruit, celery, or carrots.
Chew gum or spices such as ginger, cinnamon bark, or cloves.
Use nicotine replacements if necessary, such as lobeline sulphate tablets (unless you have an ulcer) or nicotine-containing gum.
Perform moderately strenuous physical activity, such as bicycling, jogging, or swimming (if the person's heart and lungs are not too damaged).
Spend as much time as possible in places where smoking is prohibited, such as movie theaters, libraries, and so on.
Use mouthwash after each meal.

We add a tip from personal experience (Venturelli):

Chew or slowly dissolve sugarless minted candy all day long.

And we might add: Get rid of drug paraphernalia, such as ashtrays and lighters. How serious a person is about quitting can often be gauged by how willing he or she is to give up an expensive ashtray, cigarette box, or engraved lighter.

Stop Smoking Aids

Nicorette Gum Besides self-help books and videotapes on smoking cessation, Nicorette, a nicotine chewing gum, has been developed. The purpose of this gum is to lessen the desire to smoke by substituting a cigarette for nicotine gum so that small amounts of nicotine can be absorbed in the mouth's lining and into the bloodstream ("Gum to Help You Stop Smoking" 1984; Krough 1992).

How successful is Nicorette in stopping smoking? When used with behavior programs, Nicorette's success is greatly increased (Grabowski and Hall 1985). Furthermore, the smoker's desire to quit and perseverance in adhering to a behaviorally based treatment program greatly increases the likelihood of quitting smoking.

The Nicotine Patch Another more recent medical approach to smoking cessation is the *nicotine patch,* which contains Nicoderm and Habitrol (see photo). The patch, directly applied and worn on the skin releases a continuous flow of small doses of nicotine to quell the desire for nicotine. The method of delivering nicotine to the skin reduces the nicotine withdrawal symptoms as the smoker attempts to quit.

The Motivation Not to Smoke

Although behavioral modification treatments are more effective than earlier methods, rates of 50% recidivism and 33% long-term abstinence leave considerable room for improvement. When relapse rates for heroin users, cigarette smokers, and alcoholics were plotted on graph paper, the curves for the percentage of relapse over a one-year period were virtually identical. However, these data were taken from people who sought treatment. Heroin users and alcoholics who quit drugs on their own have much higher success rates.

We actually know very little about the success rate for the estimated 30 million American smokers who have quit on their own. It could be that those who seek treatment have a more severe form of dependence (Jaffe and Kanzler 1979). Mark Twain once said that he could give up smoking with ease and had in fact done so, "hundreds of times."

Many pleasant changes take place within a few weeks after you stop smoking. There is a reduction in coughing, nasal discharge, and saliva production. Shortness of breath usually improves rapidly. Food tastes better, sleep is sounder, fatigue diminishes, breath odor improves, and tobacco stains on the teeth and fingers disappear.

More effective methods of motivating smokers to quit and of discouraging teenagers from starting are clearly needed. Changing social attitudes toward smoking are proving to have a strong effect on prevalence rates.

Although in 1993, 71% of respondents report having used cigarettes during their lifetime (Johnston et al. 1993), 26% of the current population continues to smoke. In comparing 1988 with 1992, the following percentages are encouraging:

Combined percentages of cigarette smokers and users of smokeless tobacco in U.S. population

	Percentages	
Age	**1988**	**1992**
12–17	15%	12%
18–25	41	38
26–34	40	38
35 and older	30	29

From these comparison percentages, we can see that across all age groups the use of nicotine continues to diminish, ever so slowly.

Social Issues: Looking to the Future

Economic Interests

The tobacco industry spends approximately $2.5 billion a year on advertising (Davis 1987)—more than any other industry. In fact, when the total spent on print and billboard advertising is broken down, the tobacco industry spends approximately $40 annually on every smoker in the United States (Liska 1990).

Although cigarette advertising was banned on

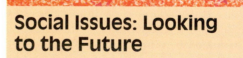

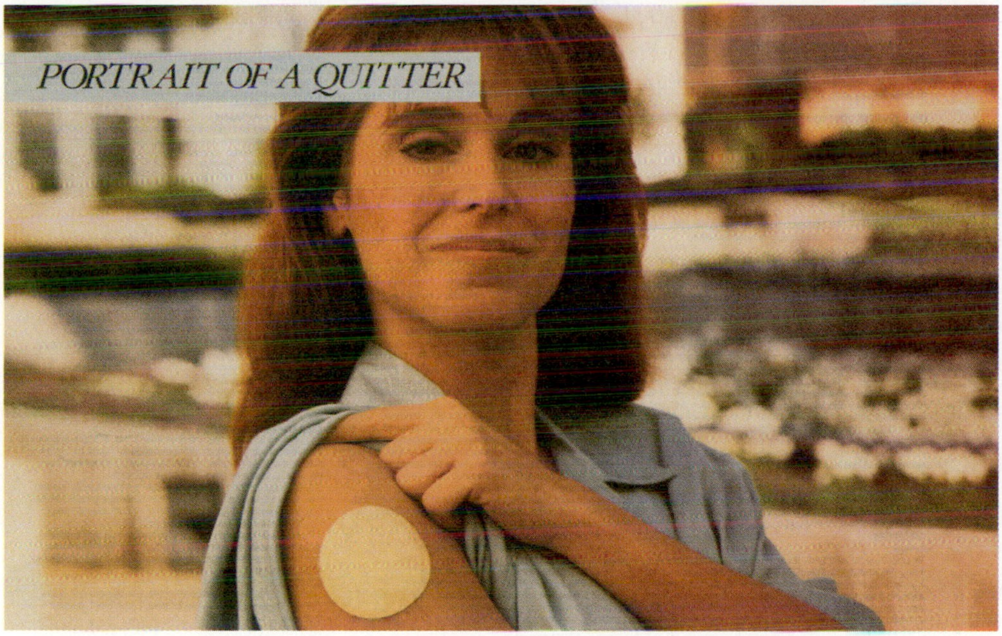

A transdermal patch, an example of a popular recent remedy for quitting smoking.

television in 1971, it has increased in magazines oriented to youth and women. Ads portray smokers to be sexy, healthy, and adventurous, enjoying recreation and close relationships with lovers and friends. All these themes are especially appealing to youth (Altman et al. 1987). Furthermore, the journal of the American Medical Association *(JAMA)* reported that the Camel cartoon character, popularly known as Joe Camel, is as recognizable to 6-year-olds as the Mickey Mouse silhouette that denotes the Disney Channel. In fact, the character is even familiar to many 3-year-olds and is generally more identifiable to children than to adults, according to the research (Rovner 1991).

Interestingly, as the consumption of cigarettes has declined in the United States, new markets abroad have increased. Western nations like the United States and Canada have been fairly successful in broadcasting that the use of tobacco is hazardous to your health. Per capita consumption in primarily nonindustrialized Third World countries has steadily increased with the availability of tobacco produced in the United States (see the Here and Now box).

American-brand cigarettes hold prestige for middle- and lower-class groups in many foreign societies. In India, for example, along with English cigarettes, U.S. cigarettes are considered superior in quality and are a status symbol for those who can afford to purchase such luxury items.

In some countries, such as China, approximately 90% of the male population smokes. Such nations represent an incredibly appealing market to U.S. cigarette manufacturers. Given the shrinking market in the United States as well as in most modern industrialized nations, U.S. manufacturers feel compelled to look overseas. They find lucrative markets in many Third World nations. Tobacco sales are becoming stronger in certain foreign markets while becoming weaker in others.

Here and Now

Should the United States Stop Peddling Its Cigarettes?

Americans have had access to considerable research showing the health-related hazards of smoking. The U.S. government has responded to this research with attempts to protect or at least warn the public about the dangers of smoking. The result has been a steady decline in the number of Americans who smoke.

Should the U.S. government extend its warning to those Third World nations in which smoking is on the rise? What responsibility does the United States have as a world leader to protect humanity, particularly those who are uneducated and oppressed? What responsibility does the federal government have to U.S. business interests, such as cigarette manufacturers?

Tobacco as a "Gateway" Drug

Just recently, conclusive research findings have indicated that tobacco is more of a serious **"gateway" drug** than previously expected. For example, nearly all heroin addicts initially began using "gateway" drugs such as alcohol and/or tobacco products. (Granted, most people who drink alcohol and use tobacco do not become heroin addicts!)

Biochemical evidence proving that the use of "gateway" drugs leads to the abuse of others is currently weak. But other findings are quite interesting. "The decisions to use tobacco or other gateway drugs set up **patterns of behavior** that make it easier for a user to go on to other drugs" ("Non-Smoking Youth" 1991). In other words, smokers have developed the behavioral patterns that may lead them to experiment and use other licit and illicit drugs.

How strong is this evidence? Figure 11.4 illustrates that daily smokers as opposed to nonsmokers are much more likely to engage in the use of controlled substances such as marijuana and cocaine. The University of Michigan's Institute for Social Research (NIDA 1990b) found that, of the high school seniors surveyed, cigarette smokers were 10 times more likely to use cocaine regularly than seniors who did not smoke. Also, the more a student smoked, the greater the likelihood of marijuana and cocaine use.

"GATEWAY" DRUGS drugs whose use leads to the use of other drugs: alcohol, cigarettes, and marijuana are considered "gateway" drugs

PATTERNS OF BEHAVIOR consistent and related behaviors that occur together, such as marijuana use and euphoria, alcohol abuse and intoxication

Smoking Prohibition Versus Smokers' Rights

In response to the percentage of the U.S. population that has effectively banned smoking from certain

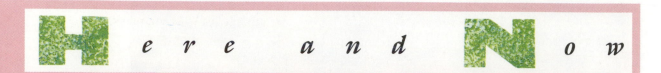

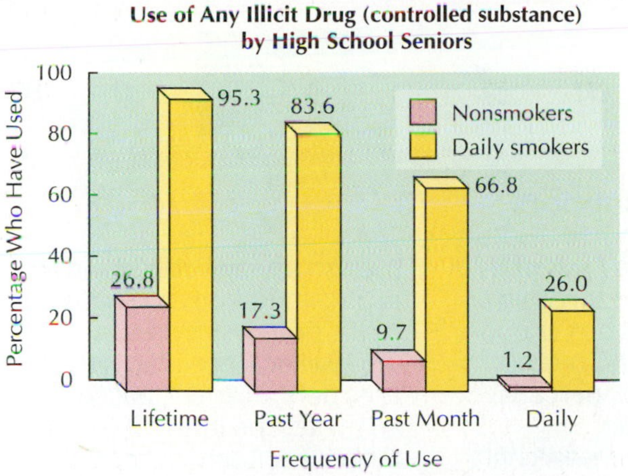

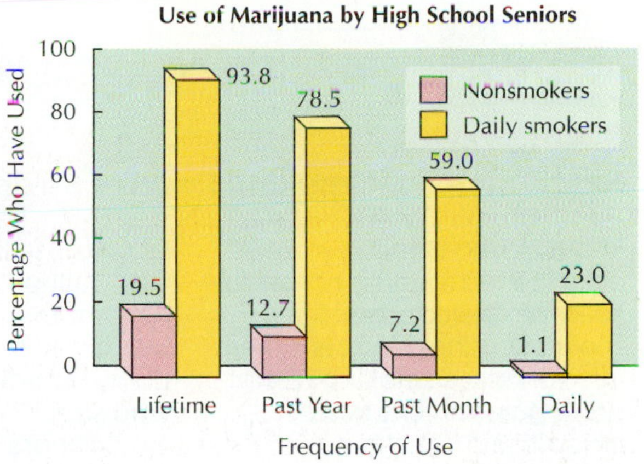

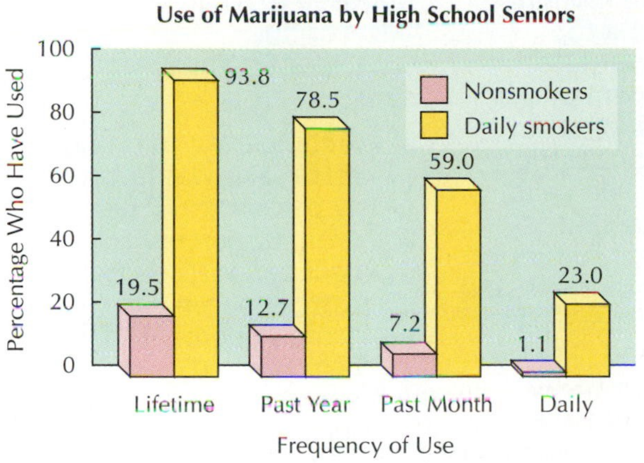

FIGURE 11.4 Use of illicit substances by daily nonsmokers and smokers. *Source:* In "Focus on 'Gateway Drugs' Non-Smoking Youth Better Resist Other Drugs." *Prevention Newsline* (Indiana Prevention Resource Center, Indiana University, Bloomington) 4, no. 3 (Spring 1991):4. Reprinted from L. D. Johnston, P. M. O'Malley, and J. G. Bachman, *National Trends in Drug Use and Related Factors Among American High School Students and Young Adults, 1975–1986*. Rockville, MD: National Institute on Drug Abuse, 1987.

public facilities, people who desire to continue smoking have formed action groups to press their right to smoke. These groups have largely been organized by several tobacco companies. Through mailing lists, newsletters, and slick magazine promotions, the groups advocate and report on

1. How the rights of smokers have been eroded in public and private places
2. How to write to members of Congress, and other political leaders, urging them to uphold smokers' rights
3. How to effectively lobby for smoking in the workplace
4. How the harmful effects of secondhand smoke have been exaggerated or remain unproven
5. How people who enjoy smoking have won major battles, preserving their right to smoke

Although some modest gains have been made by these groups, the trend to restrict and ban cigarette smoking continues to be very strong. Antismoking groups have been highly successful in their efforts (see the Here and Now box). Responding to a Gallup poll in July 1988, 60% of the population indicated they would like to see laws that ban smoking in public places. This view was supported by 26% of the smokers and 75% of the nonsmokers (Bezilla 1988). In yet other research findings, in response to the question "Would you favor or oppose a complete ban on smoking in all public places?" in 1987, 55% favored the idea and 43% were opposed to banning smoking in public places

Here and Now

Restrictions on Smoking Receive Strong Support

ATLANTA (AP)–Surveys from 10 U.S. cities—including one in the heart of tobacco country—show overwhelming sentiment for workplace smoking restrictions, government health officials said Thursday.

These surveys also found widespread support for outlawing tobacco advertising, the Centers for Disease Control reported.

Support for restricting smoking in the workplace ranged from 90 percent to 95 percent, the CDC said. From 47 percent to 73 percent of respondents called for a total ban on tobacco advertising.

But while large majorities favored restricting smoking in private workplaces, only 10 percent to 29 percent called for a total smoking ban there.

"The really compelling thing . . . is that we consistently got the same results. It shows this belief is nationwide," said Russell Sciandra, a Buffalo, N.Y., cancer researcher working with the survey project.

The survey results are similar to those in previous polls. A 1990 Gallup Poll report said 94 percent of Americans support workplace smoking restrictions, including 25 percent who support a ban.

Sciandra said researchers were particularly surprised by the numbers from Raleigh, N.C., the capital of a top tobacco-producing state.

There, 92 percent of the adults surveyed supported workplace smoking restrictions, including 14 percent who wanted it stopped entirely; 98 percent supported restrictions in restaurants; and 47 percent supported a ban on tobacco advertising.

"In the heart of tobacco country, even though the numbers tend to be lower than the rest of the country, we have strong support for smoking restrictions and restrictions on tobacco marketing," said Sciandra, associate director of the smoking control program at the Roswell Park Cancer Institute of Buffalo, N.Y.

"When you get almost a majority of the people in Raleigh saying tobacco advertising should be eliminated, that's pretty strong."

Walker Merryman, vice president of the Tobacco Institute, the industry's trade association, said other polls have shown most Americans opposed to a ban on cigarette advertising.

Other findings from the 10 surveys:

- A complete ban on cigarette sales was favored by 17 percent to 49 percent.
- From 62 percent to 74 percent supported smoking restrictions in bars.
- From 77 percent to 93 percent favored fining merchants selling tobacco to minors.
- And 31 percent to 56 percent thought tobacco companies should not be allowed to sponsor cultural or sports events.

Source: Associated Press. "Restrictions on Smoking Receive Support." *Vidette Messenger* (Valparaiso, IN), (31 May 1991):C1.

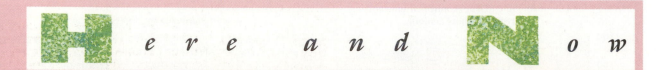

(Hugick and Leonard 1991). Increased sentiment in favor of more restrictions has even touched the heart of tobacco country, Raleigh, North Carolina! In short, the willingness of nonsmokers to speak up as firmly as necessary against being exposed to secondhand smoke is affecting smoking habits.

A complete network of state laws restricts smoking. From a regional perspective, many states in the south (especially the "Deep South") are least restrictive, while many northeastern states are more restrictive. As of March 1989, 44 states restricted smoking in any public places, 27 limited smoking in restaurants, 32 limited smoking in public worksites, and 19 limited smoking in private worksites—(Foster et al. 1989, 135). Currently, all domestic airline flights ban smoking.

Several organized groups of nonsmokers have made quite an impact, including Action on Smoking and Health (ASH), the Group Against Smokers' Pollution (GASP), the American Lung Association, the American Cancer Society, and medical and dental associations. These groups have been instrumental in passing legislation restricting or banning smoking in public places; banning cigarette commercials on television; and prohibiting smoking on commercial aircraft, interstate buses, and in some restaurants, elevators, indoor theaters, libraries, art galleries, and museums.

Future Smokers

Not much research addresses who future smokers are likely to be. One study predicted that smokers will change because some subpopulations are not quitting (Coambs et al. 1988). This study surveyed 736 **"die-hard"** smokers, those who are defined as "least likely to quit." The respondents were divided into two groups: more and less likely to continue smoking. Based on a series of questions about attitudes toward smoking, the reluctant quitters had the following characteristics:

1. They started smoking at a younger age; 36% started between ages 16 and 18, and 4% began under 16 (Hugick and Leonard 1991).
2. They smoked the strongest brands.
3. They were not particularly concerned with the health-related effects of smoking.
4. Smokers over the age of 40 were more physically dependent on nicotine than those under 40.

"Die-hard" smokers were believed to continue smoking because of denial rather than ignorance. Apparently, they either refuse to admit the health consequences of smoking, or they simply avoid the health warnings by subscribing to the view that "It won't happen to me."

Review Questions

1. If smoking is the most preventable cause of disease and premature death in the United States, why do people continue to smoke?
2. How effective are the health warning labels on cigarette packages? Interview two or three smokers about the warning labels.
3. List and define the diseases cigarette smokers are most likely to contract.
4. What effects do cigarettes have on the fetus?
5. Why is smokeless tobacco perceived as safer than other forms of tobacco?
6. What behavioral treatments are available for smoking cessation?
7. Who is more likely to smoke, and why?
8. Why do people who smoke become dependent on tobacco?
9. As tobacco markets in the United States have shrunk, what has happened abroad?

"DIE-HARDS" slang term for drug users who strongly resist quitting

10. Explain why tobacco is a gateway drug.
11. Explain the differences between smoking prohibition groups and smokers' rights groups.
12. How do you feel about tobacco advertising? How about tobacco advertising at sporting events?

Key Terms

Nicotiana tabacum
tobacco chewing
snuff dipping
emphysema
sudden infant death syndrome (SIDS)
secondhand smoke
smokeless tobacco
"sidestream" smoke
"gateway" drugs
patterns of behavior
"die-hards"

Summary

1. Nicotine is by far one of the most addictive drugs.
2. Tobacco farming is the sixth largest cash crop in the United States. Ranking ahead of it are corn, soybeans, hay, wheat, and cotton.
3. The quality of leaf tobacco has changed throughout years of production. Since 1956, the amount of leaf tobacco in a cigarette has gone down by approximately 25%. Most cigarettes today are low-tar and low-nicotine types, and 90% are filtertips.
4. Cigarette consumption in the United States is declining while the exportation and use of cigarettes abroad is increasing. Latest surveys indicate that, while the percentage of teenagers who first use tobacco is slowly declining, a high percentage continue to try tobacco.
5. National health surveys found that gender, education, and race and ethnicity strongly affect who is most likely to smoke. Findings show that, the more education you have, the less likely you are to smoke. Men are more likely to smoke than women, and African Americans are more likely to smoke than whites.
6. Users of such "gateway" drugs as alcohol and cigarettes are more easily allured than nonusers into experimenting with other licit and illicit drugs.
7. Tobacco products classified as *smokeless tobacco* include chewing tobacco and snuff. *"Sidestream" smoke* comes directly from the lighted tip of a cigarette between puffs and has much higher concentrations of irritating and hazardous substances. *Secondhand smoke* includes all smoke from tobacco products released into the air.
8. Nicotine is the substance in tobacco that causes dependence. This drug initially stimulates and then depresses the nervous system.
9. Research clearly shows that the tar and nicotine contents of cigarettes affect mortality rates. Cigarette smokers tend to die at an earlier age than nonsmokers. They also have a greater probability of contracting various illnesses: types of cancers; chronic bronchitis and emphysema; diseases of the cardiovascular system; and peptic ulcers. Finally, smoking also has adverse effects on pregnancy and may harm the fetus.
10. Because of all the negative publicity regarding cigarette smoking, prohibitionists versus smokers' rights groups are challenging one another.
11. The main types of behavioral treatment for the cessation of smoking are (a) punishment and aversive therapy, (b) stimulus control, and (c) substitute smoking procedures.

References

Altman, D. G., M. D. Slater, C. L. Albright, and N. Maccoby. "How an Unhealthy Product Is Sold: Cigarette Advertising in Magazines, 1960–1985." *Journal of Communication* 37 (1987): 95–106.

American Cancer Society. *Cancer Facts and Figures.* Atlanta, GA: American Cancer Society, 1990.

Armitrage, A. K., C. T. Dollery, C. F. George, T. H. Houseman, P. J. Lewis, and P. M. Turner. "Absorption and Metabolism of Nicotine from Cigarettes." *British Medical Journal* 4 (1985): 313–16.

Associated Press. "Restrictions on Smoking Receive Support." *Vidette Messenger* (Valparaiso, IN), (31 May 1991): C1.

Austin, G. A. *Perspectives on the History of Psychoactive Substance Use.* Washington, DC: National Institute on Drug Abuse, 1978.

Benowitz, N. L. "Pharmacological Aspects of Cigarette Smoking and Nicotine Addiction." *New England Journal of Medicine* 319 (1988): 1318–30.

"Beware Those Spicy Cigarettes." *Consumer Reports* 50 (1985): 641.

Bezilla, R., ed. *America's Youth 1977–1988.* Princeton, NJ: Gallup Organization, 1988.

Callahan, M. "How Smoking Kills You." *Parade Magazine* 213 (December 1987): 209–11.

CBS Evening News (8 February 1994), New York, NY.

Centers for Disease Control (CDC). "The Surgeon General's 1989 Report on Reducing The Health Consequence of Smoking: 25 Years of Progress (Executive Summary)." *Morbidity and Mortality Weekly Report* 38, Supplement 5-2 (1989): 1.

Centers for Disease Control (CDC). "Cigarette Smoking Among Adults—United States." *MMWR* 41 (1990): 354–55, 361–62.

"Cigarette Smoking Among Adults—United States, 1991." *Morbidity and Mortality Weekly Report* 42, no. 12 (2 April 1993): 230–33.

"Cigars." *Encyclopedia Americana.* Danbury, CT: Grolier, 1988.

Coambs, R., L. James, F. Fliger, and S. Li. "Characterizing Future Smokers." In *Problems and Drug Dependence, 1988,* edited by L. S. Harris. Washington, DC: National Institute on Drug Abuse, 1988.

Cook, Paddy Shannon, Robert C. Petersen, and Dorothy Tuell Moore. "Alcohol, Tobacco, and Other Drugs May Harm the Unborn." Rockville, MD: U.S. Department of Health and Human Services, 1990.

Corti, E. C. *A History of Smoking.* London: Harrap, 1931.

Davis, R. M. "Current Trends in Cigarette Advertising and Marketing." *New England Journal of Medicine* 316 (1987): 725–32.

DeAngelis, T. "Behavior Is Included in Report on Smoking." *APA Monitor* 20, no. 3 (1989): 1, 4.

Degnan, Susan Miller, Miami *Herald,* 9 October 1993: LIVING Section.

Fiore, M. C., T. E. Novotny, J. P. Pierce, E. J. Hatziandreau, K. M. Patel, and R. M. Davis. "Trends in Cigarette Smoking in the U.S.—The Changing Influence of Gender and Race." *JAMA* 261 (January 1989): 49–56.

"Focus on 'Gateway Drugs' Non-Smoking Youth Better Resist Other Drugs." *Prevention Newsline* 4, no. 3 (Spring 1991): 4.

Fort, Joel. *The Pleasure Seekers.* Indianapolis: Bobbs-Merill, 1969.

Foster, Carol D., N. R. Jacobs, and M. A. Siegel, eds. *Illegal Drugs and Alcohol—America's Anguish.* Wylie, TX: Information Plus, 1989.

Gonzales, M., and B. Edmonson. "The Smoking Class." *American Demographics* 10, no. 11. (November 1988): 34–37.

Grabowski, Hon, and Sharon M. Hall, eds. *Pharmacological Adjuncts in Smoking Cessation.* Washington, DC: U.S. Government Printing Office, 1985.

Heimann, R. K. *Tobacco and Americans.* New York: McGraw-Hill, 1960.

Hugick, Larry, and Jennifer Leonard. "Despite Increasing Hostility, One in Four Americans Still Smokes." *Gallup Poll News Services* 56, no. 29 (1 December 1991): 1–7.

Jaffe, J. H., and M. Kanzler. "Smoking as an Addictive Disorder." In *Cigarette Smoking as a Dependence Process,* Research Monograph 23, edited by N. A. Krasnegor, 4–23. Washington, DC: National Institute on Drug Abuse, U.S. Department of Health, Education, and Welfare, 1979.

Johnston, L. D., P. M. O'Malley, and J. G. Bachman. *National Survey Results from the Monitoring the Future Study, 1975–1992.* Vol. 1: *Secondary School Students.* Rockville, MD: National Institute on Drug Abuse, 1993.

Kilbourne, Jean. "Advertising Addiction: The Alcohol Industry's Hard Sell." *Multinational Monitor* (June 1989): 13–16.

Krasnegor, N. A. "Introduction." In *The Behavioral Aspects of Smoking,* Research Monograph 26, edited by N. A. Krasnegor, 1–6. Washington, DC: National

Institute on Drug Abuse, Department of Health, Education, and Welfare, 1979.

Krough, David. "Smoking—Why Is It so Hard to Quit? Priorities of the American Council on Science and Health," New York, NY (Spring 1992): 29–32.

Langton, P. A. *Drug Use and the Alcohol Dilemma.* Boston: Allyn and Bacon, 1991.

Liska, Ken. *Drugs and the Human Body.* New York: Macmillan, 1990.

Morris, D. "Gum to Help You Stop Smoking." *Consumer Reports* 49, no. 8 (August 1984): 37–39.

National Institute on Drug Abuse (NIDA). *Facts About Teenagers and Drug Abuse.* NIDA Capsule 17, 2. Rockville, MD: NIDA, U.S. Department of Health and Human Services, January 1990a. Photocopy.

National Institute on Drug Abuse (NIDA). *Monitoring the Future Study.* Ann Arbor, MI: Institute for Social Research, 1990b.

National Institute on Drug Abuse (NIDA). *Drug Use Among Youth: Findings from the 1988 Household Survey on Drug Abuse.* DHHS Pub. no. (ADM) 91-1765. Rockville, MD: NIDA, 1991a.

National Institute on Drug Abuse (NIDA). "Population Estimates of Lifetime and Current Drug Use, 1991." Capsule 22. Rockville, MD: NIDA, 1991b.

"Non-Smoking Youth Better Resist Other Drugs." *Prevention Newsline* 4, no. 3 (Spring 1991): 5.

Office of Smoking and Health, U.S. Department of Health and Human Services, *Reducing the Health Consequences of Smoking: 25 Years of Progress: A Report of the Surgeon General.* DHHS Pub. no. (CDC) 89-8411. Washington, DC: USDHHS, 1989.

Palfai, T., and H. Jankiewicz. *Drugs and Human Behavior.* Dubuque, IA: Brown, 1991.

Perry, S. "Recognizing Everyday Addicts." *Current Health* 2, no. 16 (May 1990): 20–23.

Pierce, J. J., et al. "Trends in Cigarette Smoking in the United States—Educational Differences Are Increasing." *Journal of the American Medical Association* 261 (6 January 1989): 23–32.

Pomerleau, O. F. "Behavioral Factors in the Establishment, Maintenance, and Cessation of Smoking." In *The Behavioral Aspects of Smoking,* Research Monograph 26, edited by N. A. Krasnegor, 47–67. Washington, DC: National Institute on Drug Abuse, U.S. Department of Health, Education, and Welfare, 1979.

Rovner, Sandy. "Up in Smoke: Why Do So Many Kids Ignore All the Evidence Condemning Cigarettes?" *Washington Post,* National Weekly Edition, (16–22 December 1991).

Schultes, R. E. "Ethnopharmacological Significance of Psychotropic Drugs of Vegetal Origin." In *Principles of Psychopharmacology,* 2d ed., edited by W. G. Clark and J. del Giudice, 41–70. New York: Academic Press, 1978.

"Smokeless Tobacco, Think Before You Chew." Leaflet. Chicago, IL: American Dental Association, 1990.

Stellman, S. D., and L. Garfinkel. "Smoking Habits and Tar Levels in a New American Cancer Society Prospective Study of 1.2 Million Men and Women." *Journal of the National Cancer Institute* 76 (1986):1057–63.

Substance Abuse and Mental Health Services Administration (SAMHSA), Office of Applied Studies. *1992 National Household Survey on Drug Abuse.* Rockville, MD: U.S. Department of Health and Human Services, June 1993.

Taylor, P. "Ganglionic Stimulating and Blocking Agents." In *The Pharmacological Basis of Therapeutics,* 6th ed., edited by A. G. Gilman, L. S. Goodman, and A. Gilman, 211–19. New York: Macmillan, 1980.

Tobacco Institute. "About Tobacco Smoke." Washington, DC: Tobacco Institute, 1982.

Tobacco Industry Profile. Washington, DC: Tobacco Institute, 1988.

Tolchin, M. "Surgeon General Asserts That Smoking Is an Addiction." *New York Times,* 17 May 1988, pp. 1, 26.

U.S. Bureau of the Census, *Statistical Abstract of the United States, 1993.* 113th ed. Washington, DC: U.S. Government Printing Office, 1993.

U.S. Department of Health and Human Services (USDHHS) and Centers for Disease Control (CDC). *Smoking, Tobacco and Health: A Fact Book.* DHHS Publication no. (CDC) 87-8397, October 1989. Washington, DC: USDHHS.

U.S. Department of Health and Human Services (USDHHS) and Centers for Disease Control (CDC). "Current Trends: Use of Smokeless Tobacco Among Adults—United States, 1991." *Morbidity and Mortality Weekly Report,* 42, no. 14 (16 April 1993): 263–66.

U.S. Department of Agriculture. *Annual Report on Tobacco Statistics, and the Tobacco Outlook and Situation Report.* Washington, DC: 1988, chapter 10.

U.S. Surgeon General. *Smoking and Health: A Report of the Surgeon General.* Publication no. (PHS) 79-50066. Washington, DC: U.S. Department of Health, Education, and Welfare, 1979.

U.S. Surgeon General. *The Changing Cigarette.* Publication no. (PHS) 81-51056. Washington, DC:

U.S. Department of Health, Education, and Welfare, 1981.

U.S. Surgeon General. *The Health Consequences of Smoking*. Washington, DC: 1984.

U.S. Surgeon General. *The Health Consequences of Smoking: Cancer and Chronic Lung Disease in the Workplace*. Washington, DC: U.S. Government Printing Office, 1985.

Volle, R. L., and G. B. Koelle. "Ganglionic Stimulating and Blocking Agents." In *The Pharmacological Basis of Therapeutics*, 6th ed., edited by L. S. Goodman and A. Gilman, 565–74. New York: Macmillan, 1975.

Wolfe, R. "Smokeless Tobacco, the Fatal Pitch." *Multinational Monitor* (July–August 1987): 20–21.

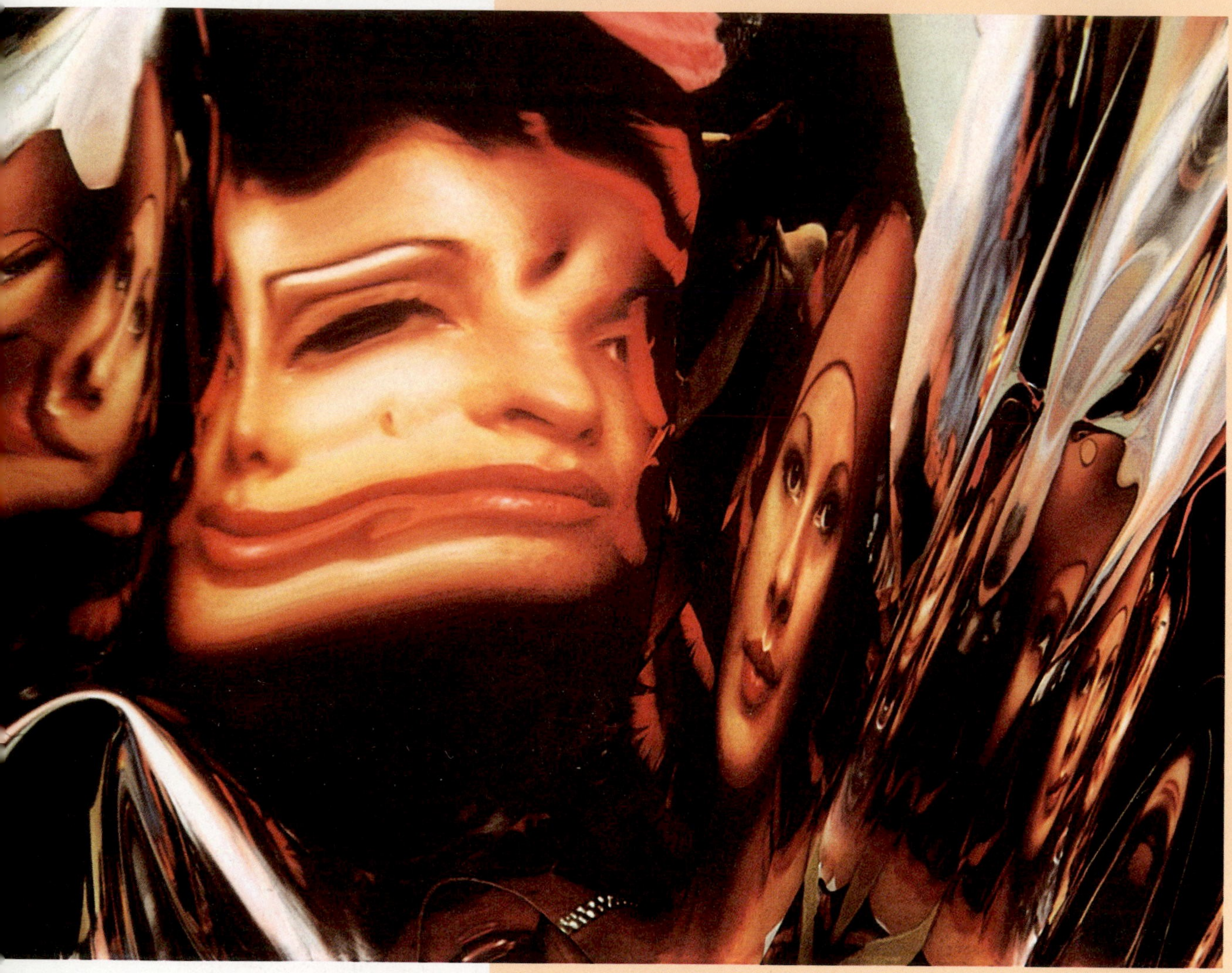

Chapter 12

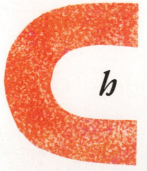

DID YOU KNOW THAT . . .

- Many of the ancient mystics used hallucinogens as part of their religious ceremonies.
- Hallucinogens were abused by relatively few people in the United States until the social upheaval of the 1960s.
- The Native American Church in the United States can legally use the psychedelic mescaline as part of its religious ceremonies.
- Some hallucinogens—such as LSD, MDA, and "Ecstasy"—have been used by psychiatrists to assist in psychotherapy with certain patients.
- Hallucinogens such as LSD do not tend to cause physical dependence.
- The senses are grossly exaggerated and distorted under the influence of hallucinogens.
- For some users, hallucinogens can cause frightening, nightmarish experiences called "bad trips."
- PCP was originally developed as a general anesthetic.
- PCP is commonly used as an additive in "street" hallucinogens.
- Intense use of PCP can cause psychotic episodes accompanied by tremendous strength, making management of users by medical or law enforcement personnel very dangerous.
- Inhalant drugs of abuse can cause permanent damage to the brain, the heart, and other organs.

Hallucinogens

LEARNING OBJECTIVES

On completing this chapter, you will be able to

1. Identify the three principal types of hallucinogens and their four principal hallucinogenic effects.
2. Explain why hallucinogens became so popular during the 1960s but are less commonly used today.
3. Describe the nature of the sensory changes that occur due to the influence of hallucinogens.
4. Outline how psychedelic, stimulant, and anticholinergic effects are expressed in the three principal types of hallucinogens.
5. Describe the rationale for using hallucinogens in psychotherapy.
6. Explain how the abuse liability of hallucinogens differs from that associated with other commonly abused drugs.
7. Describe what effects environment and personality have on the individual's response to hallucinogens.
8. Discuss the occurrence of psychosis and "flashbacks" following LSD use.
9. Identify the problems of purity with "street" LSD.
10. Characterize how PCP differs from other hallucinogens.
11. Identify the abused inhalants, who uses them, and what hazards they cause.

Healthy People 2000

Reduce drug abuse-related hospital emergency department visits by at least 20%.

We have drunk the Soma and become immortal!
We have attained the light, we have found the Gods!
What can the malice of mortal man
or his spite, O Immortal, do to us now?

—Rig Veda, Book VII, 48 (in Panikkar 1977)

This ancient Sanskrit hymn dates back to 1500 B.C. Some researchers believe Soma may have been the mushroom *Amanita muscaria,* which causes hallucinations. Others believe Soma was hashish or even nutmeg preparations. People have known and written about drug-related hallucinations for centuries. Throughout the ages, individuals who saw visions or experienced hallucinations were perceived as being holy or sacred, receiving divine messages, or possibly as being bewitched and controlled by the devil. There are many indications that medicine men, shamans, witches, oracles, and perhaps mystics and priests of various groups were familiar with drugs and herbs that caused such experiences and today are known as *hallucinogens.*

In this chapter, we will begin with a brief historical review of the use of hallucinogens, tracing the trend in the United States from the 1960s to today. Next, the nature of hallucinogens and the effects they produce will be examined. The rest of the chapter addresses the various types of psychedelic agents: LSD types, phenylethylamines, anticholinergics, and other miscellaneous substances.

HALLUCINOGENS substances that alter sensory processing in the brain, causing perceptual disturbances, changes in thought processing, and depersonalization

PSYCHOTOMIMETIC substances that cause psychosis-like symptoms

The History of Hallucinogen Use

Probably the oldest record of **hallucinogens** in the Western hemisphere is a 4,500-year-old grave of a South American Indian, which contained a snuff tube and some snuff (see Figure 12.1). This type of snuff—called *cohoba snuff*—is still being used today by some native tribes in that region. Its active ingredient is dimethyltryptamine (DMT), which is a fairly potent hallucinogen.

Prior to the 1960s in the United States, several psychedelic substances, such as mescaline from the peyote cactus, could be obtained from chemical supply houses with no restriction. Abuse of hallucinogens did not become a major social problem in this country until this decade of racial struggles, the Vietnam War, and violent demonstrations. Many individuals frustrated with the hypocrisy of "the establishment" tried to "turn on and tune in" by using hallucinogens as pharmacological crutches.

Psychedelic drugs became especially popular because some medical professionals such as Harvard psychology professor, Timothy Leary, reported that these drugs allowed users to get in touch with themselves and achieve a peaceful inner serenity. At the same time, it became well publicized that the natural psychedelics (such as mescaline and peyote) were and had been for many years used routinely by some religious organizations of Native Americans for enhancing spiritual experiences. This contributed to the mystical, supernatural aura associated with hallucinogenic agents and added to their enticement to a so-called dropout generation.

However, with widespread use of LSD, it was observed that this and similar drugs may induce a form of psychosis like schizophrenia (American Psychiatric Association 1994). The term **psychotomimetic** was coined to describe these compounds; it means "psychosis mimicking" and is still used in medicine today. The basis for the designation is the effects of these drugs that induce mental states that impair ability to recognize and respond appropriately to reality.

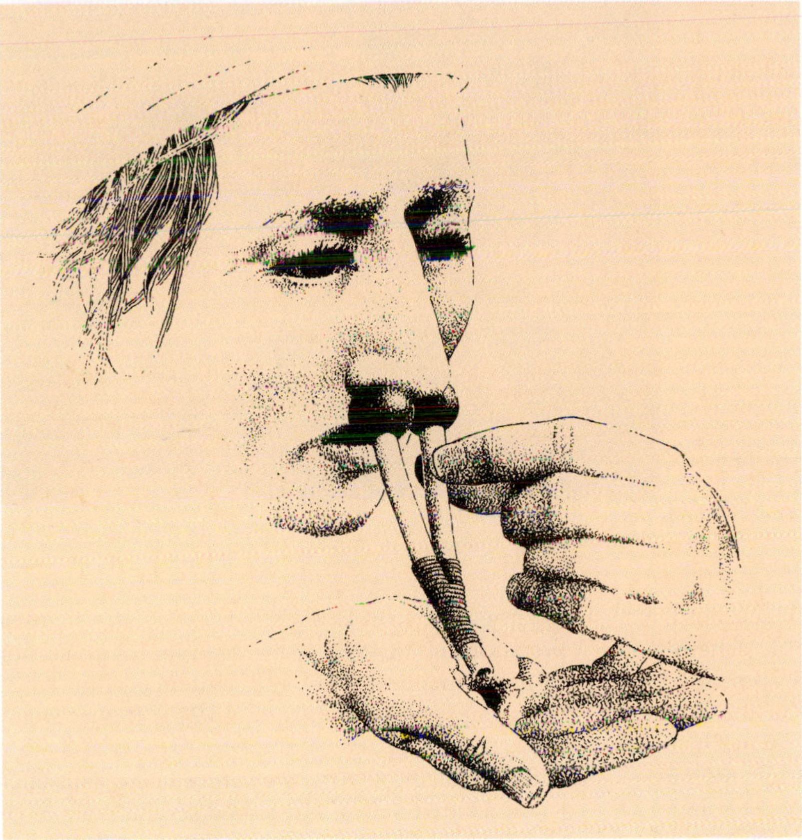

FIGURE 12.1 A South American Indian using a *tabaco,* or snuff tube.

By the mid-1960s, federal regulatory agencies became concerned with the misuse of hallucinogens and the potential emotional damage caused by these drugs. Access to hallucinogenic agents was restricted, and laws against their distribution were passed. Despite the problems of the psychedelics, some groups demanded that they be allowed to use these substances.

The Native American Church

Peyote plays a central role in the ceremonies of Native Americans who follow a religion that is a combination of Christian doctrine and Native American religious rituals. They are located as far north as Canada. They believe that God made a special gift of this sacramental plant to them so that they might commune more directly with him. The first organized peyote church was the First-Born Church of Christ, incorporated in 1914 in Oklahoma. The Native American Church of the United States was chartered in 1918 and is the largest such group at present (approximately 100,000 to 200,000 members).

Because of the religious beliefs of the members of the Native American Church concerning the powers of peyote, when Congress legislated against its use in 1965, it allowed room for religious use of this psychedelic plant. The American Indian Religious Freedom Act of 1978 made clear the intent of Congress was that the members of the Native American Church should be allowed access to peyote due to constitutional guarantees of religious freedom. The Drug Enforcement Administration (DEA) acknowledged the intent of the Congress and issued permits to church members to buy and distribute small, legal quantities of peyote. These arrangements continued unquestioned until 1990, when a decision by the U.S. Supreme Court ruled that users of peyote for religious purposes are not

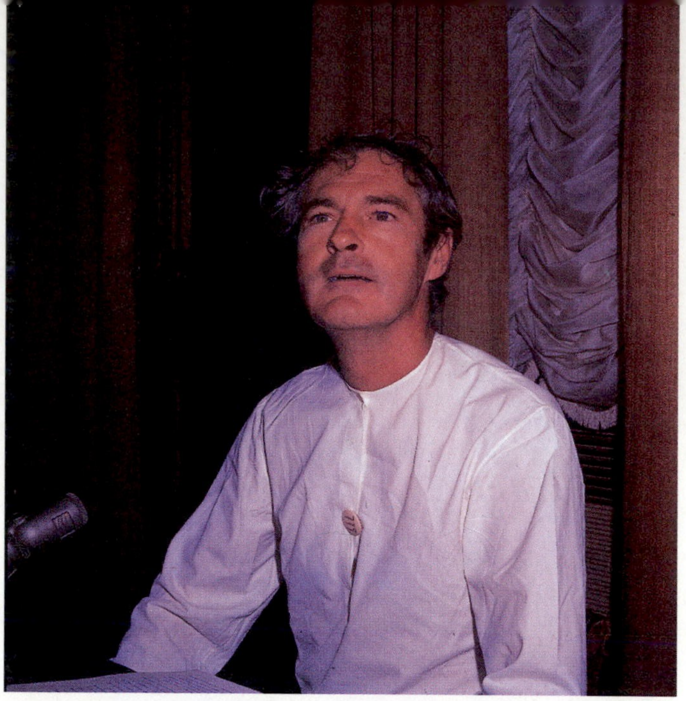

Timothy Leary attempted to legalize LSD in the 1960s

excluded from rules or regulations required by employers concerning the use of scheduled substances. This decision removed some of the constitutional protection enjoyed by the Native American Church and again has brought into question the use of peyote by church members ("Indian Religion" 1990). However, the religious use of peyote by members of the North American Church continues to be allowed by the DEA.

Timothy Leary and the League of Spiritual Discovery

In 1966, three years after being fired by Harvard because of his controversial involvement with hallucinogens, Timothy Leary also attempted a constitutional strategy to retain legitimate access to LSD. He began a religion called the League of Spiritual Discovery; LSD was the sacrament. This unorthodox religious orientation to the LSD experience was presented in a manual called *The Psychedelic Experience* (Leary et al. 1964), which was based on the Tibetan Book of the Dead. It became the "bible" of the psychedelic drug movement.

The movement grew, but most members used "street" LSD and did not follow Leary's directions. Leary believed that the hallucinogenic experience was only beneficial under proper control and guidance. But the members of this so-called religion merely used the organization as a front to gain access to an illegal drug. Federal authorities did not agree with Leary's *freedom of religion* interpretation and in 1969 convicted him for possession of marijuana and LSD and sentenced him to 20 years imprisonment (Stone 1991). Before being incarcerated, Leary escaped to Algeria and wandered for a couple of years before being extradited to the United States. He served several years in jail and was released in 1976.

Even though Leary claims to no longer be actively involved in a "drug movement," he continues to believe that U.S. citizens should be able to use hallucinogens without governmental interference. Although actively involved in developing computer software, he still preaches that "psychedelic drugs allow (the user) to exit the repetitious world processes of your mind to boot up limitless programs, directories and files in your brain. All of which . . . are technicolor, multi-media and moving at the speed of light" ("Mind Expansion," 1991).

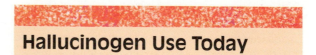

Hallucinogen Use Today

Today, the use of hallucinogens (excluding marijuana) is primarily a young adult phenomenon (Johnston et al. 1993) and has not returned to the high rate seen in the late 1960s and early 1970s. In 1993, 10.9% of high school seniors reported having ever used hallucinogens, compared to 16% in 1975 (Johnston 1994). Several factors have likely contributed to the decline of hallucinogen popularity in the United States.

1. In 1970, federal agencies included LSD in the same regulatory category as heroin (Jaffe 1990), making access to these drugs more difficult.
2. Relatively pure psychedelics do not tend to cause physical dependence, although minor psychological dependence might occur. Because severe addiction does not occur, discontinuation of hallucinogen use is not particularly problematic.
3. Social conditions in America are very different today from conditions 20 to 30 years ago, when these agents were extremely popular. In the 1960s, there was great public agitation and discontentment concerning social and political issues. These frustrations encouraged many members of a socially conscious generation to turn to hallucinogens for relief. Recent generations appear to be less likely to feel alienated from social institutions and their government; as a result, they may have less inclination to turn to hallucinogens.
4. Concern about health issues relative to the use of the hallucinogens has contributed to the depopularization of these agents. For example, research conducted in the late 1960s suggested that LSD use caused chromosome breakage that could result in fetal damage if pregnancy were to occur. Federal agencies trying to control consumption of hallucinogens used these reports as part of their "education program" to convince young people to avoid using these compounds. On closer scrutiny of this early work and additional research, the validity and reliability of the initial studies have been seriously questioned (Dishotsky et al. 1971). Even so, the reports served their purpose and frightened many potential hallucinogen users (see later in this chapter). Another health concern for the potential user has been the presence of dangerous adulterant chemicals such as strychnine that are frequently used to "cut" hallucinogens.

Even though hallucinogen use is down considerably from the 1960s and 1970s, there was a trend of increased use in the early 1990s by high school students and young adults (see Table 12.1). This increase was observed particularly in the use of LSD, although its significance has been questioned by some observers (Negin 1993). It has been speculated that this relatively small increase reflects the ignorance of a new generation about the potential problems of the hallucinogens and a shift from using the widely publicized drugs of abuse such as cocaine and heroin (Johnston 1994).

The Nature of Hallucinogens

Agreement has not been reached on what constitutes a hallucinogenic agent (Glennon 1987), for several reasons. First, a variety of seemingly unrelated drug groups can all produce hallucinations, delusions, or sensory disturbances under certain conditions; for example, besides the traditional hallucinogens (such as LSD), anticholinergics, cocaine, amphetamines, and steroids can cause hallucinations.

What's more, responses to even the traditional hallucinogens can vary tremendously from person to person and experience to experience. It is apparent that multiple mechanisms are involved in the actions of these drugs, which contributes to the array of responses that they can cause. These drugs most certainly influence the complex inner workings of the human mind and have been described as **psychedelic, psychotogenic,** or (as already mentioned) *psychotomimetic*. The features of hallucinogens that distinguish them from other drug groups are their

PSYCHEDELIC substances that expand or heighten perception and consciousness

PSYCHOTOGENIC substances that initiate psychotic behavior

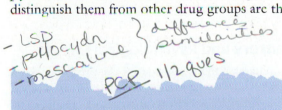

TABLE 12.1 Trends in the use of inhalants, LSD and all hallucinogens (for this survey, inhalants and marijuana were not considered as hallucinogens) by eighth-graders through young adults from 1991 to 1993

	Used during lifetime			Used during year			Used during month		
	1991	1992	1993	1991	1992	1993	1991	1992	1993
Eighth-graders									
Inhalants	17.6%	17.4%	19.4%	9.0%	9.5%	11.0%	4.4%	4.7%	5.4%
LSD	2.7	3.2	3.5	1.7	2.1	2.3	0.6	0.9	1.0
All hallucinogens	3.2	3.8	3.9	1.9	2.5	2.6	0.8	1.1	1.2
Tenth-graders									
Inhalants	15.7	16.6	17.5	7.1	7.5	8.4	2.7	2.7	3.3
LSD	5.6	5.8	6.2	3.7	4.0	4.2	1.5	1.6	1.6
All hallucinogens	6.1	6.4	6.8	4.0	4.3	4.7	1.6	1.8	1.9
Twelfth-graders									
Inhalants	17.6	16.6	17.4	6.6	6.2	7.0	2.4	2.3	2.5
LSD	8.8	8.6	10.3	5.2	5.6	6.8	1.9	2.0	2.4
All hallucinogens	9.6	9.2	10.9	5.8	5.9	7.4	2.2	2.1	2.7
Young adults									
Inhalants	14.1	13.9	n.a.	3.5	3.1	n.a.	0.9	1.1	n.a.
LSD	13.5	13.8	n.a.	3.8	4.3	n.a.	0.8	1.1	n.a.
All hallucinogens	16.0	15.9	n.a.	4.6	5.1	n.a.	1.2	1.6	n.a.
Ecstasy	3.2	3.9	n.a.	0.8	1.0	n.a.	0.1	0.3	n.a.

Note: n.a., not available.

Source: L. Johnston. "Drug Use Rises Among Teenagers." University of Michigan News Release, 27 January 1994. L. Johnston, P. O'Malley, and J. Bachman. *National Survey Results on Drug Use from Monitoring the Future Study,* Vol. 1. Washington, DC: National Institute on Drug Abuse, 1993.

ability to alter perception, thought, and feeling in such a manner that does not normally occur except in dreams or during experiences of extreme religious exaltation (Jaffe 1990). We will examine these characteristics throughout this chapter.

Sensory and Psychological Effects

In general, LSD is considered the prototype agent by which other hallucinogens are evaluated. Typical users experience several stages of sensory experiences; they can go through all stages during a single "trip" or more likely, they will only pass through some. These stages include (1) heightened, exaggerated senses, (2) loss of control, (3) self-reflection, and (4) loss of identity and a sense of cosmic merging.

The following illustrations on the stages of the LSD experience are based primarily on an account by Solomon Snyder (1974), a highly regarded neuroscientist (one of the principal discoverers of endorphins; see Chapter 5), who as a young resident in psychiatry personally experienced the effects of LSD.

Altered Senses In his encounter with LSD, Snyder used a moderate dose of 100 to 200 micrograms and observed few discernible effects for the first 30 minutes except some mild nausea. After this time had elapsed, objects took on a purplish tinge and appeared to be vaguely outlined. Colors,

Case in Point

Taking a Trip

The following description was shared with Dr. Glen Hanson by one of his students in 1992. The student describes a psychedelic "trip" caused by consuming a slurry of grain grown with a hallucinogen-producing fungus.

> "The effect started about 45 minutes after drinking the slurry and was extraordinary. While it lasted (about three hours), the trip caused by consuming the fungus was the most sublime, ineffable experience I've ever had. Unlike cocaine, this experience could easily have been considered religious. Indeed, it was the closest thing to the Beatific Vision I can imagine. The intoxication I experienced was truly singular. I tasted colors, I saw beautiful lights with my eyes closed, my hands could pass through solid objects, I felt extraordinary compassion for other living things. I laughed and cried over a tomato I ate, for giving its life so that I might sustain mine. I looked at my little daughter crawling on the floor and could remember being a toddler, surrounded by a vast floor and large objects towering above me. The antics of my 2-year-old son made me laugh till I had to leave the room for fear of going into hysterics. . . .
>
> "Then it wore off. I didn't have any particular hangover or headache afterward—I just slid back into reality. Easy come, easy go, I guess."

This experience appears to have been pleasant for the user and not a threat to anyone. How can drug-induced experiences such as this cause problems?

*flashbacks

textures, and lines achieved a richness Snyder had never before experienced. Perception was so exaggerated that individual skin pores "stood out and clamored for recognition" (p. 42). Objects became distorted; when Snyder focused on his thumb, it began to swell, undulate, and then moved forward in a menacing fashion. Visions filled with distorted imagery occurred when his eyes were closed. The sense of time and distance changed dramatically; "a minute was like an hour, a week was like an eternity, a foot became a mile" (p. 43). The present seemed to drag on forever, and the concept of future lost its meaning. The exaggeration of perceptions and feelings gave the sense of more events occurring in a time period, giving the impression of time slowing.

An associated sensation described by Snyder is called **synesthesia,** a crossover phenomenon between senses. For example, sound takes on visual dimensions and vice versa, enabling you to see sounds and hear colors. These altered sensory experiences are described as a heightened sensory awareness (see Case in Point), and relate to the first component of the psychedelic state (Jaffe 1990).

Loss of Control The second feature of LSD also relates to altered sensory experiences and a loss of control (Jaffe 1990). The user cannot determine whether the psychedelic trip will be a pleas-

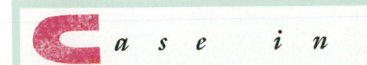

SYNESTHESIA a subjective sensation or image of a sense other than the one being stimulated, such as an auditory sensation caused by a visual stimulus ant, comfortable experience or a "bad trip," with recollections of hidden fears and suppressed anxieties that can precipitate neurotic or psychotic responses. The frightening reactions may persist a few minutes or several hours and be mildly agitating or terrifyingly threatening. Some bad trips can include feelings of panic, confusion, suspiciousness, helplessness, and a total lack of control. Replays of these frightening experiences can occur at a later time, even though the drug has not been taken again; such recurrences are referred to as **"flashbacks."**

It is not clear what determines the nature of the sensory response. Perhaps it relates to the state of anxiety and personality of the user or of the nature of his or her surroundings. It is interesting that Timothy Leary tried to teach his "drug disciples" that "turning on correctly means to understand the many levels that are brought into focus; it takes years of discipline, training and discipleship" ("Celebration #1" 1966). He apparently felt that, with experience and training, you could control the sensory effects of the hallucinogens. This is an interesting possibility but has never been well demonstrated.

Self-Reflection Snyder (1974) makes reference to the third component of the psychedelic response in his LSD experience. During the period when sensory effects predominate, self-reflection also occurs. While in this state, Snyder explains, the user "becomes aware of thoughts and feelings long hidden beneath the surface, forgotten and/or repressed" (p. 44). As a psychiatrist, Snyder claims that this new perspective can lead to valid insights that are useful psychotherapeutic exercises.

Some psychotherapeutists have used or advocated the use of psychedelics for this purpose since the 1950s, as described by Sigmund Freud, to "make conscious the unconscious" (Snyder 1974, 44). It should be noted that, while a case can be made for the psychotherapeutic use of this group of drugs, the Food and Drug Administration (FDA) has not approved any of these agents for psychiatric use. The psychedelics currently available are considered to be too unpredictable in their effects and possess substantial risks. Not only is their administration not considered to be significantly therapeutic, but their use is deemed a great enough risk that the principal hallucinogenic agents are scheduled as controlled substances.

Loss of Identity and Cosmic Merging The final features that set the psychedelics apart as unique drugs are described by Snyder (1974) as the "mystical-spiritual aspect of the drug experience." He claims, "It is indescribable. For how can anyone verbalize a merging of his being with the totality of the universe? How do you put into words the feeling that 'all is one,' 'I am of the all,' 'I am no longer.' One's skin ceases to be a boundary between self and others" (p. 45). Because consumption of hallucinogen–containing plants has often been part of religious ceremonies, it is likely that this sense of cosmic merging and union with all humankind correlates to the exhilaratingly spiritual experiences described by many religious mystics.

The loss of identity and personal boundaries caused by hallucinogens is not viewed as being so spiritually enticing by all. In particular, for individuals who have rigid, highly ordered personalities, the dissolution of a well-organized and -structured world is terrifying because the drug destroys the individual's emotional support. Such an individual finds that the loss of a separate identity can cause extreme panic and anxiety. During these drug-induced panic states, which in some ways are schizophrenic-like, people have committed suicide or homicide. These tragic reactions are part of the risk of using hallucinogenics and explains some of the FDA's hesitancy to legalize or authorize them for psychotherapeutic use.

Mechanisms of Action

As with most drugs, hallucinogens represent the proverbial "two-edged sword." These drugs may cause potentially useful psychiatric effects for many people. However, the variability in positive versus negative responses, coupled with lack of understanding as to what factors are responsible for the

"FLASHBACK" The recurrence of an earlier drug-induced sensory experience in the absence of the drug

ERGOTISM poisoning by toxic substances from the ergot fungus *Claviceps purpurea*

variables, have made these drugs dangerous and difficult to manage.

Some researchers have suggested that all hallucinogens act at a common central nervous system (CNS) site to exert their psychedelic effects. Although this hypothesis has not been totally disproven, there is little evidence to support it. The fact that so many different types of drugs can cause hallucinogenic effects suggests that multiple mechanisms are likely responsible.

The most predictable and typical psychedelic experiences are caused by LSD or similar agents. Consequently, these agents have been the primary focus of studies intended to elucidate the nature of hallucinogenic mechanisms. Although LSD has effects at several CNS sites, from the spinal cord to the cortex of the brain, its effects on the neurotransmitter serotonin most likely account for its psychedelic properties (Strassman 1992). That LSD and similar drugs alter serotonin activity has been proven; how they affect this transmitter is not so apparent.

Although many experts believe changes in serotonin activity are the basis for psychedelic properties of most hallucinogens, a case can be made for the involvement of norepinephrine, dopamine, acetylcholine, and perhaps other transmitter systems as well. Only additional research will be able to sort out this complex but important issue.

Types of Hallucinogenic Agents

Due to recent technological advancements, understanding of hallucinogens has advanced; even so, the classification of these drugs remains somewhat arbitrary. Many agents produce some of the pharmacological effects of the traditional psychedelics, such as LSD and mescaline.

A second type of hallucinogen includes those agents that have amphetamine-like molecular structures (referred to as *phenylethylamines*) and possess some stimulant action; this group includes drugs such as DOM (dimethoxymethyl*amphetamine*), MDA (methylenedioxy*amphetamine*), and MDMA (methylenedioxy*methamphetamine*). These agents vary in their hallucinogen or stimulant properties. MDA is more like an amphetamine (stimulant), while MDMA is more like LSD (hallucinogen). However, in large doses, each of the phenylethylamines causes substantial CNS stimulation.

The third major group of hallucinogens is the anticholinergic drugs, which block some of the receptors for the neurotransmitter, acetylcholine (see Chapter 5). Almost all drugs that antagonize these receptors cause hallucinations in high doses. Many of these potent anticholinergic hallucinogens are naturally occurring and have been known, used, and abused for millennia.

Traditional Hallucinogens: LSD Types

The LSD-like drugs are considered to be the prototypical hallucinogens and are used as comparison for other types of agents with psychedelic properties. Included in this group are LSD itself and some hallucinogens derived from plants, such as mescaline from the peyote cactus, psilocybin from mushrooms, dimethyltryptamine (DMT) from seeds, and myristicin from nutmeg. Because LSD is the principal hallucinogen, its origin, history, and properties will be discussed in detail, providing a basis for understanding the other psychedelic drugs.

Lysergic Acid Diethylamide (LSD) LSD is a relatively new drug, but similar compounds have existed for a long time. For example, accounts from the Middle Ages tell about a strange affliction that caused women to abort and others to develop strange burning sensations in their extremities. Today, we call this condition **ergotism** and know that it is caused by eating grain contaminated by the ergot fungus. This fungus produces compounds related to LSD called the *ergot alkaloids* (Goldstein 1994). Besides the sensory effects, the ergot substances can also cause hallucinations, delirium, and psychosis.

In 1938, Albert Hofmann, a scientist for Sandoz Pharmaceutical Laboratories of Basel, Switzerland, worked on a series of ergot compounds in search for active chemicals that might be of medical value. Lysergic acid was similar in structure to a compound called *nikethamide,* a stimulant, and

Case in Point

Albert Hofmann's Discovery

Following synthesis of the diethylamide derivative of lysergic acid in 1938, Hofmann noted nothing unusual about the product, so he stored it in a bottle on the laboratory shelf. In 1943, he checked over some of the synthetic compounds he had worked on and started making further tests of LSD. Most likely due to carelessness, a small amount must have entered his blood. Hofmann noted that

> Last Friday, April 16, 1943, I was forced to stop my work in the laboratory in the middle of the afternoon and to go home, as I was seized by a peculiar restlessness associated with a sensation of mild dizziness. Having reached home, I lay down and sank in a kind of drunkenness which was not unpleasant and which was characterized by extreme activity of imagination. As I lay in dazed condition with my eyes closed (I experienced daylight as disagreeably bright), there surged upon me an uninterrupted stream of fantastic images of extraordinary plasticity and vividness and accompanied by an intense, kaleidoscope-like play of colors. This condition gradually passed off after about two hours.

Hofmann realized the experience was probably caused by the chemical he had been working with and decided to try a measured amount on himself. If the minute amount he had unwittingly taken caused the sensations he recorded, he thought 250 micrograms might be enough to prove the chemical's effects. Hofmann was to find out that LSD is one of the most potent drugs known. As low a dose as 50 micrograms can affect some people.

This is Hofmann's record of the first known deliberate LSD trip:

> 4:20 P.M.: 0.5 cc (0.25 mg LSD) ingested orally. The solution is tasteless.
>
> 4:50 P.M.: No trace of any effect.
>
> 5:00 P.M.: Slight dizziness, unrest, difficulty in concentration, visual disturbances, marked desire to laugh . . . [At this point, the laboratory notes are discontinued.]
>
> The last words could only be written with great difficulty. I asked my laboratory assistant to accompany me home as I believed that my condition would be a repetition of the disturbance of the previous Friday. While we were still cycling home, however, it became clear that the symp-

Hofmann tried to create slight chemical modifications that might be worth further testing. The result of this effort was the production of lysergic acid diethylamide, or LSD. Hofmann's experience with this new compound gave insight to the effects of this drug and are detailed in the Case in Point box.

Soon after LSD was discovered, the similarity of LSD experiences to the symptoms of schizophrenia were noted, which prompted researchers to investigate correlations between the two. The hope was to use LSD as a tool for producing an artificial psychosis to aid in understanding the biochemistry of psychosis. Interest in this use of LSD has declined because it is now generally accepted that LSD effects are different from natural psychoses.

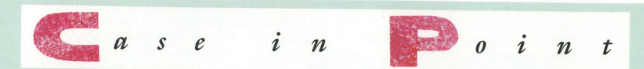

The use of LSD in psychotherapy has also been tried in the treatment of alcoholism, autism, paranoia, schizophrenia, and various other mental and emotional disorders. Therapeutic use of LSD has not increased to any great extent over the years because of its limited success, legal aspects, diffi-

toms were much stronger than the first time. I had great difficulty in speaking coherently, my field of vision swayed before me, and objects appeared distorted like images in curved mirrors. I had the impression of being unable to move from the spot, although my assistant told me afterwards that we had cycled at a good pace.

By the time the doctor arrived, the peak of the crisis had already passed.

As far as I remember, the following were the most outstanding symptoms: vertigo; visual disturbances; the faces of those around me appeared as grotesque, colored masks; marked motor unrest, alternating with paresis; an intermittent heavy feeling in the head, limbs and the entire body, as if they were filled with metal; cramps in the legs, coldness and loss of feeling in the hands; a metallic taste on the tongue; dry, constricted sensation in the throat; feeling of choking; confusion alternating between clear recognition of my condition, in which state I sometimes observed, in the manner of an independent, neutral observer, that I shouted half insanely or babbled incoherent words. Occasionally I felt as if I were out of my body.

Six more hours after ingestion of the LSD, my condition had already improved considerably. Only the visual disturbances were still pronounced. Everything seemed to sway and the proportions were distorted like the reflections in the surface of moving water. Moreover, all objects appeared in unpleasant, constantly changing colors, the predominant shades being sickly green and blue. When I closed my eyes, an unending series of colorful, very realistic and fantastic images surged in upon me. A remarkable feature was the manner in which all acoustic perceptions (for example, the noise of a passing car) were transformed into optical effects, every sound causing a corresponding colored hallucination constantly changing in shape and color like pictures in a kaleidoscope. At about 1 o'clock I fell asleep and awakened next morning somewhat tired but otherwise feeling perfectly well.

Source: Quotes from Albert Hofmann. "Psychotomimetic Agents." In *Drugs Affecting the Central Nervous System*, vol. 2, edited by A. Burger, 169–235. New York: Dekker, 1968.

culty in obtaining the pure drug, adverse reactions to the drug ("bad trips" can occur under controlled as well as uncontrolled conditions), and the problems of rapid tolerance buildup in some patients.

Nonmedical interest in LSD and related drugs began to grow during the 1950s and peaked in the 1960s, when LSD was used by millions of young Americans for chemical escape. Occasionally a "bad trip" would cause a user to feel terror and panic and resulted in well-publicized accidental deaths due to jumping from building tops or running into the pathway of oncoming vehicles (U.S. Department of Justice 1991b).

As with other hallucinogens, the use of LSD declined somewhat over the past two decades but began to rise again in the early 1990s (Johnston 1994). Of high school seniors sampled in 1975 11.3% had used LSD sometime during their life; that number declined to 8.7% in 1990 and rebounded to 10.3% in 1993 (Johnston et al. 1993; Johnston 1994). Similar patterns were also ob-

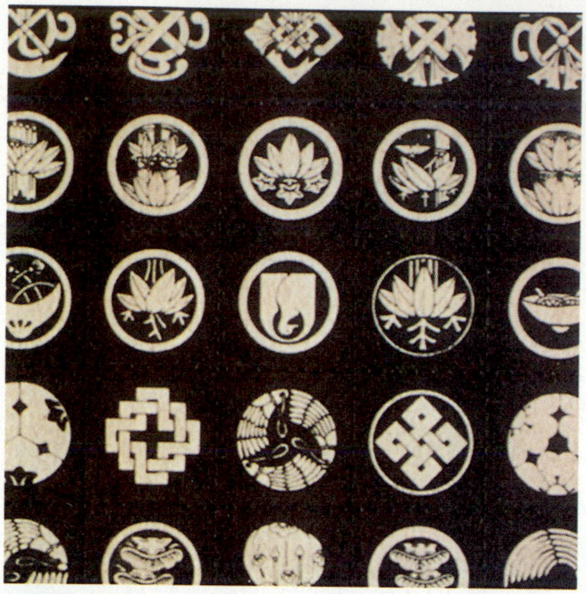

FIGURE 12.2 LSD blotter paper. Small amounts of LSD are added to decorated, absorbent paper, such as this. Each small square represents a single dose to be chewed or swallowed. The designs on the paper have no drug function.

served in college and young adult populations (Johnston et al. 1993).

Synthesis and Administration. LSD is a complex molecule that requires about one week to be synthesized. Because of the sophisticated chemistry necessary for its production, LSD is not manufactured by local illicit laboratories. It appears that an illegal operation in San Francisco is the principal source of LSD for the United States and even much of the world. Because of LSD's potency, it has been difficult to locate the illicit LSD labs; small quantities of LSD are sufficient to satisfy the demand and can be easily transported without detection (U.S. Department of Justice 1991a).

The physical properties of LSD are not distinctive. In its purified form, LSD is colorless, odorless, and tasteless. It can be purchased in several forms, including tiny tablets (about 1/10 the size of aspirins, called "microdots"), capsules, and occasionally even a liquid. The street names of LSD include *acid, blotter acid, microdot,* and *white lightning* (U.S. Department of Justice 1991b). Although LSD usually is taken by mouth, it is sometimes injected (Mathias 1993).

LSD often is added to absorbent paper, such as blotter paper, that can be divided into small decorated squares. Each square is swallowed or chewed and represents a single dose (see Figure 12.2). When LSD is added to tiny, thin squares of gelatin, it is called "windowpanes," which are administered orally (U.S. Department of Justice, 1991a).

Physiological Effects. Like many hallucinogens, LSD is remarkably potent (Goldstein 1995). The typical dose today is 20–30 micrograms compared to a typical dose of 150–300 micrograms in the 1960s. This difference in dose likely explains why today fewer users of LSD are experiencing severe side effects (U.S. Department of Justice 1991a). In monkeys, the lethal dose has been determined to be about 5 milligrams (mg) per kilogram (kg) of body weight. In rats, the lethal dose (expressed as LD-100, which means it kills 100% of the test animals) is about 20 mg/kg of body weight. The LD-50 (lethal dose for 50%) for humans is estimated at 150 to 200 times the hallucinogenic dose.

When taken orally, LSD is readily absorbed and diffused into all tissues. It will pass through the placenta into the fetus and through the blood–brain barrier. The brain receives about 1% of the total dose.

Within the brain, LSD is particularly concentrated in the hypothalamus, the limbic system, and the auditory and visual reflex areas. Electrodes placed in the limbic system show an "electrical storm," or a massive increase in neural activity, which might correlate with the overwhelming flood of sensations and the phenomenon of synesthesia reported by the user (Goldstein 1995). LSD also activates the sympathetic nervous system; shortly after the drug is taken, body temperature, heart rate, and blood pressure rise, the person sweats, and the pupils of the eyes become dilated. Its effects on the parasympathetic nervous system cause an increase in salivation and nausea (Mathias 1993). These systemic effects do not appear to be related to the hallucinogenic properties of the drug.

Pharmacokinetic experiments with LSD show that about half of the substance is cleared from the body within 3 hours, and more than 90% is excreted within 24 hours (Goldstein 1995). The effects of this hallucinogen can last 2–12 hours depending on the dose and previous experience with the drug (U.S. Department of Justice 1991). Tolerance to the effects of LSD develops more rapidly and lasts longer than tolerance to other hallucinogens. Tolerance develops very quickly to repeated doses, probably because of a change in sensitivity of the target cells in the brain rather than a change in its metabolism. Tolerance wears off within a few days after the drug is discontinued. Because there are no withdrawal symptoms, a person does not become physically dependent, but some psychological dependency on LSD can occur (Mathias 1993).

Behavioral Effects. Because LSD alters a number of systems in the brain, its behavioral effects are many and variable between individuals (Goldstein 1995). The following sections address common CNS responses to this drug.

Creativity and Insight. A question often raised by researchers interested in experimenting with LSD is "Does it help expand the mind, increasing insight creativity?" This is an extremely difficult question to answer because no one has ever determined the origin of insight and creativity. Moreover, each of us views these qualities differently.

Generally, subjects under the influence of LSD often express the feeling of being more creative, but creative acts such as drawing and painting are hindered by the motor impairment caused by LSD. The products of artists under the influence of the drug usually prove to be inferior to those produced prior to the drug experience. Paintings done in LSD creativity studies have been described as reminiscent of "schizophrenic art."

In an often cited study, creativity, attitude, and anxiety tests on 24 college students found that LSD had no objective effect on creativity, although many of the subjects said they felt they were more creative (McGlothin et al. 1967). This paradox is noted in several studies of LSD use: The subjects feel they have more insight and provide better answers to life's problems, but they do not or cannot demonstrate this increase objectively. Overt behavior is not modified, and these new insights are short-lived unless they are reinforced by modified behavior (Cohen 1978).

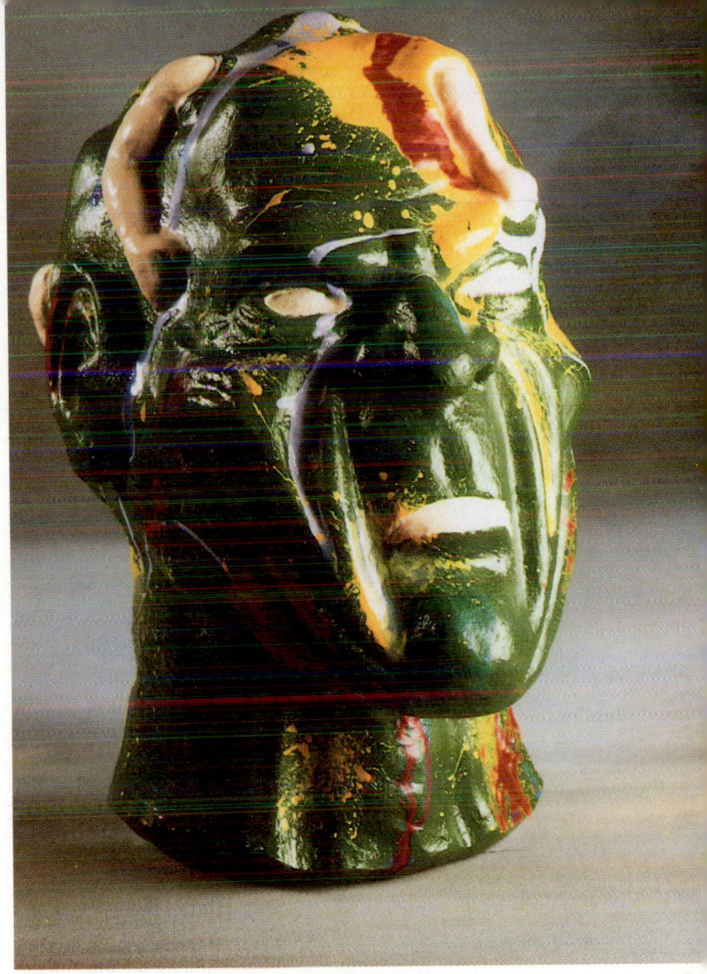

This piece of sculpture was done by a university student while under the influence of LSD.

In spite of these results, some researchers still contend that LSD can enhance the creative process. For example, Oscar Janigar, a psychiatrist at the University of California, Los Angeles, claims to have determined that LSD does not produce a tangible alteration in the way a painter paints; thus, it does not turn a poor painter into a good one. However, Janigar claims that LSD does alter the way the painter appraises the world and allows the artist to "plunge into areas where access was restricted by confines of perceptions" and consequently becomes more creative (Tucker 1987, 16).

Adverse Psychedelic Effects. It is important to remember that there is no typical pattern of response to LSD. It varies for each user as a function of the person's set, or expectations, and setting, or environment, during the experience. Two of the major negative responses are described as follows (Pahnke et al. 1970):

1. *The psychotic adverse reaction,* or *"freakout,"* is an intense, nightmarish experience. The subject may have complete loss of emotional control, and experience paranoid delusions, hallucinations, panic attacks, psychosis, and catatonic seizures. In rare instances, some of these reactions are prolonged, lasting days. In 1991, 4,000 episodes were reported in U.S. emergency rooms due to adverse LSD reactions (Mathias 1993).
2. *The nonpsychotic adverse reaction* may involve varying degrees of tension, anxiety, fear, depression, and despair but not as intense a response as the "freakout." A person with deep psychological problems or a strong need to be in conscious control or one who takes the drug in an unfavorable setting is more likely to have an adverse reaction than a person with a well-integrated personality.

Severe LSD behavioral toxicity can be treated with tranquilizers or a benzodiazepine (Jaffe 1990).

Perceptual Effects. Because the brain's sensory processing is altered by a hallucinogenic dose of LSD, many kinds of unusual illusions can occur. Some users report seeing shifting geometrical patterns mixed with intense color perception; others observe the movement of stationary objects, such that a speck on the wall appears as a large blinking eye or an unfolding flower. Interpretation of sounds can also be scrambled; a dropped ashtray may become a gun fired at the user, for instance. In some cases, LSD alters perceptions to the extent that people feel they can walk on water or fly through the air. The sensation that the body is distorted and even coming apart is another common effect, especially for novice users. Thoughts of suicide and sometimes actual attempts can be caused by use of LSD, as well (U.S. Department of Justice 1991b).

Many LSD users find their sense of time distorted, such that hours may be perceived as years or an eternity. As discussed earlier, users may also have a distorted perception of their own knowledge or creativity; for instance, they may feel their ideas or work are especially unique, brilliant, or artistic. When analyzed by a person not on LSD, however, or explained after the "trip" is over, these ideas or creations are almost always quite ordinary.

In sum, LSD alters perception such that any sensation can be perceived in the extreme. An experience can be incredibly beautiful and uplifting or completely foul and disgusting.

The "flashback" is an interesting and poorly understood phenomenon of LSD use. Although usually thought of as being adverse, sometimes flashbacks are pleasant and even referred to as "free trips" (Nadis 1990). During a flashback, sensations caused by previous LSD use return, although the subject is not using the drug at the time.

There are three broad categories of LSD-related flashbacks:

1. *The "body trip"*—the recurrence of an unpleasant physical sensation
2. *The "bad mind trip"*—the recurrence of a distressing thought or emotion
3. *Altered visual perception*—the most frequent, consisting of seeing dots, flashes, trails of light, halos, false motion in the peripheral field, and other sensations (see the accompanying Case in Point box for an example)

Flashbacks are most disturbing because they come on unexpectedly. Some have been reported as long as 5 years after use of LSD (Goldstein 1994); for most people, however, flashbacks usually subside within weeks or months after taking LSD (Nadis 1990). The duration of a flashback is variable, lasting from a few minutes to several hours.

Although the precise mechanism of flashbacks is unknown, physical or psychological stresses and some drugs such as marijuana may trigger the experience (Goldstein 1995). It has been proposed that flashbacks are an especially vivid form of memory that becomes seared into the subconscious mind due to the effects of LSD on the brain's transmitters. Treatment consists of reassurance that the condition will go away and use of Valium if necessary to treat the anxiety or panic that can accompany the flashback experience (Nadis 1990).

Genetic Damage and Birth Defects. Experiments conducted in the mid-1960s suggested that LSD could cause birth defects, based on the observation that, when LSD was added to a suspension

Case in Point

The "After Flash"

As a teenager, John Doe took LSD approximately 30 times. Some 15 years later, he still sees grainy, photographic dots. He also sees "trails," blurred images associated with a moving object, such as a waving arm. "It's as if the lens of a camera were left open taking a time-lapse photograph." Doe also complains that the visual distortions also bring twinges of fear. "I have the feeling of coming on, a rush. It hits me in the gut, like going over the top of a hill. I take Valium, which stops it in its tracks" (Nadis 1990, 24).

Why do you think the effects of LSD persisted in this previous LSD user?

of human white blood cells in a test tube, the chromosomes of these cells were damaged. From this, it was proposed that, when LSD was consumed by humans, it could cause damage to the chromosomes of the male sperm, female egg, or the cells of the developing infant. Such damage theoretically could result in congenital defects in offspring (Dishotsky et al. 1971).

Carefully controlled studies conducted after news of LSD's chromosomal effects were made public have not supported this hypothesis. Experiments have revealed that, in contrast to the test tube findings, there is no chromosomal damage to white blood cells or any other cells when LSD is given to a human being (Dishotsky et al. 1971).

Studies have also shown that there are no carcinogenic or mutagenic effects from using LSD in experimental animals or humans, with the exception of the fruit fly. (LSD is a mutagen in fruit flies if given in doses that are equivalent to 100,000 times the hallucinogenic dose for humans.) Teratogenic effects occur in mice if LSD is given early in pregnancy. LSD may be teratogenic in rhesus monkeys if it is injected in doses (based on body weight) exceeding at least 100 times the usual hallucinogenic dose for humans. In other studies, women who took "street" LSD but not those given pure LSD had a higher rate of spontaneous abortions and births of malformed infants; this suggests that contaminants in adulterated LSD were responsible for the fetal effects and not the hallucinogen itself (Dishotsky et al. 1971).

Early Human Research. In the 1950s, the U.S. government—specifically, the Central Intelligence Agency (CIA) and the army—became interested in reports of the effects of mind-altering drugs, including LSD. Unknown to the public at the time, these agencies conducted tests on humans to learn more about such compounds and determine their usefulness in conducting military and clandestine missions. These activities became public when a biochemist, Frank Olson, killed himself in 1953 after being given a drink laced with LSD. Olson had a severe psychotic reaction and was being treated for the condition when he jumped out of a tenth-story window. His family was told only that he had committed suicide. The connection to LSD was not uncovered until 1975. The court awarded Olson's family $750,000 in damages in 1976.

In 1976, the extent of these studies was revealed: nearly 585 soldiers and 900 civilians had been given LSD in poorly organized experiments in which participants were coerced into taking or not told that they were being given this drug. Powerful hallucinogens such as LSD can cause serious psychological damage in some subjects, especially when they are unaware of what is happening.

The legal consequences of these LSD studies

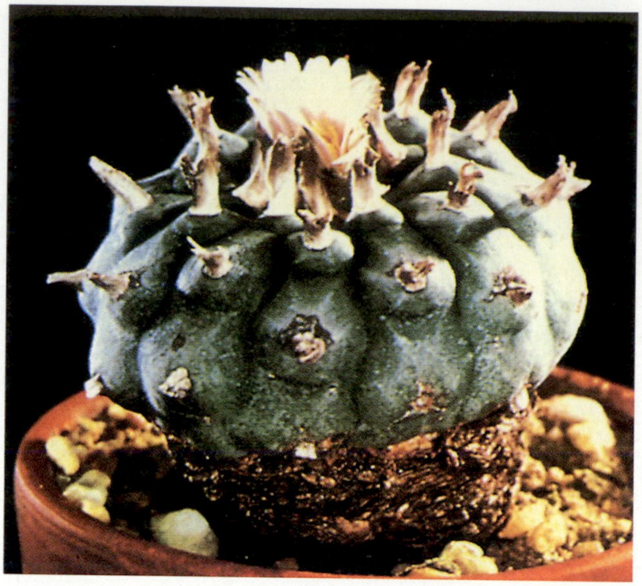

FIGURE 12.3 The peyote cactus contains a number of drugs; the best known is mescaline.

continued for years. As recently as 1987, a New York judge awarded $700,000 to the family of a mental patient who killed himself after having been given LSD without an explanation of the drug's nature. The judge said that there was a "conspiracy of silence" between the army, the Department of Justice and the New York State Attorney General to conceal events surrounding the death of the subject, Harold Blauer.

Mescaline (Peyote) Mescaline is one of approximately 30 psychoactive chemicals that have been isolated from the peyote cactus (see Figure 12.3) and used for centuries in the Americas. One of the first reports on the peyote plant was made by Francisco Hernandez of the court of King Philip II of Spain. King Philip was interested in reports from the earlier Cortés expedition about strange medicines the natives used and sent Hernandez to collect information about herbs and medicines. Hernandez worked on this project from 1570 to 1575 and reported the use of more than 1,200 plant remedies, as well as the existence of many hallucinogenic plants. He was one of the first to record the eating of parts of the peyote cactus and the resulting visions and mental changes.

In the seventeenth century, Spanish Catholic priests asked their Indian converts to confess to the use of peyote, which they believed was used to conjure up demons. However, nothing stopped its use. There is evidence that, by 1760, use of peyote had spread into what is now the United States.

Peyote has been confused with another plant, the mescal shrub, which produces dark red beans that contain an extremely toxic alkaloid called *cytisine*. This alkaloid may cause hallucinations, convulsions, and even death. There is also a mescal liquor, made from the agave cactus. Partly because of misidentification with the toxic mescal beans, the U.S. government outlawed the use of peyote and mescaline.

Mescaline is the most active drug in peyote; it induces intensified perception of colors and euphoria in the user. However, as Aldous Huxley said in *The Doors of Perception* (1954), his book about his experimentation with mescaline, "Along with the happily transfigured majority of mescaline takers there is a minority that finds in the drug only hell and purgatory." After Huxley related his experiences with mescaline, it was used by an increasing number of people.

Physiological Effects. The average dose of mescaline that will cause hallucinations and other physiological effects is from 300 to 600 mg. It may take up to 20 peyote (mescal) buttons (ingested orally) to get 600 mg of mescaline.

Based on studies of animals, it is estimated that

from 10 to 30 times the lowest dose that will cause behavioral effects in humans may be lethal. (About 200 mg is the lowest mind-altering dose.) Death in animals results from convulsions and respiratory arrest. Mescaline is perhaps 1,000 to 3,000 times less potent than LSD and 30 times less potent than another common hallucinogen, psilocybin (Mathias 1993)—see later in this chapter.

Effects include dilation of the pupils **(mydriasis),** increase in body temperature, anxiety, visual hallucinations, and alteration of body image. The last effect is a type of hallucination in which parts of the body may seem to disappear or to become grossly distorted. Mescaline induces vomiting in many people and some muscular relaxation (sedation). Apparently, there are few after effects or drug hangover at low doses. Higher doses of mescaline slow the heart and respiratory rhythm, contract the intestines and the uterus, and cause headache, difficulty in coordination, dry skin with itching, and hypertension (high blood pressure).

Mescaline users report that they lose all awareness of time. As with LSD, the setting for the "trip" influences the user's reactions. Most mescaline users prefer natural settings, most likely due to the historical association of this drug with Native Americans and their nature-related spiritual experiences (often under the influence of this drug). The visual hallucinations achieved depend on the individual. Colors are at first intensified and may be followed by hallucinations of shades, movements, forms, and events. The senses of smell and taste are enhanced. Some people claim (as with LSD) that they can "hear" colors and "see" sounds, such as the wind. Synesthesia occurs naturally in a small percentage of cases.

At low to medium doses, an ecstatic state of euphoria is reported, often followed by a feeling of anxiety and less frequently by depression. Occasionally, users observe themselves as two people and experience the sensation that the mind and body are separate entities. A number of people have had cosmic experiences that are profound, almost religious, in which they discover a sense of unity with all creation. People who have this sensation often believe they have discovered the meaning of existence.

Mechanism of Action. Within 30 to 120 minutes after ingestion, mescaline reaches a maximum concentration in the brain and may persist for up to 9 or 10 hours. Hallucinations may last up to 2 hours and are usually affected by the dose level. About half the dose is excreted unchanged after 6 hours and can be recovered in the urine for reuse (if peyote is in short supply). A slow tolerance builds up after repeated use, and there is cross-tolerance to LSD. As with LSD, mescaline intoxication can be alleviated or stopped by taking a dose of chlorpromazine (Thorazine, a tranquilizer) and to a lesser extent with diazepam (Valium). Like LSD, mescaline probably exerts much of its hallucinogenic effects by altering serotonin systems (Jaffe 1990).

Analysis of "street" samples of mescaline in a number of U.S. cities over the past decade shows that the chemical sold rarely is authentic. Regardless of color or appearance, these street drugs are usually other hallucinogens, such as LSD, DOM, or PCP. If a person decides to take hallucinogenic street drugs, "let the buyer beware." Not only is the actual content often different and potentially much more toxic than bargained for (they are frequently contaminated), but the dosage is usually unknown even if the drug is genuine.

Psilocybin The drug psilocybin has a long and colorful history. Its principal source is the *Psilocybe mexicana* mushroom of the "magic" variety (Goldstein 1994). It was first used by some of the early natives of Central America more than 2,000 years ago. In Guatemala, statues of mushrooms that date back to 100 B.C. have been found. The Aztecs later used the mushrooms for ceremonial rites. When the Spaniards came into Mexico in the 1500s, the natives were calling the *Psilocybe mexicana* mushroom "God's flesh." Because of this seeming sacrilege, they were harshly treated by the Spanish priests.

Gordon Wasson identified the *Psilocybe mexicana* mushroom in 1955 (see Figure 12.4). The active ingredient was extracted in 1958 by Albert Hofmann, who also synthesized LSD. Doing research, Hofmann wanted to make certain he

MYDRIASIS pupil dilation

FIGURE 12.4 The psilocybe mushroom, source of psilocybin and psilocin.

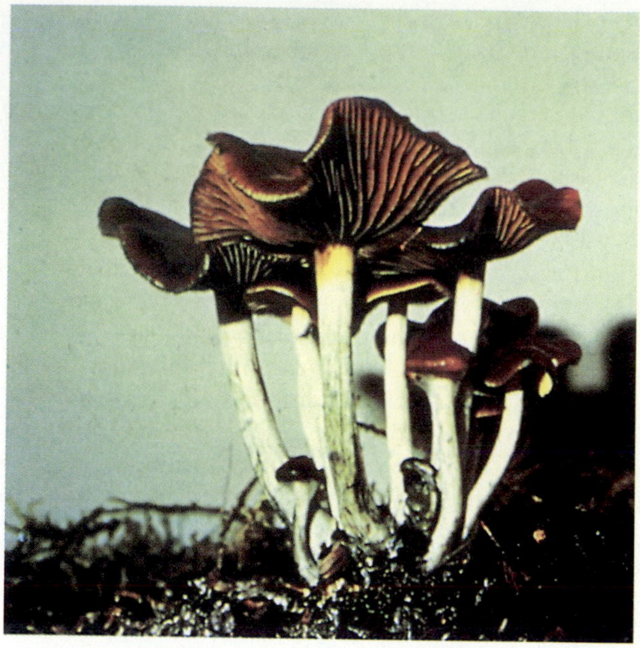

would feel the effects of the mushroom, so he ate 32 of them, weighing 2.4 grams (a medium dose by Indian standards) and then recorded his hallucinogenic reactions (Burger 1968).

Timothy Leary also tried some psilocybin mushrooms in Mexico in 1960; apparently the experience influenced him greatly. On his return to Harvard, he carried out a series of experiments using psilocybin with student groups. Leary was careless in experimental procedures and did some work in uncontrolled situations. This caused a major administrative upheaval, ending in his departure from Harvard.

One of Leary's questionable studies was the "Good Friday" experiment in which 20 theological students were given either a placebo or psilocybin in a double-blind study (that is, neither the researcher nor the subjects know who gets the placebo or the drug), after which all attended the same 2.5-hour Good Friday service. The experimental group reported mystical experiences whereas the control group did not (Pahnke and Richards 1966). Leary believed that the experience was of value and that, under proper control and guidance, the hallucinatory experience could be beneficial.

Psilocybin is not very common on the street. Generally, it is administered orally and is eaten either fresh or dried. Accidental poisonings are common for those who mistakenly consume poisonous mushrooms rather than the hallucinogenic variety.

The dried form of these mushrooms contains from 0.2 to 0.5% psilocybin. The hallucinogenic effects produced are quite similar to those of LSD, and there is a cross-tolerance between psilocybin, LSD, and mescaline. The effects caused by psilocybin vary with the dosage taken. Up to 4 mg will cause a pleasant experience, relaxation, and some body sensation. In some subjects, higher doses cause considerable perceptual and body image changes, accompanied by hallucinations. Psilocybin stimulates the autonomic nervous system, dilates the pupils, and increases the body temperature. There is some evidence that psilocybin is metabolized into psilocin, which is more potent and may be the principal active ingredient. Psilocin is found in the mushroom but in small amounts. Like the other hallucinogens, psilocybin apparently causes no physical dependence.

Dimethyltryptamine (DMT) DMT is a short-acting hallucinogen found in the seeds of certain leguminous trees native to the West Indies and parts of South America (Schultes 1978). It is also prepared synthetically in illicit laboratories. For centuries, the powdered seeds have been used as a snuff called *cohoba* in pipes and snuffing tubes. The Haitian natives claim that, under the influence of the drug, they can communicate with their gods. Its effects may last under one hour, which has earned it the nickname "the businessman's lunch break" drug.

DMT has no effect when taken orally; it is inhaled either as smoke from the burning plant or in vaporized form. DMT is sometimes added to parsley leaves or flakes, tobacco, or marijuana in order to induce its hallucinogenic effect. The usual dose is 60 to 150 mg. In structure and action, it is similar to psilocybin although not as powerful. Like the other hallucinogens discussed, DMT does not cause physical dependence.

Nutmeg High doses of nutmeg can be quite intoxicating, causing symptoms such as drowsiness, stupor, delirium, and sleep. Prison inmates have known about this drug for years, so in most prisons, use of spices such as nutmeg is restricted.

Nutmeg contains 5 to 15% myristica oil, which is responsible for the physical effects. Myristicin (about 4%), which is structurally similar to mescaline, and elemicin are probably the most potent psychoactive ingredients in nutmeg. Myristicin blocks release of serotonin from brain neurons. Some scientists believe that myristicin can be converted in the body to MMDA (a close relative of MDA, discussed later), which also affects the central nervous system. Mace, the exterior covering of the nutmeg seed, also contains the hallucinogenic compound myristicin.

Two tablespoons of nutmeg (about 14 g) taken orally cause a rather unpleasant "trip" with a dreamlike stage; rapid heartbeat, dry mouth, and thirst are experienced, as well. Agitation, apprehension, and a sense of impending doom may last about 12 hours, with a sense of unreality persisting for several days (Claus et al. 1970).

Phenylethylamine Hallucinogens

The phenylethylamine drugs are chemically related to amphetamines. Phenylethylamines have varying degrees of hallucinogenic and CNS stimulant effects, which are likely related to their ability to release serotonin and dopamine, respectively. Consequently, the phenylethylamines that predominantly release serotonin are dominated by their hallucinogenic action and are LSD-like, while those more inclined to release dopamine are dominated by their stimulant effects and are cocainelike.

Dimethoxymethylamphetamine (DOM or STP) The basic structure of DOM is amphetamine. Nonetheless, it is a fairly powerful hallucinogen that seems to work through mechanisms similar to those of mescaline and LSD. In fact, the effects of DOM are similar to those caused by a combination of amphetamine and LSD, with the hallucinogenic effects of the drug overpowering the amphetaminelike physiological effects.

DOM produces a higher incidence of acute and chronic reactions than any of the other commonly used hallucinogens, with the possible exception of PCP (see later in this chapter). As with LSD and mescaline, the tranquilizer chlorpromazine (Thorazine) will rapidly ease the effects of the long "trip" but may also interfere with breathing. Use of Valium has been recommended because it causes fewer reactions than chlorpromazine (Bourne 1976).

"Designer" Amphetamines "Designer" amphetamines were discussed in Chapter 10 but are presented again here due to their hallucinogenic effects. Their hybrid actions as psychedelic stimulants not only make them a particularly fascinating topic for research but also provide a unique experience described by drug abusers as a "smooth amphetamine." This characterization likely accounts for the recent popularity of the designer amphetamines.

3,4-Methylenedioxyamphetamine (MDA). MDA, first synthesized in 1910, is structurally related to both mescaline and amphetamine. Early research found that MDA is an anorexiant (causing loss of appetite) as well as a mood elevator in some persons. Further research has shown that the mode of action of MDA is similar to that of amphetamine. It causes extra release of the neurotransmitters serotonin, dopamine, and norepinephrine.

MDA has been used as an adjunct to psychotherapy. In one study, eight volunteers who had previously experienced the effects of LSD under clinical conditions were given 150 mg of MDA. Effects of the drug were noted between 40 and 60 minutes following ingestion by all eight subjects. The subjective effects following administration peaked at the end of 90 minutes and persisted for approximately 8 hours. None of the subjects experienced hallucinations, perceptual distortion, or closed-eye imagery, but they reported that the feelings the drug induced had some relationship to those previously experienced with LSD. The subjects found that both drugs induced an intensification of feelings, increased perceptions of self-insight, and heightened empathy with others during the experience. Most of the subjects also felt an increased sense of aesthetic enjoyment at some point during the intoxication. Seven of the eight subjects said they perceived music as "three dimensional" (Naranjo et al. 1967).

On the "street," MDA has been called the "love drug" because of its effects on the sense of touch and the attitudes of the users. Users often report experiencing a sense of well-being (likely a stimulant effect) and heightened tactile sensations (like a hallucinogenic effect) and thus increased pleasure through sex and expressions of affection. Those under the influence of MDA frequently focus on interpersonal relationships and demonstrate an overwhelming desire or need to be with or talk to people. Some users say they have a very pleasant "body high"—more sensual than cerebral and more emphatic than introverted.

The unpleasant side effects most often reported are nausea, periodic tensing of muscles in the neck, tightening of the jaw and grinding of the teeth, and dilation of the pupils. "Street" doses of MDA range from 100 to 150 mg. Serious convulsions and death have resulted from larger doses, but in these cases, the quantity of MDA was not accurately measured. Ingestion of 500 mg of pure MDA has been shown to cause death. The only adverse reaction to moderate doses seems to be marked physical exhaustion, lasting as long as two days (Marquardt et al. 1978).

An unpleasant MDA experience should be treated the same as a "bad trip" with any hallucinogen. The person should be "talked down" (reassured) in a friendly and supportive manner. Usually, the use of other drugs is not needed, although medical attention may be necessary. Under the Comprehensive Drug Abuse Prevention and Control Act of 1970 (see Chapter 3), MDA is classified as a Schedule I substance; illegal possession is a serious offense.

Methylenedioxymethamphetamine (MDMA). MDMA is a modification of MDA and in comparison is thought to have more psychedelic but less stimulant (for example, euphoria) activity. MDMA is also structurally similar to mescaline. This drug has become known as "Ecstasy," "XTC" and "Adam" (U.S. Department of Justice 1991b).

MDMA was synthesized in 1912, but it only became widely used in the 1980s (Shulgin 1990). This "designer" amphetamine can be produced easily; the reaction can literally be set up in a "cookie jar" using a coffee filter. The synthesis is often done sloppily by illicit labs and causes contaminants in the final product (Randall 1992a). The unusual psychological effects it produces are part of the reason for its popularity. The drug produces euphoria, increased sensitivity to touch, and lowered inhibitions. Many users claim it intensifies emotional feelings without sensory distortion and that it increases empathy and awareness both of your body and of the aesthetics of the surroundings (Creighton et al. 1991; Taylor 1994). Some consider MDMA an aphrodisiac. Because MDMA lowers defense mechanisms and reduces inhibitions, it has even been used during psychoanalysis (Creighton et al. 1991; Grob et al. 1992).

MDMA has also been popularized by articles in *Newsweek* (Adler 1985), *Time* (Toufexis 1985), and other magazines, which have mentioned the euphoric effects, potential therapeutic value, and lack of serious side effects. MDMA is still popular with college-age students and young adults (Johnston et al. 1993)—see Table 12.1. Because of its effect to enhance sensations, MDMA has been used as part of a countercultural "rave" scene, including high-tech music and laser light shows. Observers report that MDMA-linked "rave" parties are reminiscent of the "acid parties" of the 1960s and 1970s (Randall 1992b).

Because of the widespread abuse of MDMA, the DEA prohibited its use by placing it on Schedule I in 1985 (Greenhouse 1992). At the time of the ban, it was estimated that up to 200 physicians were using the drug in psychotherapy (Greer and Tolbert 1990) and an estimated 30,000 doses a month were being taken for recreational purposes

CROSSCURRENTS

Because of its ability to help people retrieve hidden thoughts and feelings, the use of MDMA (Ecstasy) for psychotherapy has been debated since it was classified as a Schedule I drug in 1985. Select one of the following positions:

1. MDMA has been proven to be a useful adjunct in psychotherapy. Because some psychiatric patients may be able to benefit from the use of this drug, it should not be classified as a Schedule I drug.
2. MDMA has been proven to be potentially dangerous and unreliable in its therapeutic action. Consequently, this drug should never be used for treatment of psychiatric patients and should remain as a Schedule I drug.

Defend your position with information contained in this text or other reputable sources.

(*American Medical News* 1985). See the Crosscurrents box.

MDMA is usually taken orally, but it is sometimes snorted or even occasionally smoked (Taylor 1994). After the "high" starts, it may persist for minutes or even an hour, depending on the person, the purity of the drug, and the environment in which it is taken. When "coming down" from an MDMA-induced high, people will often take small oral doses known as "boosters" to get high again. If they take too many boosters, they become very fatigued the next day. The average dose is about 75–150 mg; a number of cases of toxic effects have been reported at higher doses (Randall 1992a).

There is disagreement as to the possible harmful side effects of MDMA. Some negative physiological responses caused by recreational doses include dilated pupils, dry mouth and throat, clenching of teeth (in 76% of users), muscle aches and stiffness (in 28% of users), fatigue (in 80% of users), insomnia (in 38% of users), agitation, and anxiety. Some of these reactions can be intense and unpredictable. Under some conditions, death can be caused by *hyperthermia* (elevated body temperature), instability of the autonomic nervous system and kidney failure (Randall 1992a; Greenhouse 1992).

Several studies have demonstrated long-term damage to serotonin neurons in the brain following a single high dose of both MDMA and MDA (Stone et al. 1987; Gibb et al. 1990; Ricaurte 1992). Although the behavioral significance of this damage in humans is not clear, at the present time caution using this drug is warranted.

Anticholinergic Hallucinogens

The anticholinergic hallucinogens include naturally occurring alkaloid (bitter organic base) substances that are present in plants and herbs found around the world. These drugs are often mentioned in folklore and in early literature as being added to "potions." They are thought to have killed the Roman Emperor Claudius and to have poisoned Hamlet's father. Historically, they have been the favorite drugs used to eliminate inconvenient people. Hallucinogens affecting the cholinergic neurons also have been used by South American Indians for religious ceremonies (Schultes and Hofmann 1980) and were probably used in witchcraft to give the illusion of flying, to prepare sacrificial victims, and even to give some types of marijuana ("superpot") its kick.

The potato family of plants (Solanaceae) contains most of these mind-altering drugs. Three potent anticholinergic compounds are commonly found in these plants: (1) scopolamine, or hyoscine; (2) hyoscyamine; and (3) atropine. Scopolamine may produce excitement, hallucinations, and delirium even at therapeutic doses; with atropine, doses bordering on toxic levels are usually required to obtain these effects (Schultes and Hofmann 1973). All these active alkaloid drugs block some acetylcholine receptors (see Chapter 5).

These alkaloid drugs can be used as ingredients in cold symptom remedies because they have a drying effect and block production of mucus in the nose and throat (see Chapter 14). They also prevent salivation, so that the mouth becomes uncommonly dry and perspiration may stop. Atropine may increase the heart rate by 100% and cause the pupils to dilate markedly, causing inability to focus on nearby objects. Other annoying side effects of these anticholinergic drugs include constipation and difficulty in urinating. These inconveniences usually discourage excessive abuse of these drugs for their hallucinogenic properties.

Anticholinergics can cause drowsiness by affecting the sleep centers of the brain. At large doses, a condition occurs that is similar to a psychosis, characterized by delirium, loss of attention, mental confusion, and sleepiness (Carlini 1993). Hallucinations may also occur at higher doses. At very high doses, paralysis of the respiratory system may cause death.

Although hundreds of plant species naturally contain anticholinergic substances and consequently can cause psychedelic experiences, only a few of the principal plants will be mentioned here.

Atropa Belladonna: The Deadly Nightshade Plant Knowledge of this plant is very old, and its use as a drug is reported in early folklore. The name of the genus, *Atrop,* is the origin for the drug name *atropine,* and indicates the reverence the Greeks had for the plant. Atropos was one of the three Fates in Greek mythology, whose duty it was to cut the thread of life when the time came. This plant has been used for thousands of years by assassins and murderers. In the *Tales of the Arabian Nights,* unsuspecting potentates were poisoned with atropine from the deadly nightshade or one of its relatives. Fourteen berries of the deadly nightshade contain enough drug to cause death.

The species name, *belladonna,* means "beautiful woman." The early Roman and Egyptian women knew that girls with large pupils were considered attractive and friendly. To create this condition, they would put a few drops of an extract of this plant into their eyes, causing the pupils to dilate. Belladonna has also had a reputation as a love potion.

Mandragora Officinarum: The Mandrake The mandrake contains several active psychedelic alkaloids: hyoscyamine, scopolamine, atropine, and mandragorine. Mandrake has been used as a love potion for centuries but has also been known for its toxic properties. In ancient folk medicine, mandrake was used to treat many ailments in spite of its side effects. It was recommended as a sedative, to relieve nervous conditions, and to relieve pain (Schultes and Hofmann 1980).

The root of the mandrake is forked and, viewed with a little imagination, may resemble the human body. Because of this resemblance, it has been credited with human attributes, which gave rise to many superstitions in the Middle Ages about its magical powers. Shakespeare referred to this plant in *Romeo and Juliet.* In her farewell speech, Juliet says, "And shrieks like mandrakes torn out of the earth, that living mortals hearing them run mad."

Hyoscyamus Niger: Henbane Henbane is a plant that contains both hyoscyamine and scopolamine. In A.D. 60, Pliny the Elder spoke of henbane: "For this is certainly known, that if one takes it in drink more than four leaves, it will put him beside himself" (Jones 1956). Henbane was also used in the orgies, or *bacchanalias,* of the ancient world:

> Thus at the Bacchanalia, when the wide-eyed Bacchantes with their flowing locks flung themselves naked into the arms of the eager men, one can be reasonably certain that the wine which produced such sexual frenzy was not a plain fermented grape juice. Intoxication of this kind was almost certainly a result of doctoring the wine with leaves or berries of belladonna or henbane. The orgiastic rites were never totally suppressed by the Church and persisted in secret forms through the Middle Ages. Being under the shadow of the Church's displeasure, they are inevitably associated with the devil, and those who took part in them were considered to be either witches or wizards. (De Ropp 1975)

Although rarely used today, henbane has been given medicinally since early times. It was frequently used to cause sleep, although hallucinations often occurred if given in excess. It was likely included in witches' brews and deadly concoctions during the Dark Ages (Schultes and Hofmann 1980).

Datura Stramonium: Jimsonweed The Datura group of the Solanaceae family (see earlier discussion) includes a large number of related plants found worldwide. The principal active drug in this group is scopolamine; there are also several less active alkaloids.

Throughout history, these plants have been used as hallucinogens by many societies. They are mentioned in early Sanskrit and Chinese writings and were revered by the Buddhists. There is also some indication that the priestess (oracle) at the ancient Greek temple of Apollo at Delphi was under the influence of Datura when she made prophecies (Schultes 1970). Prior to the supposed divine possession, she appeared to have chewed leaves of the sacred laurel. A mystic vapor was also reported to have risen from a fissure in the ground. The sacred laurel may have been one of the Datura species, and the vapors may have come from burning these plants.

Datura stramonium, or *jimsonweed,* was used by the Algonquin Indians of the eastern woodlands of North America during a ceremony of entry into manhood (see Figure 12.5):

> The youths are confined for long periods, given no other substance but the infusion or concoction of some poisonous, intoxicating roots. . . . They became stark, staring mad, in which raving condition they were kept eighteen or twenty days. . . . Thus they unlive their former lives and commence manhood by forgetting that they ever have been boys. (Schultes and Hofmann 1973)

Jimsonweed gets its name from an incident that took place in seventeenth-century Jamestown. British soldiers ate this weed while trying to capture Nathaniel Bacon, who had made seditious remarks about the king (see the Case in Point box). Although still abused occasionally by adventuresome young people, the anticholinergic side effects of "jimsonweed" are so unpleasant that it rarely becomes a long-term problem.

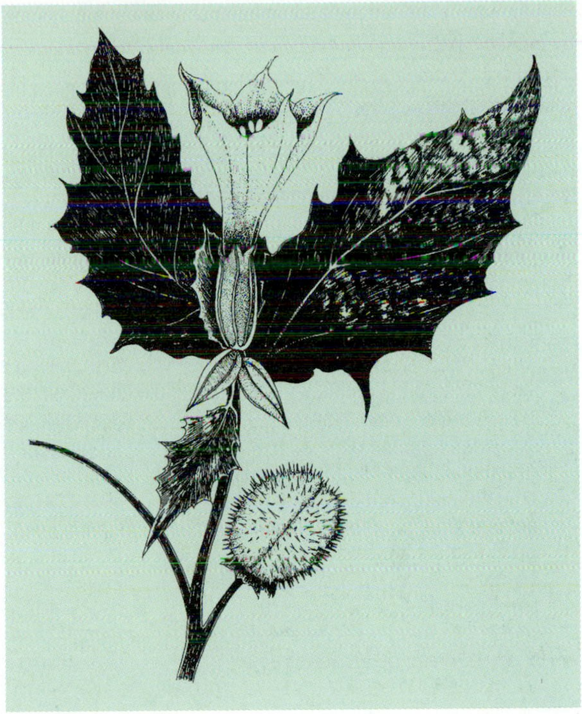

FIGURE 12.5 *Datura stramonium*, or jimsonweed, a common plant that contains the hallucinogenic drug scopolamine.

Other Hallucinogens

Technically, any drug that alters perceptions, thoughts, and feelings in a manner that is not normally experienced but in dreams can be classified as a hallucinogen. Because the brain's sensory input is complex and involves several neurotransmitter systems, drugs with many diverse effects can cause hallucinations. For example, CNS stimulants (for example, amphetamines and cocaine), CNS depressants (for example, sedatives/hypnotics or general anesthetics), and drugs that influence endocrine systems (for example, steroids), under certain circumstances can all be hallucinogens (Jaffe 1990).

These major drug groups have already been discussed in detail. Three other agents that do not conveniently fit into the principal categories of hallucinogens will be discussed in the following sections.

Case in Point

Jimsonweed in Jamestown

The following account tells of the intoxicated antics of a group of British soldiers who ate some of the "JamesTown Weed," or *jimsonweed:*

> The James-Town Weed . . . is supposed to be one of the greatest Coolers in the World. This being an early Plant, was gather'd very young for a boil'd Salad, by some of the Soldiers sent thither, to pacifie the Troubles of Bacon; and some of them eat plentifully of it, the Effect of which was a very pleasant Comedy; for they turn'd natural Fools upon it for several Days: One would blow up a Feather in the air; another wou'd dart Straws at it with much Fury; and another stark naked was sitting up in a Corner, like a Monkey, grinning and making Mows at them; a Fourth would fondly kiss, and paw his Companions, and snear in their Faces, with a Countenance more antick, than any in a Dutch Droll. In this frantick Condition they were confined, lest they should in their Folly destroy themselves; though it was observed, that all their Actions were full of Innocence and good Nature. Indeed, they were not very cleanly; for they would have wallow'd in their own Excrements, if they had not been prevented. A thousand such simple Tricks they play'd, and after Eleven Days, return'd to themselves again, not remembering any thing that had pass'd. (Beverly 1947, 139)

Phencyclidine (PCP) PCP is considered by many experts as the most dangerous of the hallucinogens (U.S. Department of Justice 1991b). PCP was developed in the late 1950s as an intravenous anesthetic. Although it was found to be effective, it had serious side effects that caused it to be discontinued for human use. Sometimes when people were recovering from PCP anesthesia, they experienced delirium and manic states of excitation lasting 18 hours (Jaffe 1990). PCP is currently a Schedule II drug, legitimately available only as an anesthetic for animals. However, it has been banned from veterinarians since 1985 because of its high theft rate. Most, if not all, PCP used in the United States today is produced illegally (U.S. Department of Justice 1991b).

"Street" PCP is mainly synthesized from readily available chemical precursors in clandestine laboratories. Within 24 hours, "cooks" (the makers of street PCP) can set up a lab, make several gallons of the drug, and destroy the lab before the police can locate them. Liquid PCP is then poured into containers and ready for shipment (Sanchez 1988).

PCP first appeared on the street drug scene in 1967 as the *"PeaCe Pill."* In 1968, it reappeared in New York as a substance called "hog." By 1969, PCP was found under a variety of guises. It was sold as "angel dust" and sprinkled on parsley for smoking. It has sold on the streets under at least 50 different slang names, including *loveboat, lovely, key to street E, greed, wacky weed, supergrass, rocket fuel, elephant tranquilizer, snorts, cyclone, cadillac, earth, killer weed, embalming fluid,* and *flying saucers* (Sanchez 1988; U.S. Department of Justice 1991b).

It was in the late 1960s that PCP began to find its way into a variety of street drugs sold as psychedelics. By 1970, authorities observed that phencyclidine was used widely as a main ingredient in psychedelic preparations. It is still frequently substituted for and sold as LSD, mescaline, marijuana, and cocaine (Goldstein 1995).

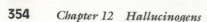

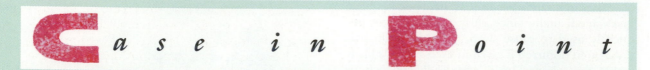

One difficulty in estimating the effects or use patterns of PCP is caused by variance in drug purity. Also, there are about 30 **analogs** of PCP, some of which have appeared on the street. PCP has so many other street names that people may not know they are using it or they may have been deceived when buying what they thought was LSD or mescaline. Users may not question the identity of the substances unless they have a bad reaction.

PCP is available as a pure, white crystalline powder, as tablets, or as capsules. However, because it is usually manufactured in makeshift laboratories, it is frequently discolored by contaminants from a tan to brown with consistency ranging from powder to a gummy mass (U.S. Department of Justice 1991b). PCP can be taken orally, smoked, sniffed, or injected (American Psychiatric Association 1994). In the late 1960s through the early 1970s, PCP was mostly taken orally, but it is now commonly snorted or applied to dark brown cigarettes, leafy materials such as parsley, mint, oregano, marijuana, or tobacco and smoked (U.S. Department of Justice 1991b). By smoking PCP, the experienced user is better able to limit his or her dosage to a desired level. After smoking, the subjective effects appear within 1 to 5 minutes and peak within the next 5 to 30 minutes. The "high" lasts about 4 to 6 hours, followed by a 6- to 24-hour "comedown."

In the 1979 national drug survey taken by the National Institute on Drug Abuse, about 7% of the U.S. high school seniors had used PCP in a 12-month period; however, in 1993 that rate declined to 1.4% (Johnston 1994).

Physiological Effects. Although PCP may have hallucinogenic effects, it can also cause a host of other physiological actions, including stimulation, depression, anesthesia, and analgesia. The effects of PCP on the central nervous system vary greatly. At low doses, the most prominent effect is similar to that of alcohol intoxication, with generalized numbness. As the dose of PCP is increased, the person becomes even more insensitive and may become fully anesthetized. Large doses can cause coma, convulsions, and death (American Psychiatric Association 1994).

The majority of peripheral effects are apparently related to activation of the sympathetic nervous system (see Chapter 5). Flushing, excess sweating, and a blank stare are common, although the size of the pupils is unaffected. The cardiovascular system reacts by increasing blood pressure and heart rate. Other effects include side-to-side eye movements, called *nystagmus;* muscular incoordination; double vision; dizziness; nausea; and vomiting (U.S. Department of Justice 1991b). These symptoms occur in many people taking medium to high doses.

ANALOGS drugs with similar structures

Psychological Effects. PCP has unpleasant effects most of the time it is used. Why, then, do people use it repeatedly as their drug of choice?

PCP has the ability to alter markedly the person's subjective feelings; this may be reinforcing, even though the alteration is not always positive. There is an element of risk, not knowing how the "trip" will turn out. PCP may give the user feelings of strength, power, and invulnerability. One user describes the effects of PCP as follows: "I felt like I didn't have a care in the world. It made me feel like God, like I was powerful. I felt superhuman" (Sanchez 1988). Other positive effects include heightened sensitivity to outside stimuli, a sense of stimulation and mood elevation, and dissociation from surroundings. Also, PCP is a social drug; virtually all users report taking it in groups rather than during a solitary experience (Petersen and Stillman 1978).

PCP also causes serious perceptual distortions. Users cannot accurately interpret the environment and as a result may walk in front of moving cars or jump off buildings, feeling indestructible or weightless (Goldstein 1995). In California, when many people were experimenting with PCP, drownings were frequent. A study found that, in 19 cases of death where PCP was present, 11 were due to drowning (one in the shower). Apparently, some PCP users lose their orientation while swimming or immersed in water and drown, sometimes in small amounts of water (Petersen and Stillman 1978). High oral doses have been used to commit suicide; respiratory depression is the specific cause of death.

Chronic users may take PCP in "runs" extending over two to three days, during which time they do not sleep or eat. In later stages of chronic administration, users may develop outright paranoia and unpredictable violent behavior, as well as auditory hallucinations (American Psychiatric Association 1994). Law enforcement officers claim

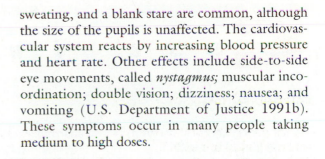

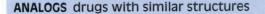

Case in Point

The PCP Explosion

The following account relays a horrible incident involving a woman on PCP and law enforcement personnel who tried to subdue her:

> Before the Prince George's County police officer pumped three bullets into her, 26-year-old Sharon Araoye horrified neighbors in a Riverdale Hills apartment complex in July. Walking toward the officer in the parking lot, Araoye, who was nude, repeatedly plunged a butcher knife into her body—including her eye, chest abdomen, and groin. She continued to stab herself even after the officer fired at her. She died five hours later.
>
> The reason for the fatal outburst; phencyclidine. PCP. (Sanchez 1988)

How justified are law officers to resort to violence when they believe they are dealing with suspects under the influence of PCP?

to be more fearful of suspects on PCP than of suspects on other drugs of abuse. Often such people appear to have superhuman strength and are totally irrational and very difficult, even dangerous, to manage (see Case in Point box).

"PCP" has no equal in its ability to produce brief psychoses similar to schizophrenia. The psychoses—induced with moderate doses given to normal, healthy volunteers—last about two hours and are characterized by changes in body image, thought disorders, estrangement, autism, and occasionally rigid inability to move (**catatonia,** or catalepsy). Subjects report feeling numb, have great difficulty differentiating between themselves and their surroundings, and complain afterward of feeling extremely isolated and apathetic. They are often violently paranoid during the psychosis (American Psychiatric Association 1994). When PCP was given experimentally to hospitalized chronic schizophrenics, it made them much worse not for several hours but for six weeks. "PCP is not just another hallucinogen, to be warned about in the same breath as LSD. . . . PCP is far more dangerous to some individuals than the other abused drugs" (Luisada 1978; Goldstein 1995).

Medical Management. The diagnosis of a PCP overdose is frequently missed because the symptoms often closely resemble those of an acute schizophrenic episode.

Simple, uncomplicated PCP intoxication can be managed with the same techniques used in other psychedelic drug cases. It is important to have a quiet environment, limited contact with an empathic person capable of determining any deterioration in the patient's physical state, protection from self-harm, and the availability of hospital facilities. "Talking down" is not helpful; the patient is better off isolated from external stimuli as much as possible.

Valium is often used for its sedating effect to prevent injury to self and to staff and also to reduce the chance for severe convulsions. An antipsychotic agent (for example, Haldol) is used to make the patient manageable (Jaffe 1990).

The medical management of a comatose or convulsing patient is more difficult. The patient may need external respiratory assistance and external cooling to reduce fever. Blood pressure may have to be reduced to safe levels and convulsions controlled. Restraints and four to five strong hospital aides are often needed to prevent the patient from injuring himself or herself or the medical staff. After the coma lightens, the patient typically becomes delirious, paranoid, and violently assaultive (Petersen and Stillman 1978).

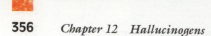

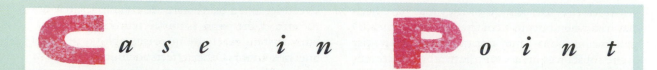

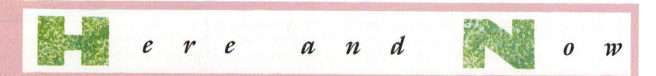

Here and Now

Sniffing Out the Inhalants: Signs of Abuse

The following are common signs found in children who are frequent users of inhalants (see photo):

1. Collect an unusual assortment of chemicals (such as glues, paints, thinners and solvents, nail polish, liquid eraser, and cleaning fluids) in bedroom or with belongings.
2. Breath occasionally smells of solvents.
3. Often has sniffles similar to a cold, but without other symptoms of the ailment.
4. Appears drunk for short periods of time (15–60 min.), but recovers quickly.
5. Doesn't do well in school and usually is unkempt.
6. Smell of inhalants or solvents in unusual containers around the house, such as soda cans and plastic bags or on rags and bandannas.
7. If sniffing continues for extended time, there may be physical signs such as a rash around the mouth and nose, frequent headaches, nausea, slurred speech, nose bleeds, and loss of weight (U.S. Department of Justice, 1991b).

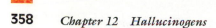

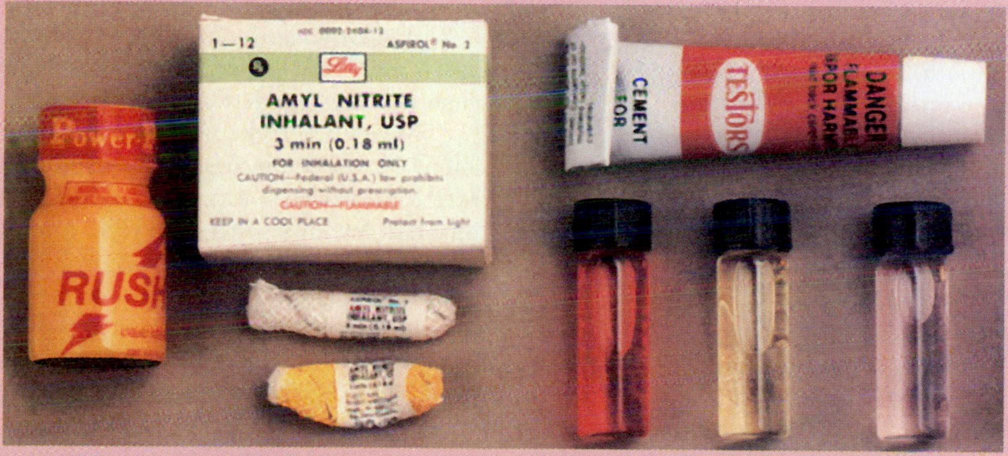

Inhalants. These volatile chemicals, which include many common household substances, are often the most dangerous drug, per dose, a person can take. In addition, inhalants are most often used by young children.

Effects of Chronic Use. Chronic PCP users may develop a tolerance to the drug; thus, a decrease in behavioral effects and toxicity can occur with frequent administration. Different forms of dependence may occur when tolerance develops. Users may complain of vague cravings after cessation of the drug. In addition, long-term difficulties in memory, speech, and thinking persist for 6 to 12 months in the chronic user (Jaffe 1990). These functional changes are accompanied by personality deficits such as social isolation, states of anxiety, nervousness, and extreme agitation (American Psychiatric Association 1994).

Marijuana In high doses, marijuana use can result in image distortions and hallucinations (Abood and Martin 1992). Some users claim that marijuana can enhance hearing, vision, and skin sensitivity, although these claims have not been confirmed in controlled laboratory studies.

Although typical marijuana use does not appear to cause severe emotional disorders like the other hallucinogens, some experts suggest it can aggravate underlying mental illness such as depression. Each month, an estimated 5,000 people seek professional treatment due to marijuana-related problems (Brown 1991). In contrast to other hallucinogens that have a combination of stimulant and psychedelic effects, high doses of marijuana cause a combination of depression and hallucinations and enhances the appetite (Goldstein 1995). Marijuana is discussed thoroughly in Chapter 13.

Inhalants Many adolescents (eighth to twelfth grades) in the United States will at some time during their young lives experiment with inhalants (U.S. Department of Justice 1991b). In fact, during 1993 almost 20% of the eighth-graders in this country had used these substances (Johnston et al. 1993; Johnston 1994). Inhalants are gases that can be introduced into the body through the pulmonary (lungs) route. This category of drugs includes an array of different compounds and can be classified into three major groups: **volatile** solvents, anesthetics, and nitrites (Swan 1993). Most of the inhalants can cause hallucinations as well as create intoxicating and euphorigenic effects.

Volatile Solvents. Many of these substances were never intended to be used by humans as drugs; consequently, they are often not thought of as having abuse potential. For example, these inhalants include some solvents, glue, paint thinner, aerosols from paints, hairsprays, cookware coating agents, liquid paper correction fluid, nail polish remover, felt-tip marking pens, lighter and cleaning fluids, and gasoline (U.S. Department of Justice 1991b). These chemicals are not regulated like other drugs of abuse, so they are readily available to young people. Consequently, children and teenagers (7 to 17 years) are most likely to abuse the volatile solvents (Swan 1993). Parents should be particularly cautious about making sure their children are not inadvertently exposed to these chemicals (see the Here and Now box).

The effects of the volatile chemicals that are commonly abused include initial nausea with some irritation of airways causing coughing and sneezing. With low doses there is often a brief feeling of light-headedness, mild stimulation followed by a loss of control, lack of coordination, and disorientation accompanied by dizziness and possible hallucinations (Goldstein 1995). With higher doses, there can be relaxation and depression leading to sleep or coma. The depression effects resemble those caused by alcohol but of a shorter duration: 15–60 min. (U.S. Department of Justice 1991b; American Psychiatric Association 1994).

Several potential toxicities may result from inhaling large quantities of these substances. Some of these chemicals can cause heart arrhythmia, the principal cause of death from acute inhalant exposure (Jaffe 1990). In some cases, the abuser inhales the vapors from containers such as plastic bags or soda cans (called "sniffing," "snorting," or "huffing") to maximize the dose as well as from old rags or bandannas soaked in a solvent fluid (U.S. Department of Justice 1991b). If inhalation is continued, dangerous **hypoxia** may occur and cause

CATATONIA a condition of physical rigidity, excitement, and stupor

VOLATILE readily evaporated at low temperatures

HYPOXIA a state of oxygen deficiency

brain damage or death (Swan 1993). Other potential toxic consequences of inhaling such substances include hypertension and damage to the cardiac muscle, peripheral nerves, brain, and kidneys (American Psychiatric Association 1994).

The potential harm from chronic use of the volatile inhalants has not been well studied. However, it appears that repeated exposure to these chemicals can cause (1) permanent brain damage, which interferes with reasoning, memory, and problem-solving ability; (2) impairment of motor behavior, which results in frequent falls and accidents and an inability to do simple motor tasks; (3) severe psychological problems, which cause a withdrawn personality frequently accompanied with severe depression; (4) other serious health consequences such as damage to airways, lungs, kidneys, and liver. In addition, chronic users of inhalants frequently lose their appetite, are continually tired, and experience nose bleeds. If use of inhalants persists, some of the damage becomes irreversible (U.S. Department of Justice 1991b; American Psychiatric Association 1994).

Why do children and teenagers sniff the fumes of these dangerous chemicals? Most often a friend or sibling encourages the initial exposure. Chronic inhalant users frequently have a profile like that associated with other substance abusers; that is, often they live in unhappy surroundings with severe family or school problems, they have poor self-images, and sniffing gives them a readily available escape (U.S. Department of Justice 1991b).

As with most substances of abuse, the fewer times volatile inhalants are used, the easier it is to stop and the less likely it is that severe physiological damage has been done. Although the inhalants do not tend to cause dangerous physical dependence, their chronic use can cause an addiction, which requires professional counseling or even hospitalization (American Psychiatric Association 1994). Frequently, the young inhalant users resist treatment for their addiction, because of peer pressure (U.S. Department of Justice 1991b).

Anesthetics. When used properly, other forms of inhalants with abuse potential are important therapeutic agents. Included in this category are the general anesthetics. Although all the anesthetic gases work much like the CNS depressants, only nitrous oxide (laughing gas) is available enough to be a significant abuse concern (Swan 1993). Nitrous oxide is frequently used for minor outpatient procedures in offices of both physicians and dentists. Consequently, the most likely abusers of this substance are health professionals themselves or their staff. For the most part, nitrous oxide does not pose a significant abuse problem for the general public. However, occasionally college students also abuse nitrous oxide via small cylindrical cartridges used as charges for whipped cream dispensers and referred to as "whippets" (Goldstein 1995). Although significant abuse problems are infrequent, there are occasional reports of severe hypoxia or death due to acute overdoses with nitrous oxide or psychosis and neuronal disorders developing after chronic abuse (Dohrn 1993).

Nitrites. Historically, nitrites have been abused by only a few, selective groups, such as gay men, to enhance "sexual stamina and pleasure." The nitrite products are referred to as "poppers" or "rush" and used to contain butyl and propyl nitrites. However, their use has dramatically declined since these chemicals were banned in 1991 (Swan 1993).

Patterns of Inhalant Abuse. Inhalant abuse is typically a problem of younger adolescents. Older teenagers often view use of inhalants with disdain and consider it unsophisticated and a "kid's" habit. There has been a recent disturbing trend of increasing inhalant abuse by younger kids (for example, approximately 20% more eighth-graders abused inhalants in 1993 than in 1991; see Table 12.1). Much of this increase in abuse is thought to be due to more young girls starting to sniff the volatile solvents. At present, it appears that in most parts of the country, males use solvents at only a slightly higher rate than females (Swan 1993).

Survey results suggest that patterns of inhalant abuse are more dependent on socioeconomic than ethnic factors. For example, use by Hispanic adolescents is high in some low-income neighborhoods; however, their patterns of abuse are similar to other ethnic groups in intermediate- and high-income neighborhoods. Consequently, it is not surprising that Native Americans, who on average live in the worst socioeconomic conditions, also have the highest solvent abuse rates (Swan 1993).

The extent of solvent abuse in the United

States is very difficult to determine accurately. Typically, inhalant abuse has an episodic pattern, with short-term outbreaks occurring at single schools or in a limited region. These isolated incidents reflect the faddish nature of inhalant use and result in a continually fluctuating level of abuse. Consequently, results from regional surveys for solvent abuse frequently are distorted and do not accurately represent the national abuse patterns for these substances. However, despite the problems of accurately determining the extent of inhalant use it is apparent that these products are being frequently abused by many adolescents, and the result can be deadly (Swan 1993).

Review Questions

1. Why were substances with hallucinogenic properties so popular with ancient religions and cults?
2. Why would a drug with both stimulant and hallucinogenic effects be a popular drug of abuse?
3. Why do some users find a psychedelic experience terrifying?
4. Do you think the federal government was justified in lying to the public about the dangers of LSD to get people to stop using this drug? Defend your answer.
5. How do the side effects of LSD compare to those of the CNS depressants?
6. Why is PCP more dangerous than LSD?
7. How do the effects of MDMA differ from those of LSD?
8. Why is the use of inhalants by kids especially disturbing?
9. What is the best way to convince people that hallucinogenic drugs of abuse should not be used?

Key Terms

hallucinogens
psychotomimetic
psychedelic
psychotogenic
synesthesia
"flashback"
ergotism
mydriasis
analogs
catatonia
volatile
hypoxia

Summary

1. Many drugs can exert hallucinogenic effects. The principal hallucinogens include LSD-types, phenylethylamines, and anticholinergic agents. The four major effects that occur from administering LSD include (a) heightened senses, (b) a loss of sensory control, (c) self-reflection or introspection, and (d) a loss of identity or sense of cosmic merging.
2. The popularity of the classical hallucinogens, such as LSD, has diminished substantially since the turbulent times of the 1960s. Some of the explanations for their diminished popularity include increased federal regulation, lack of physical dependence resulting from their use, changes in social climate, and concern about dangerous side effects.
3. Hallucinogens exaggerate sensory input and cause vivid and unusual visual and auditory effects.
4. The classical hallucinogens, such as LSD, cause predominantly psychedelic effects. Phenylethylamines are related to amphetamines and cause varying combinations of psychedelic and stimulant effects. Anticholinergic drugs are also psychedelic in high doses.
5. One of the prominent effects of hallucinogens is to cause self-reflection. The user becomes aware of thoughts and feelings that had been

forgotten or repressed. Some experiences help to clarify motives and relationships and cause periods of greater openness. These effects have been claimed by some psychiatrists to provide valid insights useful in psychotherapy.

6. The classical hallucinogens do not cause physical dependence. Although some tolerance can occur to the hallucinogenic effects of drugs like LSD, withdrawal effects are usually minor. Consequently, hallucinogens tend to be less abused than other scheduled drugs.
7. The environment plays a major role in determining the sensory response to hallucinogens. Environments that are warm, comfortable, and hospitable tend to create a pleasant sensory response to the psychedelic effects of these drugs. In contrast, threatening, hostile environments are likely to lead to intimidating, frightening "bad trips."
8. In some users, high doses of LSD can cause a terrifying destruction of identity, resulting in panic and severe anxiety that resembles schizophrenia. Another psychological feature commonly associated with LSD is the "flashback" phenomenon. LSD use can cause recurring, unexpected visual and time distortions that last a few minutes to several hours. Flashbacks can occur months to years after use of the drug.
9. Hallucinogens purchased on the "street" are usually poorly prepared and contaminated with adulterant substances. This practice of cutting with other substances also makes use of street hallucinogens very dangerous.
10. PCP differs from the other traditional hallucinogens in several ways: (a) It is a general anesthetic in high doses. (b) It causes schizophrenia-like psychosis. PCP can cause incredible strength and extreme violent behavior, making users very difficult to manage. (c) Management of the severe psychological reactions to PCP requires drug therapy, whereas treatment of other hallucinogens often only requires reassurance, "talking down," and supportive therapy. (d) Reactions to overdoses include fever, convulsions, and coma.
11. The commonly abused inhalants are volatile substances that can cause hallucinations, intoxication, and euphoria. These substances include the volatile solvents, the anesthetics, and the nitrites. These chemicals are typically abused by children and teenagers due to their availability. The effects of inhalant drugs are mild stimulation, lack of motor control, dizziness, and hallucinations. High doses can cause violent behavior, heart arrhythmia, unconsciousness, and even death.

References

Abood, M., and B. Martin, "Neurobiology of Marijuana Abuse." *Trends in Pharmacological Sciences* 13 (May 1992): 201–06.

Adler, J. "Getting High on Ecstasy." *Newsweek* (15 April 1985): 15.

American Medical News (14 June 1985).

American Psychiatric Association. "Substance-Related Disorders." *Diagnostic Statistical Manual of Mental Disorders*, 4th ed. *[DSM-IV]*, A. Frances, Chairperson, 175–272. Washington, DC: American Psychiatric Association 1994.

Bourne, P. G., ed. *Acute Drug Emergencies: A Treatment Manual.* New York: Academic Press, 1976.

Brown, M. *Guide to Fight Substance Abuse.* Nashville, TN: International Broadcast Services, 1991.

Burger, A., ed. "Quotes from Albert Hofman," *Drugs Affecting the Central Nervous System.* Psychotomimetic Agents, Vol. 2. New York: Dekker, 1968.

Carlini, E. "Preliminary Note: Dangerous Use of Anticholinergic Drugs in Brazil." *Drug and Alcohol Dependence* 32 (1993): 1–7.

"Celebration #1." *New Yorker* 42 (1966): 43.

Claus, E. P., V. E. Tyler, and L. R. Brady. *Pharmacognosy,* 6th ed. Philadelphia: Lea & Febiger, 1970.

Creighton, F., D. Black, and C. Hyde, "'Ecstasy' Psychosis and Flashbacks." *British Journal of Psychiatry* 159 (1991): 713–15.

De Ropp, R. S. *Drugs and the Mind.* New York: Grove, 1975.

Dishotsky, N. I., W. D. Loughman, R. E. Mogar, and W. R. Lipscomb. "LSD and Genetic Damage." *Science* 172 (1971): 431–40.

Dohrn, C., J. Lichtor, D. Coalson, A. Uitvlugt, H. deWit, and J. Zachny. "Reinforcing Effects of Extended Inhalation of Nitrous Oxide in Humans." *Drug and Alcohol Dependence* 31 (1993): 265–80.

Gibb, J. W., D. Stone, M. Johnson, and G. R. Hanson. "Neurochemical Effects of MDMA." In *Ecstasy: The*

Clinical, Pharmacological and Neurotoxicological Effects of the Drug MDMA, edited by S. J. Peroutka. Boston: Kluwer, 1990.

Glennon, R. "Psychoactive Phenylisopropylamines." In *Psychopharmacology,* edited by H. Meltzer. New York: Raven Press, 1987.

Goldstein, A. In *Addiction from Biology to Drug Policy.* New York: Freeman, 1994.

Goldstein, F. "Pharmacological Aspects of Substance Abuse." In *Remington's Pharmaceutical Sciences,* 19th ed., edited by A. R. Genaro. Easton, PA: Mack, 1995.

Greenhouse, C. "NIDA Lays Plans for Quicker Response to Drug Crises." *NIDA Notes* 7 (January–February 1992): 20–22.

Greer, G., and R. Tolbert. "The Therapeutic Use of MDMA." In *Ecstasy: The Clinical, Pharmacological and Neurotoxicological Effects of the Drug MDMA,* edited by S. J. Peroutka. Boston: Kluwer, 1990.

Grob, C., G. Bravo, R. Walsh, and M. Liester, "The MDMA-Neurotoxicity Controversy: Implications for Clinical Research with Novel Psychoactive Drugs." *Journal of Nervous and Mental Disease* 180 (1992): 355–56.

Hofmann, A. "Psychotomimetic Agents." In *Drugs Affecting the Central Nervous System,* vol. 2, edited by A. Burger, 169–235. New York: Dekker, 1968.

Huxley, A. *The Doors of Perception.* New York: Harper, 1954.

"Indian Religion, Must Say No." *Economist* 317 (6 October 1990): 25.

Jaffe, J. "Drug Addiction and Drug Abuse." In *The Pharmacological Basis of Therapeutics,* 8th ed., edited by A. Gilman, T. Rall, A. Nies, and P. Taylor. New York: Pergamon: 1990.

Johnston, L. "Drug Use Rises Among Teen-agers." University of Michigan News Release, January 27, 1994.

Johnston, L., P. O'Malley, and J. Bachman. *National Survey Results on Drug Use from Monitoring the Future Study,* 1975–1992. Vol. 1. University of Michigan, NIDA, NIH Publication no. 93-3597. National Institute on Drug Abuse, Washington, DC: 1993.

Jones, W. H. S. *Natural History.* Cambridge, MA: Harvard University Press, 1956.

Leary, T., R. Metzner, and R. Alpert. *The Psychedelic Experience.* New Hyde Park, NY: University Books, 1964.

Luisada, P. V. "The Phencyclidine Psychosis: Phenomenology and Treatment." In *Phencyclidine (PCP) Abuse: An Appraisal,* edited by R. C. Petersen and R. C. Stillman. NIDA Research Monograph no. 21. Washington, DC: National Institute on Drug Abuse, U.S. Department of Health, Education, and Welfare, 1978.

Marquardt, G. M., V. DiStefano, and L. L. Ling. "Pharmacological Effects of (±)-, (S)-, and (R)-MDA." In *The Psychopharmacology of Hallucinogens,* edited by R. C. Stillman and R. E. Willette. New York: Pergamon, 1978.

Mathias, R. "NIDA Research Takes a New Look at LSD and Other Hallucinogens." *NIDA Notes* 8 (March–April 1993): 6.

McGlothin, W., S. Cohen, and M. S. McGlothin. "Long-Lasting Effects of LSD on Normals." *Archives of General Psychiatry* 17 (1967): 521–32.

"Mind Expansion." *Compute* (October 1991): 160.

Nadis, S. "After Lights." *Omni* (February 1990): 24.

Naranjo, C., A. T. Shulgin, and T. Sargent. "Evaluation of 3, 4-Methylenedioxyamphetamine (MDA) as an Adjunct to Psychotherapy." *Medicina et Pharmacologia Experimentalis* 17 (1967): 359–64.

Negin, E. "CBS '48 Hours' Fails Acid Test." *American Journalism Review* 15 (March 1993): 10.

Pahnke, W. N., A. A. Kurland, S. Unger, C. Savage, and S. Grof. "The Experimental Use of Psychedelic (LSD) Psychotherapy." In *Hallucinogenic Drug Research: Impact on Science and Society,* edited by J. R. Gamage and E. L. Zerkin. Beloit, WI: Stash, 1970.

Pahnke, W. N., and W. A. Richards. "Implications of LSD and Experimental Mysticism." *Journal of Religion and Health* 5 (1966): 175–208.

Panikkar, R., trans. *Rig Veda, Book VIII,* 48. [Sanskrit Hymns, 1500 B.C.] Los Angeles: University of California Press, 1977.

Petersen, R. C., and R. C. Stillman. "Phencyclidine: An Overview." In *Phencyclidine (PCP) Abuse: An Appraisal,* edited by R. C. Petersen and R. C. Stillman. NIDA Research Monograph no. 21. Washington, DC: National Institute on Drug Abuse, U.S. Department of Health, Education, and Welfare. 1978.

Randall, T. "Ecstasy-Fueled 'Rave' Parties Becomes Dances of Death for English Youth." *JAMA* 268 (1992a): 1505.

Randall, T. "'Rave' Scene, Ecstasy Use, Leap Atlantic," *JAMA* 268 (1992b): 1505.

Ricaurte, G., A. Martello, M. Katz, and M. Martello. "Long-lasting Effects of MDMA on Central Serotonergic Neurons in Nonhuman Primates: Neurochemical Observations." *Journal of Pharmacology and Experimental Therapeutics* 261 (1992): 616.

Sanchez, E. "PCP Users Are Courting Fire." *Washington Post* (7 March 1988): A-1.

Schultes, R. E. "The Plant Kingdom and Hallucinogens (Part III)." *Bulletin on Narcotics* 22, no. 1 (1970): 25–53.

Schultes, R. E. "Ethnopharmacological Significance of Psychotropic Drugs of Vegetal Origin." In *Principles of Psychopharmacology,* 2d ed., edited by W. G. Clark and J. del Giudice. New York: Academic Press, 1978.

Schultes, R. E., and A. Hofmann. *The Botany and Chemistry of Hallucinogens.* Springfield, IL: Thomas, 1973.

Schultes, R. E., and A. Hofmann. *The Botany and Chemistry of Hallucinogens,* 2d ed. Springfield, IL: Thomas, 1980.

Shulgin, A. "History of MDMA." In *Ecstasy: The Clinical, Pharmacological, and Neurotoxicological Effects of the Drug MDMA,* ed. by S. J. Peroutka. Boston: Kluwer, 1990.

Snyder, S. H. *Madness and the Brain.* New York: McGraw-Hill, 1974.

Stone, D., M. Johnson, G. R. Hanson, and J. W. Gibb. "A Comparison of the Neurotoxic Potential of Methylenedioxyamphetamine (MDA) and N-Methylated and N-Ethylated Derivatives." *European Journal of Pharmacology* 134 (1987): 245–48.

Stone, J. "Turn On, Tune In, Boot Up." *Discover* 12 (June 1991): 32–33.

Strassman, R. "Human Hallucinogen Interactions with Drugs Affecting Serotonergic Neurotransmission." *Neuropsychopharmacology* 7 (1992): 241–43.

Swan, N. "Inhalant Abuse and Its Dangers Are Nothing to Sniff at." *NIDA Notes* 8 (July–August 1993): 15.

Taylor, J. "All-New MDMA FAQ." *Internet* (computer networking service), usenet News, sci.med.pharmacy (27 May 1994).

Toufexis, A. "A Crackdown on Ecstasy." *Time* (10 June 1985): 64.

Tucker, R. "Acid Test." *Omni* (November 1987): 16.

U.S. Department of Justice. "It Never Did Go Away—LSD, A Sixties Drug, Attracts Users in the Nineties." Pamphlet from DEA, Washington, DC, 1991a.

U.S. Department of Justice. "Let's All Work to Fight Drug Abuse." Pamphlet from DEA published by L.A.W. Publications and distributed with permission by International Drug Education Association, 1991b.

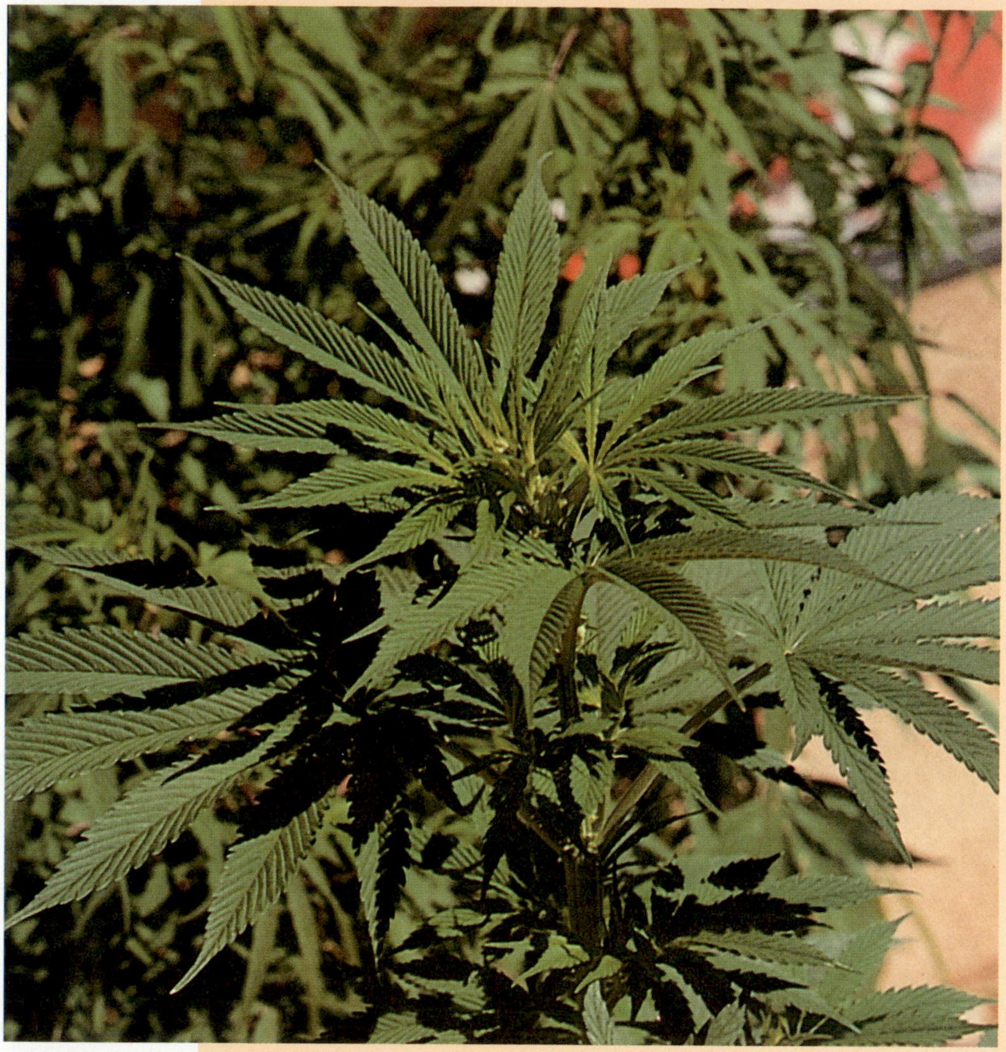

Chapter 13

Marijuana

DID YOU KNOW THAT . . .

- More than 20 million Americans are current marijuana users, making this the most frequently used illicit substance of abuse.
- In some states, marijuana is one of the largest cash-producing crops.
- The first known record of marijuana use is in the *Book of Drugs,* written in 2737 B.C. in China.
- An early use of marijuana plants was to make rope and cloth.
- THC, the main psychoactive chemical in marijuana, is what produces the "high," and is available by prescription in a drug called Marinol.
- THC remains stored for a long period in body fat; complete elimination can take up to 30 days.
- THC, the active ingredient in marijuana, reaches the brain within 14 seconds after inhalation.
- A typical "high" from one marijuana cigarette lasts two to three hours.
- Findings from surveys indicate that 60 to 80% of marijuana users sometimes drive when "high."
- Cannabis has been used to treat extreme nausea, glaucoma, pain, and convulsions.
- George Washington grew marijuana plants at Mount Vernon for medicine and to make rope.

LEARNING OBJECTIVES

On completing this chapter, you will be able to

1. Explain what marijuana is.
2. Describe the effects that high and low doses of marijuana have on the body.
3. Define *hashish* (or *hasheesh*), *ganja, sinsemilla,* and *bhang.*
4. Summarize how THC affects the body overall and in particular, the respiratory system, blood pressure, sexual behavior, and growth and development.
5. Describe how tolerance and dependence affect the response to marijuana and its use.
6. Describe how marijuana has been prescribed for therapeutic purposes.
7. Summarize the effects of marijuana on motor functions.
8. Define the "amotivational syndrome" for marijuana.
9. Explain the patterns of marijuana use in the United States.
10. Discuss the link between marijuana use and progression to other more serious drugs.

Healthy People 2000

Increase by at least one year the average age of first use of . . . marijuana by adolescents aged 12 through 17.

Reduce the proportion of young people who have used . . . marijuana . . . in the past month.

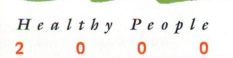

"So how to get over, how to get by?/I wish I had a joint to get me high." These lyrics from the song "I Need a Joint," by the rap group Basehead, reflect the psychological dependence many users have developed on the plant known as *marijuana*. Perhaps no other substance has been the object of so much research and controversy as marijuana. It is a vegetable substance called *Cannabis sativa,* the hemp plant, and grows wild in most temperate and tropical climates. It is also a money-making cash crop in parts of the world, including the United States. When prepared as a drug, marijuana consists of dried and crushed leaves, flowers, stems, and seeds. At low dose levels, usually when smoked or eaten, marijuana has sedative effects; at higher doses, the effects are similar to those of mind-expanding hallucinogens. The potency of marijuana varies tremendously, depending on the source and parts of the cannabis plant used.

Marijuana has a long, controversial history of use and abuse, and the pharmacological and social impact of its recreational administration has been somewhat trivialized in Western industrialized countries since the 1960s (Nahas and Latour 1992). This substance is remarkable for its wide-ranging effects on human behavior and its wide-ranging street names, such as *hashish, weed, hay, hash, pot, grass, reefer, joint, stick, Mary Jane, Acapulco gold, rope, bhang, jive, loco weed, dope, Thai sticks, ganja,* and *herb* (Spence 1991). Because of its potential therapeutic benefits, relatively wide margin of safety and minor abuse potential, legalization of marijuana has become a major issue in the debate over decriminalizing drugs of abuse.

In this chapter, we begin with a review of current attitudes toward marijuana use. The history of marijuana use is considered next, tracing its roots to ancient civilizations. The physiological and behavioral effects of marijuana are examined in some detail, along with known therapeutic uses. The chapter concludes with a look at use trends. The role of marijuana as a "gateway" drug is considered, as well.

Attitudes Toward Marijuana Use

There are interesting ironies connected with marijuana use. One is that marijuana continues to be perceived as a mild substance. Despite the fact marijuana is considered to be one of the least seriously addicting of the drugs of abuse, it is the most widely used illicit (illegal) substance in the United States. It is currently used by almost 20 million Americans (Gardner 1992).

However, as with most substances of abuse, there was a significant decline in marijuana use by teenagers from the mid-1980s to 1991; a pattern that appeared to reverse in 1993 (Table 13.1). The 1993 reversal in the decline of marijuana use is of great concern to experts and may suggest that there has been a recent increase in general acceptance of this illicit substance by adolescents (Johnston et al. 1994; Epidemiology Report 1994). There is also evidence that increased marijuana use is occurring because some established drug abusers

TABLE 13.1 Trends in prevalence of marijuana use by high school seniors in the United States from 1979 to 1993 (values are percentages of usage by those who were involved in the survey)

	1979	1986	1991	1992	1993
Lifetime	60.4%	50.9%	32.7%	32.6%	35.3%
Within Past Year	50.8	38.8	23.9	21.9	26
Daily Use	10.3	4.0	2.0	1.9	2.4

Source: L. Johnston, P. O'Malley, and J. Bachman. *National Survey Results from The Monitoring the Future Study, 1975–1992 (1993)*. Rockville: MD: National Institute on Drug Abuse, 1993 and 1994.

CROSSCURRENTS

Use of marijuana in the United States is much greater than that for any of the other illicit drugs; in fact, it approaches the rate of use that occurred for alcohol during prohibition. Interestingly, this and other similarities between marijuana and alcohol are the basis for arguments both for and against legalization of cannabis. Consider the following opposing views:

1. As with alcohol, prohibition against marijuana is ineffective. Also as with alcohol, marijuana should be legalized and its sale should be controlled and taxed by the government.
2. Even though alcohol is legal, its excessive use is a much greater problem than that caused by all the illicit substances combined. Thus it is likely that legalization of cannabis would have a tremendously negative social impact.

Choose a side, and support your argument with factual information from this text and other authoritative sources.

have turned to marijuana to replace harder drugs such as cocaine and heroin (Farley 1993).

Another irony is that in some states, despite being illegal, marijuana is one of the largest cash-producing crops. Law enforcement efforts to eliminate the production and distribution of this illicit substance have been so unsuccessful that some highly regarded governmental authorities, such as the surgeon general of the United States (Dr. Joycelyn Elders) and federal and local judges have recommended legalizing marijuana (Kearns 1993; Knight-Ridder News Service 1992). The rationale for such an action would be to reduce the social problems caused by this weed, although the actual consequences of such an action are unclear (see Crosscurrents box).

The History of Marijuana Use

In many societies, marijuana has historically been a valued crop. It is called *hemp* because the woody fibers of the stem yield a fiber that can be made into cloth and rope. The term *cannabis* comes from the Greek word for *hemp*.

Cannabis was apparently brought to the Western hemisphere by the Spaniards as a source of fiber and seeds. For thousands of years, the seeds have been pressed to extract a red oil used for medicinal and euphorigenic purposes (Iversen 1993; Abood and Martin 1992). The plant (both male and female) also produces a resin with active ingredients that affect the central nervous system (CNS). Marijuana contains hundreds of chemical compounds, but only a few found in the resin are responsible for producing the euphoric "high."

The first known record of marijuana use is the *Book of Drugs* written about 2737 B.C. by the Chinese Emperor Shen Nung; he prescribed marijuana for treating gout, malaria, gas pains, and absent-mindedness. The Chinese apparently had much respect for the plant. They obtained fiber for clothes and medicine from it for thousands of years. The Chinese named the plant *ma (maw)*, which means "valuable" or "endearing." The term "ma" was still used as late as 1930.

Around the year 500 B.C., another Chinese book of treatments referred to the medical use of marijuana. Nonetheless, the plant got a bad name from the moralists of the day, who claimed that

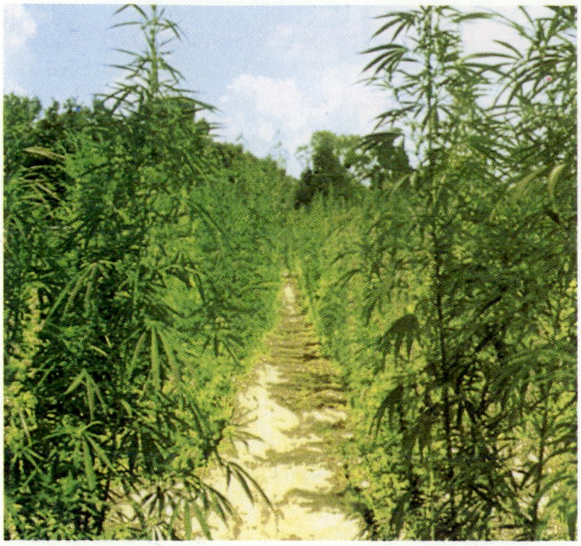

Marijuana can be grown almost anywhere.

A manicured marijuana plant.

youngsters became wild and disrespectful from the recreational use of *ma*. They called it the "liberator of sin" because under its influence, the youngsters refused to listen to their elders and did other scandalous things. Marijuana was banned in China but because of rampant use was later legalized.

India also has a long and varied history of marijuana use. It was an essential part of Indian religious ceremonies for thousands of years. The well-known Rig Veda and other chants describe the use of *soma,* which some believe was marijuana. (As mentioned earlier, in Chapter 12, others believe it was the Amanita mushroom.) Early writings describe a ritual in which resin was collected from the plants. After fasting and purification, certain men ran naked through the cannabis fields. The clinging resin was scraped off their bodies, and cakes were made from it and used in feasts. For centuries, missionaries in India tried to ban the use of marijuana, but they were never successful; its use was heavily ingrained in the culture.

Records for Assyria in 650 B.C. refer to a drug called *azulla* that was used for making rope and cloth and was consumed to experience euphoria. The ancient Greeks also knew about marijuana. Galen described the general use of hemp in cakes, which when eaten in excess were narcotic. Herodotus described the Scythian custom of burning marijuana seeds and leaves to produce a narcotic smoke in steambaths. It was believed that breathing the smoke from the burning plants would cause frenzied activity. Groups of people stood in the smoke and laughed and danced as it took effect.

One legend about cannabis is based on the travels of Marco Polo in the twelfth century. Marco Polo told of the legendary Hasan Ibn-Sabbah, who terrorized a part of Arabia in the early 1100s. His men were some of the earliest political murderers and were supposed to kill under the influence of hashish, a strong, unadulterated cannabis derivative. The cult was called the *hashishiyya,* from which came the word *hashish.* (The word *assassin* may be derived from the name of *Sheik Hasan,* who was a political leader in the tenth century.)

It is unlikely, however, that using hashish can turn people into killers. Experience suggests that people tend to become sleepy and indolent rather than violent after eating hashish or another of the strong cannabis preparations available in Arabia (Abel 1989).

Napoleon's troops brought hashish to France after their campaign in Egypt at the beginning of the nineteenth century, despite Napoleon's strict

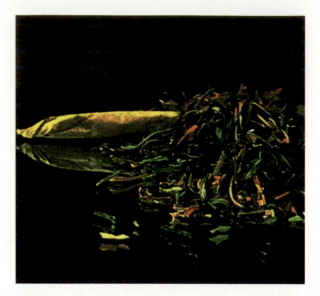

orders to the contrary. By the 1840s, the use of hashish, as well as opium, was widespread in France, and efforts to curb its use were unsuccessful.

In North America, hemp was planted near Jamestown in 1611 for use in making rope. By 1630, half the winter clothing at this settlement was made from hemp fibers. There is no evidence that hemp was used medicinally at this time. Hemp was also valuable as a source of fiber for clothing and rope for the Pilgrims at Plymouth. To meet the demand for fiber, a law was passed in Massachusetts in 1639, requiring every household to plant hemp seed. However, it took much manual labor to get the hemp fiber into usable form, resulting in a chronic shortage of fiber for fish nets and the like (Abel 1980).

George Washington had a field of hemp at Mount Vernon, and there is some indication that it was used for medicine as well as for making rope. Washington once mentioned that he forgot to separate the male and female plants, a process usually done because the female plant gave more resin if unpollinated.

In the early 1800s, U.S. physicians used marijuana extracts to produce a tonic intended for both medicinal and recreational purposes. This changed in 1937 with passage of the Marijuana Tax Act, which prohibited its use as an intoxicant and regulated its use as a medicine.

Most of the abuse of marijuana in the United States during the early part of the twentieth century occurred near the Mexican border and in the ghetto areas of major cities. Cannabis was mistakenly considered a narcotic, like opium, and legal authorities treated it as such (Abood and Martin 1992). In 1931, Harry Anslinger, who was the first appointed head of the Bureau of Narcotics and later would become responsible for the enforcement of marijuana laws, thought that the problem was slight. But by 1936, he claimed that the increase in the use of marijuana was of great national concern (Anslinger and Cooper 1937). Anslinger set up an informational program that finally led to the federal law that banned marijuana. The following sensationalized statement was part of Anslinger's campaign to outlaw the drug:

> What about the alleged connection between drugs and sexual pleasure? . . . What is the real relationship between drugs and sex? There isn't any question about marijuana being a sexual stimulant. It has been used throughout the ages for that: in Egypt, for instance. From what we have seen, it is an aphrodisiac, and I believe that the use in colleges today has sexual connotations. (Anslinger and Cooper 1937)

Also during this time, some usually accurate magazines reported that marijuana was partly responsible for crimes of violence. In 1936, *Scientific American* reported that "marijuana produces a wide variety of symptoms in the user, including hilarity, swooning, and sexual excitement. Combined with intoxicants, it often makes the smoker vicious, with a desire to fight and kill" ("Marijuana Menaces Youth" 1936). A famous poster of the day, called "The Assassination of Youth," was effective in molding attitudes against drug use (see Figure 13.1).

Largely because of the media's effect on public opinion, Congress passed the Marijuana Tax Act in 1937. However, it was declared unconstitutional in 1969. Marijuana has not been classified as a narcotic since 1971.

Marijuana still grows wild in many American states today. Curiously, one reason for this is that, during World War II, the fiber used to make rope (sisal) was hard to import, so the government subsidized farmers to grow hemp. Much of today's crop comes from these same plants. Another reason for the spread of the plants is that, until recently, the seeds were used in birdseed. Canaries sing better after eating a little marijuana. Leftover seed was discarded in the garbage and thus spread to landfill dumps, where it sprouted. Birdseed containing marijuana seeds is still available, but the seeds are sterilized so they cannot germinate.

The Indian Hemp Drug Commission Report in the 1890s and the 1930 Panama Canal Zone Report on marijuana stressed that available evidence did not prove marijuana to be as dangerous as it was popularly thought; these reports were given little publicity, however, and for the most part disregarded. In 1944, a report was issued by the LaGuardia Committee on Marijuana, which consisted of 31 qualified physicians, psychiatrists, psychologists, pharmacologists, chemists, and sociologists appointed by the New York Academy of Medicine. They stated in one key summary that marijuana was not the killer many thought it to be:

> It was found that marijuana in an effective dose impairs intellectual functioning in general. . . .

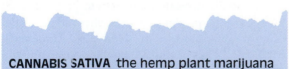

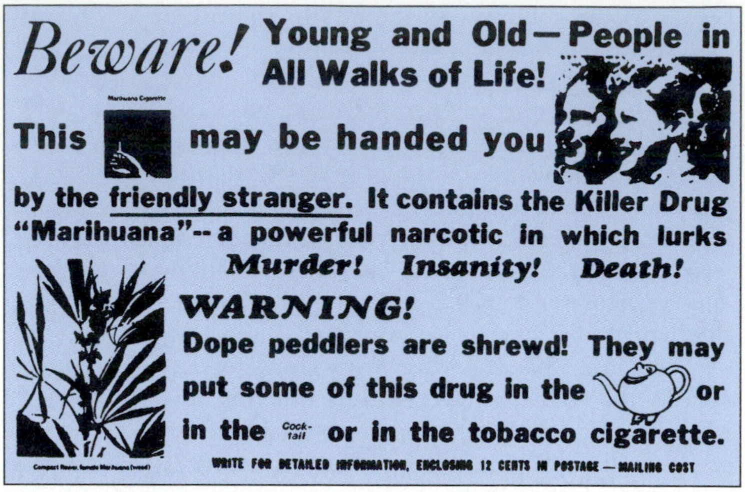

FIGURE 13.1 This anti-marijuana poster was distributed by the Federal Bureau of Narcotics in the late 1930s.

> Marijuana does not change the basic personality structure of the individual. It lessens inhibition and this brings out what is latent in his thoughts and emotions but it does not evoke responses that would otherwise be totally alien to him. . . . Those who have been smoking marijuana for years showed no mental or physical deterioration that may be attributed to the drug. (Solomon 1966)

Much of the early research conducted did not consider the potency of marijuana. As a result, findings from various studies are often conflicting and difficult to compare (Chait and Pierri 1992). Because the quality of marijuana varies so greatly, it is impossible to know the amount of drug taken without analyzing the original material and the leftover stub, or "roach." Conditions such as soil moisture and fertility, amount of sunlight, and temperature all have an effect on the amounts of active ingredients found in the resulting marijuana plant.

Characteristics of Cannabis

In 1753, Carolus Linnaeus, a Swedish botanist, classified marijuana as ***Cannabis sativa.*** *Cannabis sativa* is a plant that grows readily in many parts of the world. Most botanists agree that there is only one species *(sativa)* and that all the variants *(indica, americana,* and *africana)* belong to that species; others believe that the variants are three distinct species (Schultes 1978). *Indica* is considered to have the most potent resin, but climate, soil, and selective plant breeding all influence potency.

Cannabis is *dioecious,* meaning that there are male and female plants (see Figure 13.2). After the male plant releases its pollen, it usually dies. Cultivators of marijuana often eliminate or remove the male plants once the female plant has been pollinated. The world's record marijuana plant was 39 feet tall, and its woody stem was nearly 3 inches in diameter.

There are more than 400 different chemicals in the cannabis plant, many of which have not yet been identified. Delta-9-tetrahydrocannabinol, or THC, is the primary mind-altering (psychoactive) agent in marijuana (Abood and Martin 1992) and appears to be important for the reinforcing prop-

CANNABIS SATIVA the hemp plant marijuana

SINSEMILLA one of the most potent types of marijuana available; means "without seeds"

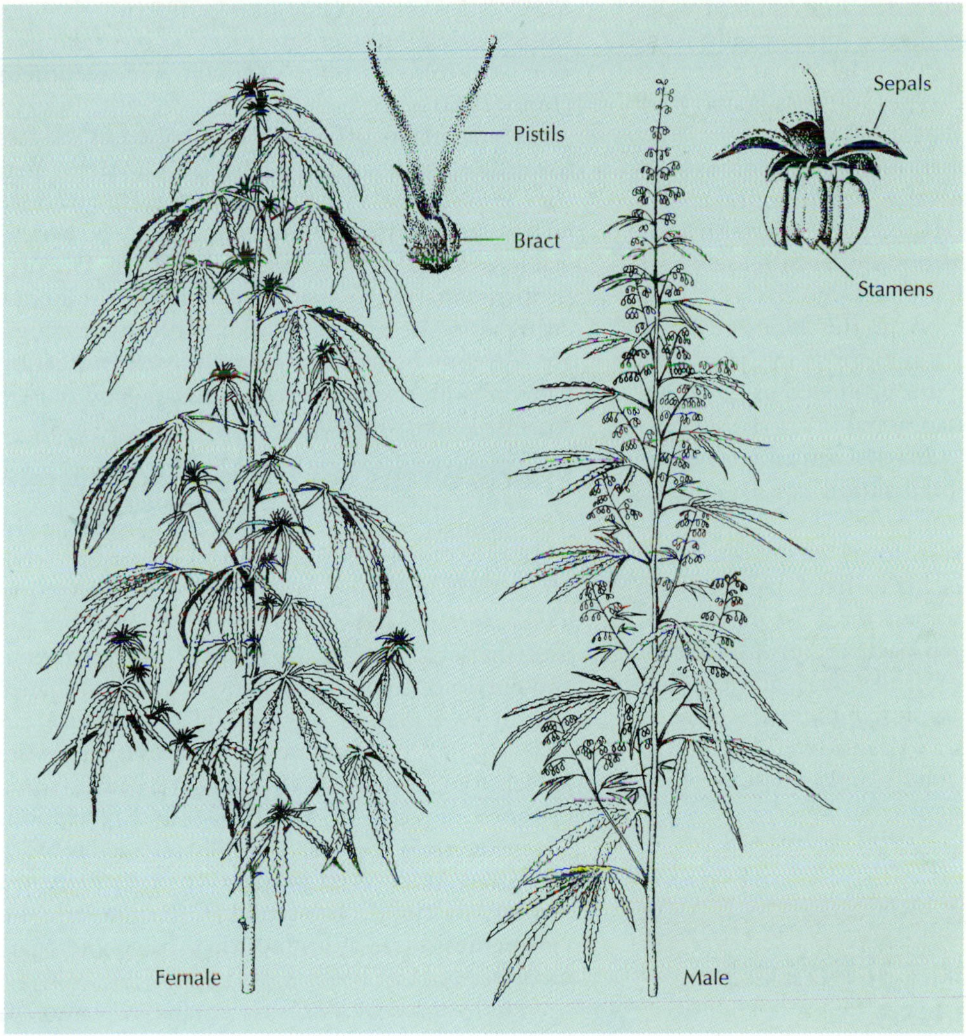

FIGURE 13.2 Male and female marijuana plants.

erties of this substance (Kelly et al. 1994). THC is most highly concentrated in the flowering tops and upper leaves of the female plant. When crushed or eaten, these flowering tops produce a resin in which the psychoactive ingredient THC is found.

In cultivated marijuana crops, male plants are eradicated from the growing fields so that they cannot pollinate the female plants. The lack of pollination makes the potency of female plants increase dramatically. In the United States, this method produces a type of marijuana known as **sinsemilla** (meaning "without seeds" in Spanish). This type of marijuana is one of the most potent varieties available.

Native U.S. cannabis is considered inferior because of a low concentration of THC, usually less than 0.5%. THC levels in Jamaican, Colombian, and Mexican varieties range between 0.5% and 7%.

In the United States, the amount of THC found in "street"-sold marijuana ranges broadly from 0.5 to 11%. Reports that the amount of THC in marijuana has risen dramatically since the 1960s appear to be false (Mijuriya and Aldrich 1988).

Rather, the quantities of other more potent types of marijuana like sinsemilla are more readily available in illegal drug markets. The actual potencies of the more generic types of marijuana have remained the same in the last 30 years.

As mentioned earlier, *hashish* (or *hasheesh*), is another cannabis derivative that contains the purest form of resin. THC content in hashish averages from 7 to 14%. Historically, hashish users have represented a somewhat small percentage of the cannabis user population in the United States. Generally, this derivative is more widely used outside the United States; it is produced in Lebanon, Afghanistan, and Pakistan.

A third derivative of the cannabis plant is *ganja* in India. This preparation consists of the dried tops of female plants.

Finally, the weakest form of marijuana is known as *bhang;* it is made from parts of the cannabis plant that contain the least amount of THC. Often these dried parts are ground into a powder and mixed into drinks, teas, and candies. Bhang is rarely found in the United States, largely because it is very weak and considered low grade, usually containing less than 1 or 2% THC.

The Physiological Effects of Marijuana Use

When marijuana smoke is inhaled into the lungs, THC, the psychoactive ingredient, leaves the blood rapidly through metabolism and through efficient uptake into the tissues. THC and its metabolites tend to bind to proteins in the blood and remain stored for long periods in body fat. Five days after a single injection of THC, 20% remains stored, whereas 20% of its metabolites remain in the blood. Complete elimination of a single dose can take up to 30 days. Measurable levels of THC in blood from chronic users can often be detected for several days or even weeks after their last marijuana cigarette.

In smokers, lung absorption and transport of THC to the brain are rapid; THC reaches the brain within as little as 14 seconds after inhalation. Marijuana is metabolized more efficiently through smoking than intravenous injection or oral ingestion. It is also three to five times more potent (Jones 1980).

Some effects of cannabis described in the following sections are unquestionably toxic in that they can either directly or indirectly produce adverse health effects. Other effects may be beneficial in treating some medical conditions. The uses of marijuana, THC, and synthetic cannabinoids, either alone or in combination with other drugs, are currently being investigated for use in treating pain, inflammation, glaucoma, nausea, and muscle spasms (Iversen 1993).

Effects on the Central Nervous System

The primary effects of marijuana—specifically, THC—are on CNS functions. The precise CNS effects of consuming marijuana or administering THC can vary according to the expectations of the user, the social setting, the route of administration, and previous experiences (Jaffe 1990; Abood and Martin 1992). Smoking a marijuana cigarette can alter mood, coordination, memory, and self-perception. Usually, such exposure causes some euphoria, a sense of well-being, and relaxation. Marijuana smokers often claim heightened sensory awareness and **altered perceptions** (particularly a slowing of time), associated with hunger (**the "munchies"**) and a dry mouth (Abood and Martin 1992).

High doses of THC or greater exposure to marijuana can cause hallucinations, delusions, and paranoia (American Psychiatric Association 1994; Goldstein 1995). Some users describe anxiety developing into panic after high-dose exposure. Due to the availability and widespread use of marijuana, extreme dysphoria and psychiatric emergencies from marijuana overdose are becoming somewhat common. Long-term users often show decreased interest in personal appearance or goals (part of the "amotivational syndrome" discussed later in this chapter) as well as an inability to concentrate, make appropriate decisions, and remember (Abood and Martin 1992).

The precise classification of THC is uncertain because the responses to marijuana are highly variable and appear to have elements of all three major groups of drugs of abuse. Consequently, marijuana use can cause euphoria and paranoia (like stimulants), drowsiness and sedation (like depressants), and hallucinations (like psychedelics). It is possible that THC alters several receptor or transmitter systems in the brain; this would account for its diverse and somewhat unpredictable effects. However, the recent dramatic discovery of a specific receptor site in the brain for THC, called the "cannabinoid" receptor, suggests that a selective endogenous marijuana system exists in the brain and is activated by THC when marijuana is consumed (Hudson 1990). Some researchers speculate that an endogenous fatty-acid–like substance called **anandamide** naturally works at these marijuana sites; efforts are being made to characterize this substance, which perhaps is a neurotransmitter (Iversen 1993). It is possible that, from this discovery, a group of new therapeutic agents will be developed that can selectively interact with the marijuana receptors, resulting in medical benefits without the side effects that generally accompany marijuana use (Iversen 1993; Swan 1993).

Effects on the Respiratory System

Marijuana is often smoked like tobacco, and like tobacco can cause serious damage to the lungs (Consroe and Sandyk 1992). In smoking tobacco, for example, nearly 70% of the total suspended particles in the smoke are retained in the lungs. There is reason to believe that, because marijuana smoke is inhaled more deeply than tobacco smoke, even more tar residues are retained.

Smoke is a mixture of tiny particles suspended in gas, mostly carbon monoxide. These solid particles combine to form a residue called *tar.* Cannabis produces more tar (up to 50% more) than an equivalent weight of tobacco and is smoked in a way that increases the accumulation of tar (Jones 1980).

Over 150 chemicals have been identified in marijuana smoke and tar. A few are proven carcinogens; however, many have not yet been tested for carcinogenicity. The carcinogen benzopyrene, for example, is 70% more abundant in marijuana smoke than in tobacco smoke. When cannabis tar is applied to the skin of experimental animals, it causes precancerous lesions similar to those caused by tobacco tar. Similarly, whenever isolated lung tissue is exposed to these same tars, precancerous changes result (Jones 1980; Turner 1980; Hollister 1986).

Special white blood cells in living lung tissue—*alveolar macrophages*—play a role in removing debris from the lungs. When exposed to smoke from cannabis, these cells are less able to remove bacteria and other foreign debris.

Smoking only a few marijuana cigarettes a day for six to eight weeks can significantly impair pulmonary function. Laboratory and clinical evidence often indicates that heavy use of marijuana causes cellular changes and that users have a higher incidence of such respiratory problems as laryngitis, pharyngitis, bronchitis, asthmalike conditions, cough, hoarseness, and dry throat (Jones 1980; Hollister 1986; Goldstein 1995). Recent reports emphasize the potential damage to pulmonary function that can occur from chronic marijuana use (National Institute on Drug Abuse [NIDA] 1991). Evidence suggests that many 20-year-old smokers of both hashish and tobacco have lung damage comparable to that of heavy tobacco smokers over 40 years of age. It is believed that the tar from tobacco and marijuana have damaging effects, but it is not known whether smokers who use both products suffer synergistic or additive effects (Jones 1980; Hollister 1986).

Effects on the Cardiovascular System

In humans, cannabis causes both vasodilation (enlarged blood vessels) and an increase in heart rate related to the amount of THC consumed (Abood and Martin 1992). The vasodilation is responsible for a reddening of the eyes often seen in the marijuana smoker. In physically healthy users, these effects, as well as slight changes in heart rhythm, are transitory and do not appear to be significant. In patients with heart disease, however, the increased oxygen requirement due to the

ALTERED PERCEPTIONS changes in the interpretation of stimuli, resulting from marijuana use

THE "MUNCHIES" hunger experienced while under the effects of marijuana

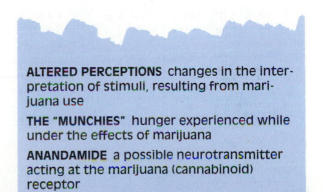

ANANDAMIDE a possible neurotransmitter acting at the marijuana (cannabinoid) receptor

accelerated heart rate may have serious consequences. The effect of cannabis on people with heart rhythm irregularities is not known.

Because of vasodilation caused by marijuana use, abnormally low blood pressure can occur when standing. In addition, if a user stands up quickly after smoking, a feeling of lightheadedness or fainting may result. Chronic administration of large doses of THC to healthy volunteers shows that tolerance develops to the increase in heart rate and vasodilation.

People with cardiovascular problems seem to be at an increased risk when smoking marijuana (Hollister 1986). Marijuana products also bind hemoglobin, limiting the amount of oxygen that can be carried to the heart tissue. This deficiency could trigger heart attacks in susceptible people (Palfai and Jankiewicz 1991). The National Academy of Science's Institute of Medicine recommends that people with cardiovascular disease avoid marijuana use because there are still many unanswered questions about its effects on the cardiovascular system.

Effects on Sexual Performance and Reproduction

Drugs may interfere with sexual performance and reproduction in several ways. Drugs may alter sexual behavior, affect fertility, damage the chromosomes of germ cells in the male or female, or adversely affect fetal growth and development.

The Indian Hemp Commission, which wrote the first scientific report on cannabis, commented that it had a sexually stimulating effect, like alcohol. However, the report also said that cannabis was used by Asian Indian ascetics to destroy the sexual appetite. This apparent discrepancy may be a dose-related effect. Used occasionally over the short term, marijuana may act as an **aphrodisiac** by releasing CNS inhibitions. In addition, the altered perception of time under the influence of the drug could make the pleasurable sensations appear to last longer than they actually do.

APHRODISIAC a substance that stimulates or intensifies sexual desire

Marijuana affects the sympathetic nervous system to increase vasodilation in the genitals and to delay ejaculation (Harclerode 1980). High doses over a period of time lead to depression of libido and impotence, possibly due to the decreased amount of testosterone, the male sex hormone.

Cannabis has several effects on semen. The total number of sperm cells and the concentration of sperm per unit volume is decreased during ejaculation. Moreover, there is an increase in the proportion of sperm with abnormal appearance and reduced motility. These qualities are usually associated with low fertility and a higher probability of producing an abnormal embryo should fertilization take place.

Despite these effects, there are no documented reports of children with birth defects in which the abnormality was linked to the father's smoking marijuana. It is possible that damaged sperm cells are incapable of fertilization (so that only normal sperm cells reach the egg) or that the abnormal sperm appearance is meaningless in terms of predicting birth defects. When marijuana use stops, the quality of the semen gradually returns to normal over several months (Harclerode 1980; Institute of Medicine 1982).

Less reliable data are available on the effects of cannabis on female libido, sexual response (ability to respond to sexual stimulation with vaginal lubrication and orgasm), and fertile reproductive (menstrual) cycles ("Marijuana" 1987; Consroe and Sandyk 1992). Preliminary data from the Reproductive Biology Research Foundation show that chronic smoking of cannabis (at least three times per week for the preceding six months) adversely affects the female reproductive cycle. Results with women were correlated with work in rhesus monkeys; it was found that THC blocks ovulation (due to effects on female sex hormones).

Data on effects of marijuana use during pregnancy and lactation are inconclusive. Some evidence suggests that the use of this drug by pregnant women can result in intrauterine growth retardation, which is characterized by prolonged labor, low birthweight, and behavioral abnormalities in newborns and increased fetal mortality (see Case in Point) (Roffman and George 1988, Nahas and Latour 1992; Fernandez-Ruiz et al. 1992).

Pregnant rhesus monkeys treated with THC levels equivalent to those associated with moder-

Case in Point

The Link Between Marijuana Use and Pregnancy

How does the use of marijuana affect fetal growth and development? Findings from Zuckerman et al. (1989) indicate that infants born to mothers using marijuana weighed an average of 79 g less and were an average of 0.5 cm shorter than infants of nonusers. Another finding is that children born to women who smoked marijuana just prior to or during pregnancy were 10 times more likely to develop a rare form of leukemia than were children born to drug-free women (Robison et al. 1989).

Pregnant women should be warned that high doses of marijuana impair fetal growth. In addition, heavy marijuana use may retard fetal growth, increase the likelihood of stillbirth and interfere with the development of organs in the fetus (Murphy and Bartke 1992).

ately heavy marijuana use (according to U.S. standards) had an abortion and fetal death rate about four times higher than the drug-free control monkeys. THC and other cannabinoids pass through the blood–placenta barrier and concentrate in the fetus's fatty tissue, including its brain. Ethical considerations prevent duplication of the experiment in humans.

Women who smoke marijuana during pregnancy also often use other drugs—such as alcohol, tobacco, and cocaine—that are known to have adverse effects on the developing fetus. Because multiple drugs are used, it is difficult to isolate the specific effects of marijuana during pregnancy. Like many other substances, THC is taken up by the mammary glands in lactating females and is excreted in the milk. Effects on human infants due to the presence of marijuana in the maternal milk have not been determined (Petersen 1980; Murphy and Bartke 1992).

In studies on mice and rats (but not humans), the addition of THC to pregnant animals lowered litter size, increased fetal reabsorption, and increased the number of reproductive abnormalities in the surviving offspring (Dewey 1986). The offspring of the drug-treated animal mothers had reduced fertility and more testicular abnormalities. The dose of cannabinoids used in these studies was proportionally higher than that used by humans. Clearly, pregnant women should be advised against using marijuana, even though there is little direct data on its prenatal effects in humans (Dewey 1986; Murphy and Bartke 1992).

Tolerance and Dependence

It has been known for many years that tolerance to some effects of cannabis builds rapidly in animals; namely, the drug effect becomes less intense with repeated administration. Frequent use of high doses of marijuana or THC in humans produces similar tolerance. For example, increasingly higher doses must be given to obtain the same intensity of subjective effects and increased heart rate that occur initially with small doses (Abood and Martin 1992).

Frequent high doses of THC also can produce mild physical dependence. Healthy subjects who smoke several "joints" a day or who are given comparable amounts of THC orally experience irritability, sleep disturbances, weight loss, loss of appetite, sweating, and gastrointestinal upsets when drug use is stopped abruptly. This mild form of withdrawal is not experienced by all subjects, however. It is much easier to show psychological dependence in heavy users of marijuana (Hollister 1986; Abood and Martin 1992).

Psychological dependence involves an attachment to the euphoric effects of the THC content in marijuana and may include "craving." The subjective effects of marijuana intoxication include a heightened sensitivity to and distortion of sight, smell, taste, and sound; mood alteration; and diminished reaction time.

In general, outright cannabis addiction, with obsessive drug-seeking and compulsive drug-taking behavior, is relatively rare with low-dose cannabis preparations, but much more common with high-dose products, such as hashish (Gardner 1992). Because the less potent forms of marijuana are used in the United States, most chronic users in this country would have little problem controlling or eliminating their cannabis habit if they so desired (Abood and Martin 1992).

Therapeutic Uses

Cannabis was used to treat a variety of human ills in folk and formal medicine for thousands of years in South Africa, Turkey, South America, and Egypt as well as such Asian countries as India, the Malays, Burma, and Siam. As recently as 1937, tinctures of cannabis were still cited in the *U.S. Pharmacopeia and National Formulary,* which listed current therapeutic drugs.

After marijuana was legally classified as a narcotic and the Marijuana Tax Act of 1937 required that its use be reported, medical use effectively ceased. Only in the past decade has there been organized renewed interest in possible medical uses for cannabis. A few therapeutic applications have been demonstrated, and others are being investigated to a limited extent. Because of potential clinical uses for marijuana, enforcement of laws prohibiting the use of this substance can be awkward and very controversial (see the Here and Now box). One of the problems with trying to determine the clinical usefulness of cannabis is that the effectiveness of this substance decreases with repeated use (tolerance develops). In addition, effective doses vary according to routes of administration (smoking versus oral ingestion), and responses are highly variable among users (Goldstein 1995).

The use of marijuana, THC, or related drugs for treatment of the extreme nausea and vomiting that often accompany cancer chemotherapy is an example of a beneficial application of this drug. Consequently, the FDA has approved the use of purified THC as the drug called **Marinol** (dronabinol) for antiemetic treatment in cancer patients (Sewester 1993). Although the use is not FDA-approved, some have argued that administration of THC by smoking a marijuana product is a particularly useful form of administering this drug in nauseated and vomiting patients receiving chemotherapy (Gavzer 1994). Another FDA-approved application for THC is to stimulate appetite in patients with advanced AIDS who are suffering from severe anorexia (Sewester 1993).

Marijuana has been shown to be effective in the treatment of several other medical conditions; however, because other medicines are available that are at least as effective and without abuse potential, none of these applications are currently FDA sanctioned. According to researchers (Iversen 1993; Abood and Martin 1992; Consroe and Sandyk 1992), the unauthorized therapeutic benefits for marijuana include

1. *Reduction in intraocular (eye) pressure.* Marijuana lowers **glaucoma**-associated intraocular pressure, even though it does not cure the condition or reverse blindness (Goldstein 1995). Use of marijuana to treat this eye disease is not widespread.
2. *Antiasthmatic effect.* Some research indicates that short-term smoking of marijuana has improved breathing for asthma patients. Marijuana smoke dilates the lung's air passages (bronchodilation). Findings also show, however, that the lung-irritating properties of marijuana smoke seem to offset its benefits. Regardless, marijuana may still prove useful

MARINOL FDA-approved THC in capsule form (dronabinol)

GLAUCOMA an eye disease manifested by increased intraocular pressure

Here and Now

The Dilemma of Brownie Mary

Mary Rathbun of San Francisco is known locally as "Brownie Mary" because of her unique use of marijuana in her legendary brownie batter. Mary, an advocate of the medical use of marijuana since the 1960s, bakes her unusual confectionaries for AIDS patients. She claims her brownies help to relieve the pain and nausea of the disease and its treatment. Although she has been indicted for felony marijuana possession in Sonoma County Municipal Court, in 1991 a San Francisco supervisor proposed a "Brownie Mary Day" to honor her efforts to relieve the suffering of AIDS victims. In 1989, she was named "Volunteer of the Year" for San Francisco General Hospital's outpatient AIDS Ward.

What is the result of such mixed signals concerning marijuana use and how do you think this will be eventually resolved?

Source: E. Herscher. "'Brownie Mary' Is Cheered During Testimony at City Hall." *San Francisco Chronicle* 173 (August 1992):A-1.

when other drugs are not effective because of a different mode of action in causing bronchodilation.

3. *Muscle-relaxant effect.* Some studies also indicate that muscle spasms are relieved when patients with muscle disorders, such as multiple sclerosis, use marijuana.
4. *Antiseizure effect.* Marijuana has both convulsant and anticonvulsant properties and has been considered for use in preventing seizures associated with epilepsy. In animal experimentation, the cannabinoids reduced or increased seizure activities, depending on how the experiments were conducted. One or more of the marijuana components may be useful in combination with other standard antiseizure medication, although at present their value seems limited. A survey of young epileptics who smoked marijuana did not show a change in their seizure patterns, but caution is advised ("Pot Kills Motivation" 1981).
5. *Antidepressant effect.* Cannabis and the synthetic cannabinoid synhexyl have been used successfully in Great Britain as specific euphoriants for the treatment of depression.
6. *Analgesic effect.* Published testimonials have reported that marijuana can relieve the intense pain associated with migraine and chronic headaches or inflammation. In South Africa, native women smoke cannabis to dull the pain of childbirth (Solomon 1966). The pain-relieving potency of marijuana has not been carefully studied and compared with other analgesics such as the narcotics or aspirin-type drugs.

Whether THC or a similar drug is accepted as a legitimate medicine depends on several considerations. For example, it must be determined whether the pharmaceutically desirable effects are useful for treating chronic conditions because tolerance develops rapidly to many of the actions of THC. Like any other medication, marijuana and related products must be carefully tested for toxicity and therapeutic effectiveness. This process is time consuming, expensive, and is not worthwhile if other drugs are already available, which are as good, or better, therapeutically than the marijuana substances. In addition, concerns about abuse potential and the social stigmas associated with marijuana need to be considered.

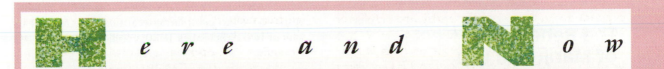

The Behavioral Effects of Marijuana Use

In the 1930s, it was believed that the acute effects of marijuana were very devastating and that marijuana use could suddenly lead to violent and even promiscuous behavior. Publications forecasted that marijuana use would lead to madness (Rowell and Powell 1939) and that it was the "assassin of youth" (Anslinger and Cooper 1937).

These concerns are no longer considered valid for casual or occasional use. In most individuals, low to moderate doses of cannabis produce euphoria and a pleasant state of relaxation (Goldstein 1994). This state is usually mild and short-lived; a typical "high" from one "joint" may last from two to three hours. The user experiences altered perception of space and time, impaired memory of recent events, and impaired physical coordination (Abood and Martin 1992). An occasional "high" is not usually hazardous unless the person attempts to drive a car, operate heavy machinery, fly a plane, or function in similar ways requiring coordination, good reflexes, or quick judgment (Nahas and Latour 1992). Even low doses of marijuana adversely affect perception, such as being able to judge the speed of an approaching vehicle or how much to slow down on an exit ramp.

An acute dose of cannabis can produce adverse reactions, ranging from mild anxiety to panic and paranoia in some users. A few rare cases exhibit psychoses characterized by detachment from reality, delusional and bizarre behavior, and hallucinations (Abood and Martin 1992). These reactions occur most frequently in individuals who are under stress, or who are anxious, depressed, or borderline schizophrenic (Nahas and Latour 1992); such effects may also be seen in normal users who accidentally take much more than their usual dose.

Extreme reactions also can occur as a result of ingesting marijuana treated (or "laced") with such things as LSD, PCP, or other additives, like datura (jimsonweed) leaves. Based on limited evidence from survey studies, mild adverse reactions are experienced on one or more occasions by more than one-half of regular users; they are mainly self-treated and usually go unreported. The small number of users who experience severe adverse reactions usually respond well to psychiatric treatment and recover in one or two days (Jones 1980; Hollister 1986).

Driving Performance

Evidence shows that the ability to perform complex tasks, such as driving, is strongly impaired while under the influence of marijuana (Goldstein 1994). This effect has been demonstrated in laboratory assessments of driving-related skills such as eye–hand coordination and reaction time, in driver simulator studies, in test course performance, and in actual street-driving situations (Chait and Pierri 1992).

In limited surveys, from 60 to 80% of marijuana users indicate that they sometimes drive while high! A study of drivers involved in fatal accidents in the greater Boston area showed that marijuana smokers were overrepresented in fatal highway accidents as compared to a control group of nonusers of similar age and gender. A 1989 study found that, of nearly 1,800 blood samples taken from drivers arrested for driving while intoxicated, 19% tested positive for marijuana.

One study tested subjects on the effects of known amounts of marijuana, alcohol, or both on driving. The subjects drove a course rigged with various traffic problems. There was a definite deterioration in driving skills among those who had used either drug, but the greatest deterioration was in subjects who had taken both. In another test, 59 subjects smoked marijuana until they were high and then were given sobriety tests on the roadside by highway patrol officers. Overall, 94% of the subjects didn't pass the test 90 minutes after smoking, and 60% failed at 150 minutes, even though the blood THC was much lower at this time (Hollister 1986). Other studies on driving show this same inability to drive for as long as 12 to 24 hours after marijuana use.

Because some perceptual or other performance deficits resulting from marijuana use may persist for some time after the high, users who attempt to drive, fly, operate heavy machinery, and so on may not recognize their impairment because they do not feel intoxicated (NIDA 1980). States such as California have established testing procedures to detect the presence of THC in urine or blood samples from apparently intoxicated drivers.

If the use of marijuana becomes more socially

Here and Now

Specific Signs of Marijuana Use

1. A sweet odor similar to burnt rope in room, on clothes, etc.
2. Roach—small butt end of a marijuana cigarette.
3. Joint—looks like a hand-rolled cigarette, usually the ends are twisted or crimped.
4. Roach clips—holders for the roach. These could be any number of common items such as paper clips, bobby pins or hemostats. They could also be of a store-bought variety in a number of shapes and disguises.
5. Seeds or leaves in pockets or possession.
6. Rolling papers or pipes, usually hidden somewhere.
7. Eye drops—for covering up red eyes.
8. Excessive use of incense, room deodorizers or breath fresheners.
9. Devices for keeping the substance such as boxes, cans, or even concealed containers like a soft drink can with a screw-off lid.
10. Eating binges—an after effect in some marijuana users.
11. Appearance of intoxication yet no smell of alcohol.
12. Excessive laughter.
13. Yellowish stains on finger tips from holding the cigarette.

Source: L.A.W. Publications, "Let's All Work To Fight Drug Abuse," rev. ed. Addison, TX: C&L Printing, 1985, p. 39. Used with permission of the publisher.

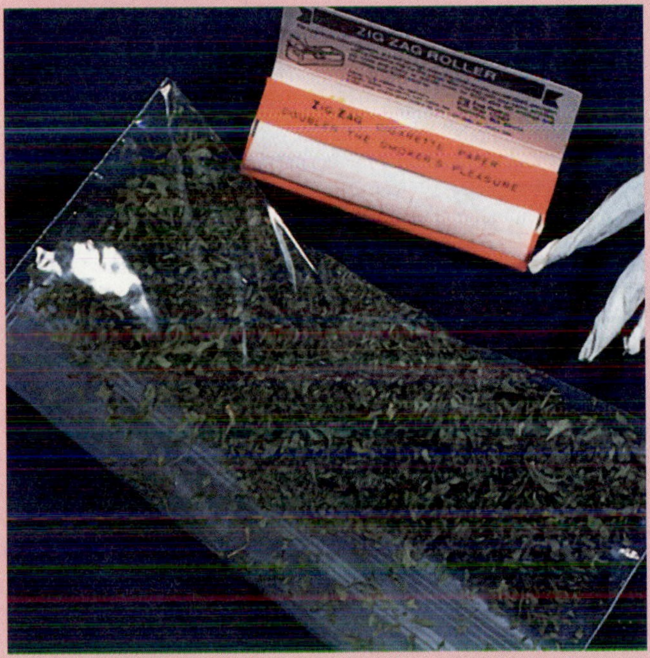

Marijuana paraphernalia.

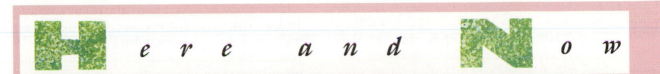

acceptable (or perhaps even legal) and penalties for simple possession become more lenient, it is likely that individuals will feel less inclined to hide their drug use. Unfortunately, it follows that these individuals may also be more inclined to drive while high, endangering themselves and others.

Chronic Use

With regard to the physiological effects of chronic use of marijuana, early research findings reported (1) chromosomal damage (Stenchever et al. 1974), (2) cerebral atrophy (shrinking of the brain) (Campbell et al. 1971), and (3) lowered capacity of white blood cells to fight disease (Nahas et al. 1974). To date, these findings have all been contradicted or otherwise refuted by subsequent research. The only finding that appears credible is that chronic use of marijuana impairs lung capacity (Oliwenstein 1988; Bloodworth 1987).

Other evidence indicates that chronic, heavy use of cannabis can lead to persistent and troublesome behavioral changes in some users (see the Case in Point box). Apathy, such as a lack of concern for the future and a general loss of motivation, has been observed in some heavy users. This condition has been referred to as the **amotivational syndrome** and also includes general dullness, impaired judgment and memory, and an inability to concentrate (Abood and Martin 1992), (discussed further in the next section). Psychotic and paranoid symptoms have been seen in others (Nahas and Latour 1992). These symptoms usually disappear when regular drug use is discontinued and recur when use is resumed.

In fact, such reactions are somewhat rare, although case studies suggest that certain cannabis users may be more susceptible than others (Institute of Medicine 1982; Peterson 1980; Hollister 1986). Many psychiatrists are concerned about such reactions in youthful drug users (11 to 15 years of age) because of the possibility that regular use may produce adverse effects on psychological as well as physical maturation. (This concern involves all psychoactive drugs, including alcohol.)

AMOTIVATIONAL SYNDROME a lack of motivation and reduced productivity caused by regular marijuana use

A few cannabis users experience spontaneous recurrences of the symptoms of acute intoxication days or weeks later, similar to LSD "flashbacks." These recurrences are not common and do not require treatment. Because THC is stored in body fat, it is possible that flashbacks might be triggered by something that causes THC to be released from the fat cells where it has accumulated. This has not been proven, however.

Do other changes in brain function persist after a marijuana-induced high? Limited clinical evidence suggests that some long-term users do not recover completely when they discontinue drug use. Psychological functioning—which includes perception, coordination, intelligence, and other factors—has been tested in heavy users in Jamaica, Costa Rica, Greece, Egypt, and India. The conclusions from these studies conflict and in some cases are difficult to interpret accurately because of poor experimental methods and possibly biased investigators. Studies with the largest groups of subjects done in Egypt and India show significant differences between users and matched nonusers, whereas the studies using much smaller samples in Jamaica and Costa Rica do not show any significant differences between users and nonusers (Jones 1980; Hollister 1986).

We are led to the conclusion that with regard to chronic effects, there is very little reliable information. Although high doses of cannabis have been associated with adverse psychological effects, cannabis appears to be a relatively safe substance. Even in large doses there is no evidence that anyone has ever died from an acute overdose of marijuana alone.

The Amotivational Syndrome

Amotivational syndrome characterizes regular users of marijuana who experience a lack of motivation and reduced productivity. Specifically, users show apathy, difficulty in concentration, and a lingering disinterest in pursuing goals.

Case in Point

Chronic Marijuana Use

The following comments show how marijuana use can become a disturbing habit:

> I guess you could say it was peer pressure. Back in 1969, I was a sophomore in college, and everyone was smoking "dope." The Vietnam War was in progress, and most students on college campuses were heavily involved in the drug scene. I first started smoking marijuana when my closest friends did. I was taught by other students who already knew how to enjoy the effects of "pot."
>
> I recall that one of my fellow students used to supply me with "nickel bags," and many users nicknamed him "God." How did he get such a name? Because he sold some very potent marijuana that at times caused us to hallucinate.
>
> I used pot nearly every day for about a year and a half, and hardly an evening would pass without smoking dope and listening to music. Smoking marijuana became as common as drinking alcohol. I used it in the same manner a person has a cocktail after a long day. At first, I liked the effects of being "high," but later, I became so accustomed to the stuff that life appeared boring without it.
>
> After graduating, my college friends went their separate ways, and I stopped using marijuana for a few years. A year later, in graduate school, a neighborhood friend reintroduced me to the pleasure of smoking pot. I began using it again but not as often. Whenever I experienced some pressure, I would use a little to relax.
>
> After finishing my degree, I found myself employed at an institution that at times was boring. Again, I started using pot at night to relax, and somehow it got out of control. I used to smoke a little before work and sometimes during lunch. I thought all was going well until one day I got fired because someone accused me of being high on the job.
>
> Soon afterward, I came to the realization that the use of marijuana can be very insidious. It has a way of becoming psychologically addictive, and you don't even realize it. When I was high, I thought that no one knew and that I was even more effective with others. Little did I know, I was dead wrong and fooling no one.
>
> I do not oppose someone else using marijuana, but I learned my lesson seven years ago. Since then, I have smoked dope only three times.

Source: Interview with a 39-year-old male, Peter Venturelli, May 1990.

This syndrome has received considerable attention. People who are high, or "stoned," lack the desire to perform hard work and are not interested in doing difficult tasks (Miranne 1979). There is some evidence of this behavior in regular marijuana users (Nahas and Latour 1992). Overall, chronic users have lower grades in school, are more likely to be absent from classes, and are likely not to complete assignments and to drop out of school (Liska 1990). In terms of age, the earlier someone begins smoking marijuana, the more likely the amotivational characteristics will prevail and the more difficult it will be to cease using this drug.

While the effects of marijuana per se are somewhat responsible for creating this syndrome, other factors contribute, as well. For instance, marijuana users are more likely to associate with peers who are also users. Surveys show that members of these peer groups tend to be alienated from society and are likely to be classified as nonconformers or rebellious youths. Imagine how an entire group of marijuana users can exert a profound effect on one

TABLE 13.2 Marijuana use reported in 1991 by Americans during lifetime, past year, and past month according to age (values are expressed as percentages of those surveyed)

Age	Time Period		
	Lifetime	Past Year	Past Month
13–14 years	10.2%	6.2%	3.2%
15–16	23.4	16.5	8.7
17–18	36.7	23.9	13.8
21–22	56	27	15
25–26	67	22	13
31–32	73	20	12

Note: These are the only age groups included in the study.
Source: L. Johnston, P. O'Malley, and J. Bachman. *National Survey Results from The Monitoring the Future Study, 1975–1992.* Rockville: MD: National Institute on Drug Abuse, 1992.

another. They perpetuate a subculture emphasizing pleasure and nonconformity rather than hard work and success. The amotivational syndrome also dictates a noncaring attitude toward others and prompts subjective pleasure and alienation. Close ties with such a group desensitizes the individual about the negative aspects of drug abuse.

Subjective Experiences

How does it feel to experience a cannabis high? There is a general sense of relaxation and tranquility, coupled with heightened sensitivity toward sound, touch, and taste (a typical hallucinogenic effect). Users report that their thinking wanders and short-term memory does not function very well. A brochure from the National Institute on Drug Abuse (NIDA) states that "the effects of marijuana can interfere with learning by impairing thinking, reading comprehension, and verbal and mathematical skills. Research shows that students do not remember what they have learned when they are 'high'" (NIDA 1990, 37).

One marijuana user reported, "When I am high, things just simply flow differently. It's not like being high on alcohol. An alcohol high is a body high, while a pot high is more of a head experience" (unpublished interview by Venturelli). Users report feeling "mellow" and believe that everything is fine. Other marijuana users cite feelings of euphoria and satisfaction with themselves. Another user said, "Being high can become habit forming, simply because it feels so good" (interview by Venturelli). Marijuana is considered a recreational drug because it often intensifies pleasure and is used in conjunction with other pleasurable activities: eating, listening to music, meeting friends, and having sex.

Trends in Marijuana Use

Age Differences

The data in Table 13.2 show that marijuana use is strongly related to age. For 13- to 14-year-olds (10.2%), lifetime rates in 1991 were low. Lifetime rates were sharply higher in successive ages—23.3% among 15- to 16-year-olds and 36.7% among 17- to 18-year-olds. Lifetime rates of marijuana use steadily increased with age (Johnston et al. 1992).

Likewise, annual use (used at least once during the year) steadily increased with age until the group of 21 to 22 years (27%) and then decreased. Those 21 to 22 years old also were most likely to report marijuana use during the past month (15%) (Johnston et al. 1992).

Peer Influences

As discussed in the early chapters of this text, the mass media and parental role models have a significant impact on the attitudes that youth develop regarding drug use. However, peers may exert the most influence of all (Tec 1974; Tudor et al. 1987; Norem-Hebeisen and Hedlin 1983).

Research shows that it is very unlikely that an individual will use drugs when his or her peers do not use drugs. Marijuana use, in particular, is a group occurrence and thus strongly affected by peer pressure and influence. Learning theory (see Chapter 2) shows how peers can influence one another; drug-using peer members serve as role models, legitimizing this form of deviant behavior. Peers in such groups are in effect saying, "It's OK to use drugs," and they make drugs available. Heavy drug users are likely to belong to drug-using groups; in contrast, people who don't use drugs belong to groups where drug use is perceived as a very deviant form of social recreation.

Other Research Findings

The following recent trends regarding marijuana use were identified in a NIDA survey (Johnston et al. 1993):

1. In 1992, regular users (used marijuana within the previous 30 days) were roughly comparable in all ages from 19 to 32 years—ranged from 11.3 to 14.7% (Johnston et al. 1993).
2. Gender differences in ages 19 to 32 years were most apparent for intense marijuana use in 1992, with 3.6% males versus 1.3% females using this substance daily. However, the gender differences disappeared when all the young adults who had experienced any marijuana use were also included in the 1992 measurement. Under these conditions, 61.9 males versus 58.6% females had used marijuana sometime during their lives (Johnston et al. 1993).
3. The prevalence of intense (daily) marijuana use in populations of 19 to 32 years of age was somewhat dependent on U.S. geographical location in 1992, with the West having the highest (3.3%) and the South the lowest (2.0%) rates. A similar pattern was observed when identifying people who had used marijuana sometime during the previous year (32.2% in the West and 22.7% in the South) (Johnston et al. 1993).
4. During 1992, residents of large metropolitan areas were more likely to use marijuana (29.2%) than in small towns (25.2%) or in rural surroundings (22.3%) (Johnston et al. 1993).
5. After high school (one to four years), those who continued their education in college during 1992 and those who did not, had similar patterns of casual marijuana use, with approximately 26–28% of both groups having used the substance at least once during the year. However, intense daily marijuana use was three times higher in noncollege young adults compared to college students (3 versus 1%) (Johnston et al. 1993).
6. As the level of peer disapproval and perceived harmfulness of marijuana increased in all young adult populations from 1980 to 1992, the incidence of use decreased. Despite this reduction of use, the perceived availability of marijuana declined only slightly (see Figure 13.3), suggesting that access is not as important as peer pressure and perceived risks in determining patterns of marijuana use.

Radosevich et al. (1980) have highlighted three different factors that determine marijuana use patterns: (1) structural factors, such as age, gender, social class, and ethnicity or race; (2) social and interactional factors, such as type of interpersonal relationships, friendship cliques, and drug use within the peer group setting; and (3) attitudinal factors, personal attitudes toward the use of

A. Perceived availability: Young adults were asked if they were able to get marijuana if desired.

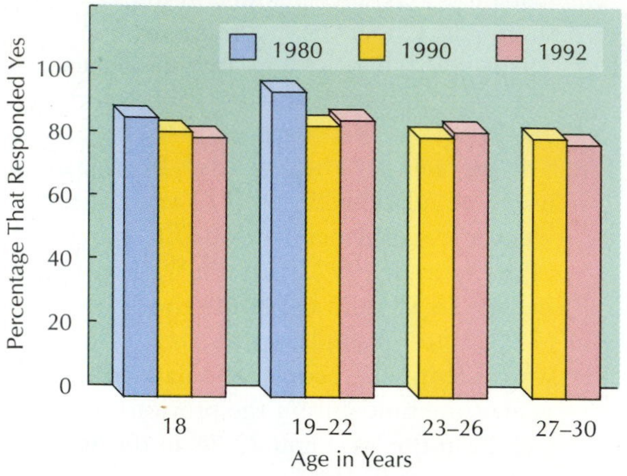

B. Marijuana experience of friends: Young adults were asked if they associated with friends who have smoked marijuana.

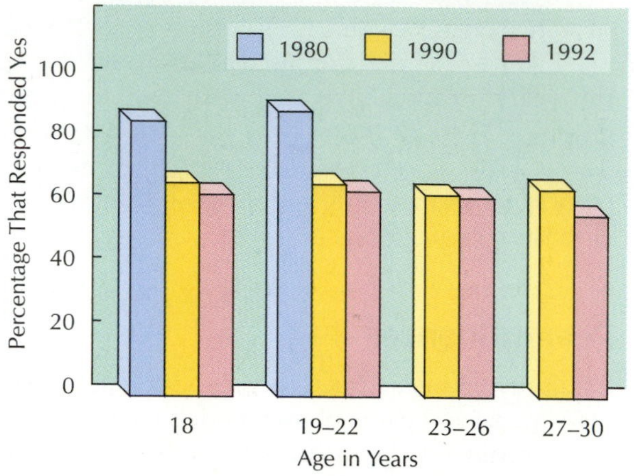

C. Negative peer pressure: Young adults were asked if they disapproved of their friends using marijuana.

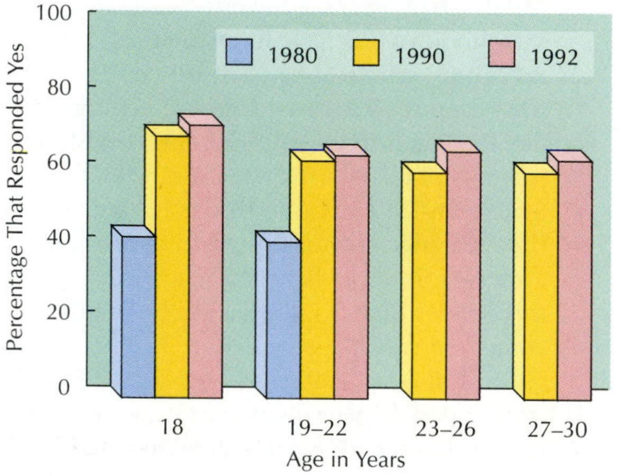

D. Perceived risk: Young adults were asked if they perceived the occasional use of marijuana as harmful.

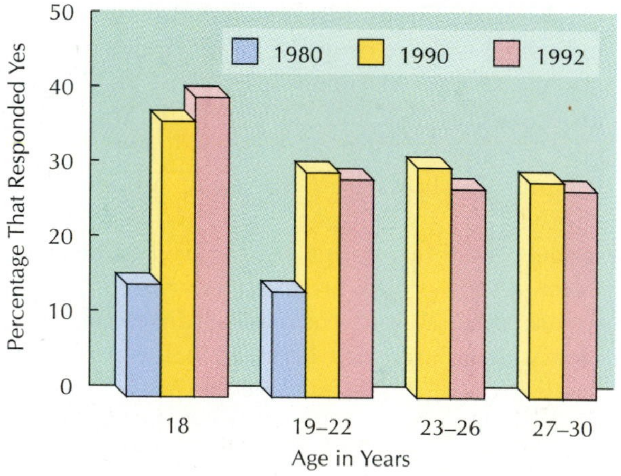

E. Annual prevalence of use: Young adults were asked if they used marijuana during the preceding year.

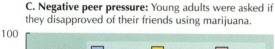

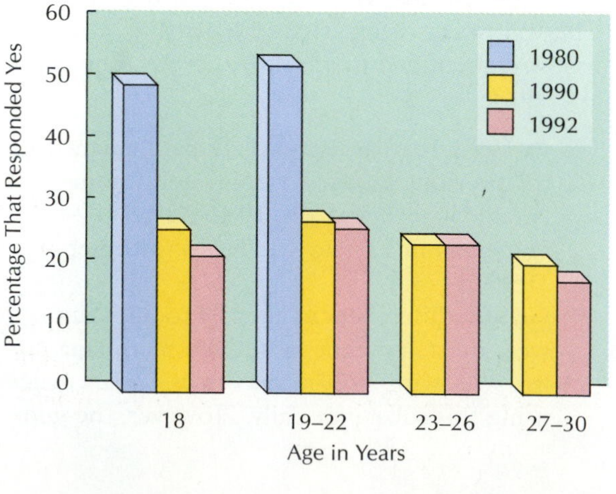

FIGURE 13.3 Changing patterns in attitudes toward the use of marijuana by young adults. As use of marijuana declined from 1980 to 1992 (E), so did association with marijuana-using friends (B). Corresponding with the declining use was an increase in perceived risk (D) and peer pressure not to use marijuana (C). However, there was no change in marijuana availability (A). *Source:* L. Johnston, P. M. O'Malley, and J. Bachman. *National Survey Results from The Monitoring the Future Study, 1975–1992.* Rockville, MD: National Institute on Drug Abuse, 1993.

drugs. Keep in mind that these factors can easily overlap; they are not separate and distinct.

The Role of Marijuana as a "Gateway" Drug

The claim that marijuana use leads to the use of other more serious drugs, such as heroin, is controversial (Gardner 1992). Although it is true that many heroin addicts began drug use with marijuana, it is also true that many, if not most, also used coffee and cigarettes. What's more, there are millions of marijuana users who never go beyond this drug. As one study reports, "There are only a few thousand opiate addicts in Great Britain, yet there are millions who have tried cannabis" (Gossop 1987).

Nevertheless, some explanation is needed for the small percentage of marijuana users who do progress to such hard drugs as heroin. It is not likely that the use of marijuana is the principal cause of moving to harder drugs, but much more important factors are the personality of the users as well as their socioeconomical environment. As described in Chapter 15, youth who turn to drugs are usually slightly to seriously alienated individuals. Thus, progression from marijuana to other drugs is more likely to depend on peer group composition, family relationships, social class, and the age at which drug use begins.

Review Questions

1. Why do you think that marijuana has become the most frequently used illicit substance in the United States?
2. Do you believe that prosecution for marijuana possession should be more or less rigid than it currently is? Why?
3. How do one's surroundings and personality affect the response to cannabis?
4. Sometimes use of marijuana can cause relaxation and sedation. How does marijuana differ from typical CNS depressants in terms of tolerance, dependence, and withdrawal?
5. Why do you think a user of cannabis can develop psychological dependence?
6. Do you believe that use of marijuana is more or less harmful than use of tobacco products? Should they be regulated differently? Please explain your response.
7. Why do you think that there is so much controversy concerning the effects of marijuana on fetal development and sexual behavior?
8. What effects does marijuana have on the cardiovascular and respiratory systems?
9. What is the drug Marinol, and what are its FDA-approved uses?
10. Why does the FDA refuse to approve marijuana for clinical uses?
11. What are the potential effects of chronic high-dose cannabis use?
12. What is the *amotivational syndrome*, and how does it occur?
13. What are the most important factors in determining the pattern of marijuana use?
14. How are the patterns of marijuana use affected by factors such as gender, geographic location, and college education?

Key Terms

Cannabis sativa
sinsemilla
altered perceptions
the "munchies"
anandamide
aphrodisiac
Marinol
glaucoma
amotivational syndrome

Summary

1. Marijuana consists of the dried and crushed leaves, flowers, stems, and seeds of the *Cannabis sativa* plant. THC (delta-9-tetrahydrocannabinol) is the primary mind-altering (psychoactive) ingredient in marijuana.
2. Effects of marijuana can vary according to expectations and surroundings. At low doses, such as when smoked or eaten, marijuana often has a sedative effect. At higher doses, it can produce hallucinations and delusions.
3. *Hashish*, *ganja*, *sinsemilla*, and *bhang* are all derivatives of the cannabis plant; of these hashish (or *hasheesh*) is the strongest derivative and *bhang* is the weakest.
4. As with tobacco, smoking marijuana can impair pulmonary function, cause chronic respiratory diseases, such as bronchitis and asthma, and promote lung cancer. Marijuana causes vasodilation and a compensatory increase in heart rate. The effects of marijuana on sexual performance and reproduction is controversial. Some studies have suggested this substance enhances sexual arousal and may retard fetal growth if smoked during pregnancy.
5. Tolerance to the CNS and cardiovascular effects of marijuana develops rapidly with repeated use. Although physical dependence and associated withdrawal are minor, psychological dependence can be significant in chronic, heavy users.
6. The active ingredient, THC, has been used as treatment for a variety of seemingly unrelated medical conditions. Because of its clinical potential, THC is available as the FDA-approved product Marinol. This drug is indicated for treatment of nausea and vomiting in cancer patients receiving chemotherapy and to treat anorexia (lack of appetite) in AIDS patients. Other potential therapeutic uses for THC include relief of intraocular pressure associated with glaucoma, as an antiasthmatic drug, for muscle relaxation, as prevention for some types of seizures, as an antidepressant, and as an analgesic to relieve migraines and other types of pain.
7. *Highs* from using marijuana can impair motor coordination and cause perceptual and performance deficits, especially when the user engages in complex activities, such as driving a motor vehicle.
8. Chronic, heavy use of marijuana can cause an "amotivational syndrome" in some users. This syndrome consists of a lack of desire to pursue goals, apathy, a noncaring attitude about others and an inability to concentrate at work, in school, or during other activities that require attention.
9. Currently, approximately 20 million Americans use marijuana. Marijuana use is related to age, with the 19 to 32 years of age group most likely to be regular users. Other trends of marijuana use include males are more likely than females to use it daily, although there is little gender difference in casual users; intense use tends to be highest in the West and lowest in the South; intense daily use is lower in college students compared to noncollege young adults. Declines in marijuana use during the past decade appear to be due to increased peer disapproval and perceived harmfulness; not due to a change in availability. However, an increase in marijuana use in 1993 by high school seniors may mean that attitudes about marijuana use are changing again.
10. No direct evidence suggests that marijuana is a "gateway" drug and leads to the use of other more addictive drugs, like heroin or cocaine. Although most hard-core drug users start with alcohol, cigarettes, and marijuana, millions of cannabis users do not progress to more serious drugs. Correlation does not mean causation.

References

Abel, E. L. *Marijuana: The First Twelve Thousand Years.* New York: Plenum, 1980.

Abood, M., and B. Martin. "Neurobiology of Marijuana Abuse." *Trends in Pharmacological Sciences* 13 (May 1992): 201–06.

American Psychiatric Association. "Substance-Related Disorders." In *Diagnostic and Statistical Manual of Mental Disorders,* 4th ed., chairman Allen Frances. Washington, DC: APA, 1994: 175–272.

Anslinger, H. J., and C. R. Cooper. "Marijuana: Assassin of Youth." *The American Magazine* 124 (July 1937): 18–19, 150–53.

Bloodworth, R. C. "Major Problems Associated with Marijuana Use." *Psychiatric Medicine* 3, no. 3 (1987): 173–84.

Campbell, A. G., M. Evans, J. L. Thomson, and M. J. Williams. "Cerebral Atrophy in Young Cannabis Smokers." *Lancet* (1971): 1219–25.

Chait, L., and J. Pierri. "Effect of Smoked Marijuana on Human Performance: A Critical Review." In *Marijuana/Cannabinoids, Neurobiology and Neurophysiology,* edited by L. Murphy and A. Bartke, 387–424. Boca Raton, FL: CRC Press, 1992.

Consroe, P., and R. Sandyk. "Potential Role of Cannabinoids for Therapy of Neurological Disorders." In *Marijuana/Cannabinoids, Neurobiology and Neurophysiology,* edited by L. Murphy and A. Bartke, 459–524. Boca Raton, FL: CRC Press, 1992.

Dewey, W. L. "Cannabinoid Pharmacology." *Pharmacological Reviews* 38, no. 2 (1986): 48–50.

Epidemiology Report. "Marijuana Use is Up Again." *NIDA Notes* 9 (February–March 1994): 12, 13.

Farley, C. "Hello Again, Mary Jane." *Time* (April 1993).

Fernandez-Ruiz, J., F. Rodriguez de Fonseca, M. Navarro, and J. Ramos. "Maternal Cannabinoid Exposure and Brain Development: Changes in the Ontogeny of Dopaminergic Neurons." In *Marijuana/Cannabinoids, Neurobiology and Neurophysiology,* edited by L. Murphy and A. Bartke, 118–64. Boca Raton, FL: CRC Press, 1992.

Gardner, E. "Cannabinoid Interaction with Brain Reward Systems: The Neurobiological Basis of Cannabinoid Abuse." In *Marijuana/Cannabinoids, Neurobiology and Neurophysiology,* edited by L. Murphy and A. Bartke, 275–335. Boca Raton, FL: CRC Press, 1992.

Garzer, B. "Should Marijuana be Legal?" *Parade* magazine, 12 June 1994: 4–7.

Goldstein, A. *Addiction from Biology to Drug Policy.* New York: Freeman, 1994: 169–177.

Goldstein, F. "Pharmacological Aspects of Substance Abuse." In *Remington's Pharmaceutical Sciences,* 19th ed. Easton, PA: Mack, 1995.

Gossop, M. *Living with Drugs,* 2d ed. Aldershot, England: Wildwood House, 1987.

Harclerode, J. "The Effect of Marijuana on Reproduction and Development." In *Marijuana Research Findings: 1980,* edited by R. C. Petersen. NIDA Research Monograph no. 31. Washington, DC: National Institute on Drug Abuse, 1980.

Herscher, E. "'Brownie Mary' Is Cheered During Testimony at City Hall." *San Francisco Chronicle* 173 (August 1992): A-1.

Hollister, L. E. "Health Aspects of Cannabis." *Pharmacological Reviews* 38 (1986): 39–42.

Hudson, R. "Researchers Identify Gene That Triggers Marijuana's 'High.'" *Wall Street Journal* (9 August 1990): B-2.

Institute of Medicine, National Academy of Sciences. *Marijuana and Health.* Washington, DC: National Academy Press, 1982.

Iversen, L. "Medicinal Use of Marijuana." *Nature* 365 (1993): 12–13.

Jaffe, J. H. "Drug Addiction and Drug Abuse." In *The Pharmacological Basis of Therapeutics,* 8th ed., edited by A. Gilman, T. Rall, A. Nies, and P. Taylor. New York: Pergamon, 1990.

Johnston, L., P. O'Malley, and J. Bachman. *National Survey Results from The Monitoring the Future Study, 1975–1992.* Rockville, MD: National Institute on Drug Abuse 1992, 1993, and 1994.

Jones, R. T. "Human Effects: An Overview." In *Marijuana Research Findings: 1980,* NIDA Research Monograph no. 31. Washington, DC: National Institute on Drug Abuse, 1980.

Kearns, R. "Legalize Drugs? Elders Sparks Firestorm." *Salt Lake Tribune* 247 (9 December 1993): A-18.

Kelly, T., R. Foltin, C. Enurian, and M. Fischman. "Effects of THC on Marijuana Smoking, Drug Choice and Verbal Report of Drug Liking." *Journal of Experimental Analysis of Behavior* 61 (1994): 203–211.

Knight-Ridder News Service. "Time to Make Drugs Legal? Many Say Yes." *Salt Lake Tribune* 244 (21 September 1992).

L.A.W. Publications. *Let's All Work to Fight Drug Abuse,* 3d ed. Addison, TX: C&L Printing, 1985.

Liska, K. *Drugs and the Human Body,* 3d ed. New York: Macmillan, 1990.

"Marijuana." *Harvard Medical School Mental Health Letter* 4, no. 5 (November 1987): 1–4.

"Marijuana Menaces Youth." *Scientific American* 154 (1936): 151.

Miranne, A. C. "Marijuana Use and Achievement Orientation." *Journal of Health and Social Behavior* 20 (1979): 194–99.

Murphy, L., and A. Bartke. "Effects of THC on Pregnancy, Puberty, and the Neuroendocrine System." In *Marijuana/Cannabinoids, Neurobiology and Neurophysiology,* 539. Boca Raton, FL: CRC Press, 1992.

Nahas, G., and C. Latour. "The Human Toxicity of Marijuana." *Medical Journal of Australia* 156 (April 1992): 495–97.

Nahas, G. G., et al. "Inhibition of Cellular Immunity in Marijuana Smokers." *Science* 183 (1 February 1974): 419–20.

National Institute on Drug Abuse (NIDA). *Drug Abuse and Drug Abuse Research.* Washington, DC: U.S. Department of Health and Human Services, 1991. DHHS Publication no. 91-1704.

National Institute on Drug Abuse (NIDA). *Marijuana and Health.* Eighth Annual Report to the U.S. Congress from the Secretary of Health and Human Services. Washington, DC: NIDA, 1980.

National Institute on Drug Abuse (NIDA). "Capsules: Facts About Teenagers and Drug Abuse." no. 17. Rockville, MD: NIDA, January 1990. Photocopy.

Norem-Hebeisen, A., and D. P. Hedlin. "Influences on Adolescent Problem Behavior: Causes, Connections, and Contexts." In *Adolescent Substance Abuse: A Guide to Prevention and Treatment,* edited by R. Isralowitz and M. Singer. New York: Haworth, 1983.

Oliwenstein, L. "The Perils of Pot." *Discover* 9, no. 6 (1988): 18.

Palfai, T., and H. Jankiewicz. *Drugs and Human Behavior.* Dubuque, IA: Brown, 1991.

Petersen, R. C. "Marijuana and Health." In *Marijuana Research Findings: 1980.* NIDA Research Monograph no. 31. Washington, DC: National Institute on Drug Abuse, 1980.

"Pot Kills Motivation, Impairs Cognitive Functioning." *U.S. Journal* 12 (May 1981): 97–103.

Radosevich, M., L. Lanza-Kaduce, R. L. Akers, and M. D. Krohn. "The Sociology of Adolescent Drug and Drinking Behavior: Part II." *Deviant Behavior* 1 (January–March 1980): 145–69.

Robison, L. J. Buckley, A. Daigle, G. Hammond, R. Wells, D. Benjamin, and D. Arthur. "Use and Risk of Childhood Nonlymphoblastic Leukemia Among Offspring." *Cancer* 63 (15 May 1989): 1904–11.

Roffman, R. A., and W. H. George. "Cannabis Abuse." In *Assessment of Addictive Behaviors,* edited by D. M. Donovan and G. A. Marlatt. New York: Guilford, 1988.

Rowell, E., and R. Powell. *On the Trail of Marijuana: The Weed of Madness.* Mountain View, CA: Pacific, 1939.

Schultes, R. E. "Ethnopharmacological Significance of Psychotropic Drugs of Vegetal Origin." In *Principles of Psychopharmacology,* 2d ed., edited by W. G. Clark and J. del Giudice. New York: Academic Press, 1978.

Sewester, S. *Drug Facts and Comparisons.* St. Louis: Kluwer, 1993: 259h–59k.

Solomon, D., ed. *The Marihuana Papers.* New York: New American Library, 1966.

Spence, W. R. "Substance Abuse Identification Guide." 1991 Health Edco Pamphlet. Waco, TX: WRS Group, 1991.

Stenchever, M. A., T. J. Kunysz, and M. A. Allen. "Chromosome Breakage in Users of Marijuana." *American Journal of Obstetrics and Gynecology* 118 (January 1974): 106–13.

Swan, N. "Researchers Make Pivotal Marijuana and Heroin Discoveries." *NIDA Notes* 8 (10 September 1993): 1.

Tec, N. *Grass Is Green in Suburbia.* Roslyn Heights, NY: Libra, 1974.

Tudor, C. G., D. M. Petersen, and K. W. Elifson. "An Examination of the Relationships Between Peer and Parental Influences and Adolescent Drug Use." In *Chemical Dependencies: Patterns, Costs, and Consequences,* edited by C. D. Chambers, J. A. Inciardi, D. M. Petersen, H. A. Siegal, and O. Z. White. Athens: Ohio University Press, 1987.

Turner, C. E. "Chemistry and Metabolism." In *Marijuana Research Findings: 1980.* NIDA Research Monograph no. 31. Washington, DC: National Institute on Drug Abuse, 1980.

Zuckerman, B., D. A. Frank, R. Hingson, H. Amaro, S. M. Levenson, H. Kayne, S. Parker, R. Vinci, K. Aboagye, L. E. Fried, H. Cabral, R. Timperi, and H. Bauchner. "Effects of Maternal Marijuana and Cocaine Use on Fetal Growth." *New England Journal of Medicine* 320 (1989): 762–68.

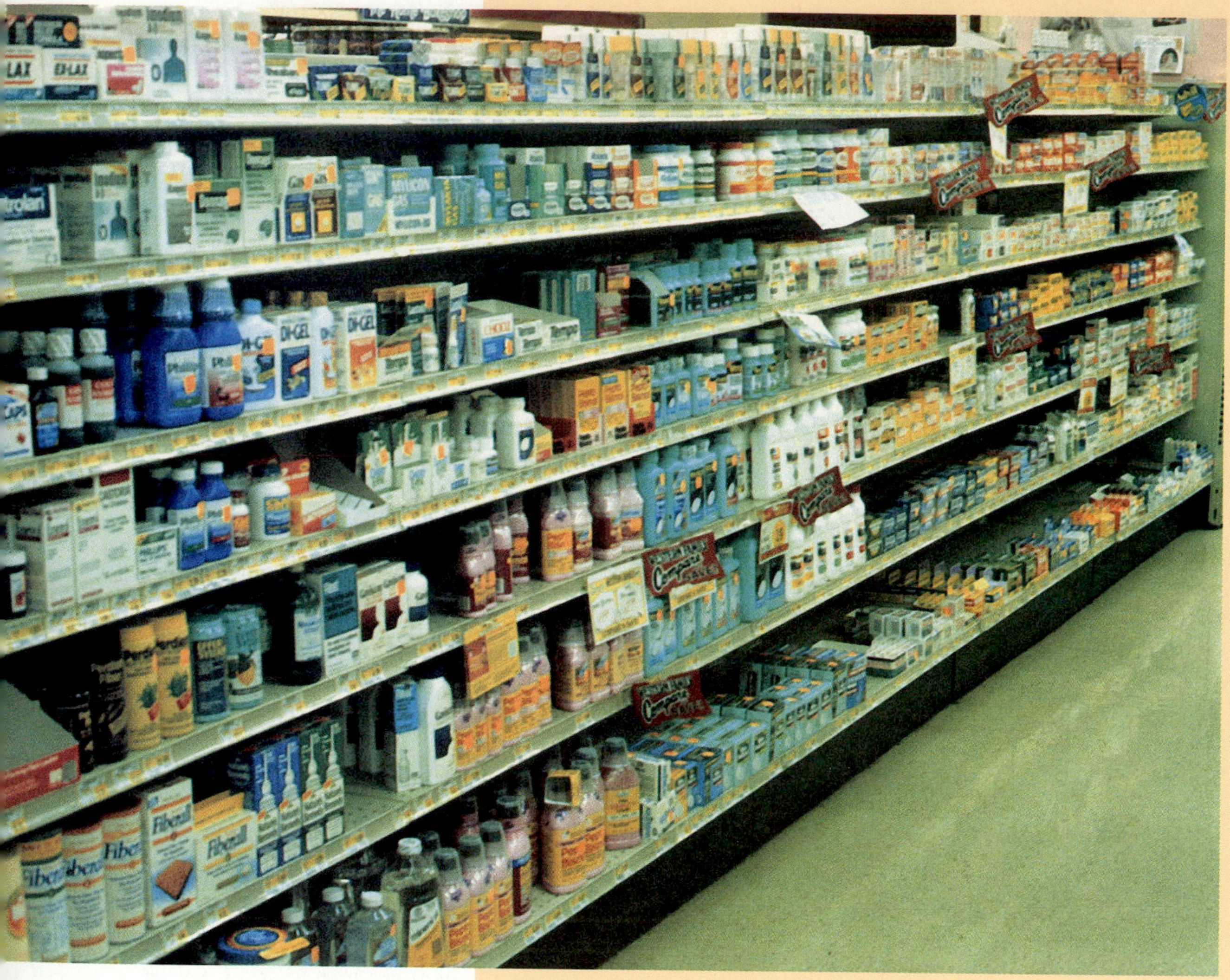

Chapter 14

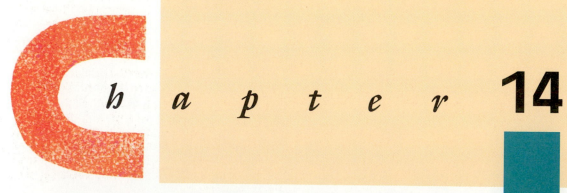

Drugs and Therapy

DID YOU KNOW THAT . . .

- The public can be much more confident of the effectiveness and safety of OTC drugs today than prior to 1972.
- The FDA is actively trying to switch safe and effective prescription drugs to OTC status. In the near future, many more drugs that are available only by prescription today will become nonprescription.
- Pharmacists can provide useful counseling in selecting appropriate OTC products.
- Excessive use of some OTC medications can cause physical dependence, tolerance, and withdrawal symptoms.
- OTC drugs can interact with prescription drugs in a dangerous and sometimes even lethal manner.
- Even though there are hundreds of different brands of OTC analgesics, there are really only three different types of active analgesic ingredients in these medications.
- OTC cold medications do not alter the course of the common cold but might relieve symptoms such as nasal congestion, muscle aches, and coughing.
- Frequent use of OTC antacids can be habit forming.
- More people die in the United States from adverse reactions to legal medications than succumb to all illegal drug use.
- Most generic drugs are as effective as, but substantially less expensive than, their proprietary counterparts.
- Pharmacists are required by law to counsel with patients concerning the use and safety of prescriptions that they fill.
- The top-selling prescription drug in 1993 was Premarin, an estrogen product used to relieve the symptoms of menopause.
- Half of the 10 best-selling prescription drugs for 1993 were for treating cardiovascular diseases.

LEARNING OBJECTIVES

On completing this chapter, you will be able to

1. Outline the general differences between prescription and nonprescription drugs.
2. Explain the rationale for the switching policy of the Food and Drug Administration (FDA).
3. Identify some of the drugs that the FDA will likely make available over the counter (OTC) in the future.
4. Discuss the potential problems of making more effective OTC drugs available to the public for self-care.
5. Describe the type of information that is included on the labels of nonprescription medicines.
6. State the rules for safe use of nonprescription drugs.

continued

Healthy People 2000

Increase to at least 75% the proportion of pharmacies and other dispensers of prescription medications that use linked systems to provide alerts to potential adverse drug reactions among medications dispensed by different sources to individual patients.

Increase to at least 75% the proportion of primary-care providers who routinely review with their patients aged 65 and older all prescribed and over-the-counter medicines taken by their patients each time a new medication is prescribed.

LEARNING OBJECTIVES

7 Classify the principal drug groups that are available OTC.
8 Discuss the type of information that should be communicated between doctor and patient to improve the quality of drug treatment.
9 Explain the differences between, as well as the advantages and disadvantages of, generic and proprietary drugs.
10 Classify the most frequently prescribed drug groups.

Prescription and nonprescription (OTC) drugs have been viewed differently by the public since these classifications were established by the Durham-Humphrey Amendment of 1951. In general, OTC medications are viewed as minimally effective and relatively free from side effects; in contrast, prescription drugs often are viewed as much more potent and frequently dangerous. However, distinctions between prescription and nonprescription drugs, which at one time appeared to be clear-cut, have become blurred by changes in public demand and federal policies. Because of escalating health costs and a growing interest in self-care, people today want access to effective medications, and governmental agencies such as the FDA are responding to their demands. Consequently, the FDA is actively involved in switching effective and relatively safe prescription medication to OTC status. It is clear that in the future, many more drugs will be removed from behind the pharmacist's counter and made available for public access as nonprescription medication. These changes underscore the arbitrary nature of classifying drugs as prescription and OTC, and remind us that similar care should be taken with all medications to achieve maximal benefit and minimal risk.

In this chapter, we begin by discussing OTC or nonprescription drugs. The first topic is policies regarding OTC drug regulation followed by a discussion of safe self-care with nonprescription drug products. A short explanation of some of the most common medications in this category concludes the section on OTC drugs. The second part of this chapter gives a general overview of prescription drugs. The consequences of misusing prescription drugs, as well as ways for the patient to avoid such problems, are discussed. A brief presentation of some of the most commonly prescribed drugs ends the chapter.

OTC Drugs

Over $12 billion is spent each year in the United States on drug products that are purchased over the counter (OTC), and this market is projected to reach $28 billion by the year 2010 (Covington 1993; Laskoski 1992). Today, more than 300,000 different OTC products are available to treat everything from age spots to halitosis and comprise 60% of the annual drug purchases in this country (McGinnis 1993). Approximately 40% of Americans use at least one OTC medication within a 2-day period, while an estimated three out of four people routinely self-medicate with these drug products (Covington 1993). The major drug classes currently approved for OTC status are shown in Table 14.1, and the most frequently used categories of OTC medications are shown in Table 14.2.

OTC substances are nonprescription drugs that may be obtained and used without the supervision of a physician or other health professional. Nevertheless, some OTCs may be dangerous when used alone or in combination with other drugs. Although some OTC drugs are very beneficial in the self-treatment of minor to moderate uncomplicated health problems, others are of questionable therapeutic value, and their usefulness is often misrepresented by manufacturers.

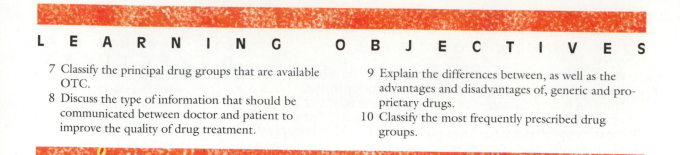

TABLE 14.1 Major drug classes approved by the FDA for OTC status

Drug Class	Effects
Analgesics and anti-inflammatories	Relieve pain, fever, and inflammation
Cold remedies	Relieve cold symptoms
Antihistamines and allergy products	Relieve allergy symptoms
Stimulants	Diminish fatigue and drowsiness
Sedatives and sleep aids	Promote sleep
Antacids	Relieve indigestion from rebound acidity
Laxatives	Relieve self-limiting constipation
Antidiarrheals	Relieve minor, self-limiting diarrhea
Emetics and antiemetics	Induce or block vomiting (respectively)
Antimicrobials	Treatment of skin infections
Bronchodilators and antiasthmatics	Assist breathing
Dentrifices and dental products	Promote oral hygiene
Acne medications	Treat and prevent acne
Sunburn treatments and sunscreens	Treat and prevent skin damage from ultraviolet rays
Dandruff and athlete's foot medications	Treat and prevent specific conditions
Contraceptives and vaginal products	Prevent pregnancy and treat vaginal infections
Ophthalmics	Promote eye hygiene and treat eye infections
Vitamins and minerals	Provide diet supplements
Antiperspirants	Promote body hygiene

Source: W. Gilbertson. "The FDA's OTC Drug Review." In *Handbook of Nonprescription Drugs,* 9th ed. Washington, DC: American Pharmaceutical Association, 1990.

Federal Regulation of OTC Drugs

The Food and Drug Administration (FDA) is responsible for regulating OTC drugs. However, many critics claim that federal agencies have not satisfactorily fulfilled their regulatory responsibility in regard to these products (Schwartz and Rifkin 1991). The history of OTC drug regulation is summarized in Table 14.3. (See also Chapter 3 for a detailed discussion.)

As discussed in Chapter 3, the active ingredients in OTC drugs have been, and continue to be, evaluated and classified according to their effectiveness and safety (Gilbertson 1993). At this time, most principal ingredients still included in nonprescription drug products are category I (that is, they are considered safe and effective) although as recently as August 1992, the FDA banned over 400 ingredients from seven categories of OTC products (Lamy 1993). In addition, the FDA is attempting to make even more drugs available to the general public by switching some frequently used and safe prescription medications to OTC status. This policy is in response to public demand to have access to effective drugs for self-medication. This policy helps to cut medical costs by eliminating the need for costly visits to health providers for treatment of minor, self-limiting ailments (Hsu 1994). A few of the more notable drugs that have been switched to nonprescription status since 1985 (Gilbertson 1993) are ibuprofen (analgesic—Advil, Nuprin); naprosyn (analgesic, anti-inflammatory—Aleve); diphenhydramine (antihistamine—Benadryl); hydrocortisone (anti-inflammatory steroid—Cortaid); loperamide (antidiarrheal—Imodium); fluoride (mouth rinses—Fluorigard);

CROSSCURRENTS

The FDA has adopted a policy of switching relatively safe, commonly used prescription drugs to OTC status. There has been substantial controversy concerning this policy as represented by the two following positions:

1. The people in this country are able to use drugs intelligently as part of self-care; thus, more effective medications for common health problems should be made available to the public. This can be done by reclassifying frequently used, and safe, prescription drugs to OTC.
2. The general public knows very little about proper drug use. If effective drugs are switched from prescription to OTC they are likely to be dangerously misused by an uninformed public. Consequently, the most effective drugs should only be administered under the supervision of a health professional to assure proper use.

Choose a side, and support your position with arguments based on the information in the text and other authoritative sources.

TABLE 14.2 The most frequently used categories of OTC medicines

Category	Percentage of Adults Who Use
Pain relievers (internal)	47%
Vitamins	46
Skin products	30
Antacids	23
Laxatives	21
Eye medications	14
External analgesics (rubs)	13
Cold remedies	11
Antihistamines	9
Cough suppressants	9

Source: "Top 200 Drugs of 1992." *Pharmacy Times* (March 1990):32.

clotrimazole (vaginal antifungal—Gyne-Lotrimin); adrenaline (bronchodilator—Bronkaid Mist); and miconazole (antifungal—Monistat 7).

A major concern of health professionals is that reclassification of safe prescription drugs to OTC status will result in overuse or misuse of these agents (see the Crosscurrents box). The switched drugs may tempt individuals to self-medicate rather than seek medical care for potentially serious health problems or encourage the use of multiple drugs at the same time, increasing the likelihood of dangerous interactions (see Case in Point). However, the FDA has proceeded cautiously and the majority of consumers support the switching policy (McCormick 1992). As of yet, no major problems have been identified and the switched products have been well received by the public; thus, of the top 10 OTC medications, 9 have been switched from prescription to OTC status since 1985 (Laskoski 1992).

It is likely that effective and safe prescription drugs will continue to be made available OTC, and it is hoped the public will be prepared to use them properly. In fact, the FDA is considering another

TABLE 14.3 History of OTC drug legislation and policy in the United States

Date	Event	Result
1906	Pure Food and Drug Act	Prohibited mislabeling and adulteration of drugs. Must list opiate, cocaine, alcohol, and cannabis contents.
1912	Sherley Amendment	Prohibited false or fraudulent therapeutic claims about a product.
1938	Food, Drug, and Cosmetic Act	New products must be judged safe before marketing.
1951	Durham-Humphrey Amendment	Drugs divided into prescription and non-prescription types.
1962	Kefauver-Harris Amendments	Required proof of safety and effectiveness of all drugs manufactured after 1938.
1966	NAS/NRC-FDA Study of Drugs	National Academy of Sciences/National Research Council evaluates 3,400 new drugs marketed between 1938 and 1962, including 512 OTC drugs. Only 15% of OTC products judged effective.
1972	FDA OTC Drug Products Evaluation Program	17 panels of experts to review all OTC drugs (over 300,000 on market).

Source: B. Berkowitz and B. Katzung. "Basic and Clinical Evaluations of New Drugs." In *Basic and Clinical Pharmacology,* 5th ed., edited by B. Katzung, 60–68. Norwalk, CT: Appleton & Lange, 1992.

Case in Point

Polydrug Use: A Therapeutic Nightmare

The use of multiple prescription and OTC drugs recently has been identified as the most prevalent factor leading to drug-induced disease. This is a particular problem in older people suffering from chronic health problems and hospitalized patients. The average number of drugs used on patients during hospitalization is 8.4. It has been demonstrated that the likelihood of adverse reactions increases disproportionately with an increase in drugs administered (Stewart 1995). What effect do you think the switching policy of the FDA would have on this problem?

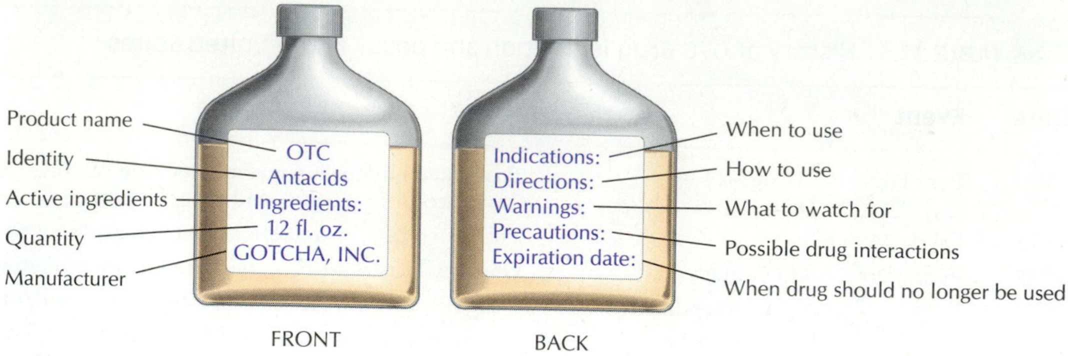

FIGURE 14.1 Label information controlled by the FDA

50 drugs or more currently available by prescription for OTC status in the next several years (Covington 1993). Included in this list of prescription drugs being evaluated for reclassification are Tagamet, Zantac, and Carafate (for treatment of ulcers), Hismanal (nonsedating antihistamine), Phenergan (sedative), Rogaine (for baldness), Retin A (for acne), Colestid (to reduce cholesterol levels), nicotine patches (to help quit smoking), and Acyclovir (antiviral for cold sores) (Covington 1993).

OTC Drugs and Self-Care

More than one-third of the time people treat their routine health problems with OTC medications in order to receive symptomatic relief from their ailments (McCormick 1992). This fact demonstrates the popularity of the OTC drugs and reflects the public enthusiasm for medical self-care. Self-care with nonprescription medications occurs because a consumer has decided that he or she has a health problem that can be adequately self-medicated without involving a health professional. Proper self-care assumes that the individual has made a correct diagnosis of the health problem and is well informed enough to select the appropriate OTC product. If done correctly, self-care with OTC medications can provide significant relief from minor, self-limiting health problems at minimal cost. However, a lack of understanding about the nature of the OTC products—what they can and cannot do—and their potential side effects can result in harmful misuse. For this reason, it is important that those who consume OTC medications be fully aware of their proper use. This usually can be achieved by carefully reading product labels and asking questions of health professionals such as pharmacists and physicians (Klein-Schwartz and Hoopes 1993).

OTC Labels Information about proper use of OTC medications is required to be cited on the drug label and is regulated by the FDA (see Figure 14.1 for an example). Required label information includes (1) approved uses of the product, (2) detailed instructions on safe and effective use, and (3) cautions or warnings to those at greatest risk when taking the medication (Gilbertson 1990).

Many consumers experience adverse side effects because they either choose to ignore the warnings on OTC labels or they simply do not bother to read them—see Case in Point (Associated Press 1992). For example, excessive or inappropriate use of some nonprescription drugs can cause drug dependence: consequently, people who are always dropping medication in the eyes "to get the red out" or popping antacids like dessert after every meal are likely addicted. They continue to use OTC products to avoid unpleasant eye redness or stomach acidity, which are actually withdrawal consequences of excessive use of these medications.

Rules for Proper OTC Drug Use The OTC marketplace for drugs operates differently than does its prescription counterpart. The use of OTC

Case in Point

Misuse of OTC Medication: Case Studies

The following cases illustrate the inappropriate use of OTC drugs and the potential problems that can result.

Case 1

Parents of a young child were going out for the evening. Their child often fussed when they were gone, so they decided to do something to keep the child from hassling the baby-sitter. They knew that cough syrup with antihistamine caused drowsiness, so they gave the child Benylin Cough Syrup (containing the antihistamine diphenhydramine) prior to the arrival of the baby-sitter in order to make the child fall asleep (Popovich 1991).

Case 2

An elderly woman experiencing delusions and hallucinations was admitted to the hospital. Laboratory tests revealed very high levels of calcium in her body. When questioned, the women explained that she consumed a few TUMS antacids each day. With further probing, it was discovered that she actually had been consuming 200 TUMS tablets every week for 9 years (Popovich 1991).

Case 3

A 4-year-old patient with juvenile rheumatoid arthritis experienced a severe chemical burn inside her mouth. It was discovered that she was given chewable aspirin every night to relieve the pain associated with her disease. One night, she fell asleep with the aspirin still in her mouth. Because of the caustic properties of this drug, the lining of her cheek was burned (Popovich 1991).

Case 4

A 34-year-old woman suffered blood clots during the delivery of her last child. She was put on the anticlotting drug warfarin to prevent additional clots. The following week, the patient experienced a headache and treated it with aspirin. She was not aware that aspirin also interferes with the formation of blood clots. The next morning, the patient slipped and fell but did not appear to be significantly injured. Later that day, she noticed large amounts of blood in her urine. Her husband rushed her to the hospital, where she was diagnosed with serious internal bleeding due to the interaction of warfarin and aspirin (Popovich 1991).

How can problems such as these be prevented?

drugs is not restricted, and consumers are responsible for making correct decisions about these products. Thus, the consumer sets policy and determines use patterns.

Because there are no formal controls over the use of OTC drugs, abuse often occurs. In extreme situations, the abuse of OTC medication can be very troublesome, even causing structural damage to the body. Proper education about the pharmacological features of these agents is necessary if consumers are to make intelligent and informed decisions about OTC drug use. To reduce the incidence of problems, the following rules should be observed when using nonprescription products:

1. *Always know what you are taking.* Identify the active ingredients in the product.
2. *Know the effects.* Be sure you know both the

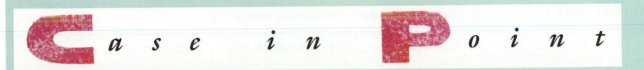

TABLE 14.4 Compositions of OTC internal analgesics (dose/unit)

Product	Salicylate (mg)	Acetaminophen (mg)	Ibuprofen (mg)	Other
Anacin	400 mg	—	—	Caffeine
Anacin (Maximum Strength)	500	—	—	Caffeine
Bayer	325	—	—	—
Empirin	325	—	—	—
Alka-Seltzer (Extra Strength)	500	—	—	Antacid
Ascriptin A/D	325	—	—	Maalox
Ecotrin	325	—	—	Coated tablet
Excedrin Extra Strength	250	250 mg	—	Caffeine
Aspirin-Free Anacin	—	500	—	—
Tylenol, Regular Strength	—	325	—	—
Tylenol, Junior Strength	—	160	—	—
Advil	—	—	200	—
CoAdvil	—	—	200	Decongestant
Haltran	—	—	200	—
Motrin IB	—	—	200	—
Nuprin	—	—	200	—

Source: Physician's Desk Reference for Nonprescription Drugs, 15th ed. Oradell, NJ: Medical Economics Data, 1994.

desired and potential undesired effects of each active ingredient.

3. *Read and heed the warnings and cautions.* The warnings are not intended to scare but to protect.
4. *Don't use anything for more than one to two weeks.* If the problem being treated persists beyond this time, consult a health professional.
5. *Be particularly cautious if also taking prescription drugs.* Serious interactions between OTC and prescription medications frequently occur. If you have a question, be sure to find the answer.
6. *If you have questions, ask a pharmacist.* Pharmacists are excellent sources of information about OTC drugs. They possess up-to-date knowledge of OTC products and can assist consumers in selecting correct medications for their health needs. Ask them to help you.
7. Most importantly: *If you don't need it, don't use it!*

Types of OTC Drugs

It is impossible to provide a detailed description of the hundreds of active ingredients approved by the FDA for OTC distribution; however, the following includes a brief discussion of the most common OTC drugs available in this country.

Internal Analgesics The U.S. public spends more than $2 billion on internal (taken by mouth) **analgesics,** the largest sales category of OTC drugs. Most of the money is for **salicylates** (aspirin products—Anacin, Bayer), acetaminophen (Tylenol, Datril, Pamprin, Panadol), and ibuprofen (Advil, Nuprin). The compositions of common OTC internal analgesics are given in Table 14.4.

Therapeutic Considerations. The internal analgesic products are effective in the treatment of several common ailments.

TABLE 14.5 Common side effects of OTC NSAIDS agents

Drugs	System Affected	Side Effects
Salicylates (aspirin-like)	Gastrointestinal	Irritation, bleeding, aggravation of ulcers
	Blood	Interference with clotting; prolongs bleeding
	Ears	Chronic high doses cause ringing (tinnitis) and hearing loss
	Pediatric	Reye's syndrome
Acetaminophen	Liver	High acute doses or chronic exposure can cause severe damage
Ibuprofen (includes other newer NSAIDS)	Gastrointestinal	Similar to salicylates but less severe
	Blood	Similar to salicylates but less severe
	Kidneys	Damage in elderly or those with existing kidney disease

Analgesic Action. The OTC analgesics effectively relieve mild to moderate somatic pain associated with musculoskeletal structures such as bones, skin, teeth, joints, and ligaments. Pains that are relieved by the use of these drugs include headaches, toothaches, earaches, and muscle strains. In contrast, these drugs are not effective in the treatment of severe pain or pain associated with internal organs, such as the heart, stomach, and intestines (Tyle 1993).

Anti-inflammatory Effects. Use of high doses (two to three times the analgesic dose) of the salicylates and ibuprofen relieves the symptoms of inflammation such as these associated with arthritis (Tyle 1993). In contrast, even high doses of acetaminophen have little **anti-inflammatory** action (Engle 1992). Because of this anti-inflammatory effect, these drugs are frequently compared to a group of natural, very potent anti-inflammatory compounds, the **steroids.** To distinguish drugs such as the salicylates and ibuprofen from steroids, these drugs are often called the **nonsteroidal anti-inflammatory drugs (NSAIDs).**

Antipyretic Effects. The OTC analgesics, such as aspirin and acetaminophen, reduce fever but do not alter normal body temperature (Tyle 1993). Such drugs are called **antipyretics.** The frequent use of these drugs to eliminate fevers is very controversial. Some clinicians believe that fever may be a defense mechanism that helps destroy infecting micro-organisms such as bacteria and viruses; thus, to interfere with fevers may hamper the body's ability to rid itself of infection-causing micro-organisms. Because no serious problems are associated with fevers of 102°F or less, they are probably better left alone (Lackner 1990).

Side Effects. When selecting an OTC analgesic drug for relief of pain, inflammation, or fever, possible side effects should be considered (Engle 1992). Although salicylates such as aspirin are frequently used, they often cause problems for both children and adults (see Table 14.5). Because of their side effects, salicylates are not recommended

ANALGESICS drugs that relieve pain while allowing consciousness

SALICYLATES aspirin-like drugs

ANTI-INFLAMMATORY relieve symptoms of inflammation

STEROIDS potent hormones released from the adrenal glands

NONSTEROIDAL ANTI-INFLAMMATORY DRUGS (NSAIDS) anti-inflammatory drugs that do not have steroid properties

ANTIPYRETICS drugs that reduce fevers

for (1) children, because of the potential for **Reye's syndrome;** (2) people with gastrointestinal problems, such as ulcers; or (3) people who have bleeding concerns, who are taking anticlot medication, who are scheduled for surgery, or who are near term in pregnancy, because salicylates interfere with clotting in the blood and prolong bleeding. For minor aches and pains, acetaminophen substitutes adequately for salicylates and it has no effect on blood clotting and does not cause stomach irritation. In addition, acetaminophen does not influence the occurrence of Reye's syndrome, a potentially deadly complication of colds, flu, and chicken pox in children (up to the age of 16 to 18 years) who are using salicylates (*Drug Facts and Comparisons* 1994).

Caffeine and Other Additives. A number of OTC analgesic products contain caffeine. There is increasing evidence that caffeine relieves some types of pain (Sawynok and Yaksh 1993). In addition, caffeine may relieve the aversion of pain due to its stimulant effect, which may be perceived as pleasant and energizing. The combination of caffeine with OTC analgesics may enhance pain relief (Abramowicz 1993) and be especially useful in treating vascular headaches because of the vasoconstrictive properties on cerebral blood vessels caused by this stimulant. In most OTC analgesic products, the amount of caffeine is less than that found in one-fourth to one-half cup of coffee (about 30 mg/tablet; for example, Anacin, Excedrin). Other ingredients—such as antacids, antihistamines, and decongestants—sometimes included in OTC pain-relieving products have little or no analgesic action and usually add little to the therapeutic value of the medication.

Cold, Allergy, and Cough Remedies The common cold accounts for 20% of all acute illness in the United States. It is also the single most expensive ailment in the country (Sause and Mangione 1991; Bryant and Lombardi 1993). More time is lost from work and school due to the common cold than from all other diseases combined. About one-half of all absences and approximately one-fourth of total work time lost each year in industry is due to cold symptoms (Sause and Mangione 1991). Americans spend nearly $2 billion annually for cough, cold, allergy, hay fever, and sinus products.

The incidence of the common cold varies with age. Children between 1 and 5 years are most susceptible; each child averages 6 to 12 respiratory illnesses per year, most of which are common colds. Individuals 25 to 30 years old average about 6 respiratory illnesses a year, and older adults average 2 or 3. The declining incidence of colds with age is due to the immunity that occurs after each infection with a cold virus; thus, if reinfected with the same virus, the micro-organism is rapidly destroyed by the body's defense and the full-blown symptoms of a cold do not occur (Sause and Mangione 1991).

Most colds have similar general symptoms: the first stage, in which the throat and nose are dry and scratchy, and the second stage, in which secretions accumulate in the air passages, nose, throat, and bronchial tubes. The second stage is marked by continuous sneezing, nasal obstruction, sore throat, coughing, and nasal discharge. There may be watering and redness of the eyes and pain in the face (particularly near the sinuses) and ears. One of the most bothersome symptoms of the common cold is the congestion of the mucous membranes of the nasal passages, due in part to capillary dilation, which causes them to enlarge and become more permeable. Such vascular changes allow fluids to escape, resulting in drainage and also inflammation due to fluid-swollen tissues (Bryant and Lombardi 1993).

Decongestants. Cold and allergy products are formulated with such drugs as decongestants (sympathomimetics), antihistamines (chlorpheniramine or pheniramine), analgesics (aspirin or acetaminophen), and an assortment of other substances (vitamin C, alcohol, caffeine, and so on). Table 14.6 lists the ingredients found in many common OTC cold and allergy products.

Antihistamines reduce congestion caused by allergies, but their effectiveness in the treatment of virus-induced colds is controversial (Consumer

REYE'S SYNDROME a potentially fatal complication of colds, flu, or chicken pox in children

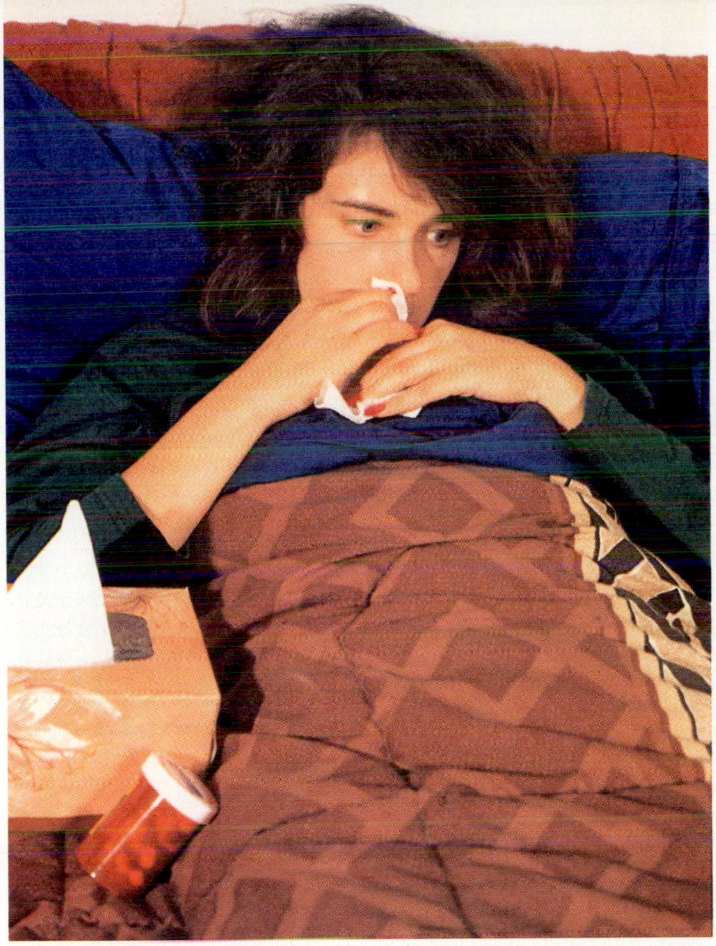

The common cold accounts for 20% of all acute illnesses in the United States.

TABLE 14.6 Compositions of common OTC cold and allergy products (dose/tablet)

Product	Sympathomimetic	Antihistamine	Analgesic
Actifed	Pseudoephedrine (60 mg)	Triprolidine (2.5 mg)	—
Allerest 12 Hour	Phenylpropanolamine (75 mg)	Chlorpheniramine (12 mg)	—
Chlor-trimeton	—	Chlorpheniramine (4 mg)	—
Contac Maximum Strength	Phenylpropanolamine (75 mg)	Chlorpheniramine (12 mg)	—
Contac Day & Night	Pseudoephedrine (60 mg)	—	Acetaminophen (650 mg)
Dimetapp Extentabs	Phenylpropanolamine (75 mg)	Brompheniramine (12 mg)	—
Dristan Cold	Phenylephrine (5 mg)	Chlorpheniramine (2 mg)	Acetaminophen (325 mg)
Sudafed Sinus	Pseudoephedrine (30 mg)	—	Acetaminophen (500 mg)

Source: Physician's Desk Reference for Nonprescription Drugs, 15th ed. Oradell, NJ: Medical Economics Data, 1994.

Report Books 1989). In high doses, the anticholinergic action of antihistamines (see Chapter 5) also decreases mucus secretion, relieving the runny nose; however, this action is probably insignificant at the lower recommended doses of OTC preparations (Sause and Mangione 1991). An anticholinergic drying action may actually be harmful because it can lead to a serious coughing response. Due to anticholinergic effects, antihistamines also may cause dizziness, drowsiness, impaired judgment, constipation, and dry mouth. Because of the limited usefulness and the side effects of antihistamine for treating colds, decongestant products without such agents are usually preferred for these viral infections (for example, Sudafed Sinus Caplets or Contac Day and Night Cold and Flu). In contrast, antihistamines are very useful in relieving allergy-related congestion and symptoms.

The sympathomimetic drugs used as decongestants cause nasal membranes to shrink because of their vasoconstrictive effect, which reduces the congestion caused by both colds and allergies. Such drugs can be used in the form of sprays or drops (topical decongestants) or systemically (oral decongestants) (see Table 14.7). FDA-approved sympathomimetics include pseudoephedrine, phenylpropanolamine, phenylephrine (probably the most effective topical), naphazoline, oxymetazoline, and xylometazoline (Bryant and Lombardi 1993).

Frequent use of decongestant nasal sprays can cause *congestion rebound* due to tissue dependence. After using a nasal spray regularly for longer than the recommended period of time, the nasal membranes adjust to the effect of the vasoconstrictor and become very congested when the drug is not present. The person becomes "hooked" and uses the spray more and more with less and less relief, until the tissue does not respond and the sinus passages become almost completely obstructed. Allergists frequently see new patients who are addicted to nasal decongestant sprays and are desperate for relief from congestion (Bryant and Lombardi 1993). This problem can be prevented by using nasal sprays sparingly and for no longer than the recommended time.

Orally ingested sympathomimetic drugs give less relief from congestion than the topical medications but do not cause rebound effects. In contrast, systemic administration of these drugs is more likely to cause cardiovascular problems (i.e., stimulate the heart, cause arrhythmia, increase blood pressure, and cause stroke; Sloan et al. 1991).

Antitussives. Other drugs used to relieve the common cold are intended to treat coughing. The cough reflex is an essential means to clear the lower respiratory tract of foreign matter, particularly in the later stages of a cold. There are two types of cough: productive and nonproductive. A *productive* cough clears mucus secretions and foreign matter so that breathing becomes easier and the infection clears up. A *nonproductive,* or dry, cough causes throat irritation; this type of cough is of little cleansing value. Some types of cough suppressant **(antitussive)** medication are useful for treating a nonproductive cough but should not be

TABLE 14.7 Compositions of OTC topical decongestants (drug concentrations)

Product	Sympathomimetic	Other
Afrin Nasal Spray	Oxymetazoline (0.05%)	—
Dristan Nasal Spray	Phenylephrine (0.5%)	Antihistamine
Neo-Synephrine, Maximum Strength	Oxymetazoline (0.05%)	—
Vicks Sinex, Long-acting	Oxymetazoline (0.05%)	—

Source: Physician's Desk Reference for Nonprescription Drugs, 15th ed. Oradell, NJ: Medical Economics Data, 1994.

TABLE 14.8 Compositions of common OTC antitussives (dose/unit)

Product	Dextromethorphan	Expectorant	Other
Cheracol plus	20 mg	—	Sympathomimetic; antihistamine; alcohol
Cheracol D	10 mg	Guaifenesin	Alcohol
Hold	5 mg	—	—
Novahistine DMX	10 mg	Guaifenesin	Sympathomimetic; alcohol
Triaminic Multisymptom	10 mg	—	Sympathomimetic; antihistamine
Robitussin CF	10 mg	Guaifenesin	Sympathomimetic
Vicks NyQuil	30 mg	—	Sympathomimetic; antihistamine; alcohol (25%)

Source: Physician's Desk Reference for Nonprescription Drugs, 15th ed. Oradell, NJ: Medical Economics Data, 1994.

used to suppress a productive cough (Sause and Mangione 1991).

Two kinds of OTC preparations are available to treat coughing:

1. *Antitussives*—such as codeine, dextromethorphan, and diphenhydramine (an antihistamine)—that act on the central nervous system (CNS) to raise the threshold of the cough-coordinating center, thereby reducing the frequency and intensity of a cough
2. **Expectorants**—such as guaifenesin and terpin hydrate—which theoretically (but not very effectively) increase and thin the respiratory tract fluids in order to soothe the irritated respiratory tract membranes and decrease the thickness of the accumulated secretions so that coughing becomes more productive.

Table 14.8 lists commonly used OTC antitussives and their compositions.

Often the tickling sensation in the throat that triggers a cough can be eased by sucking on a cough drop or hard candy, which stimulates saliva flow to soothe the irritated membranes. Unless the cough is severe, sour hard candy often works just as well as more expensive cough lozenges.

Cough remedies, like other medications, have a psychological value. Many patients with respiratory tract infections claim they cough less after using cough remedies, even when it is objectively demonstrated that the remedies reduce neither the frequency nor the intensity of the cough. Cough remedies work in part by reducing patients' anxiety about the cough and causing them to believe that their cough is lessening. If a person believes in the remedy, he or she often can get as much relief from a simple, inexpensive product as from the most sophisticated and costly one. If a cough does not ease in a few days, the person should consult a doctor.

Vitamin C. Vitamin C is found in some OTC cold remedies, although there is little evidence that it has a beneficial or preventive effect. Even so, Linus Pauling, a Nobel laureate, advocated using large doses of vitamin C (Bryant and Lombardi 1993). It should be noted that doses of 4 to 12 grams daily of this acidic vitamin (technically known as *ascorbic acid*) can cause kidney stones and that high levels can cause unreliable glucose tests in diabetics. Those who believe in taking vitamin C should use supplements instead of buying it mixed with a cold remedy. Better still, drinking lots

ANTITUSSIVES drugs that block the coughing reflex

EXPECTORANTS substances that stimulate mucus secretion and diminish mucus viscosity of orange juice may help. Even if vitamin C does not relieve the cold, the increase in liquid intake might.

What Really Works? Unfortunately, modern medicine and pharmacology have no cure for the common cold. In most cases, the best treatment is still plenty of rest, increased fluid intake to prevent dehydration and to facilitate productive coughing, humidification of the air if it is dry, gargling with diluted salt water (2 tsp. per quart), an analgesic to relieve the accompanying headache or muscle ache, and perhaps an occasional decongestant if nasal stuffiness is unbearable. Allergy symptoms, in contrast, are best relieved by antihistamines.

Sleep Aids An estimated 30% of the U.S. population experiences insomnia (the inability to get to sleep or stay asleep) annually, and 10 to 20% have serious or recurrent sleep problems (Eggert and Crismon 1992). About 1% of the adult population routinely self-medicate their insomnia with OTC sleep aids (such as Nytol, Sleep-eze, Sominex) that are advertised as inducing a "safe and restful sleep" (Eggert and Crismon 1992). Described as nonbarbiturate and non-habit forming, these low-potency products have a minimal action on the sleep and wakefulness centers of the brain.

The drugs commonly used in OTC sleep aids are antihistamines, particularly diphenhydramine (Crimson and Jermain 1993). Although antihistamines have been classified as category I sleep aid ingredients (see Chapter 3), their usefulness in treating significant sleep disorders is highly questionable. At best, some people who suffer mild, temporary sleep disturbances caused by problems such as physical discomfort, short-term disruption in daily routines (such as jet lag), and extreme emotional upset might experience temporary relief. However, even for those few who initially benefit from these agents, tolerance develops within two to four days. For long-term sleep problems, OTC sleep aids are of no therapeutic value and are rarely recommended by health professionals. Actually, their placebo benefit is likely more significant than their actual pharmacological benefit. Usually counseling and psychotherapy are more effective approaches for resolving chronic insomnia than OTC or even prescription sleep aid drugs (Eggert and Crismon 1992).

Because antihistamines are CNS depressants, in low doses, they can cause sedation and antianxiety action (see Chapter 6). Although in the past, some OTC products containing antihistamines were promoted for their relaxing effects (for example, Quietworld, Compoz), currently, no sedatives are approved for OTC marketing. The FDA decided that the earlier products relieved anxiety by causing drowsiness, so in fact, they were not legitimate sedatives (Caro and Dombrowski 1990). Because of this ruling, medications that are promoted as antianxiety products are no longer available without a prescription.

Stimulants Some OTC drugs are promoted as stay-awake (No Doz) or energy-promoting (Vivarin) products. In general, these medications contain high doses of caffeine (100 to 200 mg/tablet). (Caffeine and its pharmacological and abuse properties were discussed at length in Chapter 10.) Although it is true that CNS stimulation by ingesting significant doses of caffeine can increase the state of alertness during periods of drowsiness, the usefulness of such an approach is highly suspect (Crimson and Jermain 1993). For example, the use of these products to suppress highway fatigue following a full day of driving is frequently ineffective and can lull the user into a false sense of alertness. Routine use of stay-awake or energy-promoting products to enhance performance at work or in school can lead to dependence, resulting in withdrawal when the person stops using the drug. Most health professionals agree that there are more effective and safer ways to deal with fatigue and drowsiness; for example, get plenty of rest.

"Look-Alike" and "Act-Alike" Drugs. Mild OTC stimulants have been marketed as safe substitutes for more potent and illicit stimulants of abuse. Known as "look-alike" stimulants, these products have been made to appear as real amphetamines and are intended to give a mild lift or sense of euphoria. The principal drugs found in the look-alikes are phenylpropanolamine, ephedrine, and caffeine. The same drugs are routinely found in OTC decongestants and diet aids (Gauvin 1993).

As mentioned in Chapter 10, some states have outlawed look-alike medications, but products, called "act-alikes," have taken their place. Act-alikes do not resemble the restricted amphetamine drugs. Even so, these minor stimulants are sold on the streets as "speed" and "uppers," especially to young users, and are promoted by drug dealers as being legal and harmless.

Although much less potent than amphetamines, look-alikes and act-alikes, used in high doses, can cause anxiety, restlessness, throbbing headaches, breathing problems, and tachycardia (rapid heartbeat). There have even been reports of death due to heart arrhythmia and cerebral hemorrhaging. The availability of these drugs encourages their routine use and the development of dependence. Thus, they can serve as "gateway" drugs, leading to abuse of more potent compounds.

The manufacturers of the look-alike and act-alike drugs unscrupulously advertise in college newspapers, handbills posted at truckstops, and unsolicited literature from mail order companies (Brown 1991).

Gastrointestinal Medications The gastrointestinal (GI) system consists principally of the esophagus, stomach, and intestines and is responsible for the absorption of nutrients and water into the body, as well as the elimination of body wastes. The function of the GI system can be altered by changes in eating habits, stress, infection, and organic disorders, such as ulcers and cancers. Such problems may affect appetite, cause discomfort or pain, result in nausea and vomiting, and alter the formation and passage of stools from the intestines.

A variety of OTC medications are available to treat GI disorders such as indigestion (antacids), constipation (laxatives), and diarrhea (antidiarrheals). However, before individuals self-medicate with nonprescription drugs, they should be certain that the cause of their GI problem is minor, self-limiting, and does not require professional care. Because antacids are the most frequently used of the GI nonprescription drugs, they are discussed.

Antacids. Over $1 billion is spent annually on antacid preparations that claim to give relief from indigestion caused by excessive eating or drinking, and heartburn and for long-term treatment of chronic peptic ulcer disease (Cramer 1992). It is estimated that as much as 50% of the population has had one or more attacks of **gastritis,** often referred to as *acid indigestion, heartburn, upset stomach,* and *sour* or *acid stomach.* This gastric discomfort is most often due to acid rebound, occurring one to two hours after eating; by this time, the stomach contents have passed into the small intestines, leaving the gastric acids to irritate or damage the lining of the empty stomach.

Some cases of severe, chronic acid indigestion may progress to peptic ulcer disease. Peptic ulcers (open sores) most frequently affect the duodenum (first part of the intestine) and the stomach. Although this condition is serious, it can be treated effectively with prescription drugs such as cimetidine (Tagamet), ranitidine (Zantac), and famotidine (Pepcid), often combined with antacids. A person with acute, severe stomach pain; chronic gastritis; blood in the stools (common ulcer symptoms); diarrhea; or vomiting should see a physician promptly and not attempt to self-medicate with OTC antacids.

Most bouts of acid rebound, however, are associated with overeating or consuming irritating foods or drinks; these are self-limiting cases and can usually be managed safely with OTC antacids. Because of their alkaline (opposite of acidic) nature, the nonprescription products neutralize gastric acids and give relief.

There are four principal active ingredients found in OTC antacids:

1. *Sodium bicarbonate* is a potent and fast-acting acid neutralizer, and it is inexpensive. However, it has a high sodium content that can be harmful to those who should restrict sodium intake. In addition, frequent use of sodium bicarbonate can severely disrupt the metabolic balance of the body; this should be discouraged, especially for children. It is also of social significance to remember that bicarbonate interaction with gastric acid generates the gas carbon dioxide. Accumulation of this gas in the gastrointestinal tract can result in belching and other gaseous activities that are not socially ingratiating. Products with sodium bicarbonate include baking soda, Alka-Seltzer, and Citrocarbonate.

2. *Calcium carbonate,* an alkaline substance, is also commonly used in OTC antacid products.

GASTRITIS inflammation or irritation of the gut

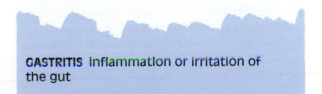

TABLE 14.9 Compositions of common OTC antacids (dose/unit)

Product (form)	Magnesium Salt	Calcium Carbonate	Aluminum Hydroxide	Other
Ascriptin	50 mg	—	50 mg	Aspirin
Di-Gel (tablets or liquid)	128 mg	280 mg	—	Simethicone
Gelusil (liquid)	200 mg	—	200 mg	—
Gaviscon	20 mg	—	80 mg	—
Maalox (tablets or liquid)	300 mg	—	600 mg	—
Mylanta Plus	200 mg	—	200 mg	Simethicone
Rolaids (tablets)	—	—	300 mg	—
Phillips Milk of Magnesia (liquid)	400 mg	—	—	—
Alka-Mints (tablets)	—	850 mg	—	—
Rolaids—Calcium Rich (tablets)	—	550 mg	—	—
TUMS (liquid or tablets)	—	500 mg	—	—
Alka-Seltzer (dissolving tablets)	—	—	—	Sodium bicarbonate

Source: Physician's Desk Reference for Nonprescription Drugs, 15th ed. Oradell, NJ: Medical Economics Data, 1994.

Calcium carbonate rapidly neutralizes acid, but it can cause a rebound effect, so that after the chemical leaves the stomach, even more gastric acid is secreted than before. Calcium carbonate may also make kidney stones worse for people who have this problem. Calcium-containing OTC antacids have been recommended for women to prevent osteoporosis. However, this practice has been questioned. Some experts argue that calcium carbonate is not the best form of calcium for treatment of this disease. OTC products containing this calcium compound are Alka-Mints, Di-Gel, and Rolaids-Calcium Rich.

3. *Aluminum hydroxide* and related compounds are used in Gaviscon, Gelusil, Maalox, and Mylanta. Because of their low neutralizing action, aluminum salts are almost always used in combination with magnesium salts. The constipating effect of aluminum salt is counterbalanced by the laxative effect of magnesium salt.

4. *Magnesium salts,* taken in low doses, are effective albeit slow antacids and safe for chronic use. In higher doses, magnesium salts stimulate the passage of feces and are even promoted as a laxative (see the label of Milk of Magnesia). Due to the slow onset of action and laxative tendency, magnesium salts are usually combined with either calcium carbonate (Mylanta Gelcaps) or aluminum hydroxide (Gelusil, Maalox, Mylanta).

Table 14.9 lists common OTC antacids and their compositions.

Some antacid products have antiflatulent ingredients to provide relief from gastric gas (for example, Di-Gel, Mylanta). The most commonly used, simethicone, breaks up gas bubbles and thus relieves pressure by facilitating belching and passing gas. Alginic acid, bismuth salts, and other substances are similarly used in some products. None of these ingredients is classified as an antacid, as they are not effective in neutralizing acid.

Generally speaking, OTC antacid preparations are safe for occasional use at low recommended doses, but some warnings must be considered (see the Here and Now box). Aluminum-magnesium hydroxide gels have low toxicity and an adequate neutralizing capacity. But all antacids can interact with other drugs; they may alter the gastrointestinal absorption or renal elimination of other med-

Here and Now

FDA Guidelines for Antacid Use

1. For relief of indigestion, antacids should not be taken for longer than two weeks. If the user still isn't relieved, a physician should be consulted.
2. The user should know that antacids may cause diarrhea (magnesium salts) or constipation (aluminum salts).
3. Patients with restricted salt intake because of blood pressure problems and the like should be aware that many antacids contain sodium; these people should select a product that does not.
4. The tablet forms of antacids are less effective than liquid preparations. If tablets are preferred, they should be chewed thoroughly and followed with a full glass of water. Effervescent tablets are supposed to be dissolved in a glass of water first; most of the bubbles should be allowed to subside before swallowing the preparation.
5. The user should be aware that significant drug interactions may occur; in such cases, a pharmacist or physician should be consulted for further information (Garnett 1990, 24).

ications. For example, some antacids inhibit the absorption of tetracycline antibiotics; thus, these products should not be taken at the same time. Consequently, patients using prescription drugs should consult with their physicians before taking OTC antacids (Pinson and Weart 1993).

Diet Aids In U.S. society, being slim and trim are prerequisites to being attractive. It is estimated that approximately 25–30% of the people in the United States are obese (with body fat in excess of 20% of normal) and 50% are overweight. Being obese is pathological and has been linked to cardiovascular disease, some cancers, diabetes, chronic fatigue, and an array of aches and pains, not to mention psychological disorders such as depression. Popular remedies for losing weight often come as fad diets advertised in supermarket journals, expensive weight loss programs, or the use of OTC diet aids.

Using drugs as diet aids is highly controversial (Doheny 1993). Most experts view them as useless or even dangerous. These drugs are supposed to depress the appetite, which helps users maintain low-calorie diets. The most effective of these are called **anorexiants.** Potent anorexiants, such as amphetamine-like drugs, can cause dangerous side effects (see Chapter 10) and are only available by prescription. The appetite suppression effects of prescription anorexiants only last for two to four weeks, after which time tolerance often occurs. Thus, even prescription diet aid drugs are usually only effective for a short period. There are no wonder drugs to help the obese lose weight permanently (Doheny 1993).

The most potent and most frequently used OTC diet aid ingredient is the sympathomimetic phenylpropanolamine (Acutrim, Dexatrim). Esti-

ANOREXIANTS drugs that suppress the activity of the brain's appetite center, causing reduced food intake

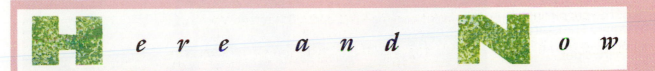

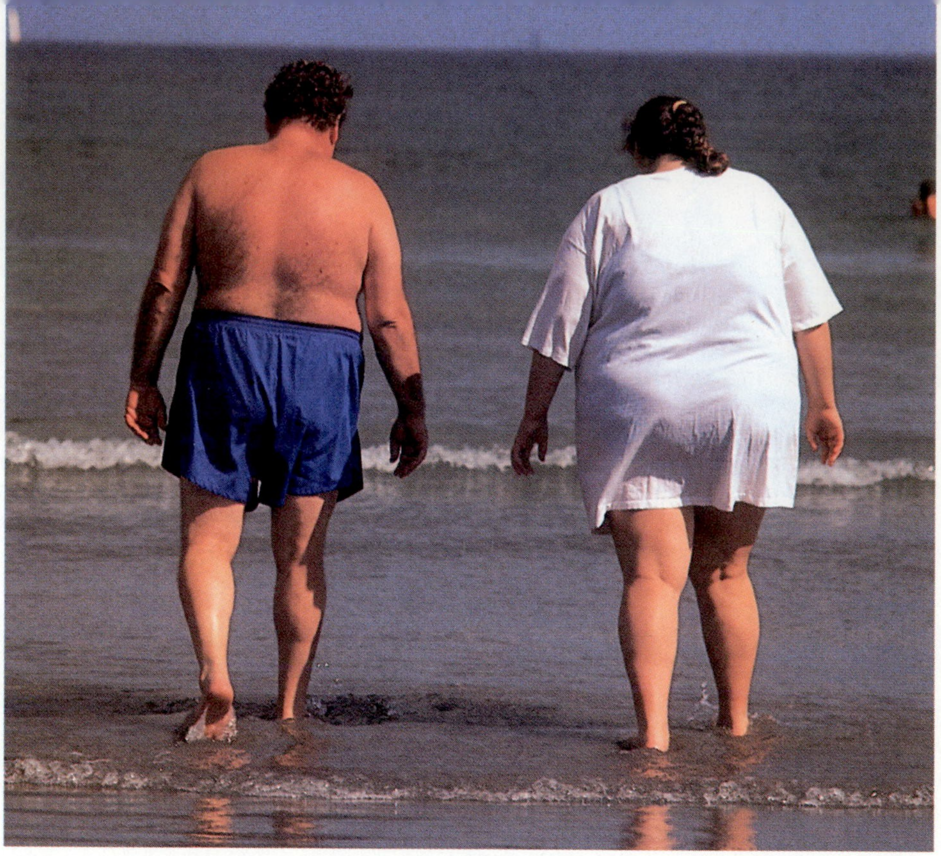

Approximately 25–30% of the people in the United States are obese and 50% are overweight.

mates show that the best of the OTC products significantly reduce appetite in less than 30% of the users, and tolerance occurs in one to three days of use (Consumer Report Books 1989). Clearly, such products are of no value in the treatment of obesity.

Skin Products Because the skin is so accessible and readily visible, most people are sensitive about its appearance. These cosmetic concerns are motivated by attempts to look good and preserve youth. Literally thousands of OTC skin products with cosmetic and health objectives are available to consumers. In this summary, only a few of the most commonly used products will be mentioned: acne medications, sun products, and basic first-aid products.

Acne Medications. Acne is a universal skin problem that occurs most frequently during puberty in response to the secretion of the male hormone androgen (both males and females have this hormone) (Zander and Weisman 1992). Acne is chronic inflammation caused by bacteria trapped in plugged sebaceous (oil) glands and hair follicles. This condition consists of whiteheads, pimples, nodules, and in more severe cases, pustules, cysts, and abscesses. Moderate to severe acne can cause unsightly scarring on the face, back, chest, and arms and should be treated aggressively by a dermatologist with drugs such as antibiotics (tetracycline) and potent **keratolytics,** such as Retin A (retinoic acid or vitamin A) or Accutane (isotretinoin). Usually, minor to moderate acne does not cause permanent skin damage or scarring and often can be safely self-medicated with OTC acne medications (Billow 1990).

Several nonprescription approaches to treating mild acne are available:

KERATOLYTICS caustic agents that cause the keratin skin layer to peel

KERATIN LAYER the outermost protective layer of the skin

1. *Sebum removal.* Oil and fatty chemicals (sebum) can accumulate on the skin and plug the sebaceous glands and hair follicles. Use of OTC products such as alcohol wipes can help remove such accumulations (for example, Stri Dex).

2. *Peeling agents.* The FDA found several keratolytic agents safe and effective for treatment of minor acne: benzoyl peroxide (Oxy 5 and Oxy 10), salicylic acid (Oxy Medicated Pads), resorcinol, and sulfur (Acnemol), alone or in combination. These drugs help to prevent acne eruption by causing the **keratin layer** of the skin to peel or by killing the bacteria that cause inflammation associated with acne. If multiple concentrations of a keratolytic are available (such as Oxy 5 and Oxy 10), it is better to start with a lower concentration and move up to the higher one, allowing the skin to become accustomed to the caustic action of these products. The initial exposure may worsen the appearance of acne temporarily; however, with continual use, the acne usually improves.

Sun Products. The damaging effects of sun exposure on the skin have been well publicized in recent years. It is now clear that the ultraviolet (UV) rays associated with sunlight have several adverse effects on the skin. It has been demonstrated that almost one million cases of skin cancer each year in the United States are a direct consequence of exposure to UV rays (Debrovner 1994b). Presently, almost 1 of 6 people will experience some form of skin cancer during his or her lifetime (Simonsen 1993).

The majority of these will be cancers of skin cells called *basal cell* or *squamous cell carcinomas* (Rigel 1991). These usually are easily excised by minor surgery and have a good prognosis for recovery. About 0.5% of the population will suffer a much more deadly form of skin cancer called *melanoma*. It is estimated that, because people today tend to spend so much time outdoors, by the year 2000, the risk of this cancer will reach 1 in 75 Americans (Ritter 1991). Melanomas are cancers of the pigment-forming cells of the skin, called *melanocytes,* and spread rapidly from the skin throughout the body, causing death in 20–25% of the cases (DeSimone 1993).

Another long-term concern (to some people worse than cancer) related to UV exposure is premature aging. Skin frequently exposed to UV rays, such as during routine tanning, experiences deterioration associated with the aging process. Elastin

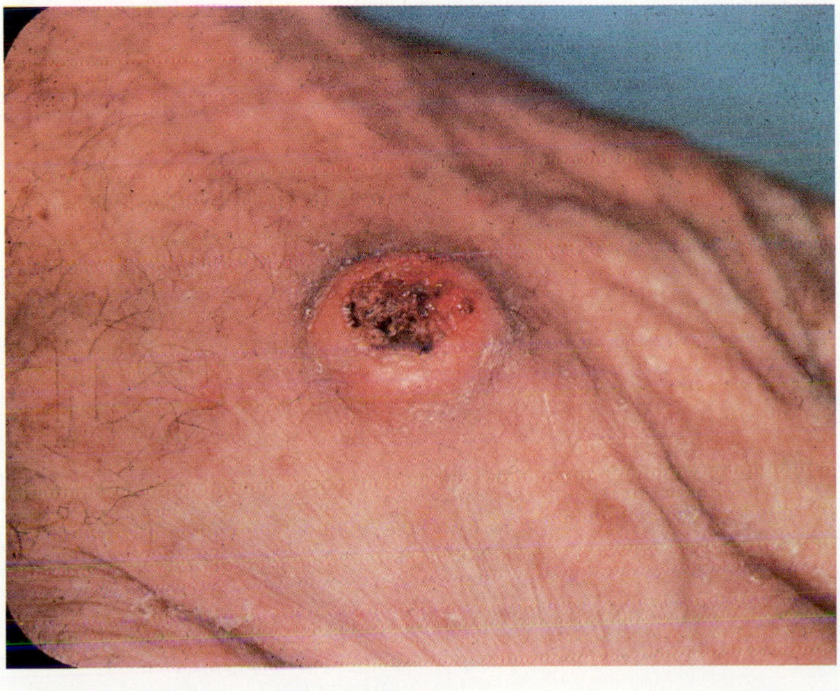

Almost all cases of skin cancer in this country are a direct consequence of exposure to ultraviolet light.

and collagen fibers are damaged, causing a loss of pliability and elasticity in the skin and resulting in a leathery, wrinkled appearance (Simonsen 1993).

Because of these damaging effects of sun exposure, an array of protective sunscreen products are available OTC. Most sunscreens are formulated to screen out the shorter UV-B rays. These products have deliberately been designed to allow passage, in varying degrees, of the UV-A rays because researchers once thought that these longer rays would help skin to tan without causing damage. Now it appears scientists were mistaken and due to deep penetration in the skin, UV-A rays likely contribute to melanoma as well as chronic skin damage, causing wrinkling, sagging skin, and loss of skin tone (Simonsen 1993; Debrovner 1994b).

The protection afforded by sunscreens is designated by an **SPF (sun protection factor) number.** This designation tells users the relative length of time they can stay in the sun before burning and varies from 2 to 46. For example, proper application of a product with an SPF of 10 allows users to remain in the sun without burning 10 times longer than if it wasn't applied. However, it is important to remember that the SPF designation does not indicate protection against UV-A rays. Although there currently is no convenient rating system to assess UV-A screening, products with SPF ratings of 15 or greater usually offer some protection against the longer UV radiation. In addition, a compound called *avobenzone* appears to offer the fullest protection against UV-A rays. Two FDA-approved products that contain avobenzone are Photoplex and Shade UVAGUARD. Both are classified as broad-spectrum screens as they also protect against UV-B and have an SPF designation of 15 ("Full Sun Protection" 1993).

Because the natural pigment in the skin affords some UV protection, people with fair skin complexion (less skin pigmentation) require products with higher SPF numbers than do dark-skinned people. Sunscreen chemicals found in these sun-protective products are shown in Table 14.10.

SPF (SUN PROTECTION FACTOR) NUMBER a designation to indicate ability to screen UV rays

People who want complete protection from UV-B exposure can use OTC sunblockers, which prevent any tanning. Sunscreen ingredients in high concentrations essentially become sunblockers (for example, Presun 46). In addition, an opaque zinc oxide ointment is a highly effective and inexpensive sun-blocking product and is available OTC.

Skin First-Aid Products. A variety of unrelated OTC drugs are available as first-aid products for the self-treatment of minor skin problems. Included in this category of agents are

1. *Local anesthetics,* such as benzocaine (such as Americaine First Aid Spray or Dermoplast) to relieve the discomfort and pain of burns or trauma
2. *Antibiotics and antiseptics,* such as bacitracin (Polysporin), neomycin (Neosporin), betadine, and tincture of iodine to treat or prevent skin infections
3. *Antihistamines* (Benadryl) or corticosteroids (hydrocortisone—Cortaid and Caldecort) to relieve itching or inflammation associated with skin rashes, allergies or insect bites

These first-aid skin products can be effective when used properly. In general, side effects to such topical products are few and minor when they occur.

Prescription Drugs

The Durham-Humphrey Amendment of 1951 established the criteria that are still used today to determine if a drug should be used only under the direction of a licensed health professional, such as a physician. According to this piece of legislation, drugs are controlled with prescriptions if they are (1) habit forming, (2) not safe for self-medication, (3) intended to treat ailments that require the supervision of a health professional, and/or (4) new and without an established safe track record. There currently are an excess of 10,000 prescription products sold commercially in the United States, representing approximately 1,500 different

TABLE 14.10 Selected approved OTC sunscreen ingredients

Ingredient	Brand
Para aminobenzoic acid (PABA), oxybenzone	PreSun
Benzophenone	Neutrogena
Oxybenzone	Vaseline Intensive Care, Aquaderm
Avobenzone	Photoplex, Shade UVAGUARD

Source: Physician's Desk Reference for Nonprescription Drugs, 15th ed. Oradell, NJ: Medical Economics Data, 1994.

drugs, with 20 to 50 new medications approved each year by the FDA (Mossinghoff 1993).

Because of specialized training, physicians, dentists, and, under certain conditions, podiatrists, physician assistants, nurse practitioners, pharmacists, and optometrists, are granted drug-prescribing privileges. The health professionals who write prescriptions are expected to accurately diagnose medical conditions requiring therapy, consider the benefit and the risk of drug treatment to the patient, and identify the best drug and safest manner of administering it. The responsibility of the health professional does not conclude with the writing of a prescription; in many ways it only just begins. Professional monitoring to ensure proper drug use and to evaluate the patient's response are crucial for successful therapy.

Proper Doctor–Patient Communication

Many unnecessary side effects and delays in proper care occur due to poor communication between the health professional and the patient when a drug is prescribed. The smaller a drug's margin of safety (difference between therapeutic and toxic doses) the greater the need for direction from a health professional to provide information concerning its proper use. The following is a brief overview of principles to help assure that satisfactory communication takes place between the health professional and the patient.

1. *Communication must be reciprocal.* We tend to think that patients listen while doctors talk when it comes to deciding on the best medication for treatment. To assure a proper diagnosis, precise and complete information from the patient is also essential. In fact, if a doctor is going to select the best and safest drug for a patient, he or she needs to know, as accurately as possible, the medical problems to be treated. In addition, the patient should provide the doctor with a complete medical and drug history particularly if there has been a problem with the patient's cardiovascular system, kidneys, liver, or mental functions. Other information that should be shared with the doctor include previous drug reactions as well as a complete list of drugs routinely being used, both prescription and nonprescription.

2. The patient needs to be educated about proper drug use, and if the doctor does not volunteer this information, the patient should insist on answers to the following questions:

- *What is being treated?* This doesn't require a long, unintelligible scientific description. It should include an easy-to-understand explanation of the medical problem.
- *What is the desired outcome?* The patient should know why the drug is prescribed and what the drug treatment is intended to accomplish. It is difficult for the patient to become involved in therapy if he or she is not aware of its objectives.
- *What are the possible side effects of the drug?* This does not necessarily include an exhaustive list of every adverse reaction ever recorded in the medical literature; however, it is important to realize that adverse drug reac-

tions to prescription drugs are very common. In the United States more people die from adverse reactions to legal medications than succumb to all illegal drug use (Fried 1994). In general, if the incidence is more than 1% of the users, it should be mentioned to the patient. In addition, the patient should be made aware of ways to minimize the occurrence of side effects (for example, an irritating drug should not be taken on an empty stomach to minimize nausea) as well as what to do if a side effect occurs (for example, if a rash occurs, call the doctor immediately).

- *How should the drug be taken to minimize problems and maximize benefit?* This should include details on how much, how often, and how long the drug should be taken.

Although it is a health professional's legal and professional obligation to communicate this information, patients frequently leave the doctor's office with a prescription that gives them legal permission to use a drug, but they do not necessarily understand how to use the drug properly. Because of this all-too-common problem, pharmacists have been mandated by legislation referred to as the Omnibus Budget Reconciliation Act of 1990 (OBRA 90), to provide the necessary information to patients on proper drug use (Zak 1993) (see the Here and Now box). Patients should be encouraged to ask questions of those who write and fill prescriptions.

Drug Selection: Generic Versus Proprietary

Although it is the primary responsibility of the doctor or health care provider to decide which drug is most suitable for a treatment, often an inexpensive choice can be as effective and safe as a more costly option. This frequently is true when choosing between generic and proprietary drugs. The germ **generic** is used by the public to refer to the common name of a drug that is not subject to trademark rights; in contrast, **proprietary** denotes medications marketed under specific brand names. For example, diazepam is the generic designation for the proprietary name Valium. Often the most common proprietary name associated with a drug is the name given when it is newly released for marketing. Because such drugs are almost always under patent restrictions for several years when first sold to the public, they become identified with their first proprietary names. After the patent lapses, the same drug often is also marketed by its less-known generic designation.

Because the pharmaceutical companies that market the generic products have not invested in the discovery or development of the drug, they often charge much less for their version of the medication. This contrasts with the original drug manufacturer, which may have invested up to $500 million for research and development (see Chapter 3). Even though the generic product frequently is less expensive, the quality usually is not inferior to the related proprietary drug; thus, substitution of generic for proprietary products rarely compromises therapy. It should be noted that occasionally an inferior generic drug product is marketed in order to increase profit margins for the manufacturer and is not therapeutically equivalent to the proprietary drug product; however, physicians and pharmacists should be aware of these differences and prescribe accordingly. If a patient alerts the physician to concerns about drug costs, less expensive generic brands often can be substituted.

Because of reduced cost, generic products have become very popular. By the mid-1990s, generic drugs will likely account for over 30% of all prescription drug sales amounting to approximately $10 billion (Simonsen 1993). Because of the great demand, all states have laws that govern the use and substitution of generic drugs; unfortunately, the laws are not all the same. Some states have positive laws that require pharmacists to substitute a generic product unless the physician gives specific instructions not to do so. Other states have negative laws that forbid substitution without the physician's permission. Some physicians use convenient prescription forms with "May" or "May

GENERIC the official, nonpatented, nonproprietary name of a drug

PROPRIETARY a brand or trademark name that is registered with the U.S. Patent Office

DRUG USE REVIEW a process conducted by pharmacists to improve the outcome of prescription drug therapy

Here and Now

OBRA 90—The Evolving Role of Pharmacists in Drug Management

In 1990 the U.S. Congress passed section 4401 of the Omnibus Budget Reconciliation Act (commonly referred to as OBRA 90), which substantially altered the role of pharmacists in drug management. This act designated the pharmacist as the key player in improving the quality of drug care for patients in this country. Because OBRA 90 is federal legislation, it can require drug-related services for Medicare patients only; however, most states have recognized that similar services should be made available to all patients and have enacted legislation to that end. OBRA 90 requires pharmacists to conduct a **Drug Use Review (DUR)** for each prescription to improve the outcome of drug therapy and reduce adverse side effects. The DUR program describes four basic professional services that a pharmacist must render whenever a drug prescription is filled:

1. Prescriptions and patients' records must be screened to avoid problems caused by drug duplications, adverse drug–drug interactions, medical complications, incorrect drug doses, and incorrect duration of drug treatment.
2. Patients should be counseled regarding
   - How to safely and effectively administer the drug
   - Common adverse effects and interactions with other drugs, food, and so forth
   - How to avoid problems with the drug
   - How to monitor the progress of drug therapy
   - How to store the drug properly
   - Whether a refill is intended
   - What to do if a dose is missed
3. Patient profiles including information on disease, a list of medications, and the pharmacist's comments relevant to drug therapy must be maintained. This information should be stored in computer files for future reference.
4. Documentation must record if the patient refuses consultation from the pharmacist, or if a potential drug therapy problem is identified and patient is warned.

Source: R. Abood, "OBRA 90: Implementation and Enforcement," NABP U.S. Pharmacists, State Boards—a Continuing Education Series. Park Ridge, IL: National Association of Boards of Pharmacy, 1992.

Not" substitution boxes that can be checked when the prescription is filled out (Consumer Report Books 1989).

Common Categories of Prescription Drugs

Of the approximately 10,000 different prescription drugs available in the United States, the top 50 drugs in sales account for almost 30% of all new and refilled prescriptions ("Top 200 Drugs of 1993" 1994). As an example, a list of the 30 top-selling prescription drugs in 1993 is shown in Table 14.11. The following includes a brief discussion of drug groups represented in the 30 most frequently prescribed medications. This list is not intended to be all inclusive, but only gives a sampling of common prescription products.

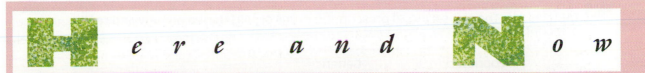

TABLE 14.11 The top-selling 30 prescription drugs of 1993 (based on new and refill prescriptions)

Ranking	Proprietary Name	Generic Name	Principal Clinical Use
1	Premarin	Estrogen	Relieve symptoms of menopause
2	Zantac	Ranitidine	Relieve ulcers
3	Amoxil	Ampicillin	Antibiotic
4	Synthroid	Levothyroxin	Replace thyroid hormone
5	Procardia	Nifedipine	Relieve angina pectoris
6	Lanoxin	Digoxin	Relieve heart failure
7	Xanax	Alprazolam	Sedation
8	Trimox	Amoxicillin	Antibiotic
9	Vasotec	Enalapril	Reduce hypertension
10	Cardizem	Diltiazem	Reduce hypertension
11	Ceclor	Cefaclor	Antibiotic
12	Augmentin	Amoxicillin	Antibiotic
13	Proventil	Albuterol	Open air passages
14	Naprosyn	Naproxyn	Analgesic
15	Provera	Medroxyprogesterone	Menstrual irregularities
16	Prozac	Fluoxetine	Antidepressant
17	Mevacor	Lovastatin	Reduce cholesterol levels
18	Seldane	Terfenadine	Nonsedating antihistamine
19	Ortho-Novum	Norethindrone Mestranol, ethynyl Estradiol	Contraceptive
20	Capoten	Captopril	Reduce hypertension
21	Tagamet	Cimetidine	Relieve ulcers
22	Cipro	Ciprofloxacin	Antibiotic
23	Ventolin	Albuterol	Open air passages
24	Amoxicillin	Amoxicillin	Antibiotic
25	Coumadin	Warfarin	Prevent blood clots
26	Lopressor	Metoprol	Reduce hypertension
27	Calan	Verapamil	Relieve angina pectoris
28	Micronase	Glyburide	Lower blood sugar
29	Dilantin	Phenytoin	Reduce seizures
30	Dyazide	Hydrochlorothiazide	Diuretic

Source: American Druggist. "Top 200." *American Druggist* (February 1994):28.

Analgesics The prescription analgesics consist mainly of the narcotic and NSAID (nonsteroidal anti-inflammatory drugs) types. The narcotic analgesics most often dispensed to patients by prescription are (1) the low-potency agents propoxyphene (Darvon) and codeine, (2) the moderate-potency agents pentazocine (Talwin) and oxycodone (Percodan), and (3) the high-potency drug meperidine (Demerol). All narcotic analgesics are scheduled drugs because of their abuse potential and are effective against most types of pain. The narcotic analgesic products are often combined with aspirin or acetaminophen (for example, Percocet is a combination of oxycodone and acetaminophen) to enhance their pain-relieving actions. For additional information on the narcotics, see Chapter 9.

The NSAIDs constitute the other major group of analgesics available by prescription. The pharmacology of these drugs is very similar to that of the OTC compound ibuprofen, discussed earlier in this chapter. All these medications are used to relieve inflammatory conditions (such as arthritis) and are effective in relieving minor to moderate musculoskeletal pain (pain associated with body structures such as muscles, ligaments, bones, teeth, and skin). These drugs have no abuse potential and are not scheduled. The principal adverse side effects include stomach irritation, kidney damage, tinnitus (ringing in the ears), dizziness, and swelling from fluid retention. About every two or three years, a new NSAID is approved for marketing by the FDA. Most prescription NSAIDs have similar pharmacological and side effects. Included in the group of prescription NSAIDs are ibuprofen (Motrin), naproxen (Anaproxyn), indomethacin (Indocin), sulindac (Clinoril), mefenamic acid (Ponstel), tolmetin (Tolectin), piroxicam (Feldene), and ketoprofen (Orudis).

Antibiotics Drugs referred to by the layperson as *antibiotics* are more accurately described by the term *antibacterials,* although the more common term will be used here. For the most part, antibiotics are effective in treating infections caused by micro-organisms classified as bacteria. Bacterial infections can occur anywhere in the body, resulting in tissue damage, loss of function, and if untreated, ultimately death. Even though bacterial infections continue to be the most common serious diseases throughout the world and in the United States today, the vast majority of these can be cured with antibiotic treatment (Carpenter 1988). There are currently close to 100 different antibiotic drugs, which differ from each other in (1) whether they kill bacteria **(bactericidal)** or stop their growth **(bacteriostatic),** and (2) the species of bacteria that are sensitive to their antibacterial action (Mills et al. 1992). Antibiotics that are effective against many species of bacteria are classified as **broad-spectrum** types, whereas those antibiotics that are relatively selective and only effective against a few species of bacteria are considered **narrow-spectrum** drugs. Although most antibiotics are well tolerated by patients, they can cause very serious side effects, especially if not used properly. For example, the penicillins have a very wide margin of safety for most patients, but 5–10% of the population is allergic to these drugs and life-threatening reactions can occur in sensitized patients if penicillins are used. The most common groups of antibiotic include penicillins (for example, ampicillin—Amoxil, Augmentin, and Trimox), cephalosporins (such as cefaclor—Ceclor), fluoroquinolones (such as ciprofloxacin—Cipro), tetracyclines (such as minocyclin—Minocin), aminoglycosides (such as streptomycin), sulfonamides (such as sulfamethoxazole—Bactrim and Septra), and macrolides (such as erythromycin—E-mycin).

Antidepressants Severe depression is characterized by diminished interest or pleasure in normal activities accompanied by feelings of fatigue, pessimism, and guilt as well as sleep and appetite disturbances and suicidal desires (Stimmel 1989). Severe depression afflicts approximately 5–6% of the population at any one time, and it is estimated that about 10% of the population will become severely depressed during their life (Debrovner

BACTERICIDAL kills bacteria

BACTERIOSTATIC stops replication and growth of bacteria

BROAD SPECTRUM effective against many species of bacteria

NARROW SPECTRUM effective against only a few species of bacteria

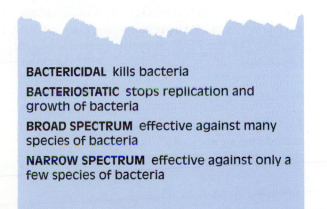

1994a). This high prevalence makes depression the most common psychiatric disorder (Hollister 1992). According to the classification of the *Diagnostic and Statistical Manual of Mental Disorders (DSM-IV)* of the American Psychiatric Association, several types of depression exist, based on their origin: (1) *endogenous major depression,* a genetic disorder that can occur spontaneously and is due to transmitter imbalances in the brain; (2) depression associated with bipolar mood disorder (that is, manic-depressive disorder); (3) reactive depression, the most common form of depression, is a response to situations of grief, personal loss, illness, or other very stressful situations. Antidepressant medication is typically used to treat endogenous major depression, although on occasion these drugs also are used to treat other forms of depression if they are resistant to conventional therapy (Hollister 1992).

Several groups of prescription antidepressant medication are approved for use in the United States. The most commonly used category is the **tricyclic antidepressants.** Included in this group are drugs such as amitryptyline (Elavil), imipramine (Tofranil), and nortryptyline (Pamelor). Although usually well tolerated, the tricyclic antidepressants can cause annoying side effects due to their anticholinergic activity. These adverse reactions include drowsiness, dry mouth, blurred vision, and constipation. The second group of drugs used to treat depression is referred to as the **monoamine oxidase (MAO) inhibitors.** Historically, these have been backup drugs for the tricyclic antidepressants. Because of their annoying and sometimes dangerous side effects as well as problems with interacting with other drugs or even food, the MAO inhibitors have become less popular with clinicians. Drugs belonging to this group include phenelzine (Nardil) and tranylcypromine (Parnate). Agents from a third, somewhat disparate, group of antidepressants have been recently approved by the FDA. Supposedly safer and with fewer side effects than the tricyclic or MAO inhibitor antidepressants, drugs in this third generation of antidepressants are rapidly gaining in popularity. Drugs belonging to this group include fluoxetine (Prozac), bupropion (Wellbutrin), and trazodone (Desyrel). Although side effects and the margin of safety of these groups of antidepressants may differ, in general they all appear to have similar therapeutic benefits (Hollister 1992).

Of this third group of antidepressants, Prozac is the best known. Ironically, Prozac is the most frequently prescribed antidepressant (in 1993 it was the sixteenth most frequently prescribed drug in the United States—see Table 14.11), as well as the most controversial (Cowley 1994). Reports began to surface in 1990 that use of Prozac caused some patients to commit suicide or murder (see Here and Now). One report described six patients who experienced intense preoccupation with suicide only after beginning treatment with Prozac (Masand et al. 1991). It was discovered that much of the early anti-Prozac propaganda was orchestrated by the "Citizens Commission on Human Rights," a nonmedical organization described by the television program "60 Minutes" as a front group for the Church of Scientology (Debrovner 1994a). However, since these early findings and anti-Prozac campaigns, close scrutiny of Prozac has not found this drug to be any more likely than other antidepressants to cause dangerous emotional problems in severely depressed patients (American Hospital Formulary Service [AHFS]

TRICYCLIC ANTIDEPRESSANTS most commonly used group of drugs to treat severe depression

MONOAMINE (MAO) INHIBITORS group of drugs used to treat severe depression

DIABETES MELLITUS disease caused by elevated blood sugar due to insufficient insulin

HYPERGLYCEMIA elevated blood sugar

DIABETES, TYPE I associated with complete loss of insulin-producing cells in pancreas

DIABETES, TYPE II usually associated with obesity; there is not a loss of insulin-producing cells

ORAL HYPOGLYCEMICS drugs taken by mouth to treat type II diabetes

EPILEPSY disease consisting of spontaneous repetitive seizures

Here and Now

Case History: A Prozac Reaction

A 58-year-old man had suffered from severe depression for 13 years. Two of his previous episodes of depression had been successfully treated with the common antidepressant drug imipramine. He did not respond to the drug after being admitted to the hospital during a third episode. Prozac treatment was started. Only three days after beginning the Prozac administration, the patient developed suicidal thoughts and tried to hang himself with a rope. Four days after stopping the Prozac treatment, suicidal thoughts abated and the patient was successfully treated with electroconvulsive therapy (Masand et al. 1991).

1994). With this reassurance of its safety, physicians prescribed in excess of $1 billion worth of Prozac for their patients in 1993 (Cowley 1994).

Antidiabetic Drugs **Diabetes mellitus** afflicts an estimated 8.3 million people in the United States and is the result of insufficient activity of insulin, a hormone secreted from the pancreas (Karam 1992). Due to the lack of insulin, untreated diabetics have severe problems with metabolism and elevated blood sugar (called **hyperglycemia**). The two major types of diabetes are type I (or juvenile type) and type II (or adult onset type). **Type I diabetes** is caused by total destruction of the insulin-producing cells in the pancreas and usually begins in juveniles, but occasionally begins during adulthood. In contrast, **type II diabetes** occurs most often after 40 years of age and is frequently associated with obesity: in these patients the pancreas is able to produce insulin, but insulin receptors no longer respond normally to this hormone (Karam 1992). In both types of diabetes mellitus, drugs are administered to restore proper insulin function.

Because of the inability to produce or release insulin in the type I diabetic, these patients are universally treated with subcutaneous injections of insulin 1–3 times a day, depending on their needs. Usually the levels of sugar (glucose) in the blood are evaluated to determine the effectiveness of treatment. Insulin products are characterized by their onset of action and duration of effects. Three types of insulin are used and include short-acting (regular and semilente), medium-acting (NPH and lente) and long-acting (PZI and ultralente) types.

The strategy for treating type II diabetics is somewhat different. For many of these patients, the symptoms of diabetes subside with proper diet, weight, and exercise management. If an appropriate change in lifestyle is insufficient to correct the diabetes-associated problems, drugs called **oral hypoglycemics** (meaning they are taken by mouth and lower blood sugar) are often prescribed. These drugs stimulate the release of additional insulin from the pancreas and include glyburide (Micronase) and tolbutamine (Orinase). If the diabetic symptoms are not adequately controlled with the oral hypoglycemic drugs, the type II diabetics are treated with insulin injections, as are the type I patients.

Antiepileptic Drugs Approximately 1% of the population in the United States has some form of **epilepsy.** Although appropriate medication can

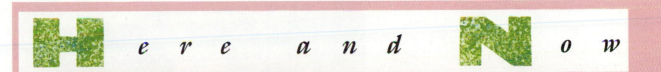

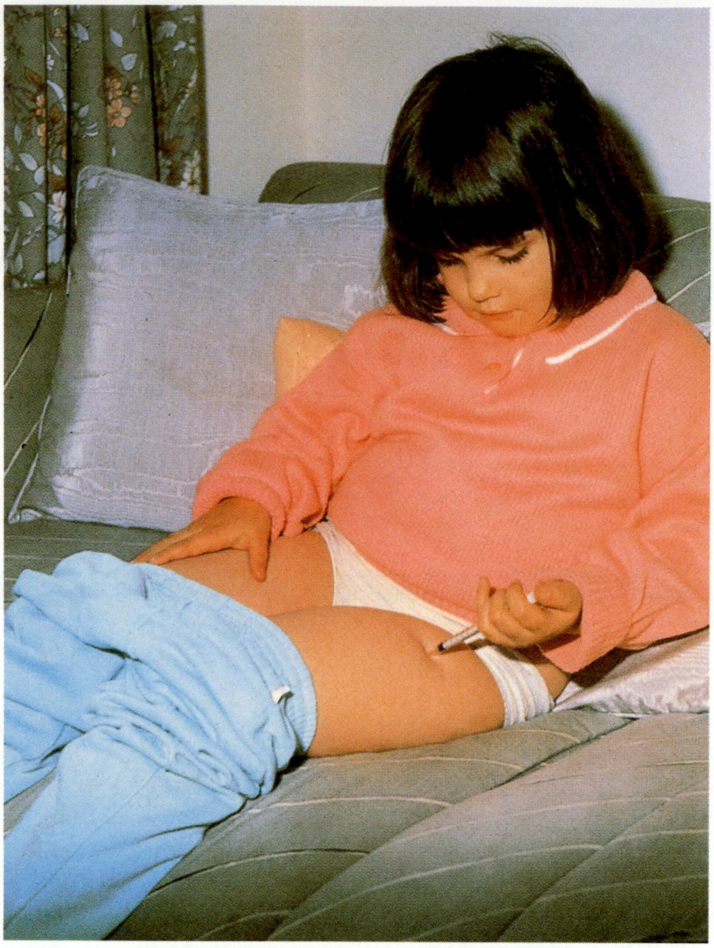

Insulin is self-administered by diabetic patients in subcutaneous injections.

control 80% of these patients, approximately 500,000 people in this country with epilepsy are inadequately treated (Porter and Meldrum 1992). Epilepsy is a neurological condition characterized by recurring seizures (that is, uncontrolled hyperactivity of the brain). Seizures are classified according to the region of the brain involved and how far the hyperactivity spreads. Thus, seizures are considered to be either partial (brain involvement stays local) or generalized (brain involvement is widespread) and can involve severe motor activity (for example, grand mal seizures) or have few motor symptoms (such as petit mal seizures). Because of the diverse nature of different types of epilepsy, several drugs are used as antiepileptics. Thus, phenytoin (Dilantin), carbamazepine (Tegretal), and phenobarbital are prescribed to control partial and grand mal seizures while ethosuximide (Zarontin) and valproic acid (Depakene) are used to treat generalized and petit mal seizures.

Antiulcer Drugs **Peptic ulcers** are sores that recur in the lining of the lower stomach (gastric ulcer) or most often in the upper portion of the small intestines (duodenal ulcer). Although the exact causes of ulcers are not known entirely, it is apparent that secretions of gastric acids and digestive enzymes are necessary for ulcer development (Altman 1992). Because gastric secretions are involved in developing peptic ulcers, several drug types are useful in ulcer treatment.

Antacids help to relieve acute discomfort due to ulcers by neutralizing gastric acidity. These drugs are discussed in greater detail in the OTC section of this chapter. Prescription drugs that block gastric secretion are the mainstay of ulcer treatment. Because the endogenous chemical histamine is important in regulating gastric secretions, drugs that selectively block the activity of gastric histamine (called H_2 blockers) substantially reduce secretion of gastric acids and digestive enzymes. The very popular prescription drugs cimetidine (Tagamet) and ranitidine (Zantac) function in this manner (Altman 1992). Because Tagamet and Zantac are used so frequently, they have been considered for switching to OTC status by the FDA.

Bronchodilators Of the top 40 prescription drugs in 1993, three (Proventil, Tenormin, and Ventolin) are drugs that widen air passages (that is, bronchi) to facilitate breathing in patients with air passage constriction or obstruction (American Druggist 1994). These drugs are called **bronchodilators** and are particularly useful in relieving respiratory difficulty associated with asthma. Asthmatic patients frequently experience bouts of intense coughing, shortness of breath, tightness in the chest, and wheezing. Many of the symptoms of asthma are due to an increased sensitivity of the airways to irritating substances (Boushey 1992) and can result in serious asthma attacks that are life threatening if not treated promptly. Two major categories of bronchodilators include sympathomimetics known as ß-**adrenergic stimulants**—for example, isoproterenol (Isuprel) and albuterol (Proventil, Ventolin) and xanthines (caffeinelike drugs) such as theophylline and its derivatives. These drugs relax the muscles of the air passages, cause bronchodilation, and facilitate breathing. In the early 1990s, some bronchial dilator medications were switched to OTC status and include products such as Bronkaid Mist and Primatene Mist.

Cardiovascular Drugs Cardiovascular disease has been the number one cause of death in the United States for the past several decades (Friedewald 1988), consequently, of the top-selling 30 drugs in this country, 9 are medications for diseases related to the cardiovascular system. The following are brief discussions of the major categories of cardiovascular drugs.

Antihypertensive Agents. It is estimated that 15% of American adults require treatment for **hypertension** (persistent elevated high blood pressure; Benowitz 1992). Because hypertension can result in serious damage to heart, kidneys, and brain, this condition needs to be treated aggressively. Treatment should consist of changes in lifestyle, including exercise and diet, but usually also requires drug therapy. There are two principal antihypertensive agents (Benowitz 1992):

1. *Diuretics*, which are drugs that lower blood pressure by eliminating sodium and excess water from the body. Included in this category is hydrochlorothiazide (Dyazide).
2. *Direct vasodilators,* which reduce blood pressure by relaxing the muscles in the walls of blood vessels that cause vasoconstriction, thereby dilating the blood vessels and decreasing their resistance to the flow of blood. Drugs included in this category are calcium channel blockers (diltiazem or Cardizem; verapamil or Calan; nifedipine or Procardia); inhibitors of the enzyme that synthesizes the vasoconstricting hormone, angiotensin II (enalapril or Vasotec; captopril or Capoten);

PEPTIC ULCERS open sores that occur in the stomach or upper segment of the small intestine

BRONCHODILATORS drugs that widen air passages

ß-ADRENERGIC STIMULANTS drugs that stimulate a subtype of adrenaline and noradrenaline receptors

HYPERTENSION elevated blood pressure

drugs that block the vasoconstricting action of the sympathetic nervous system (clonidine or Catapres; prazosin or Minipress).

Antianginal Agents. When the heart is deprived of sufficient blood (a condition called **ischemia**) the oxygen requirements of the cardiac muscle are not met and breakdown chemicals caused by the continual activity of the heart result in pain; this chest pain is described as viselike and is called **angina pectoris.** The most frequent cause of angina is obstruction of the large coronary vessels (Katzung and Chatterjee 1992). Angina pectoris frequently occurs in patients with hypertension and if left untreated, the underlying blockage of coronary vessels can result in heart attacks. All the drugs used to relieve, or prevent, angina decrease the oxygen deficit of the heart by either decreasing the amount of work required of the heart during normal functioning or by increasing the blood supply to the heart (Katzung and Chatterjee 1992). The three types of drugs prescribed for treating angina pectoris are (1) calcium channel blockers (for example, verapimil or Calan and diltiazem or Cardizem), (2) nitrates and nitrites (for example, amylnitrite or Vaporate and nitroglycerin or Transderm-nitro), and (3) blockers of the sympathetic nervous system, specifically classified as ß-adrenergic blockers (for example, atenolol or Tenormin and propranolol or Inderal).

Drugs to Treat Congestive Heart Failure. When the cardiac muscle is unable to pump sufficient blood to satisfy the oxygen needs of the body, **congestive heart failure** occurs. This condition causes an enlarged heart, decreased ability to exercise, shortness of breath, and accumulation of fluid **(edema)** in the lungs and limbs (Katzung and Parmley 1992). The principal treatment for congestive heart failure are drugs that improve the heart's efficiency, such as digoxin (Lanoxin).

Drugs that cause vasodilation are also sometimes used successfully to reduce the work required of the heart as it pumps blood through the body. Included in the drugs causing vasodilation are drugs already discussed in conjunction with other heart conditions such as hypertension and angina pectoris (for example, enalapril or Vasotec and captopril or Capoten).

Cholesterol and Lipid-lowering Drugs. Cholesterol and some types of fatty (lipid) molecules can accumulate in the walls of arteries and narrow the openings of these blood vessels. Such arterial changes cause hypertension, heart attacks, strokes, and heart failure and are the leading cause of death in the United States and other Western countries (Malloy and Kane 1992). These health problems can often be avoided by adopting a lifestyle that includes low-fat and low-cholesterol diets combined with regular, appropriate exercising. However, sometimes lifestyle changes are insufficient: in such cases, cholesterol-lowering drugs can be used to prevent the damaging changes in blood vessel walls. The drugs most often used include lovastatin (Mevacor), cholestyramine (Questran), and niacin (Vitamin B_3).

Hormone-Related Drugs As explained in Chapter 5, hormones are released from endocrine (ductless) glands and are important in regulating metabolism, growth, tissue repair, reproduction, and other vital functions. When there is a deficiency or excess of specific hormones, body functions can be impaired causing abnormal growth, imbalance in metabolism, disease, and often death. Hormones, or hormonelike substances, are sometimes administered as drugs to compensate for an endocrine deficiency and to restore normal function. This is the case for (1) insulin used to treat diabetes (see preceding discussion for more details), (2) levothyroxin (Synthroid, an artificial thyroid hormone) to treat **hypothyroidism** (insufficient activity of the thyroid gland), and (3)

ISCHEMIA tissue deprived of sufficient blood and oxygen

ANGINA PECTORIS severe chest pain usually caused by a deficiency of blood to the heart muscle

CONGESTIVE HEART FAILURE heart is unable to pump sufficient blood for the body's needs

EDEMA swollen tissue

HYPOTHYROIDISM thyroid gland doesn't produce sufficient hormone conjugated estrogens (Premarin) to relieve the symptoms caused by estrogen deficiency during menopause.

Hormones can also be administered as drugs to alter normal body processes. Thus, drugs containing the female hormones, estrogen and progesterone (norethindrone mestranol, ethynyl estradiol or Ortho Novum), can be used as contraceptives to alter the female reproductive cycles and prevent pregnancy. Another example are drugs related to corticosteroids (hormones from the cortex of the adrenal glands), which are often prescribed because of their immune-suppressing effects. In high doses, the corticosteroid drugs (for example, triamcinolone or Kenalog) reduce symptoms of inflammation and are used to treat severe forms of inflammatory diseases, such as arthritis (Goldfien 1992).

Sedative-Hypnotic Agents The sedative-hypnotics are discussed in considerable detail in Chapter 6. Because of the high incidence of anxiety and sleep disorder in the United States, drugs that encourage relaxation and drowsiness are frequently prescribed and are usually included in the list of top-selling prescription drugs (American Druggist 1994). For 1993 (Table 14.11), the benzodiazepine drug alprazolam (Xanax) was listed as the seventh most prescribed drug in the United States. Other benzodiazepines commonly prescribed are triazolam (Halcion) and diazepam (Valium).

Common Principles of Drug Use

Probably the most effective way to teach people not to use drugs improperly is to help them understand how to use drugs correctly. This can be achieved by educating the drug-using public about both prescription and OTC drug products. If people can appreciate the difference between the benefits of therapeutic drug use and the negative consequences of drug misuse or abuse, they are more likely to use medications in a cautious and thoughtful manner. To achieve this, patients must be able to communicate freely with health professionals. Before prescription or OTC drugs are purchased and used, patients should have all questions answered about the therapeutic objective, the most effective mode of administration and side effects. Education about proper drug use greatly diminishes drug-related problems and unnecessary health costs.

Review Questions

1. What types of prescription drugs would be appropriate for switching to OTC status?
2. Should the FDA use a different standard of *effectiveness* when evaluating OTC and prescription drugs?
3. What role should the pharmacists play in providing information about OTC and prescription drugs to patients?
4. What type of formal training should be required before a health professional is allowed to prescribe drugs?
5. Should health professionals other than physicians be allowed to prescribe drugs?
6. Should all physicians, regardless of their training or practice, be allowed to prescribe all drugs?
7. How can a health professional be certain that a patient has sufficient understanding concerning a drug to use it properly and safely?
8. Why are there so many different brands of OTC analgesics when there are only three basic types of drugs used in these products?
9. Should the FDA require that generic and proprietary versions of the same drug be exactly the same?
10. Even though some antibiotics have a wide margin of safety, currently there is no systemic antibiotic available OTC. Why is the FDA not willing to make some of these drugs nonprescription?

Key Terms

analgesics
salicylates
anti-inflammatory action
steroids
nonsteroid anti-inflammatory drugs (NSAIDS)
antipyretics
Reye's syndrome
antitussives
expectorants
gastritis
anorexiants
keratolytics
keratin layer
SPF (sun protection factor) number
Drug Use Review (DUR)
generic
proprietary
bactericidal
bacteriostatic
broad spectrum
narrow spectrum
tricyclic antidepressants
monoamine oxidase (MAO) inhibitors
diabetes mellitus
hyperglycemia
diabetes, type I
diabetes, type II
oral hypoglycemics
epilepsy
peptic ulcers
bronchodilators
ß-adrenergic stimulants
hypertension
ischemia
angina pectoris
congestive heart failure
edema
hypothyroidism

Summary

1. Prescription drugs are available only by recommendation of an authorized health professional, such as a physician. Nonprescription (OTC) drugs are available on request and do not require approval by a health professional. In general, OTC medications are safer than their prescription counterparts but often less effective, as well.
2. The switching policy of the FDA is an attempt to make available more effective medications to the general public on a nonprescription basis. This policy has been implemented in response to the interest in self-treatment by the public and in an attempt to reduce health care costs.
3. Drugs currently under review by the FDA for switching to OTC status include ulcer medications, such as Tagamet and Zantac; the coldsore medication Acyclovir; a nonsedating antihistamine, such as Hismanal; and a sedative, such as Phenergan.
4. Potential problems with making more effective drugs available OTC include overuse and inappropriate use, leading to dependence and other undesirable side effects. These more effective drugs could encourage self-treatment of medical problems that require professional care.
5. Information on OTC product labels is crucial for proper use of these drugs and thus regulated by the FDA. Product labels must list the active ingredients and their quantities in the product. Labels must also provide instructions for safe and effective treatment with the drug as well as cautions and warnings.
6. Although OTC drug products can be useful for treatment of many minor to moderate, self-limiting medical problems, when used without proper precaution they can cause problems. In order to optimize benefits and minimize risks when taking OTC medications, the following rules should be observed: always know what you are taking; know the effects; follow the warnings; don't use anything for a long period; be especially cautious if also taking prescription drugs; ask the pharmacist when you have questions; and don't use these drugs unless you need to.
7. The principal drug groups available OTC are used in the treatment of common, minor medical problems and include analgesics, cold remedies, allergy products, mild stimulants, sleep aids, antacids, laxatives, antidiarrheals, antiasthmatics, acne medications, sunscreens, contraceptives, and nutrients.

8. In order for drugs to be prescribed properly, patients need to provide complete and accurate information about their medical condition and medical history to their physician. In turn, the physician and/or pharmacist need to communicate to the patient what is being treated, why the drug is being used, how it should be used for maximum benefit, and what potential side effects can occur.
9. Proprietary drug names can only be used legally by the drug company that has trademark rights. Often the original proprietary name becomes the popular name associated with the drug. Because the pharmaceutical manufacturer who develops a drug is trying to recover the investment, a newly marketed proprietary drug is expensive. Once the patent rights expire, other drug companies can also market the drug, but under a different name; often the common, generic name is used because it cannot be trademarked. The generic brands are less expensive because the manufacturers do not need to recover any significant investment. Generally, the less expensive generic drug is as effective and safe as the proprietary counterpart.
10. Of the approximately 1,500 different prescription drugs currently available in the United States, the most commonly prescribed groups are analgesic, antibiotics, antidepressants, drugs used for diabetes, antiulcer drugs, antiepileptic drugs, bronchodilators, drugs used to treat cardiovascular diseases, hormone-related drugs, and sedative-hypnotics.

References

Abramowicz, M. "Drugs for Pain." *Medical Letter* 3 (8 January 1993): 6.

Altman, D. "Drugs Used in Gastrointestinal Disease." In *Basic & Clinical Pharmacology,* 5th ed., edited by B. Katzung, 888–98. Norwalk, CT: Appleton & Lange, 1992.

American Druggist. "Top 200." *American Druggist* (February 1994): 27–29.

American Hospital Formulary Service (AHFS), edited by G. McEvoy, 1401. Bethesda, MD: American Society of Hospital Pharmacists, 1994.

Associated Press. "Warning: Abusing OTC Drugs Can Be Hazardous to Health." *Salt Lake Tribune* 244 (29 April 1992): 1A.

Benowitz, N. "Antihypertensive Agents." In *Basic and Clinical Pharmacology,* 5th ed., edited by B. Katzung, 139–61. Norwalk, CT: Appleton & Lange, 1992.

Berkowitz, B., and B. Katzung. "Basic and Clinical Evaluations of New Drugs:" In *Basic and Clinical Pharmacology,* 5th ed., edited by B. Katzung, 60–68. Norwalk, CT: Appleton & Lange, 1992.

Billow, J. "Acne Products." In *Handbook of Nonprescription Drugs,* 10th ed., edited by T. Covington. Washington, DC: American Pharmaceutical Association, 1993: 511–20.

Boushey, H. "Bronchodilators and Other Agents Used in Asthma." In *Basic and Clinical Pharmacology,* 5th ed., edited by B. Katzung, 278–93. Norwalk, CT: Appleton & Lange, 1992.

Bryant, B., and J. Lombardi. "Cold, Cough and Allergy Products." In *Handbook of Nonprescription Drugs,* 10th ed., edited by T. Covington. Washington, DC: American Pharmaceutical Association, 1993: 89–115.

Carpenter, C. "Infectious Diseases." In *Textbook of Medicine,* 18th ed., edited by J. Wyngaarden and L. Smith, 1523–1852. Philadelphia: Saunders, 1988.

Consumer Report Books. *The New Medicine Show.* New York: Consumer Report Books (51 East 42nd St., New York, NY), 1989.

Covington, T. "Trends in Self Care: The Rx to OTC Switch Movement." *Drug Newsletter* 12 (February 1993): 15–16.

Covington, T. "Introduction." In *Handbook of Nonprescription Drugs,* 10th ed., edited by T. Covington. Washington, DC: American Pharmaceutical Association, 1993: XXV.

Cowley, G. "The Culture of Prozac." *Newsweek* (7 February 1994): 41.

Cramer, T. "When Do You Need an Antacid." *Pharmacy Times* (September 1992): 61–67.

Crimson, M., and D. Jermain. "Sleep Aid and Stimulant Products." In *Handbook of Nonprescription Drugs,* 10th ed., edited by T. Covington. Washington, DC: American Pharmaceutical Association, 1993: 135–46.

Debrovner, D. "Mind Menders." *American Druggist* (April 1994a): 20–26.

Debrovner, D. "Here Comes the Sun." *American Druggist* (May 1994b): 30–34.

DiSomone, E. "Sunscreen and Suntan Products." In *Handbook of Nonprescription Drugs,* 10th ed., edited by T. Covington. Washington, DC: American Pharmaceutical Association, 1993: 575–88.

Doheny, K. "The Skinny on Diet Pills." *American Druggist* (February 1993): 32–36.
Drug Facts and Comparisons. St. Louis: Lippincott, 1994.
Eggert, A., and L. Crismon. "Dealing with Insomnia." *American Druggist* (May 1992): 83–96.
Engle, J. "Internal Analgesics II." *American Druggist* (July 1992): 81–82.
Fried, S. "Prescription for Disaster." *Washington Post Magazine* (3 April 1994): 13–16.
Friedewald, W. "Epidemiology of Cardiovascular Disease." In *Textbook of Medicine,* 18th ed., edited by J. Wyngaarden and L. Smith. Philadelphia: Saunders, 1988.
"Full Sun Protection." *Wellness Letter* (June 1993): 4–5.
Garnett, W. "Antacid Products." In *Handbook of Nonprescription Drugs,* 9th ed., edited by T. Covington. Washington, DC: American Pharmaceutical Association, 1990.
Gauvin, D., K. Moore, B. Youngblood, and F. Holloway. "The Discriminative Stimulus Properties of Legal OTC Stimulants Administered Singly and in Binary and Ternary Combinations." *Psychopharmacology* 110 (1993): 309–19.
Gilbertson, W. "The FDA's OTC Drug Review." In *Handbook of Nonprescription Drugs,* 10th ed., edited by T. Covington. Washington, DC: American Pharmaceutical Association, 1993: 21–37.
Goldfien, A. "Adrenocorticosteroids and Adrenocortical Antagonist." In *Basic and Clinical Pharmacology,* 5th ed., edited by B. Katzung, 543–557. Norwalk, CT: Appleton & Lange, 1992.
Hollister, L. "Antidepressant Agents." In *Basic and Clinical Pharmacology,* 5th ed., edited by B. Katzung, 410. Norwalk, CT: Appleton & Lange, 1992.
Hsu, I. "Prescription to Over-the-Counter Switches." *American Druggist* (July 1994): 57–64.
Karam, J. "Pancreatic Hormones and Antidiabetic Drugs." In *Basic and Clinical Pharmacology,* 5th ed., edited by B. Katzung, 586–601. Norwalk, CT: Appleton & Lange, 1992.
Katzung, B., and K. Chatterjee. "Vasodilators and the Treatment of Angina Pectoris." In *Basic and Clinical Pharmacology,* 5th ed., edited by B. Katzung, 162–75. Norwalk, CT: Appleton & Lange, 1992.
Katzung, B., and W. Parmley. "Cardiac Glycosides and Other Drugs Used in Congestive Heart Failure." In *Basic and Clinical Pharmacology,* 5th ed., edited by B. Katzung, 176–89. Norwalk, CT: Appleton & Lange, 1992.
Klein-Schwartz, W., and J. Hoopes. "Patient Assessment and Consultation." In *Handbook of Nonprescription Drugs,* 10th ed., edited by T. Covington. Washington, DC: American Pharmaceutical Association, 1993: 11–20.
Lackner, T. "Antipyretic Drug Products." In *Handbook of Nonprescription Drugs,* edited by Feldman. Washington, DC: American Pharmaceutical Assoc., 1990.
Lamy, P. ". . . And on Nonprescription Products." *Elder Care News* 9 (Summer 1993): 17.
Laskoski, G. "Rx to OTC." *American Druggist* (December 1992): 47–50.
Malloy, M., and J. Kane. "Agents Used in Hyperlipidemia." In *Basic and Clinical Pharmacology,* 5th ed., edited by B. Kastung, 477–90. Norwalk, CT: Appleton & Lange, 1992.
Masand, P., S. Gupta, and M. Dewan. "Suicidal Ideation Related to Fluoxetine Treatment." *New England Journal of Medicine* 324 (1991): 420.
McCormick, E. "Rx to OTC: A Growth Industry?" *Pharmacy Times* (December 1992): 69–74.
McGinnis, T. "FDA's Bimonthly Update." *Pharmacy Times* (January 1993): 69.
Mills, J., S. Barriere, and E. Jawetz. "Clinical Use of Antimicrobials." In *Basic and Clinical Pharmacology,* 5th ed., edited by B. Katzung, 695–711. Norwalk, CT: Appleton & Lange, 1992.
Mossinghoff, G. "New Drug Arrival." *Pharmaceutical Manufacturers Association Newsletter* (January 1993): 1–12.
Physician's Desk Reference for Nonprescription Drugs, 15th ed. Oradell, NJ: Medical Economics Data, 1994.
Pinson, J., and C. Weart. "Antacid Products." In *Handbook of Nonprescription Drugs,* 10th ed., edited by T. Covington. Washington, DC: American Pharmaceutical Association, 1993: 147–79.
Popovich, N. "Not All Over-the-Counter Drugs Are Safe." *American Journal of Pharmaceutical Education* 55 (1991): 166–72.
Porter, R., and B. Meldrum. "Antiepileptic Drugs." In *Basic and Clinical Pharmacology,* 5th ed., edited by B. Kastung, 331–49. Norwalk, CT: Appleton & Lange, 1992.
Rigel, D. "Malignant Melanoma in the 1990s." *Pharmacy Times* (May 1991): 33–39.
Ritter, M. "Risk of Sometimes-Fatal Skin Cancer Rising." *Salt Lake Tribune* (13 June 1991): D10.
Sause, R., and R. Mangione. "Cough and Cold Treatment with OTC Medicine." *Pharmacy Times* (February 1991): 108–17.
Sawynok, J., and T. Yaksh. "Caffeine as an Analgesic Adjuvant: A Review of Pharmacology and Mechanisms of Action." *Pharmacology Review* 45 (1993): 43–85.
Schwartz, R., and S. Rifkin. "No More Paper Tiger."

American Druggist (June 1991): 26–34.

Simonsen, L. "Generic Prescribing and RPh Substitution Continue to Climb." *Pharmacy Times* (October 1993a): 29.

Simonsen, L. "Sun Exposure: The Stakes Are Rising." *Pharmacy Times* (May 1993b): 25–31.

Stewart, R. "Adverse Drug Reactions." In *Remington's Pharmaceutical Sciences,* 19th ed. Mack, 1995.

Stimmel, G. "Welcome Trends in Pharmacy." New York: Health Education Technologies, December 1989. Newsletter.

"Top 200 Drugs of 1993." *Pharmacy Times* (April 1994): 20.

Tyle, W. "Internal Analgesic Products." In *Handbook of Nonprescription Drugs,* 10th ed., edited by T. Covington. Washington, DC: American Pharmaceutical Association, 1993: 49–64.

Zak, J. "OBRA '90 and DUR." *American Druggist* (October 1993): 57.

Zander, E., and S. Weisman. "Self-Medication of Acne with Topical Salicylic Acid." *Pharmacy Times* (May 1992): 114–18.

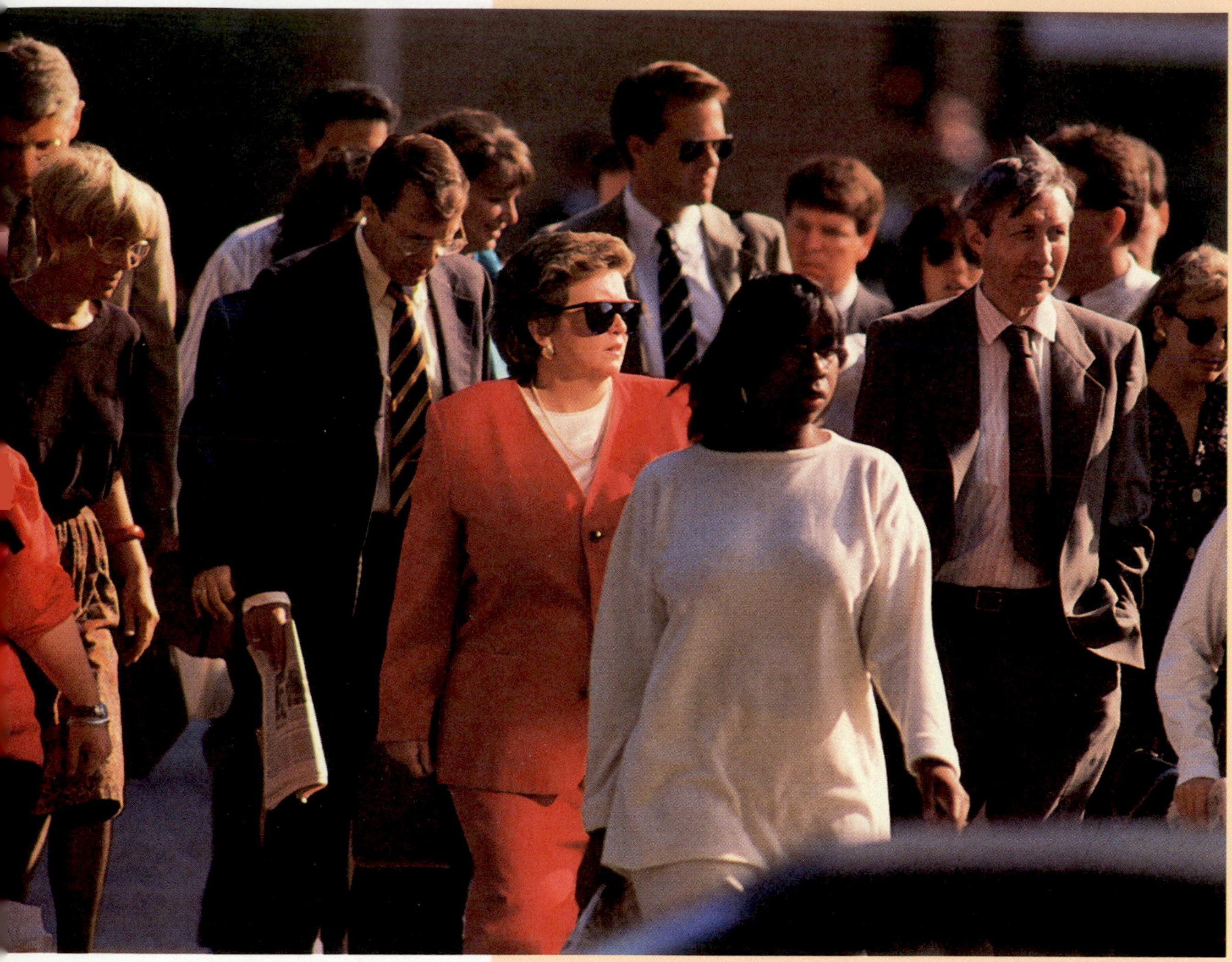

Chapter 15

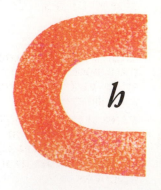

DID YOU KNOW THAT . . .

- In 1992, almost 70% of the eighth-graders in the United States had consumed alcohol, 45% had smoked cigarettes, and 11% had used marijuana sometime during their life.
- Drug abuse is more likely to be associated with criminal behavior in adolescents than in adults.
- People who were victims of incest as children are more likely to abuse drugs than the general population.
- Until recently, most drug abuse researchers excluded women from their studies.
- Women are more likely to be adversely affected by alcohol than men.
- Female college students are more likely than their male counterparts to use cigarettes daily.
- Women are less likely than men to seek therapy for their drug abuse problems.
- Athletes are no more likely than nonathletes to abuse alcohol, marijuana, or cocaine.
- If used during puberty, anabolic steroids will stunt growth.
- Those addicted to illicit drugs are currently the second largest risk group for contracting AIDS.

Drug Abuse Among Special Populations

LEARNING OBJECTIVES

On completing this chapter, you will be able to

1. Explain why adolescents use substances of abuse.
2. Describe the type of parents most likely to have drug-abusing children.
3. Identify drugs that are most likely to be abused by adolescents.
4. Explain the relationship between adolescents' involvement with drug abuse and gangs.
5. Compare patterns of drug use by females and males.
6. Explain why the unique socio-economic roles of women make them vulnerable to drug abuse problems.
7. Describe how drug treatment programs can meet the needs of female patients.
8. Know which drugs are most likely to be abused by athletes and why.
9. Be able to describe the use of drug testing for athletic competitions.
10. Explain how drug abuse contributes to the spread of AIDS.
11. Be able to list major strategies to prevent contracting AIDS.

Healthy People 2000

Reduce to no more than 3% the proportion of male high school seniors who use anabolic steroids.

Increase to at least 50% the estimated proportion of all intravenous drug abusers who are in drug abuse treatment programs.

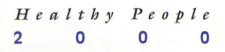

There is no such thing as a typical "drug abuser." Drug abuse problems are biased by the environmental and emotional configuration of the user; consequently, to identify effectively the nature of substance dependence and its consequences, it is essential to understand the psychosocial identity and biological makeup of those who become addicted to these drugs. This chapter examines four selective populations who, because of their unique features, present special drug abuse problems in terms of identification, prevention, and treatment. Specifically, drug abuse in adolescents, women, athletes, and AIDS victims is discussed.

Adolescents and Drugs

"It was the best of times, it was the worst of times."

Charles Dickens, *Tale of Two Cities*

This quote from Charles Dickens is an appropriate description of the psychosocial and biological turmoil experienced by many adolescents in our society. Adolescence is punctuated by emotional explosions resulting from the interaction of physiology, psychology, and culture. The adolescent's body is stretching, growing, and sometimes screaming out of control due to the hormonal changes of puberty. Adolescents are uncertain and frightened of not knowing who or what they are becoming. They are often confused as to their worth to family, peers, society, and even to themselves.

Adding to the frustration of growing up, the cultural status of adolescents is poorly defined. They find themselves trapped in a "no-man's land" between the acceptance, simplicity, and security of childhood, and the stress, complexities, expectations, independence, and responsibilities of adulthood. Not only do adolescents have difficulty deciding who and what they are, but adults are equally unsure as to how to deal with these transitional human beings. While the grownup world tries to push adolescents out of the secure nest of childhood, it isn't willing to bestow the full membership and rights of adulthood (Archambault 1992).

Because of their unique psychosocial metamorphosis, several developmental issues are particularly important to evolving adolescents (Elmen and Offer 1993):

- Discovering and understanding their distinctive identities
- Forming more intimate and caring relationships with others
- Establishing a sense of autonomy
- Coming to terms with the hormone-related feelings of puberty and expressing their sexuality
- Learning to become productive contributors to society

Due to all this developmental confusion, normal behavior for the adolescent is difficult to define precisely. However, experts generally agree that persistent low self-esteem, depression, and other severe emotional disturbances can be troublesome for teenagers. Most adolescents are relatively well adjusted and are able to cope with sociobiological changes. Emotionally stable adolescents relate well to family and peers, and function productively within their schools, neighborhoods, and communities. The majority of adolescents experience transient problems, which they are able to resolve, while others become deeply disturbed and are unable to grow out of their problems without adequate help (Elmen and Offer 1993). Those adolescents who are unable or unwilling to ask for assistance often turn to destructive devices, such as drugs, for relief from their emotional dilemmas.

Why Adolescents Use Drugs

Although there is no such thing as a "typical" substance-abusing adolescent, there are physiological, psychological, and sociological factors that are often associated with drug problems in teenagers (Lawson and Lawson 1992). However, it is important to remember that not all drug use by adolescents means therapy is necessary or even desirable. Most adolescent use of substances of abuse results from the desire to experience new behaviors and sensations, a passing fancy of maturation, an attempt to relieve peer pressure or an inclination to

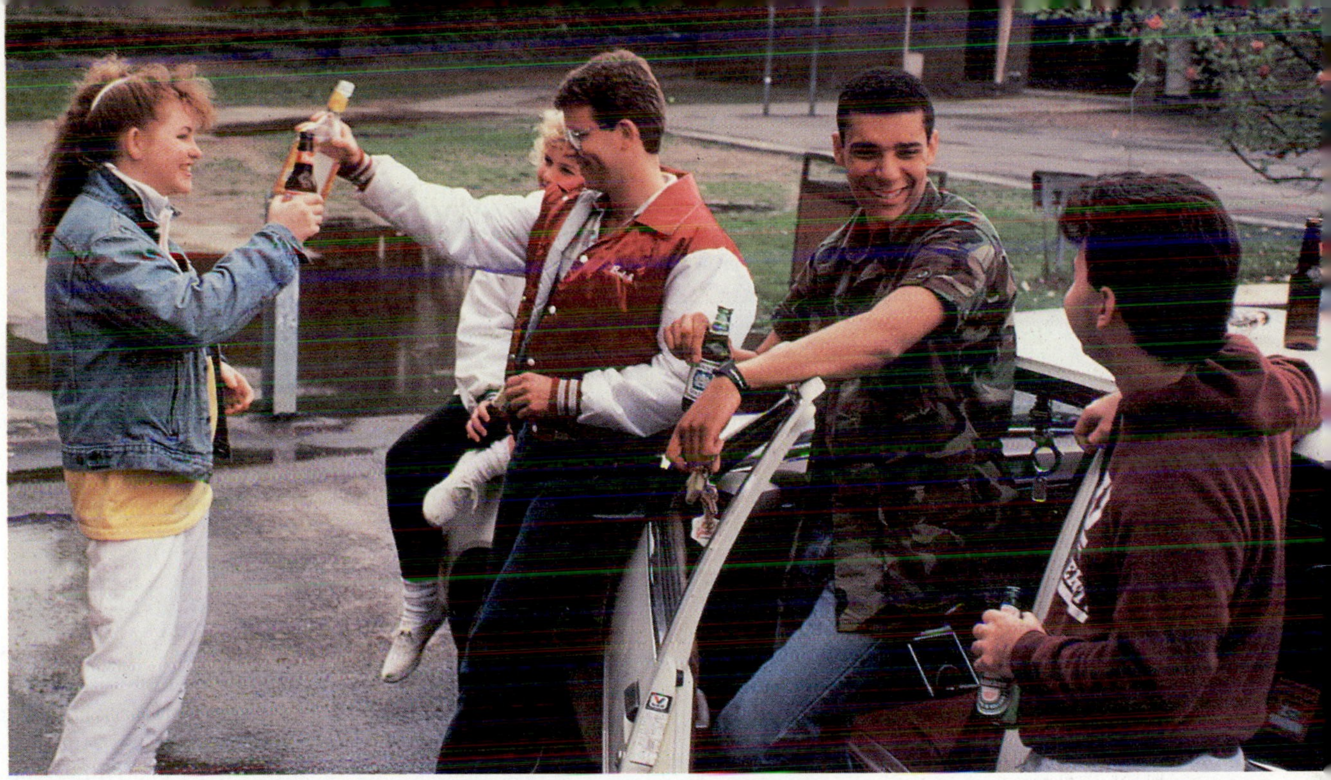

Most adolescents use substances of abuse because they want to experience new sensations, relieve peer pressure, or enhance a social setting with chemistry.

enhance a social setting with chemistry. Most of these adolescent users will not go on to develop problematic dependence on drugs and, for the most part, should be watched but not aggressively confronted or treated. The adolescents who usually have significant difficulty with drug use are those who turn to drugs for extended support as coping devices and become drug reliant because they are unable to find alternative, less destructive solutions to their problems. Several major factors can contribute to serious drug dependence in adolescents (Archambault 1992; Walsh and Scheinkman 1992).

Often adolescents use drugs to help cope with unpleasant feelings, emotions, and stress or to relieve depression and reduce tension. Psychological differences among adolescents who are frequent drug users, experimenters, and abstainers often can be traced to early childhood, the quality of parenting, and the home environment. It has been suggested that certain types of parents are more likely to raise children at high risk for substance abuse (Archambault 1992). For example, an alcoholic adolescent usually has at least one parent of the following types:

1. *Alcoholic.* This parent serves as a negative role model for the adolescent. The child sees the parent dealing with problems by consuming drugs. Even though drinking alcohol is not illegal for adults, it sends the message that drugs can solve problems. The guilt-ridden alcoholic parent is unable to provide the child with a loving supportive relationship. In addition, the presence of the alcoholic parent is often disruptive or abusive to the family and creates fear or embarrassment to the child.

2. *Nonconsuming and condemning.* This type of parent not only chooses to abstain from drinking, but is also very judgmental about drinkers and condemns them for their behavior. Such persons are often referred to as *teetotalers* and have a rigid, moralistic approach to life. Their black-and-white attitudes frequently prove inadequate and unforgiving in an imperfect, gray world. Children in these families can feel inferior and guilty when they are unable to live up to parental expectations, and they may resort to drugs to cope with their frustrations.

3. *Overly demanding.* This type of parent forces unrealistic expectations on their children. These parents often live vicariously through their children

and require sons and daughters to pursue endeavors where the parents were unable to succeed. Particular emphasis may be placed on achievements in athletics, academics, or career selections. Even though the parents' efforts may be well intended, the children get the message that their parents are more concerned about "what they are" than "who they are." These parents frequently encourage sibling rivalries to enhance performance, but in such competitions there is always a loser.

4. *Overly protective.* These parents do not give their children a chance to develop a sense of self-worth and independence. Because the parents deprive their children of the opportunities to learn how to master their abilities within their surroundings, the children are not able to develop confidence and a positive self-image. Such children are frequently unsure about who they are and what they are capable of achieving. Parents who use children to satisfy their own ego needs or are trying to convince themselves that they really do like their children, tend to be overly protective.

The principal influence for learned behavior is usually the home; therefore, several other family-related variables can significantly affect adolescents' decision to start, maintain, or cease a drug habit (Lawson and Lawson 1992). For example, adolescents usually learn their attitudes about drug use from family models. In other words, what are the drug-consuming patterns of parents and siblings? Adolescents are more likely to develop drug problems if other members of the family (1) are excessive in their drug (legal or illegal) consumption, (2) approve of the use of illicit drugs, or (3) use drugs as a problem-solving strategy.

Sociological factors that damage self-image can also encourage adolescent drug use. Feelings of rejection cause poor relationships with family members, peers, school personnel, or co-workers. In a racist society, ethnic differences sometimes contribute to a poor self-image because people of minority races or cultures are frequently socially excluded and are viewed as being inferior and undesirable by the majority population. This type of negative message is very difficult for adolescents to deal with. Sometimes to ensure acceptance, adolescents adopt the attitudes and behavior of their affiliated groups. If a peer group, or a *gang,* views drug use as *cool,* desirable, or even necessary behavior, members (or those desiring membership) feel compelled to conform and become involved in drugs.

Patterns of Drug Use in Adolescents

The first drug exposure occurs at a very early age for many adolescents in the United States. Recent surveys on 1992 drug use patterns found that by eighth grade, 17.4% of those questioned had used inhalants, 11.2% had used marijuana, 10.5% had used prescription stimulants, 69.3% had used alcohol, and 45.2% had smoked cigarettes (see Table 15.1). These findings suggest that many adolescents try drugs when they begin their teenage years. Of even more concern is that some adolescents are already using these drugs intensely by the age of 13 and 14 years and are showing signs of severe dependence (Johnston et al. 1993). For example, in 1992, 0.6% of the eighth-graders were consuming alcohol daily and 5 and 0.3% were using cigarettes and inhalants daily, respectively.

Although adolescent drug use, in general, declined from 1980 to the early 1990s, a recent rise in the use of some drugs is very troubling. For example, an annual survey of high school students revealed that in 1993 a sharp rise occurred in marijuana use throughout the country as well as increases in stimulant, LSD, and inhalant use and smoking. Experts are concerned that patterns of teenage drug abuse may be returning to those of the early 1980s (Johnston 1994).

In general, there are ethnic differences in drug use patterns among adolescents. In a 1992 survey, eighth-grade Hispanics tended to have a higher prevalence of using drugs of abuse, followed by whites, with blacks showing the lowest prevalence. Hispanics also had the highest usage rate in the senior year of high school for several of the most dangerous drugs, such as cocaine, crack, heroin, and steroids (Johnston et al. 1993). Over the past 15 years the trends for most drug use by the three major ethnic groups of adolescents have declined steadily, with some leveling from 1990 to 1992. One significant difference has been in cigarette smoking by high school seniors. Since 1981, smoking rates for whites and Hispanics declined very little, but the rates for blacks diminished steadily. Consequently, in 1992, the smoking rates for black adolescents were about one-fifth to one-third of those of whites (Johnston et al. 1993).

TABLE 15.1 Frequency of adolescent use of common drugs of abuse in 1992 (expressed as percentage using)

	Lifetime	Previous Month	Daily
Marijuana			
8th grade	11.2%	3.7%	0.2%
10th	21.4	8.1	0.8
12th	32.6	11.9	1.9
Inhalants			
8th grade	17.4	4.7	0.3
10th	16.6	2.7	0.1
12th	16.6	2.3	0.1
Stimulants			
8th grade	10.8	3.3	0.1
10th	13.1	3.6	0.1
12th	13.9	2.8	0.2
Alcohol			
8th grade	69.3	26.1	0.6
10th	82.3	39.9	1.2
12th	87.5	51.3	3.4
Cigarettes			
8th grade	45.2	15.5	7.2
10th	53.5	21.5	12.3
12th	61.8	27.8	17.2

Source: L. D. Johnston, P. O'Malley, and J. G. Bachman. *National Survey Results on Drug Use from The Monitoring the Future Study, 1975–1992.* Lansing, MI: National Institute on Drug Abuse and University of Michigan, 1993.

Adolescent Versus Adult Drug Abuse Adolescent patterns of drug abuse are very different from drug use patterns in adults (Moss et al. 1994). The uniqueness of adolescent drug abuse means that drug-dependent teenagers usually are not successfully treated with adult-directed therapy (Daily 1992b; Hoshino 1992). For example, compared to adults who abuse drugs, comparable adolescents are (1) more likely to be involved in criminal activity; (2) more likely to get involved in criminal activity at a very early age; (3) more likely to have other members of the family abusing drugs; (4) more likely to be associated with a dysfunctional family that engages in emotional and/or physical abuse of its members; and (5) more likely to begin their drug use because of curiosity or peer pressure (Segal et al. 1982; Daily 1992b; Hoshino 1992). Differences such as these need to be considered when developing adolescent-targeted treatment programs.

Consequences and Coincidental Problems

Researchers have concluded that the problem of adolescent drug use is a symptom and not a cause of personal social maladjustment. Even so, because of the pharmacological actions of drugs, routine use can contribute to school and social failures, unintended injuries (usually automobile related), criminal and violent behavior, sexual risk taking, depression, and suicide (Hernandez 1992).

However, it is important to realize that because serious drug abuse is usually the result of emotional instability, consequences of the underlying disorders may be coexpressed with chemical dependence, making diagnosis and treatment more difficult. The undesirable coincidental problems may include self-destructive, risk taking, abuse, or negative group behaviors. Some of these adolescent problems and their relationship to drug abuse are discussed in the following sections.

Adolescent Suicide Adolescents are particularly vulnerable to suicide actions; in fact, white males between 14 and 20 years are the most likely to commit suicide in the United States (Daily 1992b). Some experts have described severe chemical dependence as a form of slow drug-related suicide. Clearly, many teenagers who abuse alcohol and other drugs possess a self-destructive attitude. These adolescents often (1) feel insecure and inferior, (2) demonstrate risk-taking behaviors, and (3) have little concern for their own health or physical well-being.

Besides being a direct health threat because of their physiological effects, drugs of abuse also can precipitate suicide attempts due to their pharmacological impact. A number of studies have found a very high correlation between acute suicidal behavior and drug use (Buckstein et al. 1993). One report noted that adolescent alcoholics have a suicide rate 58 times greater than the national average. In another study, 30% of adolescent alcoholics had made suicide attempts, while 92% admitted to a history of having suicidal thoughts (Daily 1992b).

It has been speculated that the incidence of suicide behavior in drug-consuming adolescents is high because both types of behavior are the consequence of their inability to develop fundamental adult attributes of confidence, self-esteem, and independence. When drug use does not satisfy the need for these characteristics, the resulting frustrations are intensified and ultimately played out in the suicide act.

Most adolescents experiment with drugs for reasons not related to antisocial or deviant behavior but rather due to curiosity, desire for recreation, boredom, desire to gain new insights and experiences, or the urge to heighten social interactions. These are not the adolescents likely to engage in self-destructive behavior. In addition, adolescents from "healthy" family environments are not likely to attempt suicide. Specifically, families least likely to have suicidal members are those that (Daily 1992b):

- Express love and show mutual concern
- Are tolerant of differences and overlook failings
- Encourage the development of self-confidence and self-expression
- Have parents who assume strong leadership roles, but are not autocratic
- Have interaction characterized by humor and good-natured teasing
- Are able to serve as a source of joy and happiness to their members

Suicide is more likely to be attempted by those adolescents who turn to alcohol and other drugs to cope with serious emotional and personality conflicts and frustrations. These susceptible teenagers represent approximately 5% of the adolescent population (Beschner and Friedman 1985).

Wright (1985) found in his studies that four features significantly contribute to the likelihood of suicidal thought in high school students:

1. Parents with interpersonal conflicts who often use an adolescent child with drug problems as the scapegoat for family problems
2. Fathers who have poor, and often confrontational relationships with their children
3. Parents who are viewed by their adolescent children as being emotionally unstable, usually suffering from perpetual anger and depression
4. A sense of frustration, desperation, and inability to resolve personal and emotional difficulties through traditional means

Clearly, it is important to identify those adolescents who are at risk for suicide (see the Case in Point box) and to provide immediate care and appropriate emotional support.

Sexual Violence and Drugs Alcohol use has been closely associated with almost every type of sexual abuse wherein the adolescent is victimized. For example, alcohol is by far the most significant factor in date, acquaintance, and gang rapes involving teenagers (Parrot 1988). The evidence for alcohol involvement in incest is particularly overwhelming. Approximately 4 million children in America live in incestuous homes with alcoholic

Case in Point

Adolescents with severe emotional problems are inclined to make suicide attempts. Early intervention is crucial. The following signs suggest a suicidal inclination:

- Severe mental depression
- Changes in behavior, especially habitual activities
- Lack of interest in previously enjoyed activities
- Making final arrangements and giving away treasured possessions
- Talking of suicide including a fixation on the death process
- Making direct threats of suicide
- Having made previous attempts at suicide
- Not caring about one's own safety

Source: L. Wright. "Suicidal Thoughts and Their Relationship to Family Stress and Personal Problems Among High School Seniors and College Undergraduates. *Adolescence* 20 (1985):575–80.

parents. In addition, 42% of drug-abusing female adolescents have been victims of sexual abuse (Daily 1992a). It is estimated that almost half of the offenders consume alcohol before molesting a child and at least a third of the perpetrators are chronic alcoholics. Finally, 85% of child molesters were sexually abused themselves as children, usually at the same age as their victims, and the vast majority of these molesters abused drugs as adolescents (Daily 1992a).

These very disturbing associations illustrate the relationship between drugs and violent sexual behavior both in terms of initiating the act as well as a consequence of the act. The effects of such sexual violence are devastating and far reaching. Thus, incest victims are themselves more likely than the general population to abuse drugs as adolescents and engage in antisocial delinquency, prostitution, depression, and suicide (Daily 1992a).

Gangs and Drugs The very disturbing involvement of adolescents in gang organizations and gang-related activities and violence is a social phenomenon that first became widely recognized in the 1950s and 1960s. This was when Hollywood introduced America to the problems of adolescent gangs in the classic movies "Blackboard Jungle" and "West Side Story." Although the basis for gang involvement has not changed over the years, the level of violence and public concern has increased dramatically. Many communities consider gang-related problems as their number one social issue. Access to sophisticated weaponry and greater mobility has drawn unsuspecting neighborhoods and innocent bystanders into the often violent clashes of **intragang** and **intergang** warfare. Individuals and communities have been reacting angrily to this growing menace. However, to deal effectively with the threats of gang-initiated violence and crime, it is important to understand why gangs form, what their objectives are, how they are structured, and how to discourage adolescent involvement.

Why Gangs? The psychosocial deficiencies that encourage teenagers to become involved in

INTRAGANG happening between members of the same gang

INTERGANG happening between members of different gangs

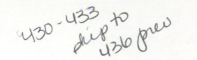

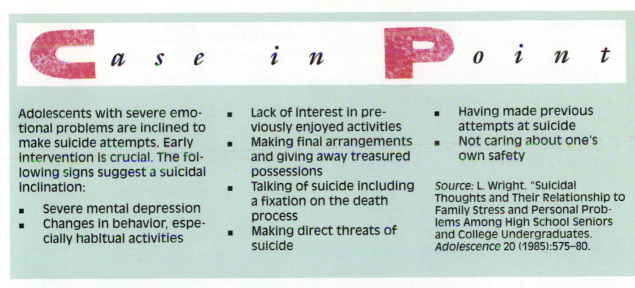

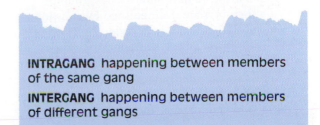

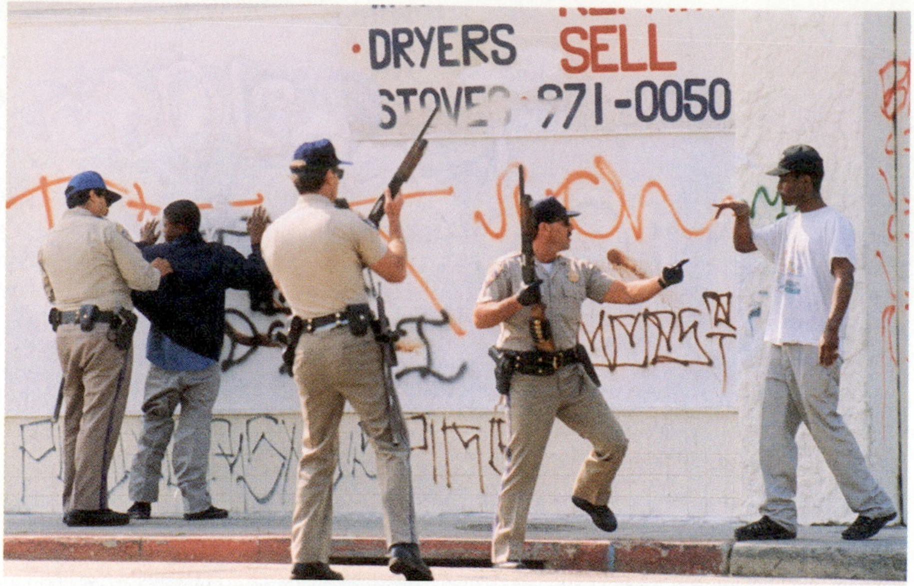

The very disturbing involvement of adolescents in gang organizations and violence is a social phenomenon that first became widely recognized in the 1950s and 1960s, but has increased dramatically in the 1990s.

gangs are those same factors that often lead to involvement with drugs. Generally, gang members lack life coping skills, self-confidence, and accountability. Gang members often are neglected by parents and are without positive role models or adequate adult supervision. Because of peer pressures and low self-esteem, members are drawn to the support and structure of gangs and the opportunity to acquire money from gang-related drug dealing and other criminal activities (Lale 1992).

In comparison to traditional, formal youth organizations, juvenile gangs appear loosely structured, but do have rules, policies, customs, and hierarchies of command that are rigidly observed. For example,

1. Gang membership is usually defined in socioeconomic, racial, and ethnic terms, and adolescents involved have similar backgrounds.
2. Gang members are distinguished by a distinctive and well-defined dress code. Violation of this code by members, or mimicking of the dress by nongang members, can result in severe physical punishment.
3. Leadership and seniority within the gang are defined by tenure, age, and achievements (often drug or crime related) (see the Here and Now box).
4. Gang members use gang slang for coded communication or a signal of membership (see the Here and Now box).

Although a stable home life does not ensure an adolescent won't become involved with gang-related activity, clearly, a strong family environment and guidance from respected parents and guardians are deterrents (Lale 1992). Many gang members are children from dysfunctional, broken, or single-parent homes. Many parents are aware of their children's gang involvement but they lack the skill, confidence, and relationship to deter the gang or drug involvement of their teenagers. To make matters worse, often ineffective parents discourage or even interfere with involvement by outside authorities due to misplaced loyalty to their children or to avoid embarrassment to their family. Sometimes families actually encourage gang participation by children, because they become economically dependent on the money gained by gang member children due to drug dealing or other illegal activities.

Because troubled adolescents are often es-

Here and Now

Gang structure is usually defined by achievements, duration of affiliation, and age. The following is a typical example of a gang's hierarchy.

HARDCORE These are the leaders and make up to 5–10% of the gang. These are the most experienced and influential members and usually have a history of arrests and imprisonments. These members are usually unemployed but often make money through drug dealing, using gang members to obtain and market illicit substances. Average age is early to mid-20s.

REGULARS Well-established, proven gang members. Usually back up the hardcores and expect to move into leadership roles. These members are frequent drug users and typically involved in gang-related violence. Average age is 14 to 17 years.

WANNA-BE'S Not official members of the gang, but want to be. They hang around gang members and try to achieve "regular" status by using drugs, writing graffiti for the gang, and carrying out assignments (often minor criminal offenses, such as shoplifting, or light drug dealing). Age 11 to 13 years.

FRINGE OR CLAIMERS Not official members, but associate with gang for protection. Tend to participate in gang-related social activities (such as parties and some drug use), but do not get involved with hard-core gang activities such as major criminal or violent acts. Age fluctuates between 11 and 15 years.

COULD-BE'S (POTENTIALS) Preadolescent children of elementary school age who have potential for gang membership. Usually live near or in a gang's neighborhood and knows or is related to a member.

Source: Adapted from T. Lale. "Gangs and Drugs." In *Adolescent Substance Abuse, Etiology, Treatment and Prevention*, edited by G. Lawson and A. Lawson, 267–81. Gaithersburg, MD: Aspen, 1992.

tranged from their families, they are particularly influenced by their peer groups. These teenagers are most likely to associate with groups who have similar backgrounds and problems, and who make them feel accepted. Because of this vulnerability, adolescents may become involved with local gangs because they offer

- Fellowship and camaraderie
- Identity and recognition
- Membership and belonging
- Family substitution and role models
- Security and protection
- Diversion and excitement
- Traditions and structure
- Money and financial gain for relatively little effort

Drug Use and Gang Involvement. Drug use and gang-related activities are often linked but are highly variable (Fagan 1990). Clearly, problems with drugs exist without gangs and gang-related activities can occur despite the absence of drugs; however, because they have common etiologies, their occurrences are often intertwined. Most adolescents who are gang associated are knowledgeable about drugs. Many gang members have experimented with drugs much like other adolescents their age. However, the hard-core gang members

classnotes
models on prevention

Here and Now

Gang members often communicate by using slang terms. The following are common gang terms and their definitions.

ACE KOOL Best friend and backup

BLOOD Family

BOOK Run, leave, get away

BUSTED, POPPED A CAP Shot at someone

CHOIAS Police

COURTING IN Initiation into a gang

DRIP A DIME Snitch on someone

GANG BANGER Gang member

GRAFFITI Coded slang used by gang to claim turf, brag, challenge rival gangs, honor fallen comrades

MAD-DOGGING Staring someone down in a challenge

PULLING YOU ON Making a fool of you

SIGNS Hand gestures that identify a gang set

Source: T. Lale. "Gangs and Drugs." In *Adolescent Substance Abuse, Etiology, Treatment and Prevention*, edited by G. Lawson and A. Lawson, 267–81. Gaithersburg, MD: Aspen, 1992.

are more likely to be engaged not only in drug use, but also in drug dealing as a source of revenue to support the gang-related activities (Lale 1992). The types of drugs used and their significance and functions varies from gang to gang (Fagan 1990). For example, many Latino gangs do not profit from drug trafficking but are primarily interested in using hard-core drugs such as heroin and PCP. In contrast, African-American gangs tend to be more interested in the illicit commercial value of drugs and often engage in dealing "crack" and other cocaine forms (Lale 1992).

Prevention and Intervention. The most effective way to prevent adolescent gang involvement is to identify, at an early age, those children at risk and provide them with lifestyle alternatives. Important components of such strategies are

- Encourage parental awareness of gangs and teach them how to address problems in their own families that encourage gang involvement.
- Provide teenagers with alternative participation in organizations or groups that satisfy their needs for camaraderie, participation, and emotional security in a constructive way. These can be groups organized around athletics, school activities, career development, or service rendering.
- Help children to develop coping skills that will enable them to deal with the frustration and stress in their personal lives.
- Educate children about gang-related problems and help them understand that like drugs, gangs are the result of problems and not the solutions.

Prevention and Treatment of Adolescent Drug Problems

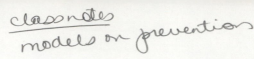

As with most health problems, the sooner drug abuse is identified in the adolescent, the greater the likelihood that the problem can be resolved. It can be difficult to recognize signs of drug abuse in teenagers because their behavior can be so erratic and unpredictable even under the best of circumstances. In fact, many of the behavioral patterns that occur coincidentally with drug problems are also present when drugs are not a problem. However, frequent occurrence or clustering of these behaviors may indicate the presence of substance abuse. The behaviors that can be warning signs are (Archambault 1992)

- Abruptly changing the circle of friends
- Experiencing major mood swings
- Continually challenging rules and regulations
- Overreacting to frustrations
- Being particularly submissive to peer pressures
- Sleeping excessively
- Keeping very late hours
- Withdrawing from family involvement
- Letting personal hygiene deteriorate
- Becoming isolated
- Engaging in unusual selling of possessions
- Manipulating family members
- Becoming easily frustrated and angered
- Developing abusive behavior to other members of the family
- Frequently coming home at night "high"

Prevention of Adolescent Drug Abuse

Logically, the best treatment for drug abuse is to prevent the problem from starting. This approach is referred to as **primary prevention** and has been typically viewed as total abstinence from drug use. Informational scare tactics are frequently used as a component of primary prevention strategies. These often consist of focusing on a dangerous (although in some cases a rare) potential side effect and presenting the warning against drug use in a graphic and frightening fashion. Although this approach may scare naive adolescents away from drugs, many adolescents today, especially if they are experienced, question the validity of the scare tactics and ignore the message (Archambault 1992).

Another form of primary prevention is to encourage adolescents to become involved in formal groups, such as structured clubs (such as athletic or fine arts teams at school) or organizations (such as outdoor or scouting groups), in order to reduce the likelihood of substance abuse (Howard 1992). Group memberships can help develop a sense of belonging and contributing to a productive, desirable objective. This involvement can also provide strength in resisting undesirable peer pressures. In contrast, belonging to informal groups such as gangs, groups with loose structure and ill-defined, often antisocial, objectives, can lead to participation in poorly controlled parties, excessive sexual involvement and nonproductive activities. Adolescent members of such poorly defined organizations tend to drink alcohol at an earlier age and are more likely to use other substances of abuse (Howard 1992).

Some experts claim that primary prevention against drug use is unrealistic for many adolescents. They believe that no strategy is likely to stop adolescents from experimenting with alcohol or other drugs of abuse, especially if these substances are part of their home environment (for example, alcohol or tobacco is routinely used), and are viewed as normal, acceptable, even expected, behavior (Howard 1992). For these adolescents, it is important to recognize when drug use goes from experimentation or a social exercise to early stages of a problem, and prevent serious dependence from developing. This approach is referred to as **secondary prevention** and consists of (1) teaching adolescents about the early signs of abuse, (2) teaching adolescents how to assist peers and family members with drug problems, and (3) teaching them how and where help is available for people with drug problems (Archambault 1992). Regardless of the prevention approach used, adolescents need to understand that drugs are never the solution for emotional difficulties nor are they useful long-term coping techniques.

Treatment of Adolescent Drug Abuse To provide appropriate treatment for adolescent drug abuse, the severity of the problem must be ascertained. The criteria for such assessments include

- Differentiating between abuse and normal adolescent experimentation with drugs
- Distinguishing between minor abuse and severe dependency on drugs
- Distinguishing between behavioral problems resulting from (1) general behavioral disorders, such as juvenile delinquency; (2) mental retardation; and (3) drugs of abuse

PRIMARY PREVENTION prevention of any drug use

SECONDARY PREVENTION prevention of casual drug use from progressing to dependence

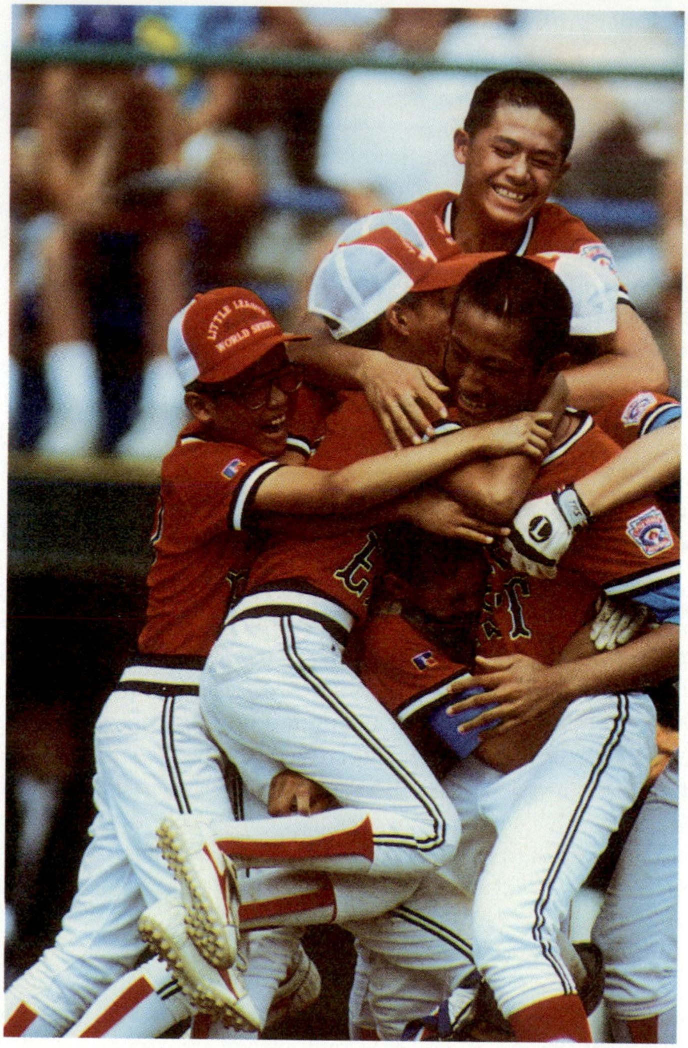

Adolescents should be encouraged to associate with healthy and supportive groups and acivities such as those found in athletics.

There is no single best approach for treating adolescent substance abuse. Occasionally the troubled adolescent is admitted to a clinic and treated on an inpatient basis. The inpatient approach is very expensive and creates a temporary "artificial" environment that may be of limited value in preparing adolescents for the problems to be faced in their real homes and neighborhoods. However, the advantage of an inpatient approach is that adolescents can be managed better and the behavior can be more tightly monitored and controlled (Hoshino 1992).

A more practical and routine treatment approach is to allow adolescents to remain in their natural environment and to help provide the necessary life skills to be successful at home, in school, and in the community. For example, adolescents being treated for drug dependence should be helped with

- Schoolwork, so appropriate progress toward high school graduation occurs
- Career skills, so adolescents can become self-reliant and learn to care for themselves and others
- Family problems and learning to communicate and resolve conflicts

If therapy is to be successful, it is important to improve the environment of the drug-abusing adolescent. This aspect of treatment includes dissociation of the adolescent from groups (such as gangs) or surroundings that encourage drug use and encourages association with healthy and supportive groups (such as a nurturing family) and experiences (such as athletics and school activities). Although desirable, such separation is not always possible, especially if the family and home environment are factors that encourage abuse: the likelihood of therapeutic success is substantially diminished under these circumstances.

Often therapeutic objectives are facilitated by positive reinforcement that encourages life changes that eliminate access to, and use of, drugs. This can frequently be done by association with peers who have similar drug and social problems, but are motivated to make positive changes in their life. Group sessions with such peers are held under the supervision of a trained therapist and consist of members sharing problems and solutions (Hoshino 1992).

Another useful approach is to discourage use of drugs by reducing their reinforcing effects. This can sometimes be achieved by substituting a stronger positive or a negative reinforcer. For example, if adolescents use drugs because they believe these substances cause good feelings and help cope with emotional problems, it may be necessary to replace the drug behavior with other activities that make the adolescent feel good without the drug (such as participation in sports or recreational activities). Negative reinforcers such as parental discovery and punishment or police apprehension may discourage drug use by teenagers who are willing to conform and respect authorities. However, negative approaches are ineffective deterrents for nonconforming, rebellious adolescents. Negative reinforcers also do not tend to discourage adolescent use of substances that are more socially acceptable, such as alcohol, tobacco, and even marijuana (Howard 1992).

A major problem with drug abuse therapy for adolescents is that most programs and facilities are not equipped to deal with the unique needs of the adolescent (Daily 1992b). Even though 20.6% of the patients being treated for drug abuse problems are teenagers, only 5% of available programs are specifically designed for adolescents.

Regardless of the treatment approach, several basic objectives must be accomplished if therapy for adolescent drug dependence is to be successful (Daily 1992b). Adolescents must

- Realize that "drugs do not solve problems"—they only make the problems worse.
- Understand why they turned to drugs in the first place.
- Be convinced that abandoning drugs grants them greater independence and control over their own lives.
- Understand that drug abuse is a symptom of underlying causes that need to be resolved.

Summary of Adolescent Drug Abuse

Drug abuse by adolescents is particularly problematic in the United States. The teenage years are filled with experimentation, searching, confusion, rebellion, poor self-image, and insecurity. These attributes, if not managed properly, can cause inappropriate coping maneuvers and lead to problems such as drug dependence, gang involvement, violence, criminal behavior, and suicide. Clearly, early detection of severe underlying emotional problems and applications of effective early preventive therapy are important for proper management. Approaches to treatment of drug abuse problems must be individualized because each adolescent is a unique product of physiological, psychological, and environmental factors.

Almost as important as early intervention for adolescent drug abuse problems is recognizing when treatment is unnecessary. We should not be too quick to label all young drug users as antisocial and emotionally unstable. In most cases, teenagers who have used drugs are merely experimenting with new emotions or exercising their new-found freedom. In such situations, nonintervention is usually better than therapeutic meddling. For the most part, if adolescents are given the opportunity they work through their own feelings, conflicts, and attitudes about substance abuse, and will develop a responsible philosophy concerning the use of these drugs.

Drug Abuse and Women

Little is known about how and why drugs are abused specifically by women. In general, most clinical drug abuse research is either conducted in male populations and the results are extrapolated

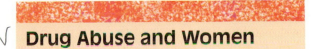

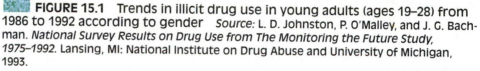

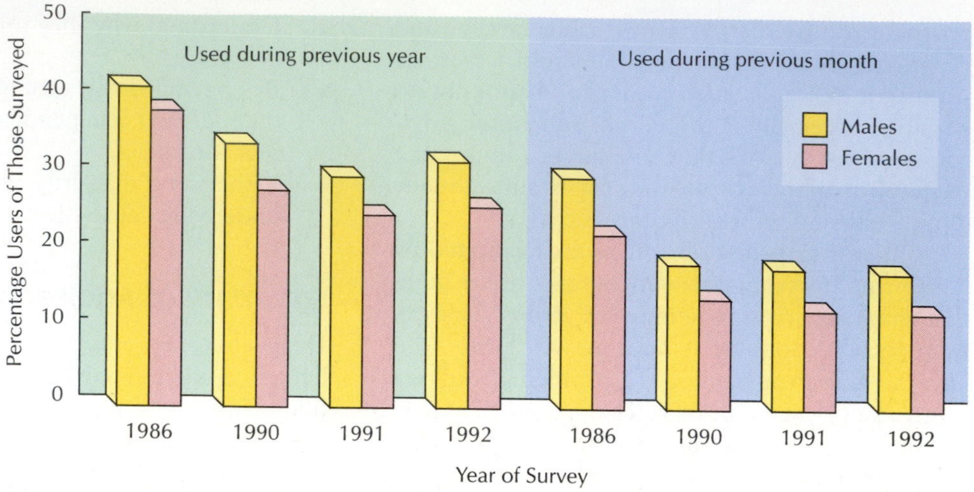

FIGURE 15.1 Trends in illicit drug use in young adults (ages 19–28) from 1986 to 1992 according to gender *Source:* L. D. Johnston, P. O'Malley, and J. G. Bachman. *National Survey Results on Drug Use from The Monitoring the Future Study, 1975–1992.* Lansing, MI: National Institute on Drug Abuse and University of Michigan, 1993.

to women, or the research is done in general populations with little regard to gender influences (Brady et al. 1993; Alexander 1994). Even basic research into drug abuse mechanisms generally prefers male animal models in order to avoid the hormonal complexities that are inherent with female laboratory animals. However, a growing concern for the importance of unique emotional, social, biochemical, and hormonal features in females has caused researchers to acknowledge the importance of gender differences; consequently, scientists now are encouraged to determine the influences of gender differences in drug abuse problems ("Ongoing Program Announcement" 1993).

Patterns of Drug Abuse by Females

Recent insightful surveys comparing male and female drug abuse patterns have demonstrated that there exist important gender differences that contribute to problems of drug addiction (Johnston et al. 1993). For example,

1. In 1992 male college students had a higher annual prevalence (that is, used drugs at least once in the preceding year) rate than comparable females for most drugs of abuse. The greatest differences were observed in the use of heroin (0.2% for men versus 0.0% for women), inhalants (4.0% for men, 2.2% for women), LSD (7.4% for males, 4.3% for females), hallucinogens in general (3.6% for men, 2.4% for women), and marijuana (30.6% for men, 25.3% for women).
2. Annual prevalence rates in 1992 were similar in college students of both genders for stimulants of abuse (3.8% for men versus 3.5% for women), barbiturates (1.4% for men, 1.5% for women), narcotics other than heroin (2.9% for men, 2.6% for women), and CNS depressants (3.0% for men, 2.7% for women).
3. Men tend to have a higher prevalence of intense drug use. Thus, in 1992 there was substantial difference in the daily use by college males versus females of marijuana (2.6 versus 0.8%) and alcohol (4.8 versus 2.8%). An exception to this trend was the daily use of cigarettes, with female college students (15.5%) having a higher prevalence than their male counterparts (12.3%).
4. In each year from 1986 to 1992 young adult females (ages 19–28 years) had a lower prevalence than comparable men for annual and

Here and Now

Women at Risk

The number of women in prison skyrocketed between 1980 and 1992 to more than 50,000; an increase of 276%. A major factor in this alarming rise has been drug offenses, accounting for 12,600 female arrests in 1991 alone. Who are the women being imprisoned? They are disproportionately women of color. These women tend to be unemployed at the time of arrest. The typical female prisoner began using drugs and alcohol at 13 years of age and has an extensive history of drug abuse. She also has problems with depression and has attempted suicide. Most female prisoners are repeat offenders, 20% are HIV positive, and 76% have children. What are the potential social consequences of imprisoning these drug-abusing mothers?

Source: M. Ragghianti. "Save the Innocent Victims of Prison." *Parade* magazine (6 February 1994):14, 15.

monthly use of illicit drugs and both showed a similar decline in illicit drug use until 1991; however, prevalence rates remained approximately the same from 1991 to 1992 in both sexes (see Figure 15.1).

5. Lifetime rates of cocaine and marijuana use show higher prevalence among white females compared to either black or Hispanic females (Alexander 1994).

As similarities and differences in the prevalence rates for the genders are observed, researchers are looking for explanations for these abuse patterns so they can better understand and deal with gender-related drug abuse problems.

Female Roles and Drug Addiction

To appreciate the impact of drug abuse on women, it is necessary to understand the uniqueness of female roles in our society. Relative to drug abuse problems, women are often judged by a double standard, and thus women suffering from drug addictions are often perceived less tolerantly than comparably addicted men (Erickson and Murray 1989). Because of these social biases, women are afraid of being condemned and are less likely to seek professional help for their drug abuse problems. In addition, family, friends, and associates are less inclined to provide drug-dependent women with important emotional support (Alexander 1994).

Due to their unique socioeconomic and family roles, women are especially vulnerable to emotional disruptions resulting from divorce, loneliness, and professional failures. Studies suggest that such stresses aggravate tendencies for women to abuse alcohol and other substances (Korolenko and Donskih 1990). In addition, drug addiction can occur in some women due to domestic adversities. Consequently, there is a high prevalence of drug dependence in women who are victims of sexual and/or physical abuse (Ladwig and Anderson 1989). These emotional traumas are the result of, or precursors to, factors leading to drug abuse, such as low self-esteem, self-condemnation, anxiety, and personal conflicts (Alexander 1994). In addition, because of their crucial nurturing roles, drug abuse problems in women can be particularly damaging to family stability (see the Here and Now Box).

Another unique role for women in drug abuse

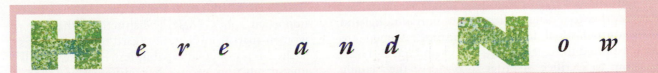

situations is that of a spouse, "significant other," or mother to a drug addict. Often, in traditional and nontraditional family relationships, women are expected to be nurturing, understanding, and willing to sacrifice in order to preserve the "family integrity." If a family member becomes afflicted by drug dependence, the wife or mother is viewed as a failure. In other words, if the woman had maintained a good home and conducted her domestic chores properly, the family member would not have been driven to drugs (Alexander 1994).

Despite the disruption and considerable stress caused by drug addiction in the home, women continue to bear the burden of raising children, performing domestic chores, and keeping the family together (Alexander 1994). In addition, women in such circumstances frequently are put at great physical risk from an addicted spouse who becomes abusive to his partner or from exposure to sexually transmitted diseases, such as HIV infection or hepatitis, transmitted by a careless infected partner. The anxiety and frustrations resulting from these stressful circumstances can encourage women themselves to become dependent as they seek emotional relief by using drugs.

Women's Unique Response to Drugs

Relatively little drug research specifically evaluates women's response to substances of abuse. Often in drug abuse studies, women populations are deliberately avoided and the effects of the drugs in men are extrapolated to females. Even when drug abuse research is conducted on women, frequently the woman's response is not of primary concern but the objective is to determine how a fetus during pregnancy or an infant during nursing, is affected (Alexander 1994). Although it generally can be assumed that the physiological and drug responses of men and women are similar, some distinctions should be recognized. For example, a recent study compared the risk for lung cancer in men and women after a lifetime of cigarette smoking. It was found that female smokers were twice as likely to get lung cancer as comparable males who had smoked an identical number of cigarettes in their lifetime ("Women Smokers Run Higher Risk for Lung Cancer" 1994). These differences suggest cigarette smoking may be more dangerous for women than men.

Drugs of Abuse and Reproduction A very important physiological distinction that sets women apart from men in regard to taking drugs is their reproductive capabilities. Because of this unique function, women have different endocrine (hormone) systems, organs and structures, and varied drug responses according to their reproductive state. These unique features can have a substantial impact on the response to drug abuse in the presence and absence of pregnancy.

Drug abuse patterns can influence the outcome of pregnancy even if they occur prior to the pregnant state. For example, women who are addicted to heroin are more likely to have poor health, including chronic infections, poor nutrition, and sexually transmitted diseases, such as human immunodeficiency virus (HIV) infection, that can damage the offspring if pregnancy occurs (American College of Obstetricians 1986). If substances are abused during pregnancy, they may directly affect the fetus and adversely alter growth and development. The incidence of substance abuse during pregnancy is not known precisely, but there is no doubt that hundreds of thousands of children have been exposed to these drugs *in utero*—while in the uterus during pregnancy (Alexander 1994). The effects of individual drugs of abuse used during pregnancy are discussed in detail in the corresponding chapters, but several specific observations merit reiteration.

1. Cocaine is a substantial threat for both the pregnant woman and the fetus. Although a number of specific claims for the fetal effects of cocaine are controversial (see Chapter 10), several observations appear legitimate. Cocaine increases the likelihood of miscarriages when used during pregnancy. Use of cocaine in the late stages of pregnancy can cause cardiovascular or CNS complication in the offspring at birth and immediately thereafter. Due to its vasoconstrictor effects, cocaine may deprive the fetal brain of oxygen, resulting in strokes and permanent physical and mental damage to the child (Alexander 1994).

2. The impact of alcohol consumption during pregnancy has been well documented and publicized. Alcohol crosses the placenta when consumed by the mother but the effect of this drug on the fetus is highly variable and depends on the

quantity of drug consumed, timing of exposure, maternal drug metabolism, maternal state of health, and the presence of other drugs (Alexander 1994). A particularly alarming consequence of high alcohol intake during pregnancy is an aggregate of physical and mental defects known as the fetal alcohol syndrome (FAS). Characteristics included in this syndrome are low birth weight, abnormal facial features, mental retardation, and retarded sensorimotor development (Alexander 1994). The incidence of FAS is thought to be 0.1 to 0.3% in the United States (U.S. Department of Health and Human Services [USDHHS] 1990). For additional details, see Chapters 7 and 8.

In addition to direct effects on the fetus, alcohol has played a major role in many unwanted pregnancies or has resulted in women's exposure to sexually transmitted diseases such as AIDS. As a CNS depressant, alcohol impairs judgment and reason, in turn encouraging sexual risk taking that normally would not be considered. The results are all too frequently tragic for the women (Alexander 1994).

3. Tobacco use during pregnancy is particularly rampant in the United States. Specifically, 25% of the smoking female adult population are pregnant (Wentz 1994). Some experts suggest smoking cigarettes during pregnancy may be a greater risk to the fetus than taking cocaine. Use of tobacco by pregnant women may interfere with blood flow to the fetus and deprive it of oxygen and nutrition and disrupt development of fetal organs, particularly the brain ("Cigarettes May Pose a Greater Risk" 1994). Also of significant concern is the possibility that exposure of nonsmoking pregnant women to secondhand tobacco smoke may be damaging to the fetus.

4. Other drugs of abuse that have been associated with abnormal fetal development when used during pregnancy include the barbiturates, benzodiazepines, amphetamines, marijuana, LSD, and even caffeine when consumed in high doses.

Clearly, women should be strongly urged to avoid all substances of abuse, especially during pregnancy.

Women and Alcohol Alcohol is the most widely used and abused drug by women in the United States. In 1992, 84.5% of U.S. women ages 19–32 years, had used alcohol sometime during their lives: 63.4% used alcohol at least once a month, and 2.6% drank daily (Johnston et al 1993). According to the National Institute on Alcohol Abuse and Alcoholism, 5% of American women have a serious drinking problem (Alexander 1994). Alcohol abuse is also a major problem for women on college campuses with a prevalence of annual use (86–89%) similar to that of males, although male college students (4.8%) are more likely than their female counterparts (2.8%) to use alcohol daily (Johnston et al. 1993).

Usually, women are less likely than men to develop severe alcohol dependence; thus, only 25% of the alcoholics in America are female. Women are also likely to initiate their drinking patterns later in life than men (Alexander 1994). Interesting ethnic patterns of alcohol consumption have been reported in females with black and white women manifesting similar drinking patterns, although white women (34%) are less likely than black women (46%) to be abstainers (USDHHS 1989). Hispanic women in the United States are even less likely to consume excessive amounts of alcohol, with 70% either abstaining or drinking less than once a month (Caetano 1989).

As for drug abuse in general, a societal double standard exists for alcoholism in women. Women who are dependent on alcohol are usually judged more harshly than men with similar difficulties (Alexander 1994). Alcoholic males are often excused because the drinking problems are caused by frustrating work conditions, family demands, economic pressures, or so-called "nagging wives and children." In contrast, the frustrations of domestic responsibilities are not considered sufficient to warrant excessive alcohol consumption by women. Thus, a male drunk is tolerated or even viewed as a comical and lovable character, while an alcoholic female is considered weak, deviant, and immoral. Such social stigmas cause women to experience more guilt and anxiety about their alcohol dependence and discourage them from admitting their drug problem and seeking professional help (Alexander 1994).

The principal reasons for excessive alcohol consumption in women range from loneliness, boredom, and domestic stress in the "housewife drinker" to financial problems, sexual harassment, boredom, lack of challenge, discrimination, and powerlessness for career women (Sandmaier 1980). Depression often is associated with alcohol problems in women, although it is not clear whether it is a cause or an effect of the excessive drug use.

Unique Physiological Response to Alcohol by Women. It appears that health consequences for excessive alcohol consumption are more severe for women than for men. For example, (1) alcoholic women are more likely to suffer premature death than alcoholic men (Lindberg and Agren 1988), with the mortality rate for female alcoholics being 4.5 times that of the general population; (2) liver disease is more common and occurs at a younger age in female versus male alcoholics (Alexander 1994); (3) in general, higher morbidity rates are experienced by alcoholic women than alcoholic men (Hasin et al. 1988).

Possible explanations for the greater adverse effects seen in female alcoholics are (1) higher blood alcohol concentrations due to smaller blood volume and more rapid absorption into the bloodstream after drinking; (2) slower alcohol metabolism in the stomach and liver, causing more alcohol to reach the brain and other organs as well as prolonging exposure to the drug following consumption (Goldstein 1995). Studies have shown that for a women of average size, one alcoholic drink has effects equivalent to two drinks in an average-sized man (Alexander 1994).

Dealing with Women's Alcohol Problems. Alcoholic consumption varies considerably in women ranging from total abstinence or an occasional drink to daily intake of large amounts of alcohol. Clearly, much is yet to be learned about the cause of excessive drinking of, and dependence on, alcohol in women. The role of genetic factors in predisposing women to alcohol-related problems is still unclear. Female alcoholics are less likely than male alcoholics to have had alcoholic parents or siblings (Alexander 1994) suggesting that heredity may be less important in female than in male alcoholics. Environment certainly is a major factor contributing to excessive alcohol consumption in women. It is well established that depression, stress, and trauma encourage alcohol consumption, because of the antianxiety and amnesic properties of this drug. Because of unreasonable societal expectations and numerous socioeconomic disadvantages, women are especially vulnerable to the emotional upheavals that encourage excessive alcohol consumption.

As with all drug dependence problems, prevention is the preferred solution to alcohol abuse by women. Alcohol usually becomes problematic when it is no longer used occasionally to enhance social events, but its consumption becomes a daily exercise to deal with personal problems. Such alcohol dependence can best be avoided by using constructive techniques to manage stress and frustrations. Because of unique female roles, women especially need to learn to be assertive with family members, associates in the workplace (including bosses), and other contacts in their daily routines. By expecting and demanding equitable treatment and consideration in personal and professional activities, stress and anxiety can often be reduced. Education, career training, and development of communication abilities can be particularly important in establishing a sense of self-worth. With these skills and confidence, women are better able to manage problems associated with their lives and less likely to resort to drugs for solutions.

Women and Prescription Drugs Women are more likely than men to suffer mental disorders such as depression, anxiety, and panic attacks (Brady 1993). Consequently, they are also more likely to take and become addicted to prescription drugs used in treating these disorders. Because these drugs are used as part of the psychiatric therapy and with the supervision of a physician, drug dependence frequently is not recognized and may be ignored for months or even years. This type of "legitimate" drug abuse occurs most often in elderly women and includes the use of sedatives, hypnotics, and antianxiety medications; thus, elderly women are prescribed these types of medications 2.5 times more often than are elderly men (Alexander 1994). Excessive use of these drugs by older women results in side effects such as insomnia, mood fluctuations, and disruption of cognitive and motor functions that can substantially compromise the quality of life (National Institute on Drug Abuse [NIDA] 1986).

Treatment of Drug Dependency in Women

As previously discussed, women are less likely than men to seek treatment for, and rehabilitation from, drug dependence (Alexander 1994). Possible reasons for their reluctance are

1. Women have unique roles with high expectations. They have demanding and ongoing responsibilities, such as motherhood, child rearing, and family maintenance, that cannot be postponed and often cannot be delegated, even temporarily, to others. Consequently, many women feel that they are too essential for the well-being of other family members to leave the home and seek time-consuming treatment for drug abuse problems.

2. Drug treatment centers often are not designed to handle the extensive and unique health requirements of females. Women have been shown to have greater health needs than men due to more frequent respiratory, **genitourinary** (associated with the sex and urinary organs), and circulatory problems (Marsh and Simpson 1986). If centers are not capable of providing the necessary physical care, women are less likely to participate in associated drug abuse programs.

3. Drug-dependent women are more inclined to be unemployed than male counterparts and more likely to be receiving public support (Alexander 1994). The implications of this difference are twofold. First, because concerns about one's job often motivate drug-dependent workers to seek treatment, this is less likely to be a factor in unemployed women. Second, without the financial security of a job, unemployed women may feel that good treatment for their drug problems is unaffordable.

The unique female requirements must be recognized and considered if women are to receive adequate treatment for drug dependence. Some considerations to achieve this objective include the following:

GENITOURINARY having to do with the reproductive and urinary systems

1. The role of motherhood needs to be used in a positive manner in drug treatment strategies. For most women, motherhood is viewed with high regard and linked to their self-esteem. Approximately 90% of the female drug abusers are in their childbearing years, and many have family responsibilities. Consequently, treatment approaches need to be tailored to allow women to fulfill their domestic responsibilities and satisfy their maternal obligations.

2. Employment and independence may be especially crucial for drug-dependent females. Helping women to gain control of their own lives by developing skills or careers and becoming financially independent can be important steps in helping them gain a sense of worth and inner strength. With self-confidence comes the belief that success and satisfaction are possible without drugs.

3. Women dependent on drugs often lack important coping skills. Because many women live restricted, almost isolated lives, which focus entirely on domestic responsibilities, they have limited alternatives for dealing with stressful situations. Under these restrictive circumstances, the use of drugs to cope with anxieties and frustrations is very appealing. In order to enhance their ability to cope, drug-dependent women need to develop communication skills and assertiveness: they need to be encouraged to control situations rather than allowing themselves to be controlled by the situation. Specific techniques useful in coping management are exercise (particularly relaxation types), relaxing visual imagery, personal hobbies, and outside interests that require active participation. Many drug-dependent women require experiences that divert their attention from the source of their frustrations while affording them an opportunity to succeed and develop a sense of self-worth.

Prevention of Drug Dependence in Women

The best treatment for drug addiction is prevention. To help prevent drug problems in women, socioeconomic disadvantages need to be recognized as factors that make women more vulnerable to drug dependence, especially from prescription medication, than men. Women need to learn that nondrug approaches are often more desirable for dealing with situational problems than prescribed medications. For example, for older women suffering loneliness, isolation, or depression, it is better to encourage participation in outside interests, such as hobbies and service activities. In addition, social support and concern should be encouraged from family, friends, and neighbors. Such nonmedicinal approaches are preferred over prescribing sedatives and hypnotics to cope with emotional distresses. Similarly, medical conditions such as obesity, constipation, or insomnia should be treated by changing lifestyle, eating, and exercise habits rather than using drug "bandage therapy."

When women are prescribed drugs, they should ask about the associated risks, especially as they relate to drug abuse potential. Frequently, drug dependency develops insidiously and is not recognized by either the patient or attending physician until it is already firmly established. If a woman taking medication is aware of the potential for becoming dependent and is instructed how to avoid its occurrence, the problems of dependence and abuse can frequently be averted.

Athletes and Drug Abuse

The Canadian sprinter, Ben Johnson, once known as the fastest human in history, was banned for life from competitive running in March 1993. Five years earlier, Johnson was stripped of a world's record for the 100-meter dash at the 1988 Seoul Olympics and forfeited the gold medal when he tested positive for steroids in his urine. Because of the first incident, Johnson was suspended from competition for two years. However, in 1992 the 31-year-old sprinter was attempting a comeback, with speeds that approached his world record times. In January 1993, a routine urine test determined Johnson was again using steroids to enhance his athletic performance (Ferrente 1993).

Widely publicized incidents such as this concerning illicit use of so-called **ergogenic** (performance-enhancing) drugs by professional and amateur athletes has created intense interest in the problems of drug abuse in sports (Merchant 1992). To understand why athletes are willing to risk using these drugs it is necessary to understand the sports mind-set. Young athletes receive exaggerated attention and prestige in almost every university or college, high school, and junior high school in the United States. Pressure to excel or "be the best" is placed on athletes by parents, peers, teachers, coaches, school administrators, the media, and surrounding community. The importance of sports is frequently distorted and even used by some to evaluate the quality of educational institutions (Lawn 1984) or the quality of living conditions in a city. Athletic success can determine the level of financial support for these institutions by local and state governments, alumni, and other private donors; thus, winning in athletics often translates into fiscal stability and institutional prosperity.

For the athlete, success in sports means psychological rewards such as the admiration of peers, school officials, family, and community. In addition, athletic success can mean financial rewards such as scholarships, paid living expenses in college, advertising endorsement opportunities, and, for a few, incredible salaries as professional athletes. With the rewards of winning, athletes have to deal with the added pressures of not winning, such as "What will people think of me if I lose?"; "When I lose, I let everybody down"; or "Losing shows that I am not as good as everyone thinks." These pressures on young, immature athletes can result in poor coping responses. Being better than competitors, no matter the cost, becomes the driving motivation, and *doing one's best* is no longer sufficient. Such attitudes may lead to serious risk-taking behavior in order to develop an advantage over the competition; this can include using drugs to improve performance.

Drugs Used by Athletes

Studies have shown that athletes are not more likely than nonathletes to use some drugs of abuse such as marijuana, alcohol, barbiturates, cocaine, and hallucinogens (Samples 1989). However, athletes are much more likely than other populations to take drugs that enhance (physically or psychologically), or are thought to enhance, competitive performance: these drugs include stimulants such as the amphetamines and an array of drugs with presumed ergogenic effects, such as anabolic

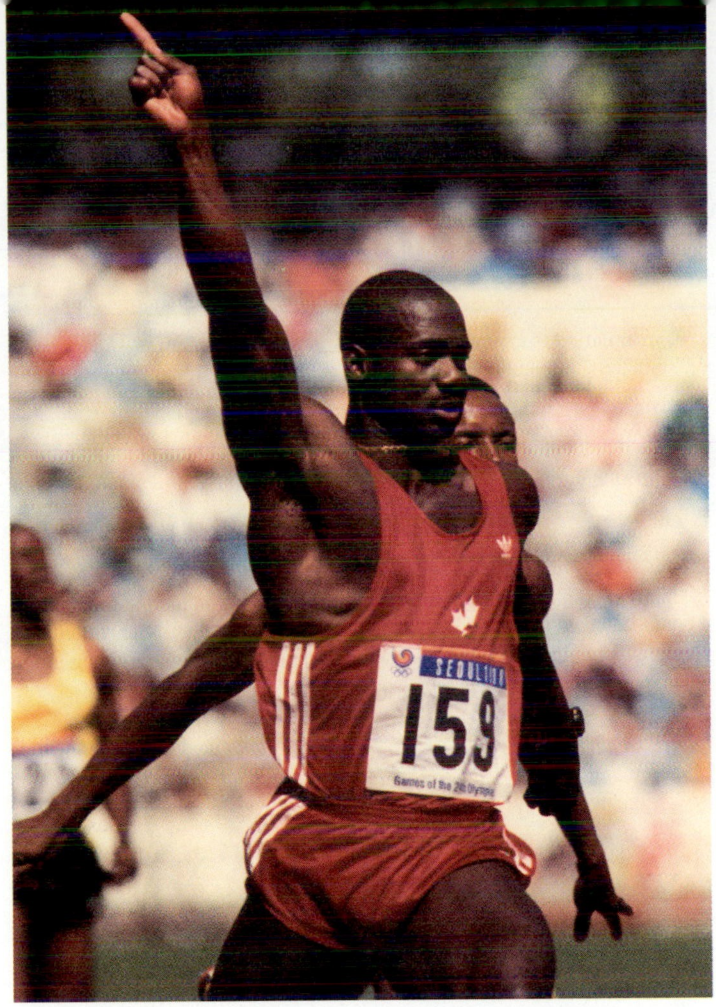

Canadian sprinter Ben Johnson at the Summer Olympics in Seoul, Korea. His gold medal was taken away because of steroid use.

steroids (Bell 1987). Some of the drugs that are abused by athletes are listed in Table 15.2 with their desired effects. The following sections discuss the drugs that are most frequently self-administered by athletes for improving their competitive performance.

Anabolic Steroids Anabolic steroids consist of a group of natural and synthetic drugs that are chemically similar to cholesterol and related to the male hormone testosterone (Lukas 1993). Naturally occurring male hormones, or **androgens,** are produced by the testes in males. These hormones are essential for normal growth and development of male sex organs as well as secondary sex characteristics such as muscular development, male hair patterns, voice changes, and fat distribution. The androgens are also necessary for appropriate growth spurts during adolescence (*Drug Facts and Comparisons* 1994). The principal accepted therapeutic use for the androgens is for hormone replacement in males with abnormally functioning testes. In such cases, the androgens are administered prior to puberty and for prolonged periods during puberty to stimulate proper male development (*Drug Facts and Comparisons* 1994).

Abuse of Anabolic Steroids by Athletes. Under some conditions, androgen-like drugs can increase muscle mass and strength; for this reason, they are

ERGOGENIC DRUGS drugs that enhance performance

ANDROGENS naturally occurring male hormones, such as testosterone

TABLE 15.2 Partial list of ergogenic substances and expected effects

Drugs	Expected Results
Amino acids	Stimulate natural production of growth hormone
Amphetamines and cocaine	Increase strength, alertness, and endurance
Anabolic steroids	Increase muscle mass and strength
B-complex vitamins	Enhance body metabolism and increase energy
Caffeine	Reduce fatigue
Chromium	Enhance carbohydrate metabolism
Ephedrine	Improve breathing
Asthma medication	Improve breathing
OTC decongestants	Increase endurance
Thyroid hormone	Enhance metabolism and energy
ß-blockers	Reduce hand tremor and stimulate growth hormone
Methylphenidate	Enhance alertness and endurance
Furosemide	Mask steroid use and enable rapid weight loss

Source: R. Harlan and M. Garcia. "Neurobiology of Androgen Abuse." In *Drugs of Abuse,* 185–201. Boca Raton, FL:CRC Press, 1992.

referred to as **anabolic** (able to stimulate the conversion of nutrients into tissue) steroids (because chemically, they are similar to the steroids produced in the adrenal glands) and are used by many athletes to improve performance (Burke and Davis 1992). It is estimated that as many as 1 million Americans have used or are currently using these drugs to achieve a "competitive edge" or for other purposes (Welder and Melchert 1993)—see Figure 15.2. Studies suggest that approximately 2% of the college men and 6.7% of male high school students use anabolic steroids (Harlan and Garcia 1992). Although the vast majority of anabolic steroid users are male, women involved in body building or strength and endurance sports also abuse these drugs. Thus, as many as 1% of the female high school students have used these drugs sometime during their life (Lukas 1993).

The first report of using anabolic steroids to improve athletic performance was in 1954 by the Russian weight-lifting team. Their performance-enhancing advantages were quickly recognized by other athletes, and it has been estimated that as many as 90% of the competitors in the 1960 Olympic games used some form of steroid (Toronto 1992). Because of the widespread misuse and associated problems with the use of these drugs, anabolic steroids were classified as Schedule III controlled drugs on 27 February 1991 (Merchant 1992).

Due to federal regulations, individuals convicted of a first offense trafficking with anabolic steroids can be sentenced to a maximum prison

ANABOLIC substances that stimulate the conversion of nutrients into tissue

STACKING use of several types of steroids together

CYCLING use of different types of steroids singly, but in sequence

PLATEAUING developing tolerance to the effects of anabolic steroids term of 5 years and a $250,000 fine. For a second offense, the prison term can increase to 10 years with a $500,000 fine. Even possession of illicitly obtained anabolic steroids can result in a 1-year term with at least a $1,000 fine (U.S. Department of Justice, 1991–1992).

Patterns of Abuse. Geographical factors appear to have little to do with the use of anabolic steroids among athletes in both inner-city and suburban schools; all are equally attracted to these drugs. However, some athletes are more inclined to abuse anabolic steroids than others; for example, football players have the highest rate of abuse, while track and field athletes have the least. In addition, the likelihood of abusing these drugs increases as the level of competition increases. Usage rates were approximately 14% in the National Collegiate Athletic Association (NCAA) division I athletes and 30–75% in professional athletes (Lukas 1993).

Usage patterns for the anabolic steroids can vary considerably according to the objectives of the athlete. The pattern usually consists of self-administering doses that are 10–200 times greater than dosages used for legitimate medical conditions (Welder and Melchert 1993)—see Table 15.3. **Stacking** is the use of several types of steroids together with the intent of maximizing their muscle-building effects and minimizing their adverse side effects; the use of different steroids taken singly but in sequence is called **cycling.** It is believed that tolerance to the effects of the anabolic steroids or **plateauing** can

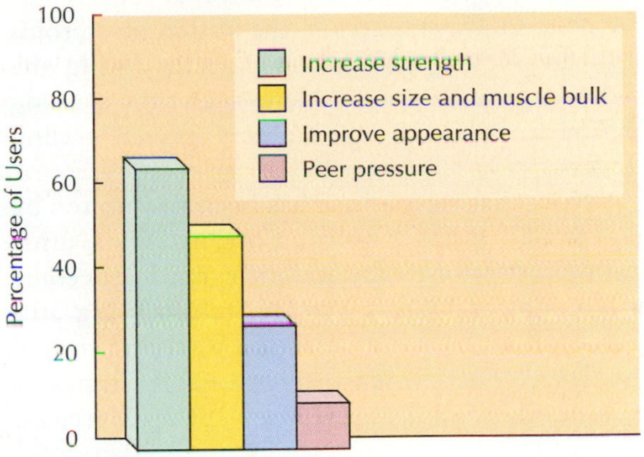

FIGURE 15.2 Reasons for nonmedicinal steroid use by college students *Source:* R. Harlan and M. Garcia. "Neurobiology of Androgen Abuse." In *Drugs of Abuse*, edited by R. Watson, 186. Boca Raton, FL: CRC Press, 1992.

TABLE 15.3 Typical patterns of anabolic steroid use

Pattern of Use	Steroid	Dosing	Duration (weeks)
Light	Methandrostenolone (Dianabol)	15 mg, oral	6
Moderate	Methandrostenolone	20 mg, oral	10
	Nandrolone decanoate (Deca-durabolin)	200 mg, intramuscular	10
	Testosterone cypionate (Depo-Testosterone)	200 mg, intramuscular	10
Intense	Methandrostenolone	40 mg, oral	16
	Oxandrolone (Anavar)	40 mg, oral	16
	Nandrolone decanoate	600 mg, intramuscular	16
	Boldenone undecylenate (Vebonol)	8 ml/week, intramuscular	16
	Methenolone enanthate	4 ml/week, intramuscular	16

Note: Moderate to intense doses are 10 to 100 times typical medical doses.

Source: R. Harlan and M. Garcia. "Neurobiology of Androgen Abuse." In *Drugs of Abuse*, edited by R. Watson, 187. Boca Raton, FL: CRC Press, 1992.

be avoided by staggering the different steroids with an overlapping dosing pattern during the cycle. In general, *power* athletes prefer the stacking approach, while body builders prefer cycling (Lukas 1993).

Now that steroid use has been prohibited by almost all legitimate sporting organizations, urine testing just prior to the athletic event has become commonplace (Lukas 1993). Steroid-using athletes attempt to avoid detection by trying to fool the tests. These highly questionable strategies include the following (Lukas 1993; Merchant 1992):

- Using the steroid only during training for the athletic events, but discontinuing its use several weeks before the competition to allow the drug to disappear from the body. Because oral steroids are cleared from the body faster than the injectable types, they are usually discontinued two to four weeks while the injection steroids are stopped three to six weeks before competition.
- Taking drugs, such as probenecid, that block the excretion of steroids in the urine.
- Using diuretics and drinking large quantities of water to increase the urine output and dilute the steroid so it cannot be detected by the test.
- Adding adulterant chemicals to the urine, such as Drano, Chlorox, ammonia, or Murine Eye Drops to invalidate the tests.

Case in Point

Lyle Alzedo Dead—Are Steroids to Blame?

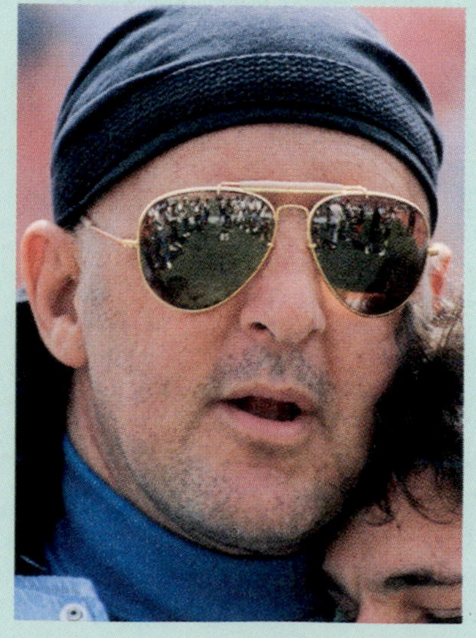

Lyle Alzedo, a former NFL all-pro defensive lineman, died at the age of 43 from a rare form of brain cancer. After the condition was diagnosed in April 1991, Alzedo admitted to having used anabolic steroids since 1969 when he was in college. He attributed his disease to prolonged use of these drugs. Although cancer specialists acknowledge there is no evidence to support Alzedo's claim, they also say that it can't be ruled out. Even though the involvement of steroids weren't proven, do you think that the Alzedo tragedy should be cited as evidence of the potentially serious consequences of using anabolic steroids?

Source: C. Burke and S. Davis. "Anabolic Steroid Abuse." *Pharmacy Times* (June 1992):35–40.

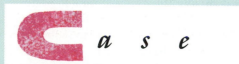

Here and Now

Although the precise effects of high doses of steroids is a controversial issue, accounts such as the following suggest that use of these drugs can be deadly in some users:

> John Kordic, a forward in the National Hockey League dies in transport to the hospital after being subdued by 9 policemen in his Quebec City motel room. Steroids and about 40 unused syringes were found in his room. During the autopsy, needle marks were found in his arm. Autopsy reports indicated that Kordic died of heart failure and an accumulation of fluid in his lungs. Although other drugs may also have been involved, the irrational rage exhibited by Kordic and the symptoms of heart failure are consistent with high-dose steroid use.
>
> (Associated Press 1992)

Although these techniques may make the analysis of steroids in the urine more difficult, they usually are not sufficient to prevent detection by carefully conducted urine drug testing.

Effects of Anabolic Steroids. Low to moderate doses of the anabolic steroids have little effect on the strength or athletic skills of the average adult. However, these drugs cause significant gains in lean body mass (that is, muscle) and strength, while decreasing fat when high doses are used by athletes during intense training programs (Lukas 1993). Because most of these effects are transient and will disappear when steroid use is stopped, athletes feel compelled to continue their use, and become psychologically *hooked* (Toronto 1992). The effect of anabolic steroids on athletic performance and skills is not clear and is difficult to measure (Lukas 1993). The drugs are most likely beneficial in contact and strength sports where increased muscle mass provides an advantage, such as weight lifting and football; but are less likely to benefit the athlete involved in sports requiring dexterity and agility, such as baseball or tennis.

The risks caused by the anabolic steroids are not completely understood (see the Case in Point on Lyle Alzedo). Most certainly, the higher the doses and the longer the use, the greater the potential damage these drugs can do to the body. Some of the adverse effects thought to occur with heavy steroid use (10 to 30 times the doses used therapeutically) include

- Increases in the blood cholesterol, which could eventually clog arteries and cause heart attacks and strokes (Burke and Davis 1992) (see the Here and Now box on John Kordic).
- Increased risk of liver disorders, such as jaundice and tumors (Lukas 1993).
- Psychological side effects including irritability, outbursts of anger ("roid rage"), mania, psychosis, and major depression (Lukas 1993; Burke and Davis 1992).
- Possible psychological and physical dependence with continual high-doses use, resulting in withdrawal symptoms such as steroid craving (52%), fatigue (43%), depression (41%), restlessness (29%), loss of appetite (24%), insomnia (20%), diminished sex drive (20%), and headaches (20%) (Lukas 1993).
- Alterations in reproductive systems and sex hormones, causing changes in sex-related characteristics (Burke and Davis 1992) such as breast enlargement in males and breast reduction in females, infertility in both sexes, and changes in genitalia in both sexes.
- Changes in skin and hair in both sexes, such

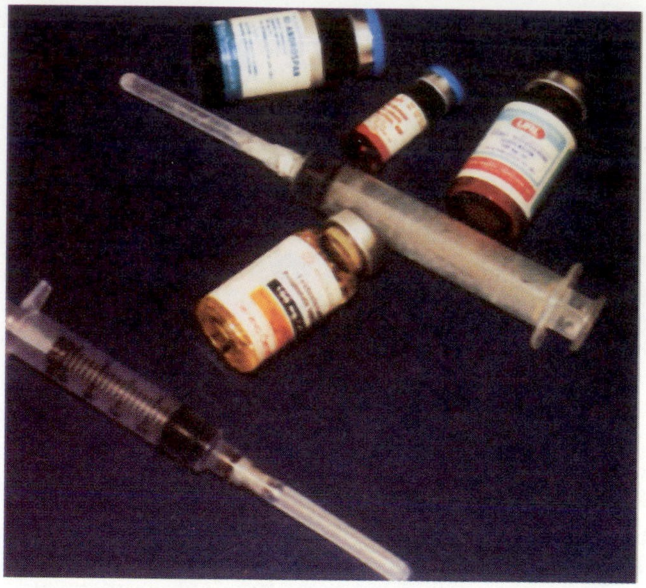

Common anabolic steroids used by athletes are Dianabol and Anavar.

as increased incidence and severity of acne, male pattern baldness, and increased body hair (Burke and Davis 1992).

- Other changes, including stunted growth in adolescents, deepening of voice in females, and water retention, causing bloating (Burke and Davis 1992).

Source of Steroids. Where do the anabolic steroids come from? About 50% of the anabolic steroids used in this country are prescribed by doctors: the other 50% are obtained from the black market. Black market sources of steroids include drugs diverted from legitimate channels, smuggled from foreign countries, designated for veterinarian use or inactive counterfeits (U.S. Department of Justice, 1991–1992). Several different types of anabolic steroids are commonly used and listed in Table 15.3. Some health food stores and mail order firms also offer products with names like the prescription anabolic steroids, such as Dynabdin, Metrobolin, and Diostero. These are "sham steroids" and only contain vitamins, amino acids, or micronutrients (Merchant 1992).

Stimulant Use in Athletes A week rarely passes in which the media do not report a football, basketball, or baseball player who has tested positive in a drug-screening evaluation or who has been suspended from competition due to stimulant abuse. Sometimes the stories are more tragic. In 1986, reports of cocaine-related deaths of sports figures included basketball star Len Bias and professional football player Don Rogers. Perhaps such sports tragedies helped convince some U.S. youth of the dangers of stimulant abuse and contributed to the decline in drug abuse in the late 1980s (Johnston et al. 1993). Clearly, no one, not even athletes, is immune from the risks of these drugs.

Amphetamine and cocaine are abused to improve athletic skills. However, it is not clear if stimulants actually enhance athletic performance or only the athlete's *perception* of performance. Many athletes believe these drugs promote quickness, endurance, delay fatigue, increase self-confidence and aggression, and mask pain. In fact, some studies have shown that stimulants can improve some aspects of athletic performance, especially in the presence of fatigue (Bell 1987). However, the risk of using stimulants in sports is substantial because these drugs mask extreme fatigue, increase the risk of heat exhaustion, and can have severe cardiovascular consequences, such as heart attacks, strokes, and failure of the cardiovascular system (Bell 1987).

Although some athletes would never consider using the *hard* stimulants, such as cocaine and the amphetamines, milder stimulants that are legal and available OTC may be thought acceptable: such stimulants include caffeine and OTC decongestants (for example, phenylpropanolamine and phenylephrine). Use of these drugs can be a two-edged sword for the athlete; their use can reduce fatigue, give a sense of energy, and even mask pain. But in high doses, especially when combined, they can cause nervousness, tremors and restlessness, impair concentration, accelerate dehydration, and interfere with sleep ("OTC Drugs and Athletes" 1992). Some athletic competitions limit permissible blood levels of caffeine (Bell 1987) and do not allow the use of OTC stimulants such as decongestant drugs (Merchant 1992).

NO **Miscellaneous Ergogenic Drugs** Most athletic organizations have banned the use of anabolic steroids and stimulants and are using more effective screening procedures to detect offenders. A result of this clamp-down has been the search for alternative performance-enhancing drugs by athletes who feel a need for such pharmacological assistance. The following are brief discussions of a few of these substitute ergogenic substances (for a more complete list, see Table 15.2).

Clenbuterol. At the 1992 Olympic Games in Barcelona, Spain, at least four athletes, including German world sprint champion Katrina Krabbe, were disqualified from competition for using the drug clenbuterol to enhance their athletic performance (Merchant 1992). Not available in the United States, this drug is known as Doper's Delight and is supposed to improve breathing and increase strength. Currently it is tested for in most athletic urine examinations.

Erythropoietin. Clinically, erythropoietin is a drug used to treat patients with anemia. Because it stimulates the production of red blood cells (the oxygen-carrying cells in the blood), it is thought this drug enhances oxygen use and causes additional energy. Erythropoietin is being used as a substitute for *blood doping*—athletes' trying to increase the number of red blood cells by reinfusing some of their own blood (which has been stored) prior to an athletic event. Erythropoietin is impossible to detect and has been reported to be used by athletes engaged in endurance activities such as long-distance cyclists. The use of erythropoietin by athletes is extremely dangerous and is thought to be responsible for several deaths. It is also very expensive, which likely has helped to limit its abuse (Merchant 1992).

Human Growth Factor (HGF). Athletes' abuse of **human growth factor (HGF),** also known as *somatotropin,* is a relatively recent phenomenon. This hormone is naturally secreted by the pituitary gland and helps to achieve normal growth potential of muscles, bones, and internal organs. Some athletes claim that release of natural HGF can be stimulated by using drugs such as levodopa (a drug used to treat Parkinson's disease), clonidine (a drug used to treat hypertension), and amino acids. Athletes use commercially prepared HGF because it cannot be distinguished from naturally occurring HGF. However, use of the hormone by athletes is limited due to its high cost. The benefits of HGF to athletic performance are very controversial, although the potential side effects are substantial and include abnormal growth patterns (called *acromegaly*), diabetes, problems with thyroid glands, heart disease, and loss of sex drive (Merchant 1992).

Beta-adrenergic Blockers. The beta-adrenergic blockers are drugs that affect the cardiovascular system and are frequently used to treat hypertension. The beta-adrenergic blockers have been used in sports because they reduce the heart rate and signs of nervousness, which in turn reduce hand tremors. Consequently, these drugs are most likely

HUMAN GROWTH FACTOR (HGF) a hormone that stimulates normal growth to be used by individuals participating in sports that require steady hands, such as competitive shooting. The use of these drugs is prohibited by most athletic organizations (Merchant 1992).

Gamma-Hydroxybutyrate (GHB). The substance gamma-hydroxybutyrate (GHB) is found naturally in the brain and has been used in England to treat insomnia. Athletes and bodybuilders have used gamma-hydroxybutyrate (GHB) to increase muscle mass and strength. Although the actual effects of the compound are not known, it has been reported to cause euphoria and increase the release of growth hormone. Acute poisoning with GHB has occurred, causing hospitalization, and can include adverse effects such as headaches, nausea, vomiting, muscle jerking, and even short-term coma; full recovery has been universal ("Bodybuilding Drug" 1992; "Multistate Outbreak" 1994). Prolonged use may cause withdrawal (insomnia, anxiety, and tremor). GHB is especially dangerous when combined with CNS stimulants such as amphetamines and cocaine.

Prevention and Treatment

If the problem of drug abuse in athletes is to be dealt with effectively, sports programs must be designed to discourage inappropriate drug use and assist athletes who have developed drug abuse problems. Coaches and administrators should make clear to sports participants that substance abuse will never give an athlete a competitive advantage in their program and will not be tolerated. The following are specific suggestions for sports leaders to discourage drug abuse in their programs (Lawn 1984):

1. Make it known publicly that you recruit non-drug-using athletes to your programs, to exert pressure on team members who use.
2. Rigidly enforce training rules and don't make exceptions, even for the "stars."
3. Select team captains and leaders who are opposed to drug use and require from them a commitment to help enforce training rules with teammates.
4. Be open about drug abuse incidents: don't avoid the subject but also communicate to the athletes your concern for users. However, be sensitive to confidentialities and the emotional and social needs of offenders.
5. Be educated about which drugs athletes typically abuse, how they are abused, and what their effects are. With such knowledge, coaches and trainers are better prepared to recognize drug abuse symptoms such as mood swings, changes in personality, impaired coordination, and sudden increases in muscle size and strength.
6. Have a definite plan in mind when an athlete gets caught abusing drugs. Ignoring the incident does not help the athlete to deal with his or her problems. The athlete should be confronted directly, and the family should be encouraged to get involved in the solution.
7. Establish and enforce a consequence or punishment for violating training rules by using drugs. However, after the rule has been enforced, the athlete should not be rejected, but encouraged.

It is essential that coaches and trainers be selected for their ability to be good role models for the athletes. They should encourage athletes to keep sports in perspective and should help the student athlete understand that many things in life are more important than success on the playing field (Lawn 1984).

Drug Abuse and AIDS

The first described case of acquired immunodeficiency syndrome (AIDS) occurred in 1981. As of 1993, over 13 million adults worldwide had been infected with the AIDS-causing human immunodeficiency virus (HIV) and more than 2 million people in the world had died from this disease (Merson 1993). The epidemic spread of HIV infection is very disturbing and is projected by the World Health Organization (WHO) to reach 30 to 50 million people by the year 2000 (Pietroski 1993).

Similar trends of rapid spread of HIV infection and AIDS-related death have been documented in

substance abuse among elderly 2-3 years

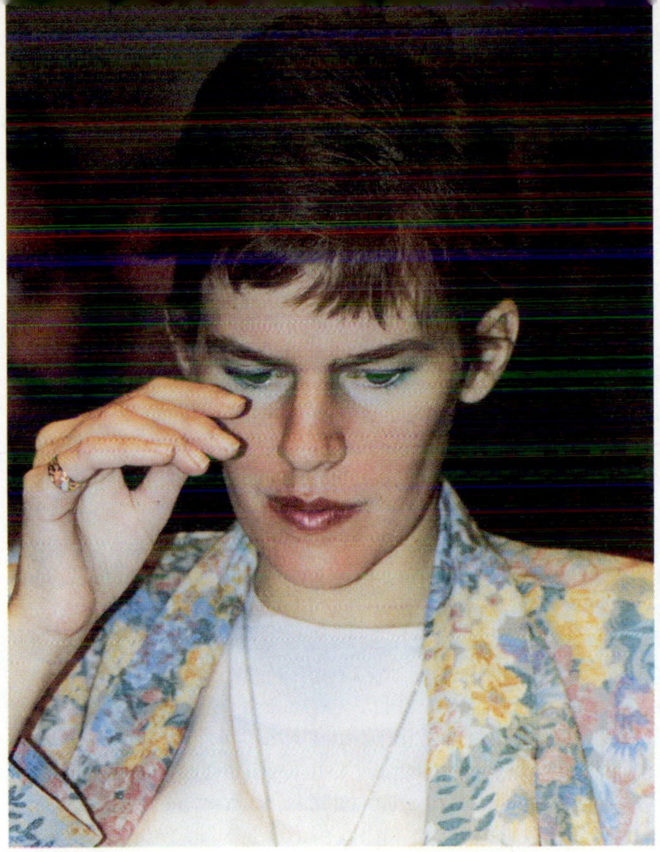

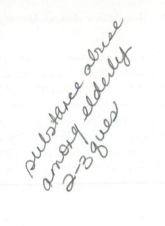

Anyone can become infected with HIV, although it is not transmitted by casual contact. Kimberly Bergalis, 23, contacted AIDS from her dentist.

the United States; as of 1993, a total of almost 1 million Americans were HIV-infected (Colthurst 1993) and 361,509 Americans were diagnosed with AIDS ("A Moving Target" 1994), with 60,000 to 70,000 new AIDS cases occurring each year (Pietroski 1993). In 1991 alone, 30,000 people died from AIDS, making it the ninth leading cause of death in the United States. By the end of 1994 it is estimated that more than 500,000 people in this country died from this disease (Grinspoon 1994).

In the early stages of the U.S. epidemic, most AIDS cases occurred in California and New York and were seen almost entirely in homosexual and bisexual men. The pattern of occurrence has changed. For example, AIDS now occurs everywhere and the incidence of AIDS in women has substantially increased (Pietroski 1993). Another emerging pattern of particular relevance to the topics of this book is that the use of substances of abuse now plays a major role in the spread of the AIDS disease; thus, 25% of all AIDS patients are IV drug users, and these people represent the second largest group at risk for the deadly AIDS disease (Pietroski 1993; National Aids Program Office 1989).

Nature of AIDS

AIDS is caused by the human immunodeficiency virus (HIV). Although much is still unknown about HIV infections, it has been determined that with time this virus severely compromises the ability of the body's immune system to fight infections; this, in turn, eventually causes AIDS (Grinspoon 1994). The damage to the immune system appears to result from the destruction of important immune cells called CD4$^+$-type helper T-lymphocytes and macrophages (Cohen 1993b). Because these immune cells are crucial in identifying and eliminating infection-causing micro-organisms, such as bacteria, fungi, and viruses, their deficiency substantially increases the likelihood and severity of infectious diseases. It is important to realize that the AIDS condition does not develop immediately following HIV infection, but is the final expression of the disease and can occur anywhere from 2 years to longer than 12 years later (Weiss 1993).

AIDS Symptoms Although the onset of AIDS-related symptoms is delayed for at least 2 years after HIV infection (10 years is the average;

Goldfinger 1994), a brief flulike illness usually occurs 6 to 12 weeks after exposure to this virus. During the latent period before AIDS develops, infected patients can enjoy a healthy, productive lifestyle although they must be made aware that they are HIV-contagious, and if they do not take appropriate cautions they can infect other people with this virus (Pietroski 1993). It is not known what determines the length of the latent period. Although unproven, it is possible that a healthy lifestyle (proper exercise, proper nutrition, and a good emotional perspective) and the use of drugs such as zidovudine (AZT, or Azidothymidine) can postpone the onset of AIDS after HIV.infection. However, the asymptomatic period eventually ends and signs of immune disorders appear. These signs include fever, weight loss, malaise, swollen lymph nodes, and CNS problems (Grinspoon 1994). With the destruction of the immune cells, infections become increasingly difficult to control with antibacterial (for example, antibiotics), antifungal, and antiviral drugs; consequently, severe *opportunistic* infections such as pneumonia, meningitis, hepatitis, tuberculosis, and Kaposi's sarcoma can occur and eventually lead to death (Pietroski 1993). The likelihood of introducing these opportunistic infections in the body increases in patients who are IV drug users because they often share injection equipment, such as needles and syringes, which are contaminated with disease-causing micro-organisms.

Diagnosis It is crucial that HIV-infected people be aware of their condition in order to avoid activities that might transmit the infection to others. Testing for the presence of infection has been available since 1985 and is done by determining if the body is producing antibodies against the HIV. The presence of these specific antibodies indicates HIV infection. If infected, it requires 6 to 12 weeks after the HIV exposure before the body produces enough antibodies to be detected in currently available tests. If the antibody is not present within six months after HIV exposure, infection likely has not occurred (Pietroski 1993).

The tests for HIV infection are very reliable, with false negatives (that is, test says no HIV present even though the individual is infected) and false positives (that is, test says individual is infected even though no HIV is present) occurring in approximately 1 out of 30,000 tests. Because AIDS is a highly emotional issue, great effort is made to assure confidentiality of the test results. The blood specimens to be tested are coded, and

CROSS CURRENTS

As more people become HIV-infected, the debate continues as to who has a right to be informed when a person tests positive for the presence of this AIDS-causing virus. Consider the following opposing views.

1. Because the human immunodeficiency virus is minimally contagious, doctors should not inform anyone except the patient when testing shows HIV infections.
2. Because the consequence of HIV infection is death, associates, family members, and involved health care personnel should be notified when an HIV infection is found in a patient.

Choose a side, and support your argument with factual information from this text and other authoritative sources.

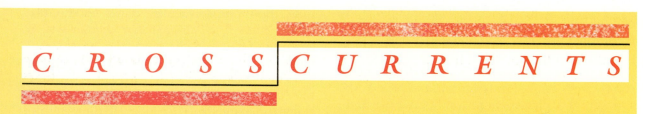

the personnel conducting the tests are not allowed to divulge the results. However, under special circumstances, the confidentiality of the results can be broken; for example, if a sexual partner is in imminent danger of becoming infected by an HIV-positive patient (Pietroski 1993). The issue of confidentiality is very controversial. It is often difficult to decide who has the right to know when an individual is found to be HIV-infected (see Crosscurrents box).

People who should be tested for HIV–infection include those who participate in high-risk activities. For example, HIV testing is recommended for (1) men who engage in sexual activity with other men, (2) people with a history of intravenous drug use or use drugs in *shooting galleries* or *crack houses,* and (3) men and women who have multiple sex partners (Pietroski 1993).

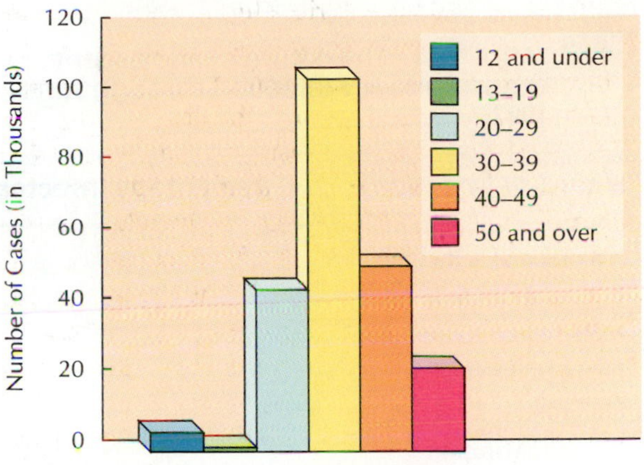

FIGURE 15.3 Cases of AIDS in the United States through June 1992 according to age (in years) *Source:* A. Novello. "Preventing the Alcohol and Other Drug Problems of HIV/AIDS." *Prevention Pipeline* 5 (September–October 1992):3–5.

Who Gets AIDS?

Although anyone can become infected with HIV, its routes of transmission are limited to blood, semen, vaginal fluid, and possibly some other body fluids (Grinspoon 1994). HIV is a virus that is not likely to survive outside of the body. Consequently, HIV is not spread by casual contact at work or school, by shaking hands, touching, hugging, or kissing. In addition, it is not spread through food or water, by sharing cups or glasses, by coughing and sneezing, or by using common toilets. It is not spread by mosquitoes or other insects. This means that infection cannot occur through ordinary social contact (Goldfinger 1994). The transmission of HIV is most often through sexual contact; the next most likely means of transmission is by exposure to contaminated blood or blood products, usually by drug addicts sharing IV needles. HIV can also be passed from an infected mother to a child either prenatally or possibly by breastfeeding (Pietroski 1993).

Because of these limited routes of HIV transmission, the populations at greatest risk for contracting AIDS are (1) men with a history of homosexual or bisexual activity, (2) injection drug users and their sexual partners, (3) infants born to HIV-infected women, and (4) people receiving contaminated blood or blood products as for transfusions or treatment of blood disorders (Pietroski 1993). Men dying from AIDS outnumber women 7 to 1. In fact, AIDS is the leading killer of black males 25 to 44 years of age and the second leading killer of white males that same age (Associated Press 1993).

Adolescents and AIDS Although people of all ages are contracting AIDS (see Figure 15.3), a particularly alarming trend is the high rate of HIV infection in the adolescent population. More than 75,000 adolescents in the United States have tested positive for the presence of HIV, and many of the 44,000 young adults (20 to 29 years of age) with AIDS were infected during their teenage years (Novello 1992). According to the Centers for Disease Control, two of the principal ways adolescents are infected with HIV are high-risk sexual activity and injecting substances of abuse (see Table 15.4). Clearly, young people must be better educated about AIDS and its transmission and consequences if this epidemic is to be controlled.

AIDS and Drugs of Abuse

During the past few years, the AIDS epidemic has become closely associated with drug abuse problems. Thus, those addicted to illicit drugs are currently the second largest risk group for contracting AIDS (Booth et al. 1993; Grinspoon 1994). AIDS

TABLE 15.4 The nature of adolescent exposure to HIV infection through June 1992

Means of Infection	Percentage Infected
Male sexual activity	24%
Injecting drugs	13
Male sexual activity plus injecting drugs	4
Hemophilia therapy	31
Heterosexual contact	14
Blood transfusion	6
Undetermined	7

Source: A. Novello. "Preventing the Alcohol and Other Drug Problem of HIV/AIDS." *Prevention Pipeline* 5 (September–October 1992):4.

in women is particularly linked to drug abuse. Nearly 70% of the female AIDS victims are infected because of IV drug use by themselves or by a sexual partner (Glave 1994). There are several reasons that account for the high incidence of this deadly infection in the drug-abusing population.

1. Intravenous drug use has become the most important factor in the spread of AIDS in the United States. One-third of the AIDS cases reported in the United States by late 1993 were associated with injecting cocaine, heroin, or both (Landau 1994). Intravenous drug use is often done with little regard to hygiene, and injection paraphernalia such as needles, syringes, and cotton are frequently shared with other drug addicts (Millstein 1993). Sharing HIV-contaminated injection equipment can result in the transmission of, and infection by, this virus. The likelihood of an intravenous drug user contracting AIDS is directly correlated with (a) the frequency of drug injections, (b) the number of partners with whom injection equipment is shared, (c) the frequency of needle sharing, and (d) the frequency of injections in locations of high AIDS infection rates, such as in shooting galleries or crack houses (Booth et al. 1993).

2. Use of drugs such as crack (Ciba Foundation 1992) and alcohol (Colthurst 1993) tend to compromise judgment and encourage high-risk activities such as IV drug use or sexual risk taking (Beard and Kunsman 1993). In particular, the use of crack has been associated with HIV infection. Crack addicts often exchange sex for drugs or money to purchase drugs (Mathias 1993). These dangerous activities frequently occur in populations with a high rate of HIV infection (Ciba Foundation 1992). Once infected, almost half the crack users continue to use sex to obtain their drugs and become a source of HIV infection for others (Diaz and Chu 1993). In general, because of the effects of cocaine on sexual activity, crack smokers also have a greater risk for HIV infection because they tend to have many sex partners during cocaine binges and frequently participate in unprotected sexual behaviors (Booth et al. 1993).

What to Do About AIDS

Although many reknowned researchers are frantically trying to identify a cure for HIV infection and AIDS, current drug therapy is only able to delay the onset of AIDS after infection with HIV or to prolong life after AIDS develops. No treatment is available that cures this deadly disease (Cohen 1993a). The lack of a cure makes prevention the most important element in dealing with the AIDS problem. Potential preventive strategies for AIDS can be divided into two main categories:

- People should be encouraged to adopt safer sexual behavior. Some of the steps to help achieve this end include (1) avoiding multiple sex partners, especially if they are strangers or only casual acquaintances; (2) avoiding risk-taking sexual behavior, which may allow HIV transmission, such as unprotected vaginal or anal intercourse; and (3) encouraging individuals who choose to continue high-risk sexual behaviors to use a condom or insist that the sexual partner use a condom (Merson 1993).
- Drug abusers should be educated about their risk of contracting AIDS. They should be encouraged to reduce their risk by (1) abstaining from use of drugs by injection; (2) not sharing injection paraphernalia or always using clean needles (if available through "needle

exchange programs"); (3) not using drugs in groups with high rates of HIV infection such as shooting galleries or crack houses; and (4) disinfecting the equipment (cleaning and boiling equipment for at least 15 minutes) between uses if they continue to share injection equipment (Millstein 1993).

One of the major difficulties in controlling the AIDS epidemic is to identify where preventive efforts should be focused. Because of limited resources, it is impossible to personally educate everyone in this country about HIV and AIDS. Consequently, we must target our most intense efforts at populations and neighborhoods with particularly high HIV infection rates. The National Research Council has declared that although anyone can be a victim of AIDS, a handful of neighborhoods have been devastated by this infection while most of the nation remains relatively unscathed (Kolata 1993). It has been speculated that some 25–30 large neighborhoods in the United States fuel the AIDS epidemic throughout the country, and if the HIV infection could be controlled in these areas the national epidemic would diminish significantly. Because of this hypothesis, it has been proposed that AIDS prevention efforts particularly be focused on gay men and IV drug users who have multiple sex partners in the high-density AIDS neighborhoods found in cities such as San Francisco, Miami, Newark, New York City, and Camden, New Jersey (Kolata 1993). Even with this focused approach, no one should be fooled into thinking the AIDS problem will be eliminated. Each person must become educated about this deadly disease and take steps to avoid HIV exposure.

Review Questions

1. Why are adolescents especially vulnerable to drug abuse problems?
2. What types of parents are most likely to have children who develop drug abuse problems?
3. Which substances of abuse are most likely to be used by adolescents, and which are most likely to be used frequently?
4. How do adolescent drug abuse patterns differ from those in adults?
5. What coincidental problems are likely to be associated with adolescent drug abuse? Why?
6. In what way are drugs of abuse associated with juvenile gang activity?
7. Should all adolescents who use drugs of abuse be treated for drug dependence? Explain your answer.
8. Describe three gender differences in use patterns for drugs of abuse. Explain why these differences occur.
9. Why do you think that in the past most drug abuse research did not study female populations? Are any of these reasons justified?
10. What factors in the unique female roles encourage the use of substances of abuse? Explain the reason for the association.
11. What factors discourage drug-dependent women from seeking treatment?
12. Why does alcohol consumption tend to cause greater physiological damage in females than in males?
13. What are some important factors that should be considered when designing drug dependence treatment and prevention programs for women?
14. What factors encourage drug use by athletes?
15. What are the principal drugs abused by athletes?
16. How are anabolic steroids used, and what are their principal effects and side effects?
17. Why are CNS stimulants used by athletes?
18. Do you think that drug testing is an effective deterrent to drug misuse in sports?
19. What type of penalties do you think should be used against athletes who abuse drugs?
20. Why are users of illicit drugs currently the second largest risk group for contracting AIDS?
21. What are the major preventive strategies to protect against contracting AIDS?
22. Do you think that it is realistic to expect drug abusers to change their habits in order to prevent the spread of AIDS?

Key Terms

intragang
intergang
primary prevention
secondary prevention
genitourinary
ergogenic drugs
androgens
anabolic
stacking
cycling
plateauing
human growth factor (HGF)

Summary

1. Most adolescents who use substances of abuse do so with normal psychosocial development and will not develop problematic dependence on these drugs. The adolescent users who have difficulty with drugs often lack coping skills to deal with their problems, have dysfunctional families, possess poor self-images, and/or feel socially and emotionally insecure.
2. Parents who are most likely to foster drug-abusing children are (a) drug abusers themselves, (b) excessively rigid and condemning, (c) overly demanding, (d) overly protective, (e) overwhelmed with their own personal conflicts, or (f) unable to communicate effectively with their children.
3. The substances adolescents are most likely to abuse are alcohol, cigarettes, inhalants, marijuana, and prescription stimulants. High-frequency use is most likely to occur with cigarettes, alcohol, and marijuana.
4. Similar problems lead to both drug abuse problems and gang involvement. In addition, gangs often use drug dealing as a means of obtaining money. Adolescent involvement in drugs and gangs can be discouraged by increasing parental awareness of the problem, providing alternative activities that help develop coping skills, and educating children about gang-related problems.
5. Most drugs of abuse are used more frequently by males than comparable females. In addition, men tend to have a higher prevalence for intense drug use. An exception to this trend is a higher daily use of cigarettes by female college students than their male counterparts.
6. Because of their traditional domestic roles, women who abuse drugs are viewed by society in general less tolerantly than men. Many women also are socioeconomically disadvantaged, which creates frustrations and stress that predispose to drug abuse. Finally, a woman's unique function in the family can create special pressures that lead to poor coping strategies such as drug dependence.
7. Drug treatment programs for women should accommodate their ongoing family responsibilities, be sensitive to their unique health needs, provide special training for employment, coping, and the development of independence.
8. The most common drugs abused by athletes are the ergogenic (performance-enhancing) substances. These include the anabolic steroids for building muscle mass and strength as well as the CNS stimulants to achieve energy, quickness, and endurance.
9. Drug testing is conducted for most athletic competitions and usually includes screens for steroids and stimulants. However, some performance-enhancing drugs, such as erythropoietin and human growth factor are undetectable. Some athletes go to great lengths to avoid detection by these drug tests.
10. Next to homosexual men, those addicted to illicit drugs are the second largest risk group for contracting AIDS. This risk is due to sharing of blood-contaminated needles and syringes and increased involvement in sexual risk taking because of the effects of drugs or in payment for drugs.
11. Major strategies to prevent contracting AIDS include (a) safer sexual behavior, (b) avoiding use of contaminated drug paraphernalia, (c) avoiding use of IV drugs, and (d) avoiding use of drugs in groups with high rates of HIV infection.

References

Alexander, L. "Alcohol and Women's Health." In *Dimensions in Women's Health.* Boston: Jones and Bartlett, 1994a.

Alexander, L. "Drug Use and Women's Health." In *Dimensions in Women's Health.* Boston: Jones and Bartlett, 1994b.

"A Moving Target: CDC Still Trying to Eliminate HIV-1 Prevalence." *Journal of NIH Research* 6 (June 1994): 25, 26.

Archambault, D. "Adolescence, a Physiological, Cultural and Psychological No Man's Land." In *Adolescent Substance Abuse, Etiology, Treatment and Prevention,* edited by G. Lawson and A. Lawson, 11–28. Gaithersburg, MD: Aspen, 1992.

Associated Press. "Shocking Death of Kordic Spurs NHL President to Clamp Down on Use of Anabolic Steroids." *Salt Lake Tribune* 244 (11 August 1992): C-4.

Associated Press. "AIDS Deaths Rise; Motor Fatalities Fall." *Salt Lake Tribune* 246 (1 September 1993): A-1.

Bell, J. "Athletes' Use and Abuse of Drugs." *The Physician and Sports Medicine* 15 (March 1987): 99–108.

Beard, B., and V. Kunsman. "A Cause for Concern: Alcohol-Induced Risky Sex on College Campuses." *Prevention Pipeline* 6 (September–October 1993): 24.

Beschner, G., and A. Friedman. "Treatment of Adolescent Drug Abusers." *International Journal of the Addictions* 20 (1985): 977–93.

"Bodybuilding Drug Yields 'High.'" *Pharmacy Times* (June 1992): 14.

Booth, R., J. Watters, and D. Chitwood. "HIV Risk-Related Sex Behaviors Among Injection Drug Users, Crack Smokers, and Injection Drug Users Who Smoke Crack." *American Journal of Public Health* 83 (1993): 1144–48.

Brady, K., D. Grice, L. Dustan, and C. Randall. "Gender Differences in Substances Use Disorders." *American Journal of Psychiatry* 150 (November 1993): 1707–11.

Buckstein, D., D. Brent, J. Perper, G. Moritz, M. Baugher, J. Schweers, C. Roth, and L. Balach. "Risk Factors for Completed Suicide Among Adolescents with a Lifetime History of Substance Abuse: A Case-Control Study." *Acta Psychiatry Scandinavia* 88 (1993): 403–8.

Burke, C., and S. Davis. "Anabolic Steroid Abuse." *Pharmacy Times* (June 1992): 35–40.

Caetano, R. "Drinking Patterns and Alcoholic Problems in a National Sample of U.S. Hispanics." In *The Epidemiology of Alcohol Use and Abuse Among U.S. Minorities.* NIAA Monograph no. 18 (DHHS Pub. no. ADM89-1435) 147–62. Washington, DC: U.S. Government Printing Office, 1989.

Ciba Foundation. "AIDS and HIV Infection in Cocaine Users." In *Cocaine: Scientific and Social Dimensions* 181–94. New York: Wiley, 1992.

"Cigarettes May Pose a Greater Risk in Developing Fetus Than Cocaine." *Prevention Pipeline* 7 (May–June 1994): 10, 11.

Cohen, J. "How Can HIV Replication Be Controlled?" *Science* 260 (May 1993a): 1257.

Cohen, J. "What Causes the Immune System Collapse Seen in AIDS?" *Science* 260 (May 1993b): 1256.

Colthurst, T. "HIV and Alcohol Impairment: Reducing Risks." *Prevention Pipeline* 6 (July–August 1993): 24.

Daily, S. "Alcohol, Incest, and Adolescence." In *Adolescent Substance Abuse, Etiology, Treatment and Prevention,* edited by G. Lawson and A. Lawson, 251–66. Gaithersburg, MD: Aspen, 1992a.

Daily, S. "Suicide Solution: The Relationship of Alcohol and Drug Abuse to Adolescent Suicide. In *Adolescent Substance Abuse, Etiology, Treatment and Prevention,* edited by G. Lawson and A. Lawson, 233–50. Gaithersburg, MD: Aspen, 1992b.

Diaz, T., and S. Chu. "Crack Cocaine Use and Sexual Behavior Among People with AIDS." *JAMA* 269 (1993): 2845–46.

Drug Facts and Comparisons, 109–109c. St. Louis: Kluwer, 1994.

Elmen, J., and D. Offer. "Normality, Turmoil and Adolescence." In *Handbook of Clinical Research and Practice with Adolescents,* edited by P. Tolan and B. Cohler, 5–19. New York: Wiley, 1993.

Erickson, P. G., and G. F. Murray. "Sex Differences in Cocaine Use and Experiences: A Double Standard Revived?" *American Journal of Drug and Alcohol Abuse* 15 (1989): 135–52.

Fagan, J. "Social Processes of Delinquency and Drug Use Among Urban Gangs." In *Gangs in America,* edited by C. R. Huff, 183–213. Newbury Park, CA: Sage, 1990.

Ferrente, R. "Ben Johnson Retires from Running After Positive Test." Morning Edition on National Public Radio, 8 March 1993.

Glave, J. "Betty Ford Got Help, but Addiction Stalks Thousands of Women." *Salt Lake Tribune* 248 (3 June 1994): A-1.

Goldfinger, S. "When HIV Hits Home." *Harvard Health Letter* 19 (April 1994): 1–3.

Goldstein, F. "Pharmacological Aspects of Substance Abuse." In *Remington's Pharmaceutical Sciences,* 19th ed. Easton, PA: Mack, 1995.

Grinspoon, L. "AIDS and Mental Health—Part 1."

Harvard Mental Health Letter 10 (January 1994): 1–4.

Harlan, R., and M. Garcia. "Neurobiology of Androgen Abuse." In *Drugs of Abuse,* edited by R. Watson, 185–201. Boca Raton, FL: CRC Press, 1992.

Hasin, D., B. Grant, and J. Weinflash. "Male/Female Differences in Alcohol-related Problems: Alcohol Rehabilitation Patients." *International Journal of the Addictions* 23 (1988): 437–48.

Hernandez, J. "Substance Abuse Among Sexually Abused Adolescents and Their Families." *Journal of Adolescent Health* 13 (1992): 658–62.

Hoshino, J. "Assessment of Adolescent Substance Abuse." In *Adolescent Substance Abuse, Etiology, Treatment and Prevention,* edited by G. Lawson and A. Lawson, 87–104. Gaithersburg, MD: Aspen, 1992.

Howard, M. "Adolescent Substance Abuse: A Social Learning Theory Perspective." In *Adolescent Substance Abuse, Etiology, Treatment and Prevention,* edited by G. Lawson and A. Lawson, 29–40. Gaithersburg, MD: Aspen, 1992.

Johnston, L. D. "Drug Use Rises Among American Teenagers." News and Information Service, the University of Michigan, 27 January 1994.

Johnston, L. D., P. O'Malley, and J. G. Bachman. *National Survey Results from The Monitoring the Future Study, 1975–1992.* Rockville, MD: National Institute on Drug Abuse, 1993.

Kolata, G. "Targeting Urged in Attack on AIDS." *New York Times* 142 (7 March 1993): 1.

Korolenko, C. P., and T. A. Donskih. "Addictive Behavior in Women: A Theoretical Perspective." *Drugs and Society* 4 (1990): 39–65.

Ladwig, G. B., and M. D. Anderson. "Substance Abuse in Women: Relationship Between Chemical Dependency of Women and Past Reports of Physical and/or Sexual Abuse." *International Journal of the Addictions* 24 (1989): 739–54.

Lale, T. "Gangs and Drugs." In *Adolescent Substance Abuse, Etiology, Treatment and Prevention,* edited by G. Lawson and A. Lawson, 267–81. Gaithersburg, MD: Aspen, 1992.

Landau, I. "Can Clean Needles Slow the AIDS Epidemic?" *Consumer Reports* (July 1994): 466–69.

Lawn, J. "Team Up for Drug Prevention with America's Young Athletes." Drug Enforcement Administration, U.S. Department of Justice, 1984.

Lawson, G., and A. Lawson, "Etiology." In *Adolescent Substance Abuse, Etiology, Treatment and Prevention,* edited by G. Lawson and A. Lawson, 1–10. Gaithersburg, MD: Aspen, 1992.

Lindberg, S., and G. Agren. "Mortality Among Male and Female Hospitalized Alcoholics in Stockholm 1962–1983." *British Journal of the Addictions* 83 (1988): 1193–1200.

Lukas, S. "Urine Testing for Anabolic-Androgenic Steroids." *Trends in Pharmacological Sciences* 14 (1993): 61–68.

Marsh, K. L., and D. D. Simpson. "Sex Differences in Opioid Addiction Centers." *American Journal of Drug and Alcohol Abuse* 12 (1986): 309–29.

Mathias, R. "Sex-for-Crack Phenomenon Poses Risk for Spread of AIDS in Heterosexuals." *NIDA Notes* 8 (May–June 1993): 8–11.

Merchant, W. "Medications and Athletes." *American Druggist* (October 1992): 6–14.

Merson, M. "Slowing the Spread of HIV: Agenda for the 1990's." *Science* 260 (May 1993): 1266–68.

Millstein, R. "Community Alert Bulletin." Rockville, MD: National Institute on Drug Abuse, U.S. Department of Health and Human Services, 25 March 1993.

Moss, H., L. Kirisci, H. Gordon, and R. Tarter. "A Neuropsychological Profile of Adolescent Alcoholics." *Alcoholism: Clinical and Experimental Research* 18 (1994): 159–63.

"Multistate Outbreak of Poisonings Associated with Illicit Use of GHB." *Prevention Pipeline* 7 (May–June 1994): 95, 96.

National AIDS Program Offices, U.S. Public Health Service. "Drug Abuse and AIDS." In *Drugs of Abuse,* 54. 1989.

National Institute on Drug Abuse. "Drugs and Drug Interactions in Elderly Women." National Institute on Drug Abuse Research Monograph 65. Washington, DC: U.S. Government Printing Office, 1986.

National Institute on Drug Abuse, U.S. Department of Health and Human Services. *National Household Survey on Drug Abuse: Population Estimates, 1989.* DHHS Pub. no. ADM789-1636. Washington, DC: U.S. Government Printing Office, 1989.

Novello, A. "Preventing the Alcohol and Other Drug Problems of HIV/AIDS." *Prevention Pipeline* 5 (September–October 1992): 3–5.

"Ongoing Program Announcement." *NIH Guide* 22 (5 November 1993): 13.

"OTC Drugs and Athletes." *Pharmacy Times* (June 1992): 16.

Parrot, A. *Date Rape and Acquaintance Rape.* New York: Rosen, 1988.

Pietroski, N. "Counseling HIV/AIDS Patients." *American Druggist* (August 1993): 50–56.

Ragghianti, M. "Save the Innocent Victims of Prison." *Parade* magazine (6 February 1994): 14, 15.

Sandmaier, M. *The Invisible Alcoholics.* New York: McGraw-Hill, 1980.

Samples, P. "Alcoholism in Athletes: New Directions

for Treatment." *The Physician and Sports Medicine* (17 April 1989): 193–202.

Segal, B., F. Cromer, H. Stevens, and P. Wasserman. "Patterns of Reasons for Drug Use Among Detained and Adjudicated Juveniles." *International Journal of Addictions* 17 (1982): 1117–30.

Toronto, R. "Young Athletes Who Use 'Enhancing' Steroids Risk Severe Physical Consequences." *Salt Lake Tribune* 244 (6 July 1992): C-5.

U.S. Department of Health and Human Services (USDHHS). *Seventh Special Report to Congress on Alcohol and Health*. Washington, DC: National Institute on Alcohol Abuse and Alcoholism, 1990.

U.S. Department of Justice. "Anabolic Steroids and You." A pamphlet from the Demand Reduction Section, Drug Enforcement Administration. Washington, DC 20537, 1991–1992.

Walsh, F., and M. Sheinkman. "Family Context of Adolescence." In *Adolescent Substance Abuse, Etiology, Treatment and Prevention,* edited by G. Lawson and A. Lawson, 149–71. Gaithersburg, MD: Aspen, 1992.

Weiss, R. "How Does HIV Cause AIDS?" *Science* 260 (May 1993): 1273–79.

Welder, A., and R. Melchert. "Cardiotoxic Effects of Cocaine and Anabolic-Androgenic Steroids in the Athlete." *Journal of Pharmacological and Toxicological Methods* 29 (1993): 61–68.

Wentz, A. "22.2 Million Women Just Don't Get IT." *Prevention Pipeline* 7 (May–June 1994): 127, 128.

"Women Smokers Run High Risk for Lung Cancer." *Prevention Pipeline* 7 (May–June 1994): 7.

Wright, L. "Suicidal Thoughts and Their Relationship to Family Stress and Personal Problems Among High School Seniors and College Undergraduates." *Adolescence* 20 (1985): 575–80.

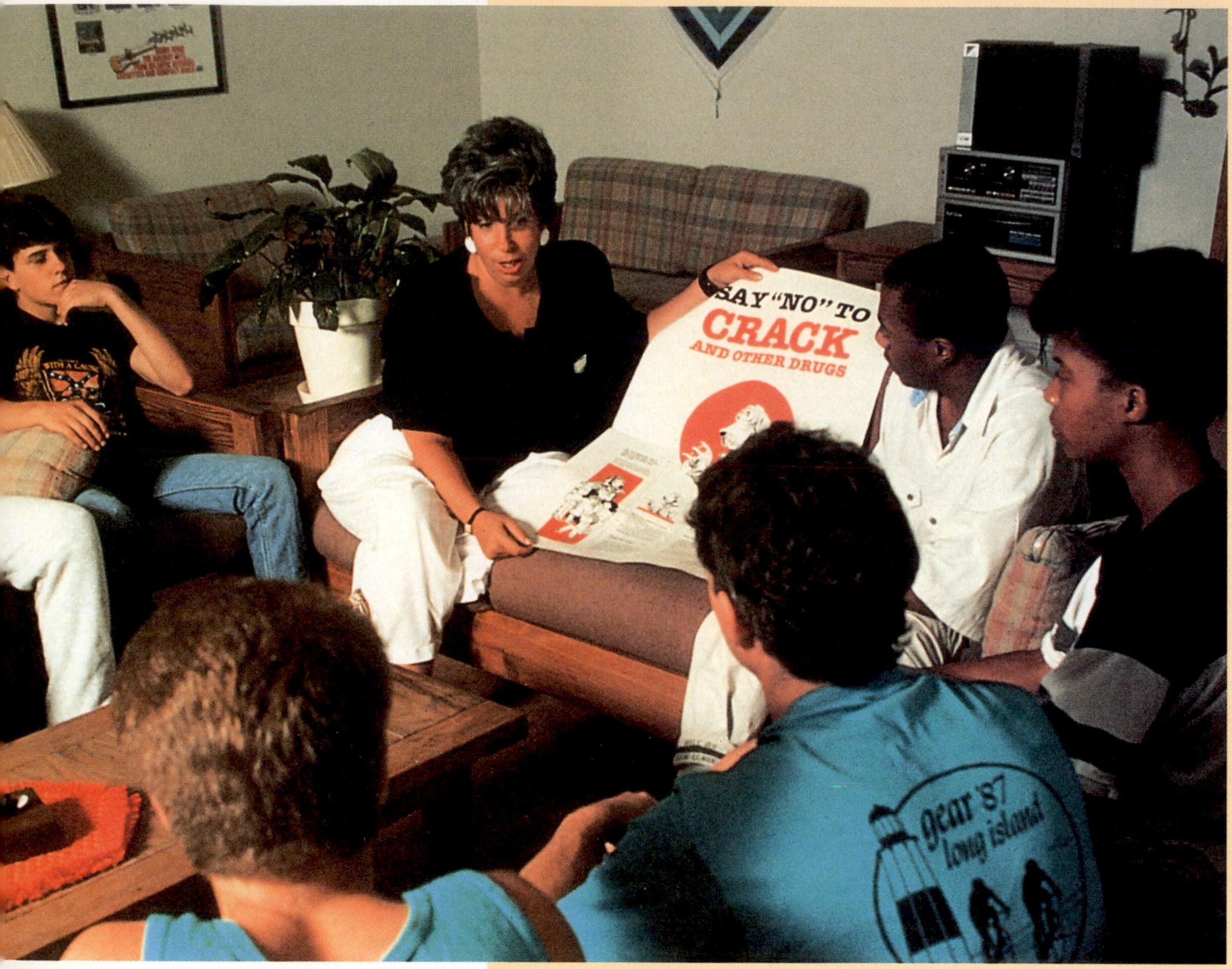

Chapter 16

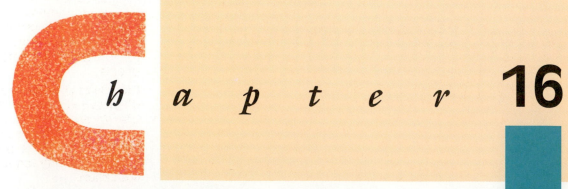

DID YOU KNOW THAT . . .

- In addition to the millions who are known drug users or abusers, there are additional millions who secretly use drugs.
- Addiction is only one phase of drug use and abuse.
- Prominent drug abuse researchers view some of the major causes of addiction as originating from poverty, affluence, racism, and dysfunctional personalities, families, and communities.
- Scare tactics used to warn against drug use have been proven to be ineffective.
- Drug treatment will never work if the user is unwilling to cease use.
- Drug education actually began in the 1800s with the temperance movement.
- Some believe that drug abuse is widespread because we have an innate need to alter our consciousness.
- Generally, people who do not use psychoactive drugs have discovered other methods of altering their consciousness.
- Rehabilitation cannot succeed if it is not specifically tailored to the type of person and the type of drug user.
- The success of a treatment program for drug dependence cannot always be based on total abstinence because, in reality, this is rarely achieved.
- The primary approaches for treating drug abuse are medical, psychotherapeutic, social, behavioral, and innovative approaches.
- Detoxification programs are aimed at reducing drug dependence to zero.
- Maintenance programs do not eliminate drug addiction; they merely stabilize it.
- Hypnosis and acupuncture are also being used by drug addicts as treatment methods.

Education, Prevention, and Treatment

LEARNING OBJECTIVES

On completing this chapter, you will be able to

1. List and briefly describe the four phases of addiction.
2. Explain the general views of addiction.
3. Describe and explain the two models of drug addiction and dependence.
4. List the five most addictive drugs.
5. Describe and briefly explain the following drug education program models: cognitive and information-based models, peer tutoring, teaching and counseling, and the social influence and resistance model.
6. Explain and give examples of the differences among primary, secondary, and tertiary prevention.
7. Describe the three approaches to prevention programs targeted to children and adolescents.

(continued)

Healthy People 2000

Establish and monitor in 50 states comprehensive plans to ensure access to alcohol and drug treatment programs for traditionally underserved people.

Provide to children in all school districts and private schools primary and secondary school educational programs on alcohol and other drugs, preferably as part of quality school health education.

LEARNING OBJECTIVES

8 Describe the alternative to drugs program.
9 Explain the difference between drug treatment and drug prevention.
10 Explain the differences among inhospital care, residential care, and day hospitals or intensive outpatient services.
11 Define the three states of consciousness—*ergotropic, normal,* and *trophotropic.*
12 List and briefly discuss the differences among the six primary approaches to drug treatment.
13 Give a brief account of how either hypnosis or acupuncture can be used to treat drug abuse.

Over 23 million Americans use drugs monthly (Senate Task Force for a Drug Free America, 1990). Although licit and illicit drug use is declining, disturbing percentages remain statistically significant. Early estimates from the latest 1992 National Household Survey on Drug Abuse (Office of Applied Studies 1993) reports that with regard to lifetime drug use by the U.S. population aged 12 and over, 36% use or have used one or more illicit-type drugs; 83% use or have used alcohol; 71% use or have used cigarettes; and 15% use or have used smokeless tobacco.

Some believe that substance abuse is one of the most serious problems facing our society and its future. To prevent and/or treat this problem, we need to understand some of the reasons why such abuse occurs. Some of the reasons include the following:

- An inability to cope with anxiety, conflict, and depression
- Physiological dependence and addiction (generally related to genetic causes)
- Psychological dependence and addiction, caused by the mental addiction associated with the belief that the drug is needed to relax and/or relieve anxiety
- Personality disturbances
- Abundance of drugs in the environment
- Peer pressure
- Faulty parental modeling and upbringing
- Dysfunctional families
- Economic factors such as unemployment and poverty
- Role strain and/or role deprivation (inability and/or unable to fulfill roles demanded by society)
- Faulty ego defense mechanisms
- Addiction to immediate, short-term pleasures
- Estrangement from the conventional values of society
- Negative accusations by family and friends (see Chapter 2, on labeling theory)
- Overly permissive—or overly strict—family relationships

Although only a small sampling is listed here, causes vary immensely. From this we can logically assume that if there is such a variety of causes, then any effective education, prevention, and treatment programs, procedures, and modalities need to vary to address these divergent causes.

In this chapter, we discuss the vast array of educational, preventive, and treatment-oriented drug use and/or abuse programs available. We also discuss the major views, controversies, strengths and weaknesses of prevention and treatment. We hope that by providing this comprehensive review of education, prevention, and treatment methods we will advance your knowledge of substance abuse issues that may occur in your life or affecting someone who has touched your life.

Chapter 1 began by outlining the scope of the substance abuse problem; Chapter 2 covered the major theories of why people use and/or abuse drugs; and Chapter 15 introduced the problems of drug use and/or abuse by the special population groups.

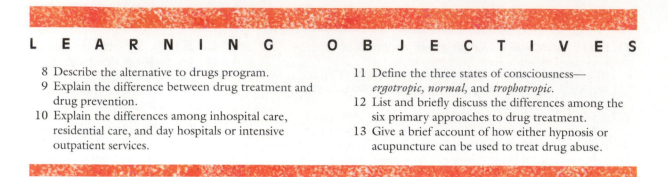

Given this context, what can be done to prevent drug abuse? Knowledge is certainly part of the answer. People must be informed about what drugs do and at what point using them becomes a problem. Equally important, people must know how to identify when a problem exists and what can be done to resolve it.

We will begin by defining *addiction,* offering several views of its meaning and social impact. A discussion of *drug education* follows; education is considered as a tool for controlling drug abuse, particularly among youth. *Drug prevention* is examined in some detail; both traditional and nontraditional approaches are presented. The final topic is *drug treatment*—namely, alternative goals, settings, and methods. A review of the effectiveness of various approaches ends the chapter.

The Nature of Drug Addiction

The American Problem

From the earliest days to the present, various types of drug dependence have plagued American society. At various times, drug dependence has been considered a moral violation, a criminal act, and an illness. Throughout history, the laws that have been passed in the United States have reflected the moral code of the times.

The history of drug addiction shows that, in the early days, alcoholism was rampant, and there were some pockets of opiate dependence. The Pilgrims and Puritans did not forbid drinking, only overindulgence. When the Revolutionary War ended in 1783, people continued to accept heavy drinking as a normal way of life, despite the belief that it was morally wrong to drink to excess. So many Americans were addicted to alcohol that Presidents Washington and Jefferson suggested that people switch from drinking distilled spirits to beer and wine, to reduce the disruptive influence of alcoholism.

Other drug addictions developed, as well. From the early 1800s to the early 1900s, opiate and cocaine addiction grew; it was legal to smoke and use these drugs, and they were widely available. Patent medicines, tonics, and elixirs contained liberal amounts of opiates and cocaine as well as alcohol, which compounded the drug dependence.

Barbiturates were also available in the early 1900s. Even though some people became addicted, little attention was given to this problem because often supplies were obtained through medical channels. Amphetamine dependence was also managed medically. Barbiturates and amphetamines were not restricted by federal laws until 1965.

The Addiction Process

In tracing the history of addiction to substances, we are left to ask, how does addition occur? What is the difference between recreational use and drug abuse? Four separate phases characterize the *process* of addiction. These four phases are **initial use, habitual use, addiction,** and **relapse** (Akers 1992, 16; see Figure 16.1). The first phase, *initial use,* involves occasional use or experimentation with drugs without prior use. Often this occurs intermittently, sporadically, or because of a unique set

INITIAL USE first phase in the addiction process, in which occasional use or experimentation with drugs without prior use occurs

HABITUAL USE second phase in the addiction process, in which a more patterned regular involvement with a particular drug(s) occurs

ADDICTION third phase in the addiction process, consisting of periodic or chronic dependence on a drug or several drugs; an insatiable desire to use drugs contrary to legal and/or social prohibitions

RELAPSE fourth phase in the addiction process, in which the user who stopped habitual use returns to regular use after having experienced some form of withdrawal symptoms

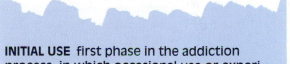

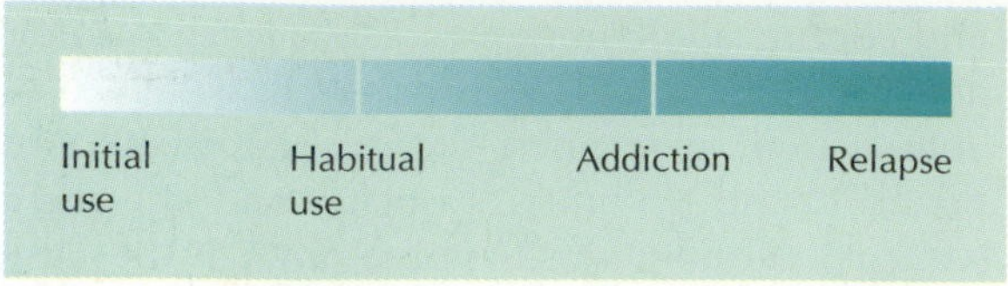

FIGURE 16.1 Processes of Addiction
Source: Deborah Franklin. "Hooked/Not Hooked. Why Isn't Everyone an Addict?" In *Health* (November—December 1990):41.

of circumstances. The second phase, *habitual use,* involves a more patterned regular involvement with a particular drug, or drugs, as with polydrug users. It is important to note that the "regular use" of drugs can vary enormously from consistent weekend use to daily use. As defined in Chapter 1, *addiction* is the third phase and it represents the higher end of habitual use. Addiction is described as a form of use characterized by repetitive and destructive use of one or more mood-altering substances. This often results from either or both a biological and/or psychological vulnerability or desirability exposed or induced by environmental forces. Addiction also includes **tolerance,** defined as a physical or biological attachment to the drug leading to physical dependence, to the point of withdrawal symptoms if the drug is stopped, and psychological dependence when mental craving for the drug follows. *Relapse* is the fourth phase when the user who stopped habitual use returns to regular use after having experienced some form of withdrawal symptoms.

Views on Addiction

In 1964, the World Health Organization of the United Nations (WHO) defined *addiction* as "a state of periodic or chronic intoxication detrimental to the individual and society, which is characterized by an overwhelming desire to continue taking the drug and to obtain it by any means" (World Health Organization 1964, 9–10; see also Eddy et al. 1965, 721–733). Today the WHO prefers the term *drug dependence,* which is indicative of changing views.

In the same definition, specific reference is made to "a particular state of mind that is termed 'psychic dependence'" (Eddy et al. 1965, 723). As we proceed in this chapter, you will notice how education, prevention, and treatment programs are geared to either educate against, prevent, or treat this psychic dependence. The word *addiction,* derived from the Latin verb *addicere,* refers to the process of binding to things. Today, the word largely refers to a chronic adherence to drugs. In our definition, we include physical and/or psychological dependence. Physical dependence is the body's need to constantly have the drug or drugs, and psychological dependence is the mental inability to stop using the drug or drugs (White 1991). Sociologists Inciardi, Horowitz, and Pottiega state that "addiction entails three characteristics: chronic use and compulsion, plus resulting problems" (1993, 83).

Others view addiction as a "career"—a series of steps or phases with distinguishable characteristics. One career pattern of addiction lists six phases: (1) experimentation or initiation, (2) escalation (increasing use), (3) maintaining or "taking care of business" (optimistic use of drugs coupled with successful job performance), (4) dysfunctional or "going through changes" (problems with constant use and unsuccessful attempts to quit), (5) recovery or "getting out of the life" (arriving at a successful view about quitting and receiving drug treatment), and (6) ex-addict (actually quitting) (Waldorf 1983; also in Clinard and Meier 1992, 206–207).

There are conflicting views on the nature of drug addiction and dependence. Two examples are the major models that prevail regarding alcohol abuse: the **moral model** and the **medical model.** The moral model believes that people abuse alco-

TOLERANCE a physical or biological attachment to a drug leading to a physical dependence

MORAL MODEL the belief that people abuse alcohol because they choose to do so

MEDICAL MODEL the belief that people abuse alcohol because of some biologically caused condition

CROSS CURRENTS

Should we illegalize all drugs that are not used for medical purposes? Look at the diagram and notice that such licit drugs as nicotine, alcohol, and caffeine are as highly addictive as many illicit drugs. From an addiction potential standpoint, why do you think the manufacture, sale, and use of these drugs are not prohibited by law? Are they "safer" than other drugs depicted in this diagram? Develop pro and con arguments for one of the following positions:

1. Alcohol and nicotine are the only two drugs that should remain legalized, because many members of our society need to be free from the shackles of the illegality of all addictive drugs. Such adages as "What a person does with his or her life is nobody's business" and "Certain people are always going to use drugs no matter what the government does" support the two positions.
2. Society is unnecessarily harmed socially and economically by the legal manufacture and sale of alcohol and nicotine. Because of these costs to society, these drugs should be prohibited.

Cite some statistics and facts from authoritative sources to support your position on this issue.

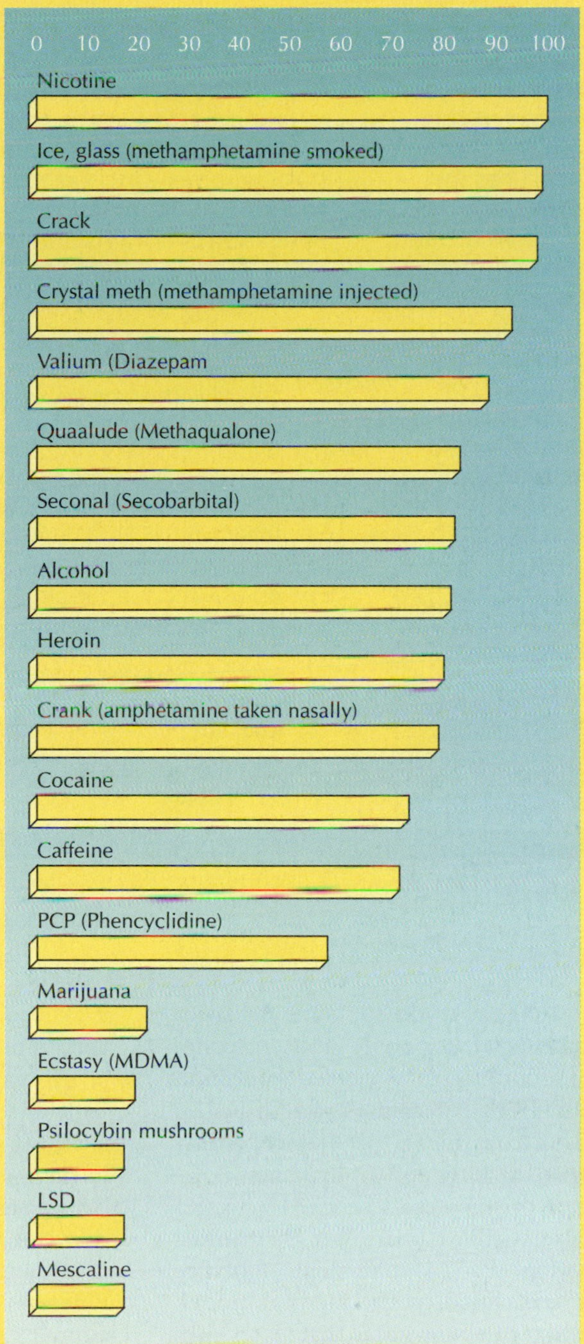

Here and Now

Harm Reduction Model

The Netherlands has put into action a new national harm reduction policy with regard to drug use. The focus of this policy is to eliminate strong punishment measures for cannabis use previously advocated by the punitive model of drug control and minimize financial costs for other citizens. Harm reduction reduces the harm facing drug users by allowing them the use of certain drugs, mainly cannabis-type drugs (marijuana and hashish), in prescribed locations such as coffeeshops and cafes and other injectable-type drugs (such as heroin) in one open-air park. S. Trebach, president of the Drug Policy foundation in Washington, D.C., says that "Harm reduction is the middle ground between traditional prohibition and full legalization" (Treaster 1993, E5). Overall, the goal is to reduce personal harm such as stiff jail sentences for drug use while simultaneously increasing the availability of the nation's education programs and treatment and prevention facilities for chronic drug users.

> In 1982, the Netherlands amended the 1928 Opium Act and gave the new drug policy the name "normalization." Under this policy, drug use, even heroin and cocaine use, is not prohibited by law. Only possession is prohibited.
>
> [Possession of] Schedule One drugs—cocaine, heroin, amphetamines, and LSD—[defined as] . . . "unacceptable risk" [-type drugs and the cannabis products], is prohibited, but possession of up to 30 grams of the cannabis products is only a misdemeanor—punishable by law, but our pragmatic prosecution policy [in the Netherlands] allows for discretion.

"Normalization [policy] does not mean everything is legal." Trafficking in drugs or stealing drugs requires punishment. How much punishing occurs in the Netherlands? Of the prison population, 30% is incarcerated for drug-related reasons, and in Amsterdam and Rotterdam, the percentage is 50%.

> The Dutch drug policy of *de facto** decriminalization of cannabis products has not encouraged more drug use. In fact, the prevalence of cannabis use in the Netherlands is low. In the age bracket between 10 and 18 years, 4.2

hol because they choose to do so, while the medical model suggests that people abuse alcohol because of some biologically caused condition (Venturelli 1994, 1–2). A recent Bureau of Justice Statistics, U.S. Department of Justice, study reports that approximately 25% of drug law violators released from prison were rearrested for a second drug offense within a year after their initial release from prison (U.S. Department of Justice 1992) could be explained by the medical model. The medical model of abuse states that alcoholism is akin to an uncontrollable disease that often subverts rational control over drinking.

Regardless of whether drug dependence is truly a disease, it is also a social problem, one that is clearly linked to social and economic conditions in the community and the nation. Granted, not all drug users turn to crime. However, drug dependence is tied to a host of social problems—from divorce to domestic violence to accidents and illnesses such as AIDS and cancer. It is a highly complex problem.

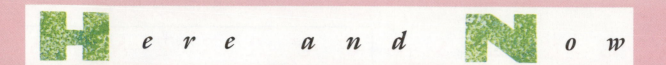

percent has ever used cannabis in their lifetime. Among this group, less than 2 percent are still using occasionally. The number of daily cannabis users appears to be one in 1,000. . . ."

Harm Reduction Policy

The Dutch drug treatment philosophy . . . attempts to focus on primary problems involved in drug abuse. The government encourages forms of treatment that are not intended to end addiction as such, but to improve addicts' physical and social well-being, and to help them function in society.

This kind of assistance may be defined as harm reduction, or, more traditionally, secondary and tertiary prevention. The effect takes the form of field-work in the street, hospital, jails and open door clinics for prostitutes. . . .

The result of Dutch health policy is that it is able to reach a very large segment of the total population of drug addicts. In Amsterdam, about 60–80 percent are being reached by some kind of assistance. . . . [In fact,] there have never been so many addicts asking for detoxification and drug free treatment. In Amsterdam, such requests doubled between 1981 and 1986.

Other results from applying this model of drug prevention are also noteworthy.

Reliable estimates on the number of drug addicts in the Netherlands, with a population of 14.5 million, vary between 15,000 and 20,000. Drug use appears to be stabilizing, even decreasing in some cities. Estimates on the number of addicts in Amsterdam, the largest city, vary from 4,000 to 7,000. The prevalence of heroin use in Amsterdam is estimated at 0.4 percent. The use of cocaine has stabilized at 0.6 percent, while crack use is still a virtual rarity. Finally, and perhaps what is most important, between 1981 and 1987 the average age of heroin and cocaine users in Amsterdam rose from 26 to 36 years.

Source: Eddy Engelsman. "The Dutch Model." *New Perspectives Quarterly* 6, no. 3 (Summer 1989), 44–45.

**De facto* refers to laws that are enforced by government.

Levels of Addiction

Drug addiction develops as a process; it is not a sudden occurrence. Several levels of addiction have been identified (Doweiko 1990, 12–13):

Level 0: Total abstinence. The individual never uses drugs for recreational purposes.

Level 1: Rare social use. The individual rarely uses chemicals during or for recreation.

Level 2: Heavy social use and drug use problems. The individual is perceived as a frequent user and abuser of drugs. Social, legal, financial, and occupational problems are likely.

Level 3: Early addiction. The individual is dependent on drugs. Some medical complications will likely occur in the early to middle stages of addiction, followed by more intense medical problems (ulcers, fatty deposits on the liver, hepatitis, pancreatitis, gastritis, and frequent blackouts). The individual at this level may continue to deny dependence.

Level 4: Mature or late addiction. The indi-

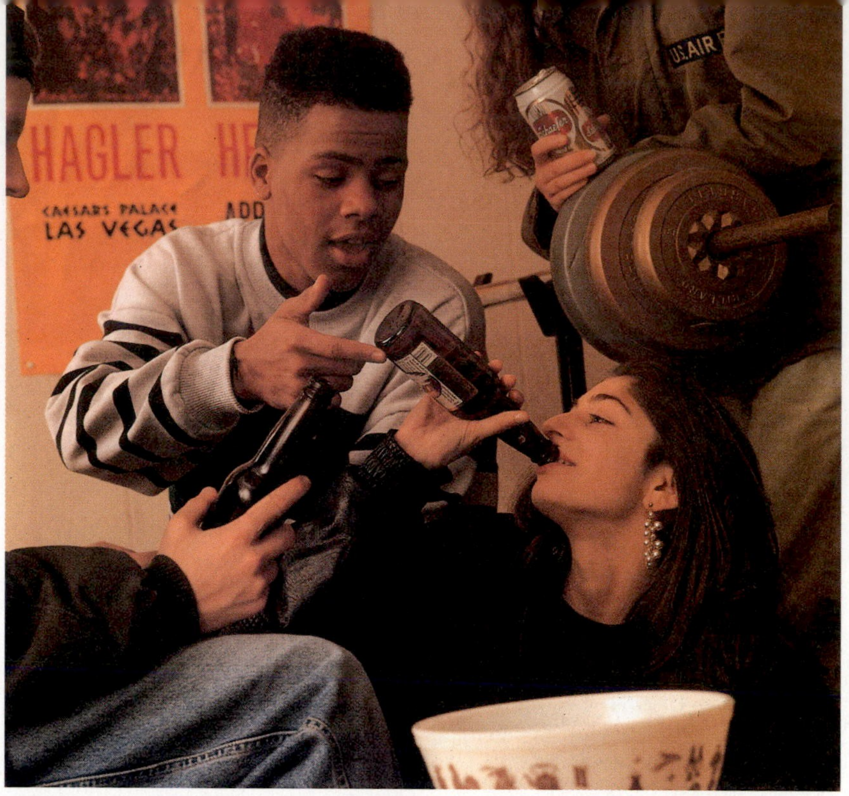

In adolescent groups, the spread of drug abuse usually involves peer influence.

vidual is affected by several medical consequences of the dependence and may even be near death. Most friends and family members have experienced a devastating deterioration in their social relations with the addict.

Drug Education

As discussed in several other chapters of this book, an important factor in drug abuse is the pervasive influence of peers. In some cases, all it takes is one person persuading another to experience the pleasure of using a particular drug.

We cannot account for all drug abuse in this manner, but we can say that most drug use begins as a result of social influence. **Social influence** is the ability to inspire, motivate, or convince others to go along with or share in novel behavior. In adolescent groups, the spread of drug abuse nearly always involves peer influence. Given that peer influence is so important, drug education is a strategy for teaching and persuading potential drug users not to abuse drugs.

Using Education to Control Drug Use

Education has been used extensively in the past to control the use and abuse of drugs, especially alcohol and tobacco. Drug education actually began in the late 1800s, when most states required that the harmful effects of certain drugs be taught. An example of an early educational attempt to curb or stop drug abuse is the temperance movement in the late nineteenth century. The Women's Christian Temperance Union (WCTU) and the Anti-Saloon League taught that alcohol consumption was harmful and against Christian morality.

Today, school programs, drug education courses, and the mass media are used extensively as

SOCIAL INFLUENCE the ability to inspire, motivate, or convince others to go along with or share in novel behavior

Here and Now

Addiction and Withdrawal

The cause of addiction or drug dependency is difficult to pinpoint. The use of many drugs causes a sense of euphoria or an escape from unpleasant realities in life. Use of the drug creates a new chemical balance in the body. Absence of the drug results in a new imbalance, which in turn causes a craving for the drug. It is hard to tell where the cycle starts and impossible to totally separate physical from psychological factors. Each drug dependency is contextual to the particular person.

Withdrawal from drug dependency is also very difficult. Drug use leads the brain and other organs to reach a new balance with the drug being present. Withdrawal of the drug then forces the brain to revert back to the balance present prior to drug use. This can be a long process. It is estimated that it takes 20–30 hours for the body to return to a normal balance following the consumption of two alcoholic drinks and 3 weeks to return to normal following 10 days of cocaine use. Once an individual has been dependent on a drug, there appears to be a "memory" of the drug-induced balance, and the body reverts back to that balance very quickly upon re-exposure to the drug.

As we learn more about the brain and how it works, we are able to learn more about how these drugs affect the brain. This knowledge will help us deal with the problem of drug dependency.

Source: Gary L. Johnson. "Addiction and Withdrawal." *HAPS News* (January 1992):12.

mediums for educating the public about the negative consequences of drug abuse. Strategies vary enormously but can be placed into three general categories:

1. Those that focus and provide information
2. Those that stress values, beliefs, and attitudes
3. Those that emphasize the consequences of drug use (namely, warnings and scare tactics about drug abuse)

Considering the Audience and Approach

The audience for drug education is composed of users and nonusers. In analyzing the population of users, categories include (1) committed users, those who abuse drugs and have no interest in stopping; (2) former users; (3) nonproblem drug users, those who abuse drugs on occasion, mostly for recreation; and (4) problem users (Kinney 1991).

It is important for people involved in drug education to know about different types of users so that programs can cater to the specific needs of these groups. For committed users, drug education should aim to prevent or delay drug abuse. Former users should be given information that will reinforce their decision to quit abusing drugs. For nonproblem users, drug education programs should examine the abuse of drugs, reinforce the importance of how uncontrolled use leads to abuse, and education on how to prevent use from escalating to abuse. Finally, for problem users, the goals should be to reduce use and change use patterns by presenting successful prevention strategies.

Professionals planning a drug education program have to decide on the type of audience they intend to pursue. A number of questions should be considered: To what type of audience should the drug information be targeted? youths or adults? peers or parents? Should information focus on knowledge, attitudes, or behavior? Should drug education emphasize and recommend abstinence *or* responsible use?

In most cases, it is appropriate for drug education to focus on knowledge, attitudes, and behavior. The three are clearly related. For instance, if the goal is to increase knowledge, should we assume that attitudes and behavior will change accordingly, or is knowledge about the harmful effects of drugs separate from attitudes and behavior? In other words, if you learn that smoking marijuana is a health hazard, equal to or more destructive than smoking cigarettes, does this knowledge change the satisfaction you derive from smoking marijuana with friends? Some would say yes. Unfortunately, many also would say no. In fact, knowledge about the harmful effects of certain types of drugs has very little effect on the personal attitudes and habits of most people. Proof of this is how many cigarette smokers are aware of the health risks involved with smoking but continue to smoke, day after day and year after year.

Drug education programs have to direct attention to a small range of behavioral objectives; they will not be effective if they address too many issues.

Finally, drug educators must decide if they will stress total abstinence or responsible use. Abstinence is radically different from responsible use. A program cannot advocate both. Consider the following: If a program is to promote abstinence, it is certain to lose compulsive users and others not convinced that drug use (or even the use of a particular drug) is bad. If the program stresses responsible use, it will lose people wanting abstinence, and, depending on the type of drug, others may or may not offer support. This decision is very complicated.

Program Models

There are a number of different education models, which accommodate various audiences. Discussions of these models follow:

The *cognitive model,* when applied separately, initially stressed the danger of drug abuse, often employing scare tactics (see Baumann's and Waterston's 1994 analysis of the televised scare tactics used by the Partnership for a Drug-Free America). Lately, however, a more rational and moderate approach has become popular because the scare tactics did not work in alleviating drug use. Recently, the cognitive model was modified to encourage the following tactics:

1. Convey the message that society is inconsistent concerning drug use. For example, certain drugs that cause serious harm to a large percentage of the population are legal, while other drugs that have less impact are illegal.
2. Convey that the reasons for drug use are complex and that drug users vary.
3. Demonstrate to youth that the young and old alike are affected by role models, in that attitudes regarding drug use are often patterned from family members who are role models.
4. That other influential role models in music, art, drama, business, and education who use and abuse drugs can affect attitudes toward drug use.

The goal of the cognitive-based model conveying these messages is to strengthen and encourage the nonuse of drugs by impressionable youth. Largely by informing and appealing to their intellect, young people are made aware that attitudes about drug use can be conveyed by significant others. Although these education-based programs have generally been effective with adults, such singularly applied programs (applied in the absence of other programs) have been ineffective with older adolescents (Forman and Linney 1988; Schups et al. 1981), but moderately effective with younger adolescents who have never tried drugs before exposure to such cognitive models.

The *cognitive model* stresses accurate, unbiased, and straightforward information on the use and effects of drugs. The model assumes that the audience is composed of rational people who can intelligently decide for themselves whether drug abuse is worth the physical and psychological risks involved.

Peer tutoring, teaching, and counseling employ peers or older youth to disseminate information on drug abuse. This includes using rehabilitated or recovering drug addicts and abusers as counselors;

they can identify with the audience and provide advice from "someone who's been there."

Social influence and resistance focuses largely on teaching how to resist peer pressure. Teachers and trainers in workshop settings teach students how to disagree, how to say no, how to be assertive without fear of reprisal, and how to respond effectively when drugs are offered in social settings. To date, this model has had much success in curtailing and alleviating drug use (Botvin 1990; Akers 1992).

Curriculum-Based Drug Education Objectives

In an effort to educate students and make them aware of the dangers in using drugs, school-based drug education programs and objectives have been implemented in most U.S. school curriculums. Specific objectives have been established for elementary, junior high, and senior high and college levels. These include

Elementary Level

Drugs versus poisons
Effects of alcohol, tobacco, and marijuana on the body
Differences between candy and drugs
Drug overdoses
Dangers of experimentation
Saying no to peers using drugs
Reasons for taking drugs: curing illness, pleasure, escape, parental use, and ceremony

Junior High Level

How peer pressure works
Saying no to peer pressure
How drugs affect the body, physiologically and psychologically
Seeking help when needed
Attitudes toward drug use
Having fun without drugs
Harmful effects of tobacco, alcohol, and marijuana on the body
How advertisers push drugs
Consequences of breaking drug laws
Differences between wine, beer, and distilled spirits
Family drug use
Identifying family drinking problems and identifying family members who may have drug addiction problems
Images of violence and drug use in rock and rap music
Teenage drug abuse and associated problems
"Just say no" programs

Senior High and College Level

Responsible use of medications
How drugs affect the body and the mind
Legal versus illegal drugs
Drinking and driving
Drug effects on the fetus
Recreational drug use
Ways of coping with problems
Detecting problem drug users
Drug education, prevention, and treatment
Positive and negative role models
Criminal sanctions for various types of drug use
"Binge" drinking
Driving and date rape
Addiction to drugs and alcoholism
"Just say no" programs

Prevention

When we speak of prevention, we are referring to efforts made to dissuade potential drug users. There are three types of prevention: primary, secondary, and tertiary. The major differences among these types of prevention are summarized in Table 16.1.

Primary prevention, defined as "persuasion against the abuse of a particular drug," seeks to avoid drug abuse. The idea of primary prevention is complex and may include alternatives to drugs, personal and social growth strategies, mental health promotion, and individual motivation to reach a high level of functioning. Theoretically, this will prevent problems associated with drug abuse from occurring.

Secondary prevention entails using immediate intervention once drug abuse has begun. Fines and

TABLE 16.1 Differences among primary, secondary, and tertiary drug abuse and addiction prevention

Timing	Activities	Terminology
Before abuse	Education Information Alternatives Personal and social growth	Primary prevention
During early stages of abuse	Crisis intervention Early diagnosis Crisis monitoring Referral	Secondary prevention
During later stages of abuse	Treatment Institutionalization Maintenance Detoxification	Tertiary prevention

Source: J. D. Swisher. "Prevention Issues." In *Handbook on Drug Abuse,* edited by R. L. DuPont, A. Goldstein, and J. O'Donnell (Washington, DC: National Institute on Drug Abuse, 1979).

incarceration are examples of secondary prevention measures for someone caught using marijuana. The goal of secondary prevention is to warn that continued drug abuse will lead to more serious consequences.

Tertiary prevention helps individuals to stop abusing drugs either immediately prior to addiction or in its early stages. Tertiary prevention is designed to help those who are already fairly dependent to cease drug use.

Three Approaches to Prevention Programs Targeted to Children and Adolescents

The cognitive and information-based drug education prevention programs that were developed in the 1970s, with their emphasis on "scare tactics," were judged to be so ineffective that the federal government created the Special Office for Drug Abuse Prevention (SODAP). SODAP determined that such programs had to be banned because federal tax dollars were being wasted.

A second approach to advancing drug prevention was to use affective education (Wallack and Corbett 1990). This approach aims at strengthening self-esteem, interpersonal skills, and logical thinking. Stress is placed on recreational activities, volunteer community services, and active participation in cultural events. (More will be said about this affective approach under alternatives to drugs.) Unfortunately, this second approach also met with little success.

The third prevention approach was heavily influenced by the "social inoculation" theory (McGuire 1969, 1985) which states that youth need to be armed against the alcohol and drug attack. Adolescents must be taught counterarguments and methods for resisting peer pressure to use alcohol and drugs. Once adolescents are equipped with such resistance skills, abstention from alcohol and drug use is more likely to result.

Because this third approach of equipping youth with resistance toward drug use was promising and bore promising results, Project DARE (Drug Abuse Resistance Education) was developed by the Los Angeles Police Department and the Los Angeles Unified School District. Project DARE targets fifth- and sixth-grade students and teaches them the art of peer pressure resistance, lessons on improving self-esteem, and the negative consequences of using alcohol and/or drugs. Furthermore, practical methods for coping with stress and having drug-free fun are also emphasized. Generally, 17 classroom sessions are taught by police officers. (See Table 16.2 for a summary of the 17 class lessons.) As of 1993, this program operates in approximately two hundred communities nationally.

Evaluations of this prevention program show that students who have completed the lessons are less likely to use and/or abuse alcohol, cigarettes, and other illicit drugs. Other longitudinal studies lasting years found that DARE graduates were less likely to either use or abuse drugs (Bangert-Downs 1988). Although Project DARE is deemed to be the most successful when comparisons are made against the other two approaches targeted at children and adolescents, the latest evaluation presented one setback. Clayton et al. (1991) report in their latest evaluation that student attitudes concerning drug use showed significant effects, while self-reports showed no change in actual drug use. Thus, there appears to be some inconsistency between general student attitudes toward drug use and personal self-assessments on individual drug use. The discrepancy between strengthening attitudes against drug use at large and personal use remains troubling, because while students indicated less approval of drug use, personal use was not as significantly affected.

The Role of Social and Personal Development

In the past several years, most drug abuse prevention specialists have adopted the idea of emphasizing personal and social development as a method for preventing the harmful consequences of drug abuse. Three issues are primary:

1. Increased self-understanding and acceptance through activities such as values clarification, sensory awareness, and decision making
2. Improved interpersonal relations through activities such as communication training, peer counseling, and assertiveness training
3. Increased ability for meeting one's needs and accomplishing goals through social institutions such as the family, church, and community affiliations

Since 1989, the federal government has spent approximately $3 billion on funding new drug education and prevention programs under the Anti-Drug Abuse Acts of 1986 and 1988 ("Measuring" 1991, 5). Moreover, the U.S. federal government directs a diverse selection of programs that are useful in helping to prevent drug abuse. These programs range from treatment of delinquency to mental health activities to a wide range of activities developed by groups funded by the National Institute on Drug Abuse (NIDA). Drug information and referrals to social help agencies are several alternatives to drug abuse.

Presently, these programs do not have a major impact in primary prevention because of inconsistent funding, duplication of services, and recent cutbacks in federal spending.

The following assumptions should be behind all primary prevention programs (U.S. Department of Education 1992):

1. A reasonable goal for drug abuse prevention should be to educate people of all ages about responsible decision making regarding the use of all drugs.
2. Responsible decisions regarding personal use of drugs should result in fewer negative consequences for individuals.
3. The most effective approach to achieve the preceding goals would be a program that increases self-esteem, interpersonal skills, and participation in alternatives to drug use and involves parents.

Many local, state, and federal agencies have similar goals for dealing with other forms of problem behavior. What is needed is a unified, governmental effort that would result in funding of the development, implementation, and evaluation of a multidimensional prevention effort.

NIDA and several individual researchers have evaluated the multitude of drug abuse prevention programs in the United States. The general conclusions of these studies are

1. Very few programs have demonstrated clear success or have been adequate in evaluating themselves.
2. The relationships among information about drugs, attitudes toward use, and actual uses of drugs are unclear in these programs.

TABLE 16.2 DARE Lessons

The DARE curriculum is organized into 17 classroom sessions conducted by the police officer, coupled with suggested activities taught by the regular classroom teacher. A wide range of teaching activities are used: question-and-answer, group-discussion, and role-play and workbook exercises, all designed to encourage student participation and response.

Each lesson is briefly summarized below, giving a sense of the scope of the DARE curriculum and the care taken in its preparation. All of these lessons were pilot tested and revised before widespread use began.

1. *Practices for Personal Safety.* The DARE officer reviews common safety practices to protect students from harm at home, on the way to and from school, and in the neighborhood.

2. *Drug Use and Misuse.* Students learn the harmful effects of drugs if they are misused as depicted in the film "Drugs and Your Amazing Mind."

3. *Consequences.* Focus in on the consequences of using and not using alcohol and marijuana. If students are aware of those consequences, they can make better informed decisions regarding their own behavior.

4. *Resisting Pressure to Use Drugs.* The DARE officer explains different types of pressure—ranging from friendly persuasion and teasing to threats—that friends and others exert on students to try tobacco, alcohol, or drugs.

5. *Resistance Techniques: Ways to Say No.* Students rehearse the many ways of refusing offers to try tobacco, alcohol, or drugs—simply saying no and repeating it as often as necessary, changing the subject, walking away, or ignoring the person. They learn that they can avoid situations in which they might be subjected to such pressures and can "hang around" with nonusers.

6. *Building Self-esteem.* Poor self-esteem is one of the factors associated with drug misuse. How students feel about themselves results from positive and negative feelings and experiences. In this session students learn about their own positive qualities and how to compliment other students.

7. *Assertiveness: A Response Style.* Students have certain rights—to be themselves, to say what they think, to say no to offers of drugs. The session teaches them to assert those rights confidently and without interfering with others' rights.

8. *Managing Stress Without Taking Drugs.* Students learn to recognize sources of stress in their lives and techniques for avoiding or relieving stress, including exercise, deep breathing, and talking to others. They learn that using drugs or alcohol to relieve stress causes new problems.

9. *Media Influences on Drug Use.* The DARE officer reviews strategies used in the media to encourage tobacco and alcohol use, including testimonials from celebrities and social pressure.

10. *Decision Making and Risk Taking.* Students learn the difference between bad risks and responsible risks, how to recognize their choices, and how to make a decision that promotes their self-interests.

11. *Alternatives to Drug Abuse.* Students learn that to have fun, to be accepted by peers, or to deal with feelings of anger or hurt, there are a number of alternatives to using drugs and alcohol.

12. *Role Modeling.* A high school student selected by the DARE officer with the assistance of the high school staff visits the class, providing students with a positive role model. Students learn that drug users are in the minority.

13. *Forming a Support System.* Students learn that they need to develop positive relationships with many different people to form a support system.

14. *Ways to Deal with Pressures from Gangs.* Students discuss the kinds of pressures they may encounter from gang members and evaluate the consequences of the choices available to them.

15. *DARE Summary.* Students summarize and assess what they have learned.

16. *Taking a Stand.* Students compose and read aloud essays on how they can respond when they are pressured to use drugs and alcohol. The essay represents each student's "DARE Pledge."

17. *Culmination.* In a schoolwide assembly planned in concert with school administrators, all students who have participated in DARE receive certificates of achievement.

Source: Office of Justice Programs, U.S. Department of Justice. *An Introduction to DARE: Drug Abuse Resistance Education,* 2d ed. NCJ 129862 (Washington, DC: U.S. Government Printing Office, October 1991), 12—13.

Here and Now

Suggestions for Making Drug Education Programs More Effective

1. *Practice deliberate planning*—Begin by matching imagined needs with real needs. Make a thorough assessment of drug information needed and problems associated with drug use. Program content should be based on this careful assessment.
2. *Review the previous history*—Don't assume that people who have been exposed to previous educational campaigns have forgotten all of what they learned. Start by considering the amount and the kind of information people have already been exposed to. If they have experience with drug education, what was successful in previous campaigns?
3. *Establish links between the messages conveyed and learned and other aspects of students' life experiences*—Involve students, teachers, administrators, and even school janitors in the drug education program. Be aware that drug use comes from many sources and that students are involved in many relationships. The drug education program must involve parents and guardians as well as the wider community.
4. *Effectively promote programs*—The information you have to convey must reach important voters and decision makers in the community. The information has to be disseminated effectively to a wide audience.
5. *Allocate resources properly*—Be mindful that, unless drug use and abuse has become a community-wide burning issue, people will tend to be interested in the drug campaign initially but be quick to lose interest. If the drug education program is to take place in schools, for example, make certain that the amounts of curriculum time and staffing are adequate and can be sustained throughout the program's duration.
6. *Evaluate constantly*—Is the program effective for the target audience? Are the goals conveyed and understood by the target population? What are the positive and negative outcomes of the strategy employed? Interview staff members of the program as well as the members of the target audience. Are they satisfied? What suggestions do they have for improving the program? These are very important questions. Their answers will reveal if the drug education program is meeting its goals (U.S. Department of Education 1992).

Some factors that are key to developing successful programs include the following:

1. *Coordinating prevention at different levels.* Successful programs involve families, schools, and communities. In most cases, these efforts are not coordinated.

2. *Integrating ongoing activities of schools, families, and community organizations.* Superficial introduction of drug prevention strategies has limited effects. For instance, door-to-door distribution of literature to households, in-class presentations of the harmful effects of drugs, and posting banners and slogans warning of the consequences of drug abuse in communities are not successful methods. Instead, programs that are integrated

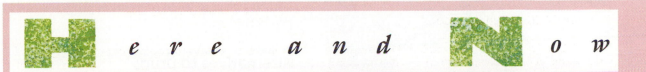

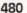

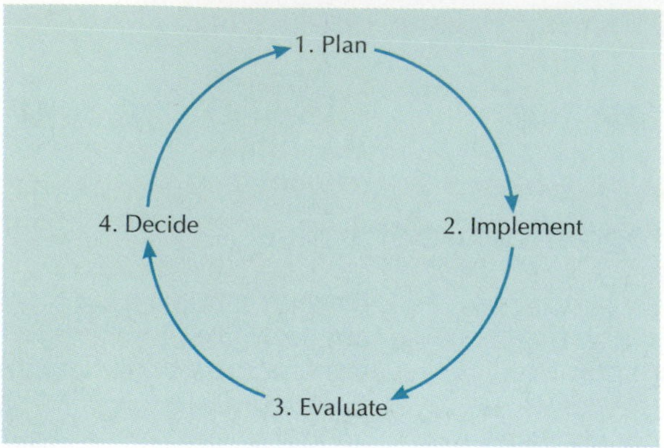

FIGURE 16.2 Preferred Prevention Model
Source: Division of Community Prevention and Training (DCPT), Office for Substance Abuse Prevention (OSAP). *The Future by Design: A Community Framework for Preventing Alcohol and Other Drug Problems Through a Systems Approach.* U.S. Department of Health and Human Services (USDHHS). DHHS Publication no. (ADM) 91-1760. Rockville, MD: Office for Substance Abuse Prevention (OSAP), 1991, p. 31.

into neighborhood clubs, organizations, and church activities are more likely to have a long-term impact on preventing drug use.

3. *Including personal autobiographical and social experience accounts of former drug abusers when distributing drug information.* Recipients of drug prevention information should be given real-life accounts of use, abuse, despair, and successful drug rehabilitation. Just getting drug information alone has little impact, either initially or over the long term.

Furthermore, when drug prevention programs are not well received, part of the reason may be the false impression on which these programs have been based. Many people still believe that only an abnormal minority abuses drugs. The truth is that all segments of the population use psychoactive drugs. Not everyone abuses what are considered illegal drugs; many people abuse legal drugs.

Finally, drug prevention programs must be responsive to the community and as a result, they must constantly undergo modification. Figure 16.2 shows a preferred model that incorporates constant change when prevention programs are in practice.

Alternatives to Drugs

It has been suggested that people have an innate need to alter their conscious state. This belief is based on the observation that, as part of their normal play, preschoolers deliberately whirl themselves dizzy and even momentarily choke each other to lose consciousness (see Wilson and Wilson 1975, 26). Some young children progress to discovering and using chemicals (such as sniffing shoe polish or gasoline) to alter consciousness and learn to be very secretive about this behavior. They learn to be circumspect or come to feel guilty and repress the desire to alter consciousness when adults catch them in these activities.

If this desire to alter the state of consciousness is inherent in human beings, then the use of psychoactive drugs legally or illegally in adulthood is natural. Drug abuse is thus a logical continuation of a developmental sequence that goes back to early childhood (Carroll 1977; Weil 1972).

Other researchers argue that, even if there is an innate desire to alter consciousness, why do only some and not all people progress to abusing chemical substances? It appears that people who do not abuse psychoactive drugs have found positive alternatives to altering consciousness. They feel no need to take chemical substances for this purpose. Involvement in such activities as Boy Scouts and Girl Scouts, youth sports teams, music groups, and the YMCA and YWCA, drug-free video game centers, drug-free dances, environmental and historical preservation projects, and social and service projects are viable alternatives to drug use. The rationale for these programs is that youth will find these activities engaging enough to forgo alcohol and drug use (Forman and Linney 1988, 555–556).

ALTERNATIVES APPROACH one approach emphasizing the exploration of positive alternatives to drug abuse, based on replacing the pleasurable feelings gained from drug abuse with involvement in social and educational activities

Here and Now

Some Good News!

The following table summarizes the percentage of high school seniors perceiving "great risk" associated with drug use, from 1980 to 1990. For most drug categories, high school seniors perceived increased risk in the use of the following drugs. The only exceptions are LSD and regular use of barbiturates, which have very low usage. Is this evidence that lately drug education programs are having an impact? Why or why not?

PERCENTAGE OF HIGH SCHOOL SENIORS EXPRESSING PERCEPTIONS OF "GREAT RISK" OF DRUG USE

Drug Use	1980	1990	Gain
Try marijuana once or twice	10.0	23.1	131%
Smoke marijuana occasionally	14.7	36.9	151
Smoke marijuana regularly	50.4	77.8	54
Try cocaine once or twice	31.3	59.4	90
Take cocaine regularly	69.2	91.1	32
Try amphetamines once or twice	29.7	32.2	8
Take amphetamines regularly	69.1	71.2	3
Try barbiturates once or twice	30.9	32.4	5
Take barbiturates regularly	72.2	70.2	–3
Try one or two drinks (alcohol)	3.8	8.3	118
Take one or two drinks nearly every day	20.3	31.3	54
Take four or five drinks nearly every day	65.7	47.1	31
Have 5+ drinks once or twice each weekend	35.9	47.1	31
Smoke 1 or more packs of cigarettes per day	63.7	68.2	7

Source: Eigen, D., and D. W. Rowden. *Prevention Works.* U.S. Department of Health and Human Services (USDHHS) and Substance Abuse and Mental Health Services Administration (SAMHSA). DHHS Publication no. (SMA) 93-246. Rockville, MD: National Clearinghouse for Alcohol and Drug Information, September 1993.

This is known as the **alternatives approach.** Workers in the drug abuse field tend to agree on its effectiveness. They note that young ex-abusers of common illicit drugs are more likely to stop when they gain satisfaction from exploring positive alternatives rather than from a fear of consequent harm. The alternatives approach assumes the following (Cohen 1971):

1. People abuse drugs voluntarily to fill a need or basic drive.
2. Most people abuse drugs for negative reasons. They may be dealing with negative feelings or situations, such as relieving boredom, anxiety, depression, tension, or other unpleasant emotional and psychological states. They may be rebelling against authority, trying to escape feelings of loneliness or inadequacy, or trying to be accepted by peers. Peer pressure is extremely important as an inducing force.
3. Some people who abuse drugs believe the experience is positive. They may feel enhance-

ment of sensual experiences or listening to music, achieve altered states of consciousness, or simply experience a sense of adventure. Some people may want to explore their own consciousness and reasons for the attraction to drug use.

Whether the reasons for drug use are positive or negative, the effects sought can be achieved through alternative, nondrug means. Such means are preferable to drug use and more constructive because the person is not relying on a psychoactive substance for satisfaction; rather, he or she is finding satisfaction based on personal achievements. Ideally, this should lead to a lifetime of self-satisfaction.

Table 16.3 lists various types of experiences, the motives for such experiences, the probable drugs of abuse that are associated, and alternatives to these drugs. As shown in the table, any constructive activity can be considered an alternative to drug abuse. For example, you can see that a young person who needs an outlet for increased physical energy might respond better to dance and movement training or a project in preventive medicine than to work on ecological projects.

In a large alternatives program in Idaho, the following activities were planned during one month: arts and crafts, karate, reforestation, backpacking, a Humane Society dog show, horseback riding, artwork for posters for various programs, astrology, camping, and volunteering in a local hospital. In southeastern Ohio, teenagers from nine area high schools researched the history of coal mining and the canal in a three-county area. Publication of their report, which they produced themselves as part of the Youth Alternatives Program, was funded by a grant from the National Endowment for the Humanities. The students were justifiably proud of a job well done and clearly got a good deal of pleasure from it as well as learning some local history.

Another example is part-time job placement. This is extremely important as one of the alternative approaches. When a first- or second-year high school student is employed on a part-time basis and begins to earn money, the probability of drug abuse is lessened because less recreation time is available. Furthermore, the extra income helps build feelings of self-worth and confidence.

Most communities offer a range of youth activities through various organizations. The problem is that the young people who readily participate in these organizations are often those who are already at low risk of becoming drug abusers. In short, they are more likely to have developed self-confidence and self-esteem, which is a factor in their not abusing drugs. Traditional organizations have few ways of reaching out to the high-risk youth who need their help. This is the irony of the alternatives approach: Much of what's needed is already in place, but it's not reaching those who need it the most. An effective drug abuse prevention program requires a leader who has community commitment to back him or her and the organizational skills to get high-risk young people involved.

Nontraditional Prevention Methods

Information about non-Western methods for preventing drug abuse is important and necessary for comprehensive coverage of this topic. Various systems of mind control have been used for thousands of years in other cultures to find peace and inner contentment, without using chemicals.

Many people are not aware that all of us have the ability to modify our conscious state of mind. Sleeping, daydreaming, meditation, anesthesia, and psychoses are examples of altered states of consciousness. The human brain is capable of processing millions of pieces (or bits) of information each minute, yet much of this processing is relegated to the unconscious. Under the influence of stress, drugs, and internal and external psychological factors, the input may be modified and the brain's interpretation may be changed. This is called *altering the conscious state*. Levels of stimulation above or below the normal range can cause such modifications and may be useful for preventing or treating drug abuse.

Examples of the ways that states of consciousness can be altered include

1. *Reducing sensory input.* Certain procedures or substances are able to reduce stimulation or motor activity, such as solitary confinement, floating on warm water in a darkened chamber, extreme muscle relaxation, biofeedback—inducing an increase in alpha or theta brain wave rhythms, meditation, and use of some depressant drugs.

2. *Increasing sensory input.* Other procedures or substances increase sensory input, including reli-

TABLE 16.3 Experiences, motives, and possible alternatives for a drug abuser

Experience	Corresponding Motives	Drugs Abused	Possible Alternatives
Physical	Desire for physical well-being: physical relaxation, relief from sickness, desire for more energy	Alcohol, sedative-hypnotics, stimulants, marijuana	Athletics, dance, exercise, hiking, diet, carpentry, outdoor work, swimming, hatha yoga
Sensory	Desire to magnify sensorium: sound, touch, taste, need for sensual/sexual stimulation	Hallucinogens, marijuana, alcohol	Sensory awareness training, sky diving, experiencing sensory beauty of nature, scuba diving
Emotional	Relief from psychological pain: attempt to resolve personal problems, relief from bad mood, escape from anxiety, desire for emotional insight, liberation of feeling and emotional relaxation	Narcotics, alcohol, barbiturates, sedative-hypnotics	Competent individual counseling, well-run group therapy, instruction in psychology of personal development
Interpersonal	To gain peer acceptance, break through interpersonal barriers, "communicate"; defiance of authority figures	Any, especially alcohol, marijuana	Expertly managed sensitivity and encounter groups, well-run group therapy, instruction in social customs, confidence training, emphasis on assisting others—for example, YMCA or YWCA volunteers
Social	To promote social change, find identifiable subculture, tune out intolerable environmental conditions—for example, poverty	Marijuana, psychedelics	Social service community action in positive social change; helping the poor, aged, infirm, young; tutoring handicapped; ecology action; YMCA or YWCA Big Brother/Sister programs
Political	To promote political change (out of desperation with the social-political order) and to identify with antiestablishment subgroup	Marijuana, psychedelics	Political service, lobbying for nonpartisan projects—for example, Common Cause; field work with politicians and public officials
Intellectual	To escape boredom, out of intellectual curiosity, to solve cognitive problems, gain new understanding in the world of ideas, research one's own awareness	Stimulants, sometimes psychedelics	Intellectual excitement through reading, debate, and discussion; creative games and puzzles; self-hypnosis; training in concentration
Creative-aesthetic	To improve creative performance, enhance enjoyment of art already produced—for example, music; enjoy imaginative mental productions	Marijuana, stimulants, psychedelics	Nongraded instruction in producing and/or appreciating art, music, drama, and creative hobbies
Philosophical	To discover meaningful values, find meaning in life, help establish personal identity, organize a belief structure	Psychedelics, marijuana, stimulants	Discussions, seminars, courses on ethics, the nature of reality, relevant philosophical literature; explorations of value systems
Spiritual-mystical	To transcend orthodox religion, develop spiritual insights, reach higher levels of consciousness, augment yogic practices, take a spiritual shortcut	Psychedelics, marijuana	Exposure to nonchemical methods of spiritual development; study of world religions, mysticism, meditation, yogic techniques

gious ceremonies (revival meetings), long periods of tension (truck driving, flying, or sentry duty, video games, long-distance running), and hallucinogen and stimulant-type drugs.

3. *Modifying body chemistry.* Such modification influences input and interpretation. Causes include dehydration, fever, sleep deprivation, anesthesia, modification of acid–base balance in the blood (for example, by hyperventilation), hypoglycemia, and drugs such as hallucinogens, depressants, and stimulants.

Treatment

Beginnings and Goals

As stated earlier, the medical view of drug abuse is that it is considered an illness. More specifically, it may be viewed as either a medical or psychological problem. The medical model views drug abuse as a biological condition that is largely uncontrollable. The user is perceived as "sick" and thus irrational about continued drug use. The psychological perspective is that drug abuse is a disease and that treatment is the method for curing the disease.

In 1966, the federal government passed the Narcotic Addict Rehabilitation Act (NARA), which established national rules for admission to treatment and rehabilitation at federal centers. Addicts were given the opportunity to have their sentences reduced or charges dismissed if they would go for treatment.

In June 1971, the first drug treatment program, the Special Action Office for Drug Abuse Prevention (SAODAP), was established. One of the roles of this office was to provide additional support for efforts to control the availability of illicit drugs. The need for drug prevention programs had become crucial. For instance, widespread use of heroin and other drugs by American servicepeople in Vietnam prompted President Nixon to direct the secretary of defense to reduce penalties for drug use, so that it would no longer be a courtmartial offense. In 1972, the Drug Abuse Office and Treatment Act provided financial backing for treatment programs.

The goal of any treatment program is to stop the abuser from taking drugs. An integral step is stabilizing the abuser's personal life and helping him or her to feel like a productive member of society.

Over the past 20 years or more that active treatment programs have been in existence, it has been difficult to determine their effectiveness. Part of the problem has been that their goals are unclear. Should the goal be to get the drug abuser completely off drugs? Should the goal be to get the ex-abuser to hold a job? How long should a person be off drugs for the treatment to be deemed a success?

There are no easy answers. If someone gets off one drug completely, he or she must not abuse other drugs as substitutes. If the criterion is to hold a job, once the job is found, the drug abuser may slide back into old habits. And if an abuser is off drugs for a few years, there is still the possibility of regression. Any of these scenarios thwarts successful treatment outcomes.

A range of possible benefits and adverse effects can be attributed to treatment programs. To evaluate a given program's success, a variety of measuring devices should be employed. To base the evaluation solely on success or failure rates is not productive, in that it ignores how these measures are achieved.

The success of a treatment program should be based on many factors. Namely, consider whether the individual has been able to accomplish the following (DeLong 1972; USDHHS 1991):

Abstinence from using illegal drugs
Abstinence from using all addicting drugs
Achieving stabilization on a maintenance drug such as methadone
Holding down a job
Decrease in criminal conduct
The ability to support a family
Improved physical and mental health
Accomplishing any or all of these could indicate partial success

Treatment Settings

A number of treatment settings are used for alleviating or eliminating addiction. The level of treatment provided at these types of facilities is based on the severity of addiction and physiological and psychological symptoms.

1. *Inhospital programs.* Intense treatment is provided within an acute care hospital program. *Acute care* refers to serious or critical care. In these settings, drug-dependent patients are continually observed and given numerous diagnostic tests, efficiently stabilized, medically supervised and made aware of their particular problem, and provided with information about drug addiction through intensive counseling. Nearly all programs run 28 days and up and many state or private facilities are costly.

2. *Residential care.* These programs focus on education and therapy, which leads to rehabilitation. This type of care is provided 24 hours per day. Although addicted patients are supervised by fewer medically trained staff members than in inhospital care programs, more counselors and mental health personnel are available. Other varieties of residential care include (a) community hospital-based programs; (b) freestanding facilities in nonhospital settings; (c) therapeutic communities, which involve intense interaction and often confrontational dialogue in groups with other addicts (see later in the chapter); (d) "halfway houses," or transition settings between 24-hour-a-day programs and independent living; and (e) detoxification centers, where short-term stay units are usually maintained by charity organizations and provide necessary shelter, clothing, food, and medical needs.

3. *Day hospitals and intensive outpatient services.* Care is usually provided three or four hours per day for patients who need additional structure while living independently. Self-help groups, seminars, and individual and group therapy are some of the programs found in day hospitals or intensive outpatient services. For example, a typical day for intensive outpatients is to go to their respective jobs in the morning, visit the hospital or treatment setting after work, and return home after work. Often patients find little time for recreational activities.

Treatment settings also can be selective or nonselective. *Selective* programs screen prospective clients and accept only those whom they judge are likely to benefit. *Nonselective* programs accept nearly all people with drug dependence problems who apply or who are sent there, except for psychotics and violent types.

Finally, treatment settings are either voluntary or involuntary. Practically all drug treatment involves some degree of coercion, if only from family or employer. However, *involuntary* usually refers to a legal requirement or a criteria for holding onto a job or staying out of jail. Most people in involuntary treatment programs sent by the courts, for example, are in treatment because they were arrested, or were referred to such facilities by law enforcement agencies such as the courts or probation agencies. The addict is required to enter some form of treatment and remain in it for some time, usually until he or she can demonstrate progress.

Next, we will discuss the following major treatment approaches: (1) medical, (2) psychological and psychotherapeutic, (3) social, (4) behavioral, and (5) innovative. We will also consider the effectiveness of some of these treatments.

Medical Treatments

There are a variety of medical approaches to drug treatment.

Detoxification and Abstinence Programs

When isolated from other treatment methods, detoxification does not have a high long-term success rate. One positive aspect is that, even if addicts don't stay off drugs, their habit is often reduced, thus lessening the need to financially support drug use. For many addicts, this is a step toward rehabilitation.

The goals and procedures of detoxification programs vary greatly. They may be residential —where the patient lives in a hospital, clinic, or therapeutic community—or ambulatory, where the addict is treated on an outpatient basis with professional help and sometimes methadone or other support drugs. Some outpatient settings require daily attendance and vary according to one-on-one or group therapy sessions (McNeece and DiNitto 1994).

Interestingly, many heroin detoxification programs do not use drugs for support. Some use methadone maintenance and a variety of drug backups, such as sedatives.

Other abstinence programs treat drug dependence by reducing intake to zero while simultaneously giving the addict mental and psychological assistance during withdrawal. Opiate addicts can be helped through the withdrawal period in 5 to 10 days. This approach is usually not used for alcohol or barbiturate dependencies because withdrawal from heavy depressant dependence can be life threatening. Instead, these addicts are stabilized on a long-acting depressant and gradually withdrawn.

Maintenance Programs Maintenance programs are based on the principle that past treatment programs have not been successful, so "incurable" addicts should be able to register and receive drugs, such as narcotics, under supervision. Proponents of these programs contend that many addicts are forced into a life of crime to support their habits but would become law-abiding and useful citizens if they received narcotics (usually a less euphoric type, such as methadone) legally. Moreover, it's argued, the illicit narcotics trade would be eliminated due to the loss of these customers. Opponents of maintenance programs say that there are sufficient treatment programs to cure many addicts and that providing addicts with substitute narcotics is not solving the basic problem causing drug dependence.

The concept of maintenance on a **noneuphoric opiate** is now widely accepted in the United States as one way to help treat drug abusers.

Morphine Maintenance After the Harrison Narcotics Act was passed in 1914, between 200,000 and 300,000 opiate addicts were no longer able to obtain drugs legally except through physicians. After 1918, more than 40 morphine maintenance clinics opened. However, public opinion was against maintenance because it was perceived as an approval of narcotic use, and the last clinic closed in 1923. The narcotics division of the federal government maintained a very tough attitude toward physicians who advocated maintenance and prescribed opiates for their patients. By 1938, approximately 25,000 doctors had been arrested for dispensing narcotics, and of these, approximately 5,000 went to jail (DeLong 1972).

Methadone Maintenance Vincent Dole and Marie Nyswander were the first doctors to use the synthetic narcotic methadone in a rehabilitation program with heroin addicts in the mid-1960s. As of 1987, an estimated 70,000 to 75,000 addicts were on methadone maintenance. The drug is used to alleviate narcotic craving and to prevent the occurrence of withdrawal symptoms. The advantages of methadone over other forms of maintenance therapy are

1. It can be administered orally.
2. It acts in the body for 24 to 36 hours, compared to heroin's action of 4 to 8 hours.
3. It causes no serious side effects at maintenance doses.
4. At sufficient dose levels, methadone will almost completely block the effects of heroin.
5. When taken orally, it does not produce substantial euphoric effects.

Disadvantages of methadone maintenance include

1. The person taking it may develop a dependence.
2. It will not prevent the addict from taking other drugs that may interfere with treatment and rehabilitation. To guard against the use of other drugs, some clinics require urine samples periodically during treatment.

Once stabilized on methadone, the addict faces a crucial period of adjustment. Once devoted to maintaining a heroin habit, 24 hours a day, 365 days a year, the addict must be transformed into a self-supporting, socially acceptable person. Methadone maintenance establishes the potential for such a change, but it is the person's motivation and capabilities that determine the success of the rehabilitation effort. A range of medical, psychiatric, social, and vocational services are usually available during this phase of treatment.

Many criticisms have been levied against the use of methadone, especially from proponents of such therapeutic communities as Synanon, Narco,

NONEUPHORIC OPIATE a drug or drugs used in maintenance programs that satisfies the craving but does not produce the euphoric effect, such as methadone

Daytop Village, Odyssey House, and others. Some critics have said that giving methadone to a heroin addict is like switching an alcoholic from bourbon to wine.

Methadone is not the ideal solution by any means. Former heroin addicts who had large habits may have to be maintained indefinitely on methadone. They are likely to relapse to heroin use if detoxified from methadone. They may never be rehabilitated in the conventional sense because their backgrounds are such that they never had a so-called normal life to begin with. To create normalcy for these people may be too much to expect.

Overall, maintenance programs provide a steady amount of a noneuphoric drug that satisfies the craving, prevents withdrawal, and eliminates the constant concern for money in order to support the habit. For a certain percentage of addicts, maintenance programs eliminate or severely curtail the amount of crime committed for supporting the drug habit.

Detoxification from methadone is possible for methadone maintenance patients who were not addicted to heroin for a long period and who did not have an extensive background of criminal activity. Detoxification is not an automatic process in methadone maintenance. Of these who completed one detoxification program, as many as 35% were narcotic free and doing well up to six years later (Sells 1979).

Use of the nonopiate drug clonidine may help those who wish to stop taking methadone. Clonidine suppresses the signs and symptoms of opiate withdrawal and reduces the anxiety and irritability experienced by patients during the difficult withdrawal step (Gold et al. 1980).

The new long-acting methadone analog levo-alpha-acetylmethadol (LAAM) need only be taken three times a week and is being used experimentally in some programs. Initially, addicts participate daily in intensive counseling. Later in the program, they come in for the maintenance drug and follow-up treatment less frequently. Addicts may be treated with daily methadone first to increase the probability that they will at least attend counseling sessions and then be switched to LAAM when they reach an appropriate point in the program. Currently, LAAM is an investigational drug and has not been approved by the Food and Drug Administration (FDA) for general clinical use.

Heroin Maintenance Great Britain set up heroin clinics to treat addicts in the early 1970s, citing both humanitarian and economic reasons. It was argued that prescription heroin for addicts would save lives, eliminate illicit narcotics dealing, and clean up the crime associated with the addict's need for money to buy heroin.

At the beginning, problems resulted due to lax controls, and heroin from the program was being sold on the "street." Eventually, better controls were established. Also, methadone began to be used in many clinics to treat heroin abuse. It was estimated that there were less than 6,000 opiate addicts in Great Britain in 1975 (Trebach 1982), with no appreciable increase by 1980.

Some have advocated the legal use of heroin in comparable maintenance programs in the United States. It is highly unlikely that this will be implemented, however, because methadone does not produce the euphoria and has other advantages over heroin. What's more, heroin use in the United States has an unsavory history.

Opiate Antagonists Recall from Chapters 5 and 9 that an *antagonist* is a compound that suppresses the actions of a drug. Narcotic antagonists have properties that make them important tools in the clinical treatment of narcotic drug dependence. For instance, they counteract the central nervous system depressant effects in opioid drug overdoses.

Antagonists were developed as a by-product of research in analgesics. Scientists were interested in dissociating the dependence-producing properties and necessary pain-relieving properties of substances that could replace morphine. This led to the development of nalorphine, the first specific opiate antagonist. Its short duration of action and frequent unpleasant side effects limited its clinical usefulness, but its properties stimulated further research on this class of drugs (Archer 1981; Palfai and Jankiewicz 1991).

Cyclazocine was the next important antagonist developed. It has a longer duration of action than nalorphine; however, it also induces some unpleasant side effects, such as sedation, visual distortions, and racing thoughts. Tolerance to the side effects develops if the drug is increased gradually over several weeks. Because of these psychotomimetic side effects, cyclazocine is not used much today.

Naloxone is a pure antagonist without analgesic properties. It does not have the unpleasant side effects that nalorphine and cyclazocine have, but it has a shorter duration of action and if taken orally is less active than desired for narcotic antagonist treatment programs. Nevertheless, it is valuable in treating toxic or near-lethal doses of narcotics. (It is five to eight times more antagonistic than nalorphine.) This drug blocks narcotics from binding the opiate receptors in the brain, thus relieving depression of breathing and heartbeat.

Naltrexone is a chemical modification of naloxone that was synthesized to find a longer-acting, more potent antagonist. It has low toxicity with few side effects, and a single dose provides an effective opiate blockade for up to 72 hours. Taking naltrexone three times a week is sufficient to maintain a fairly high level of opioid blockade. In 1971, Congress mandated a large-scale increase in research on narcotic antagonistic drugs. Naltrexone seems to be the best antagonistic developed at this point. It has been used widely in experimental narcotic antagonist treatment programs (Archer 1981).

Clinical tests with heroin addicts in treatment have shown that addicts placed on naltrexone will try heroin or methadone once or twice, early in treatment, and then stop. Addicts on placebos, on the other hand, continued to use illicit methadone or heroin sporadically. The naltrexone group also reported significantly less craving for heroin than the placebo group (Hopkins 1973).

Naltrexone is not a complete treatment (Ginzburg 1986). It is best suited to adolescent heroin users with relatively short drug experience, recently paroled prisoners who have been abstinent while incarcerated, and people who have been on methadone maintenance and with to get off but are afraid of relapsing to heroin. Unless some means of enforcing compliance can be established, such as requiring urine samples, or unless the person is highly motivated, narcotic antagonist treatment programs do not work well. Frankly, the narcotic antagonist drug does nothing positive for the user. It simply blocks the effects of heroin or methadone if the person takes these drugs up to three days after his or her last dose of naltrexone (Renault 1981).

As mentioned in Chapter 9, clonidine (Catapres) is useful in treating opiate-dependent people during the difficult withdrawal stages (Ginzburg 1986). Studies thus far show the value of this drug for withdrawal from heroin, morphine, codeine, and methadone. Clonidine is not addictive and does not cause euphoria, but it does block cravings for drugs. It also makes the person feel better compared to the depression experienced by addicts using other methods of withdrawal.

Antabuse goes by the trade name Disulfiram, which is a drug used for treating alcoholics. This drug is perceived as a deterrent drug—it makes people violently ill if alcohol is used. "Antabuse interferes with the normal metabolism of alcohol, resulting in serious physical reaction if even a small amount of alcohol is ingested" (McNeece and DiNitto 1994, 113). The greatest asset in using this drug is its ability to deter impulsive drinking (McNeece and DiNitto 1994).

Psychological and Psychotherapeutic Approaches

Psychological approaches are rooted in the premise that certain types of personalities are more prone to addiction. Namely, why do approximately 10% of all drug users become addicted? Recent research indicates that drug-dependent people are more likely to experience depression, which may be a factor (Kennedy et al. 1987).

Psychotherapeutic approaches assume that drug abusers are more likely to display antisocial personality disorders—such as coldness, aloofness, and adherence to dogmatic opinions—and that they are immature, dependent, and have difficulty in forming intimate social relationships. The general belief is that drug abuse is a symptom of deeper personality conflicts.

Within the last 20 years, psychological approaches have lost popularity. Critics charge that their success rates are low and that therapy is very time consuming and expensive, generally involving weekly hour-long sessions with a therapist over many years.

Social Approaches

Social interactions and pressures clearly play a very important role in explaining drug use. Social approaches emphasize the lack of positive role models, peer influence, depressed economic conditions, and malfunctioning families as the root of

Case in Point

AA's Twelve Steps for Recovery

1. We admitted we were powerless over alcohol—that our lives had become unmanageable.
2. Came to believe that a Power greater than ourselves could restore us to sanity.
3. Made a decision to turn our will and our lives over to the care of God *as we understood Him.*
4. Made a searching and fearless moral inventory of ourselves.
5. Admitted to God, to ourselves, and to another human being the exact nature of our wrongs.
6. Were entirely ready to have God remove all these defects of character.
7. Humbly asked Him to remove our shortcomings.
8. Made a list of all persons we had harmed, and became willing to make amends to them all.
9. Made direct amends to such people wherever possible, except when to do so would injure them or others.
10. Continued to take personal inventory and when we were wrong promptly admitted it.
11. Sought through prayer and meditation to improve our conscious contact with God *as we understood Him,* praying only for knowledge of His will for us and the power to carry that out.
12. Having had a spiritual awakening as the result of these steps, we tried to carry this message to alcoholics, and to practice these principles in all our affairs.

Source: Alcoholics Anonymous World Services, Inc., *Alcoholics Anonymous: The Story of How Many Thousands of Men and Women Have Recovered from Alcoholism,* 3rd ed. (New York: Alcoholics Anonymous, 1976):59–60. Permission to reprint this material does not mean that AA has reviewed or approved the contents of this chapter, nor that AA agrees with the views expressed herein. AA is a program of recovery from alcoholism—use of the Twelve Steps in connection with programs and activities which are patterned after AA, but which address other problems, does not imply otherwise.

drug abuse. Prevention strategies include providing positive role models, using peer intervention, improving economic conditions by increasing employment opportunities, and family counseling. Social workers are identified as the primary professionals when social approaches are implemented.

Alcoholics Anonymous (AA) Founded in the mid-1930s, AA is now an international organization. The desire to stop drinking is the sole criterion required to join. The original founders of AA were strongly influenced by a religious movement known as the Oxford Groups and the psychoanalyst Carl Jung. The "Twelve Steps for Recovery" espoused by AA are cited in the Case in Point box above.

Today, this self-help group has many professional and nonprofessional members with drinking problems. (*Self-help groups* are defined as groups not employing professionals to run the group.) The strength of AA's program as a treatment method lies in its loose organizational structure and strong interpersonal relationships. In fact, AA's success was so renowned that it led to the

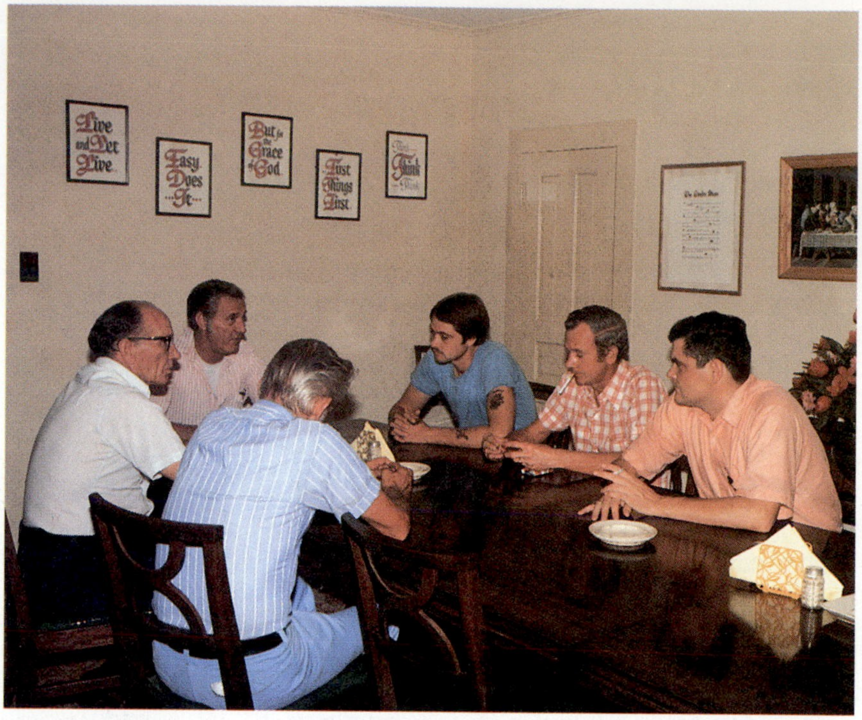

An AA meeting where common alcohol abuse–related problems are shared.

establishment of NA, Narcotics Anonymous, to help other drug abusers help themselves.

How successful is the AA program? This is a difficult assessment, for four reasons:

1. AA insists on anonymity; it does not reveal names of members.
2. Membership is strictly voluntary. Those who want to join become members when they vow to give up drinking. Controlled studies are impossible.
3. Members are a homogeneous group. They tend to be middle class and socially conservative.
4. **Alcohologists** (people who research alcohol addiction) are of the opinion that the more severe "hard core" alcoholics who refuse to seek help generally do not go to AA, while a smaller percentage of problem drinkers who come to view themselves as addicted to alcohol, do (see Rudy 1994 for further discussion of this and other related findings). In part, this may be responsible for the group's high success rate. Members are not typically hard-core alcohol addicts. Regardless, AA has been and continues to be a very important method for treating many recovering alcoholics.

AA has two types of meetings, open and closed meetings. **Open meetings** are open to anyone having an interest in attending and witnessing these meetings, and they last approximately 45 minutes to an hour. **Closed meetings** are for alcoholics having a serious desire to completely stop drinking. These meetings are not open to viewers or "shoppers." At closed meetings, recovering alcoholics address through testimonials how alcohol has diminished the quality of life.

Some outgrowths of Alcoholics Anonymous include Al-Anon, ACOA (adult children of alcoholics), and Alateen. These are parallel organizations supporting Alcoholics Anonymous. Al-Anon is for spouses and other close relatives of alcoholics and Alateen is exclusively for teenage children of alcoholic parents. Both relatives and teen members of alcoholic families learn means and methods for coping with destructive behavior(s) of alcoholic members.

√**Therapeutic Communities** Also known as self-regulating communities, **therapeutic communities (TCs)** operate on the premise that drug use is a symptom of an underlying character disorder or emotional immaturity (Klein and Miller 1986). The main goal of TCs is a complete change in lifestyle: abstinence from drugs, elimination of criminal behavior, and development of employable skills, self-reliance, personal honesty, and responsibility.

The philosophy behind TCs is that only ex-addicts can truly understand and deal effectively with addicts. Some TCs also employ professionals with training in vocational guidance, education, medicine, and mental health who are paid or who may donate their services. Residents of the traditional TC stay at least 15 months before they return to the community. Several TCs have been experimenting with shorter resident times, ranging from 2 to 9 months, based on individual client needs and progress.

The first therapeutic community for drug addicts was Synanon, which was aimed at psychiatric patients. It was founded in Santa Monica, California, in 1958. Synanon was started by Charles E. Dederich, a former alcoholic, to treat alcoholics and was later expanded to include drug addicts. When drug addicts came into the program, the alcoholics left because they felt associating with addicts was degrading.

Many branches of Synanon were founded based on the same philosophy, for example, Daytop Village and Phoenix House. They have been used as models for a number of other programs, with modifications based on the circumstances in each community. TCs have had a major impact on drug abuse treatment.

As of 1990, in the United States there were over 400 residential therapeutic communities serving drug abusers, criminal offenders, and other socially dislocated persons. These programs are quite diverse, ranging in size from 35 to 500 beds, and they serve a variety of clients.

The TC program includes encounter group therapy, educational programs, job assignments within the community, and in the later stages, conventional jobs outside the community. The primary staff are former drug addicts who have been rehabilitated in TC programs. Most TCs use self-government and group pressures, instead of relying on a professional, therapeutic personnel.

More recently, some TCs serve criminal justice clients almost exclusively (McNeece and DiNitto 1994, 190). Drug addicts referred to TCs are in appropriate settings where delinquent or criminal peers and the adverse effects of crime-ridden neighborhoods, and by extension communities, are physically distant, where the temptations of peers and environment are excluded. As a result, recent research indicates that TCs are more effective for alleviating drug use for such clients. The rate of success of TCs is higher if the patient remains in the program more than 90 days. Findings indicate that narcotic addicts who were treated with either a therapeutic community approach or methadone maintenance had about a 25% chance of relapsing to daily narcotic use if they remained in treatment for more than 90 days (Bassin 1970). Relapse back to drug use was much higher when the length of stay was less than 90 days.

Most people who apply are admitted to TCs. Only obviously psychotic or violent individuals are rejected. Some people leave without completing the program for a variety of reasons:

1. They may not be ready to deal with the complete change in lifestyle demanded by the TC.
2. They may progress to a certain point and become bored or frustrated with the TC.
3. They may relapse and return to the TC at some later point.

Treatment should not be looked on as a complete failure if the person relapses. Estimates of

ALCOHOLOGISTS people who research alcohol addiction

OPEN MEETINGS meetings to which anyone having an interest in attending and witnessing is invited

CLOSED MEETINGS meetings to which only alcoholics having a serious desire to completely stop drinking are invited

THERAPEUTIC COMMUNITIES (TCs) programs that advocate a complete change in lifestyle, such as complete abstinence from drugs, elimination of deviant behavior, and development of employable skills readmission to a TC or another form of treatment range from 30 to 60% (De Leon and Rosenthal 1979).

Family Therapy Family therapy is based on the belief that drug abuse stems from family problems. When a drug user is involved in counseling with a family therapist, the entire family is brought in during sessions. Sometimes, even extended family members—such as uncles, aunts, and grandparents—are included. The strengths of the family system are also used to develop coping skills and teach tolerance.

Behavioral Approaches

Behavioral approaches consist of operant or instrumental conditioning, counterconditioning (sensitization), biofeedback therapy, and contingency management techniques, as well as several alternative methods.

Operant or Instrumental Conditioning

This approach assumes that all behavior results from its consequences, or the rewards received when proper (acceptable) behavior is demonstrated. With regard to drug use and abuse, the belief is that the behavior is learned through **reinforcement.** The same type of conditioning that is believed to have caused the drug problem is also used to treat it. This involves rewarding appropriate behavior to change behavior.

The addictive process is shaped by conditioned responses. Drugs shape behavior by their direct, pleasant effects (positive reinforcement, which produces primary psychological dependence) or by relieving withdrawal (negative reinforcement, which produces secondary psychological dependence). It has been observed that former addicts who were free of drugs often developed tearing and yawning (opiate withdrawal signs) when they discussed drugs in group therapy. Other research has shown that conditioned withdrawal responses can be produced in animals and in humans.

These conditioned withdrawal responses are thought to be caused in part by pairing pharmacological withdrawal with environmental cues. Eventually, the environmental stimuli, such as talking about drugs or showing pictures of drugs, could elicit a conditioned withdrawal. This would explain the reactions of former addicts (yawning or forming tears) when talking about drugs or when returning to the environment in which they had previously used drugs.

Not only do addicts develop drug craving during conditioned withdrawal, but they also show actual physical signs of sickness. Some react to conditioning cues from the injection procedure alone and may even experience withdrawal relief when told they are getting an opiate, although they are actually getting a placebo. These people are sometimes called "needle freaks." When they find out the substance is a placebo, it no longer works.

Treatment methods have been developed based on our knowledge of conditioning in drug dependence (O'Brien and Ng 1979). Patients are taught how to alter the rewards derived from drug use. Often, the patient is taught how to replace or substitute drug use for behavior that elicits satisfaction or pleasure. Substituting a chemical "high" with the high experienced from intense physical exercise, such as long-distance running, is an example. Another behavioral method involves identifying and modifying conditions that create the craving for a particular drug.

Short-term goals involve eliminating or negating the reinforcing effects of drugs. Long-term goals center on eliminating drug use as an integral part of the patient's lifestyle and *reintegrating* the patient, returning him or her to a social situation where drugs are no longer an option. Such behavioral approaches have become very popular methods of treatment in the last five years.

Contingency Management Techniques

These techniques, based on operant or instrumental conditioning (discussed earlier), attempt to control behavior through a system of rewards, or schedules of reinforcement. One of the best known of these techniques is the *token economy system*, which has been used successfully to treat prisoners and mental patients. Through this system, the

REINFORCEMENT any behavior that strengthens the likelihood that a behavior will be repeated rewards and punishments in the addict's environment are identified and then manipulated to redirect his or her response. For example, subjects gain points if they perform certain tasks that are beneficial to the treatment program, such as participation in group therapy and educational programs, doing a project that benefits the group, or making a special contribution to the group. The accumulated points can be used to "buy" an early release or to get special privileges or other rewards. Addicts in such programs show greatly increased participation in therapeutic and educational activities (Pickens and Thompson 1984). They also report other socially desirable behaviors, such as improved communication and decreased hostility.

In an outpatient methadone program, it was found that "take-home" doses of methadone served as desired reinforcers. Attendance at counseling sessions increased markedly when take-home privileges were made contingent on attendance. In other programs, rewards are given if the participants' urine tests are negative for illicit drugs.

Contingency management techniques are most appropriate for structured treatment programs, such as methadone maintenance and inpatient settings. Comparisons of success rates with other techniques must still be made.

Counterconditioning (sensitization) Counterconditioning procedures involve imagining scenes during therapy. As the patient develops a craving for drugs, he or she is asked to visualize, as clearly as possible, each link in the chain of events leading to drug taking. The patient is then supposed to imagine becoming severely ill, in vivid terms, due to taking the drug. When the patient focuses on avoiding drugs, he or she is told to imagine pleasant scenes.

This method has been used in several experimental programs but not on a large scale. It is best suited for a motivated, cooperative patient who is doing well in a therapeutic community or narcotic antagonist program.

Biofeedback Relaxation Therapy Biofeedback is used to help drug addicts by stressing that the mind has the ability to control the urge or desire to ingest drugs. Therapeutic use of biofeedback is based on two distinct models: the learning theory model and the relaxation model.

In the learning theory model, the person learns to control a physiological process, such as blood pressure, with an appropriate monitoring device to let him or her know when the blood pressure is changing in the desired direction—usually down. The biofeedback is directed at general muscular or cortical relaxation, with the idea that, when in a stressful situation, the patient will use what he or she has learned.

One positive aspect of using biofeedback therapy in a treatment package is that it shifts the responsibility of "cure" from doctor to patient. The patient must become involved and actively work toward his or her own health, which should help maintain success over the long term.

Biofeedback-assisted relaxation procedures have been used as part of therapeutic approaches with alcoholics and methadone-maintenance addicts. Some patients report that they feel biofeedback has helped them. However, carefully controlled studies of addicts going through withdrawal, using muscular relaxation techniques and alpha EEG training, have not demonstrated success. Unfortunately, for many of the people who had great expectations, the various types of biofeedback methods have not proven better than general relaxation procedures (Ray et al. 1979).

Alternative Behavioral Approaches Alternative approaches consist of substituting chemically induced states of euphoria with natural "highs" brought on by altered states of consciousness.

Understanding Consciousness. Experimental psychiatrists, neurophysiologists, psychologists, and physicians are always investigating the mind. Roland Fischer is one of the researchers who has probed the ability and powers of the conscious and subconscious mind. Figure 16.3 shows his representation of the varieties of conscious states, with which he explains some abilities of the mind (Fischer 1971).

Notice in the figure that there are three major conscious states: ergotropic, normal, and trophotropic. The one in the middle, the normal waking state of mind, focuses on stimuli in normal life. This state of the conscious mind (called the *"I" portion*) is active during the daily routine. The state on the right, trophotropic, represents the lowered sensory input into the brain that occurs as

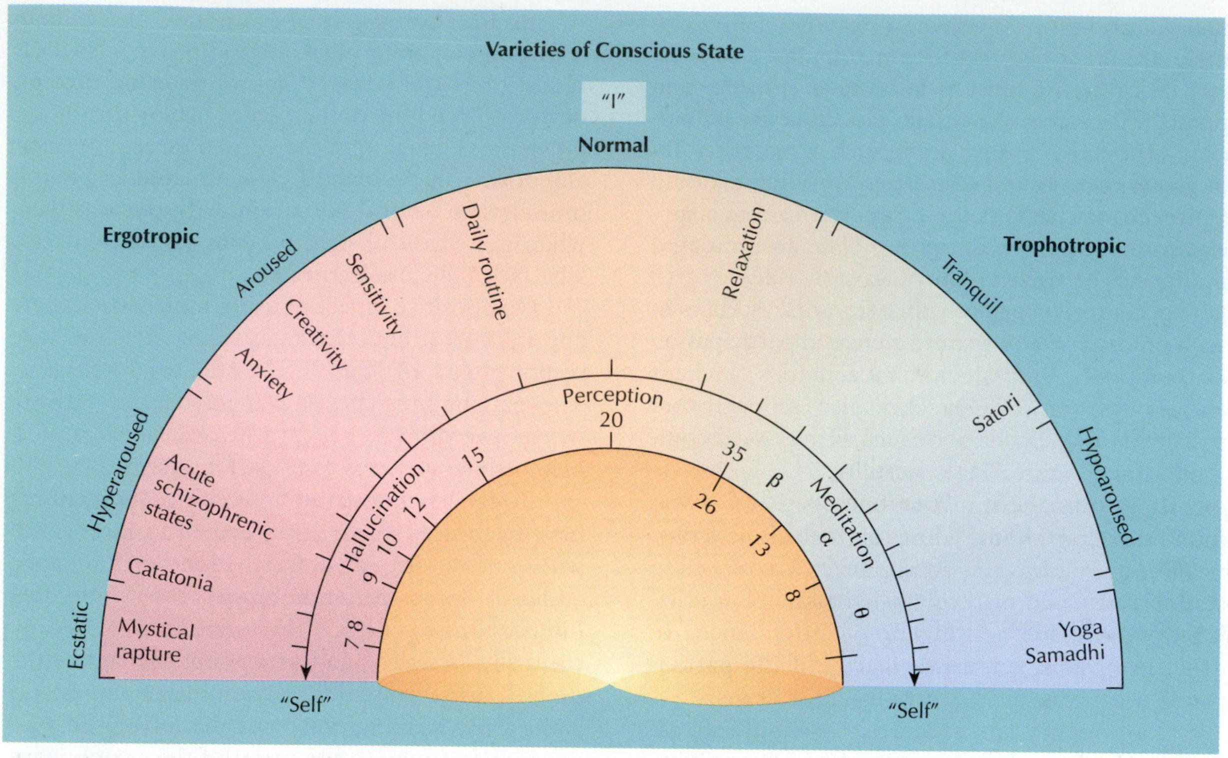

FIGURE 16.3 Fischer's map of varieties of conscious states, shown on a continuum of conscious arousal: *normal* waking consciousness ("I", middle); increased, or *ergotropic*, arousal (left); and decreased, or *trophotropic*, arousal (right). At either extreme is a state of transcendence in which the absolute "Self" is discovered; this is normally achieved only by mystics and advanced practitioners of meditation. *Source:* From R. Fischer, "A Cartography of the Ecstatic and Meditative States." *Science* 174 (26):877—904. Copyright 1971 by the American Association for the Advancement of Science. Reprinted by permission.

a person relaxes; conversely, the state on the left, ergotropic, represents increased sensory input from activity, or a removal of filters to sensory input. The change in alertness may be measured by the types of brain wave and their intensity, as may be noted on the small semicircle in the center of the diagram.

The term **ergotropic** refers to the arousal state (shown on the left in Figure 16.3) and means "inciting activity." It is characterized by increased activity of the sympathetic nervous system and an activated psychic state. During the ergotropic state, more than normal amounts of sensory input are coming into the brain. As one moves from the *aroused* to the *hyperaroused* and finally to the *ecstatic* stage, the level of stimuli coming into the brain increases, so the person's nervous system gets more excited and aroused.

This is very much like removing filters in the brain, which is probably one of the best ways to explain the increased activity. Initially, sensitivity and creativity are enhanced (aroused stage); the individual may feel inspired or have new ideas and feelings. With more stimulation, anxiety may follow (still aroused stage); the individual may now feel driven. Increased levels of stimulation may be difficult to handle, leading to psychological and physical problems. If the hyperaroused stage persists, schizophrenia or hallucinations may result, as normal processing of input fails; the person may become **catatonic.** In the ecstatic stage, **mystical rapture** is achieved. Few people are able to reach this most intense level of information processing without becoming catatonic or damaging their conscious minds. Those who can are considered to be mystics, who may be capable of visions and transcendental experiences. Some claim that they can reach this mystical stage with hallucinogenic drugs like LSD, psilocybin, and mescaline.

As the brain evolves, the sensory detection organs in and on the exterior of the body send in so much nerve impulse information that much of the information processing is delegated to the subconscious. This is a necessary function. As Aldous Huxley concluded, "The function of the brain is to protect us from being overwhelmed . . . by this mass of largely useless and irrelevant knowledge, by shutting out most . . . and leaving only that . . . special selection which is likely to be practically useful" (1954).

At the other extreme is the **trophotropic** stage, during which less sensory input enters the brain (see Figure 16.3). As the brain filters out or blocks input into the conscious mind, the individual first reaches a feeling of tranquility, or deep relaxation. Some people who meditate reach a deep state of tranquility called *satori,* after the Zen Buddhist tradition (see section "Meditation," following). The *hypoaroused* stage is achieved when sensory input has been shut out until the arousal level is very low. The highest level of the hypoaroused stage, the *yoga samadhi* stage, is the ultimate in lowered input from the senses. It takes many years to achieve the mind and body control that characterize this stage, at which the person is in complete union with the Self, or the Absolute.

Note that this stage of complete union with the Self occurs at two points—mystical rapture and yoga samadhi. There is a loop, resembling the mathematical symbol for infinity, between these extremes of the ergotropic and trophotropic states. Fischer (1971) and others believe it is possible to move from samadhi into ecstasy and vice versa. This means that an experienced meditator may spontaneously move into total ecstasy, and the person in mystical rapture may spontaneously move into total calm and peace.

One final note: Fischer's interesting map of inner space is hypothetical. It should not be interpreted as a literal representation of data obtained on the human brain.

Meditation. Some of the most intriguing research about the brain is being done on the state of the mind during **meditation.** In certain countries, like India, people have long histories of being able to achieve certain goals through meditation. The word *yoga* is derived from the Sanskrit word for *union,* or *yoking,* meaning "the process of discipline by which a person attains union with the Absolute." In a sense, it refers to the use of the mind to control itself and the body.

Meditation involves brain wave activity centered on ponderous, contemplative, and reflective thought. An individual who meditates is able to decrease oxygen consumption within a matter of minutes as much as 20%, a level usually reached only after four to five hours of sleep in the nonmeditator. However, meditation is physiologically different from sleep, based on the EEG pattern and rate of decline of oxygen consumption (although some people do fall asleep during meditation) (Pagano et al. 1976). Along with the decreased metabolic rate and changes in EEG, there is also a marked decrease in blood lactate. Lactate is produced by metabolism of skeletal muscle, and the decrease is probably due to the reduced activity of the sympathetic nervous system during meditation. Heart rate and respiration are also slowed.

Herbert Benson (1977) dubbed this sequence of changes "the relaxation response." He was interested in applying nondrug means to treat

ERGOTROPIC pertaining to the arousal state of consciousness

CATATONIC pertaining to a state of arousal characterized by trancelike consciousness; sensory input is literally jammed, and the body is rigidly fixed

MYSTICAL RAPTURE an ultimate state of consciousness similar to hallucinating

TROPHOTROPIC pertaining to a state of consciousness in which there is decreased sensitivity to external stimuli and sedation

MEDITATION a state of consciousness in which there is a constant level of awareness focusing on one object; for example, Yoga and Zen Buddhism hypertensive patients and bring down their blood pressure. With the assistance of Maharishi Mahesh Yogi with volunteers from Transcendental Meditation (TM), a Westernized form of yoga, he worked out a clinical approach he had used to treat hypertension (Benson 1977).

The four basic conditions to elicit a relaxation response are

1. A passive attitude (probably the most important condition)
2. A quiet environment
3. An object to dwell on, such as a word or sound repetition
4. A comfortable position, such as sitting, in which the person is not as likely to fall asleep during the 20-minute session as if he or she lies down

Benson recommends using the word *one* to concentrate on or a simple prayer from your own religious tradition. The relaxation response is elicited twice daily for 10 to 20 minutes each time. Benson and his co-workers recommend that the procedure works best on an empty stomach. The relaxation response is a most useful way of reducing the effects of stress on the body and mind.

The Natural Mind Approach. Some people who take drugs eventually look for other methods of maintaining the valuable parts of the drug experience. These people may learn to value the meditation "high" and abandon drugs. Long-term drug users sometimes credit their drug experiences with having given them a taste of their potential, even though continued use has diminished the novelty of drug use. Once these individuals become established in careers, they claim to have grown out of chemically induced altered states of consciousness. As Andrew Weil (1972) put it, "One does not see any long-time meditators give up meditation to become acid heads."

Although chemical "highs" are effective means of altering the state of consciousness, they interfere with the most worthwhile states of altered consciousness because they reinforce the illusion that highs come from external, material agents rather than from within your own nervous system.

Some people have difficulty using meditation as an alternative to drugs because, in order to be effective, meditation takes practice and concentration; the effects of drugs are immediate. Nevertheless, it is within everyone's potential to meditate.

Innovative Treatments

Hypnosis and acupuncture are two innovative methods of treating drug use and abuse. Although the two approaches are unconventional, they remain options of choice.

Hypnosis This procedure has been used to link drug-taking behavior to negative consequences such as nausea, anxiety, and so on. It has also been used to produce imagery of a previous "good trip," or happy drug experience. Advantages of such an approach are that they are free, under the subject's control, and not against the law. Subjects can be taught to hypnotize themselves, thus giving them further control when they feel the temptation to use drugs. Similarly to biofeedback, hypnosis can also be used to help achieve relaxation. At present the evidence for claiming that hypnosis is an effective treatment program for drug abuse remains mixed.

Acupuncture The medical use of needles has been practiced in China for 3,000 years or more and is still used there for various anesthetic purposes. Speculation about the effectiveness of acupuncture abounds

How does relaxation occur with this treatment method? Acupuncture causes the release of endorphins. Endorphins, located in the brain, are naturally occurring chemicals that mimic the painkilling effects of opiates such as heroin (Swan 1992). Experts claim that when endorphins are released, patients experience relaxation and this reduces the craving for drugs by blocking the brain mechanism responsible for addiction.

In 1972, acupuncture was used in Hong Kong on opium addicts having neurosurgery; they claimed they felt relief from withdrawal symptoms, although the acupuncture was intended only as an anesthetic. Later, a combination of acupuncture and electrical stimulation was used on heroin and opium addicts (O'Brien and Ng 1979). Fine acupuncture needles were placed subcutaneously in the outer ear and connected to an electrical stimulator for about 30 minutes. The investigators reported that symptoms of tearing, runny nose,

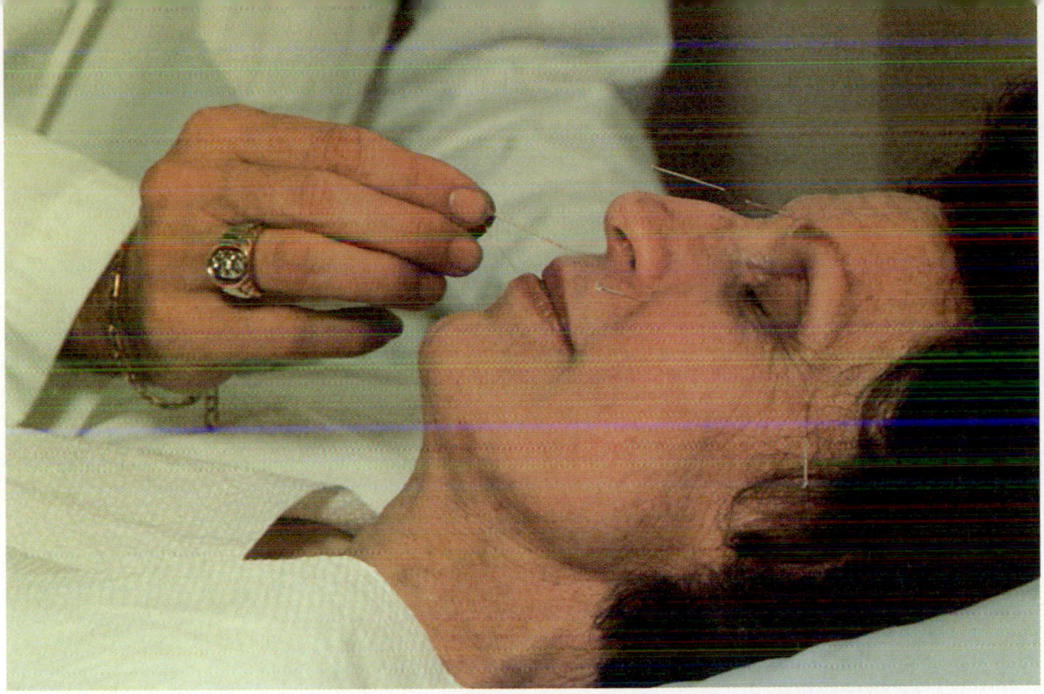

Acupuncture has been reported to temporarily relieve cravings for, and withdrawal symptoms from, narcotic drugs.

aching bones, cramps, and irritability usually disappeared after about 10 to 15 minutes. While under stimulation, the patients' craving for the narcotic drug ceased, and they began to feel more relaxed. Following this study, other researchers in the United States and abroad have given acupuncture treatments to addicts, with variation in the numbers of needles and types of needle stimulation (for example, manual, with heating, or with electricity). Encouraging results have been reported. Recently, studies at Lincoln Hospital in the Bronx, New York, have shown acupuncture to be effective. Michael Smith, director of Lincoln Hospital, says that there has been a "60 percent success rate at keeping hard-core addicts straight for a solid three months—high compared with other programs" (Findlay et al. 1991).

Evaluating Program Effectiveness

When federal funds became available to treat drug addiction in the late 1960s, four major treatment modalities evolved: methadone maintenance, therapeutic communities, outpatient drug-free programs, and short-term detoxification. These are the treatment modalities most frequently compared. Criteria for comparison include later use of narcotics and other drugs, arrest record or criminality, employment record, and follow-up treatment required.

Evaluating the success rate of a program depends on the criteria selected. "Graduates" of TCs, or those who complete the community's residential treatment program, are just a small proportion (10 to 15%) of all admissions. Five to ten years after "graduation," these former addicts have stable lifestyles, are employed, are not using opiates, and are not engaging in criminal activity. Less improvement is shown by the majority who drop out of TC programs before completion, and as might be expected, the extent of improvement is directly correlated to the length of residence in the TCs. The greatest proportion of dropouts leave during the first 30 days of residence; the rate declines rapidly thereafter. This is fairly typical of other drug abuse treatment programs as well (De Leon and Rosenthal 1979).

Methadone maintenance programs operate on an outpatient basis and are combined with a rehabilitation-oriented therapy program (USDHHS 1991). Drug-free programs, where patients are not allowed to use any drugs, are outpatient, intended primarily for nonopiate users (Akers 1992). They range from highly demanding, socialization-oriented programs, like daytime TCs, to relaxed programs that offer "rap" sessions and support on request. There is an even higher dropout rate from drug-free programs than from TCs.

As described earlier, detoxification programs are usually short term, not over 21 days, and may be inpatient or outpatient, depending on the drug and degree of dependence. Largely known as the "medical management of withdrawal," these programs are not *in themselves* treatment for alcoholism (Levin 1990); their primary goal is to eliminate physiological dependence.

Considering the variability in treatment approaches and the selection of patients, we can say that methadone maintenance, therapeutic communities, and drug-free programs have approximately the same success rates, whereas opiate antagonist and detoxification-only programs have appreciably lower success rates (Sells 1979; Akers 1992). Finally, research shows that detoxification works best for early alcohol addiction and does not have much promise for advanced alcoholics (Levin 1990).

Review Questions

1. Why use education, prevention, and treatment methods for recreational drug users?
2. Are the root causes of drug addiction more psychological than physical? Evaluate the role of mental versus the physical causes of drug abuse.
3. Since the use of drugs is nearly as old as humankind itself, should we attempt to wipe out all drug use? Why? Why not?
4. Should the use of licit gateway drugs such as tobacco and alcohol be banned and considered a criminal offense? Why or why not?
5. What aspects of the harm reduction model can be carried out in the United States? How could the "just say no" programs be modified to include aspects of the harm reduction model?
6. Which education, prevention, and treatment programs, models, or modalities can be effective against early addiction?
7. Do you think the alternatives-to-drugs approach would be effective in your community? Why or why not?
8. Only a limited amount of government funds is available for drug treatment. The government has decided to fund only two distinct types of major treatment approaches. It has a choice of five approaches, including medical, psychological and psychotherapeutic, social, behavioral, and innovative. If you were the president's appointee (our nation's drug "czar") for the nation's drug control efforts,
   a. Which two drug treatment approaches would you implement on a national basis?
   b. Why would you select these two approaches?
   c. Why would you not select the other three approaches?
9. Do you think hypnosis is effective in treating drug use and/or abuse? Why or why not?
10. Speculate on how social influence can be used to stop or curtail drug use in peer groups.
11. Outline the steps you would use in creating a drug education program for chronic drug users. Can responsible use be advocated for this group? How feasible is it to stress total abstinence for such users and abusers?
12. Scare tactics regarding drug use have lately proven to be of little value. Can you envision any redeeming value in using such tactics on certain select groups or types of drug users or potential drug users? With which groups or types of drug users would you attempt such tactics?
13. List additional topics for a junior high school drug education program in addition to the topics listed on page 475 that have been omitted but you think are important additional topics.

Key Terms

initial use
habitual use
addiction
relapse
tolerance
moral model
medical model
social influence
alternatives approach
noneuphoric opiate
alcohologists
open meetings
closed meetings
therapeutic communities (TCs)
reinforcement
ergotropic
catatonic
mystical rapture
trophotropic
meditation

Summary

1. Four phases of addiction are initial use, habitual use, addiction, and relapse. *Initial* use involves occasional use or experimentation. *Habitual* use involves regular involvement with drugs. *Addiction* represents the higher end of habitual use. *Tolerance* is defined as a physical or biological attachment to drugs leading to the point of either physical or psychological withdrawal symptoms if the drug is stopped. *Relapse* is when the user returns to regular use after having experienced some form of withdrawal symptoms.
2. Addiction can be seen as *psychic dependence* or *physical dependence*, and drug use or abuse can be seen as a *"career."*
3. Two models of drug addiction are the *moral model* and the *medical model*. The moral model assumes that drinking is a matter of choice and that alcohol abusers have lost control. The medical model views alcohol abuse as resulting from biological conditions and the loss of rational control.
4. Some evidence indicates that the five most addictive drugs are nicotine, ice, glass (methamphetamine smoked), crack, crystal meth (methamphetamine injected), and valium (diazepam).
5. The following models can be used in drug education programs: (a) cognitive, (b) information, (c) peer tutoring, (d) teaching and counseling, and (e) social influence and resistance models. In summary, the cognitive and information models rely on straightforward information about the dangers of drug use. The peer tutoring, teaching, and counseling models employ peers or older youth to disseminate information on drug abuse. The social influence and resistance model focuses on teaching how to resist peer pressure to use drugs for recreational purposes.
6. The three types of prevention are *primary*, *secondary*, and *tertiary prevention*. Primary prevention attempts to persuade against the abuse of drugs. Secondary prevention entails using immediate intervention once drug abuse has begun. Tertiary prevention helps people stop abusing drugs either immediately before addiction or in its early stages.
7. The three prevention programs targeted to children and adolescents are cognitive and information-based drug education; affective education and peer resistance programs.
8. As the name implies, the alternatives-to-drugs approach attempts to involve youths in appealing activities. Drug-free video game centers, drug-free dances and rock concerts, and social service projects are examples of alternative recreation activities.
9. Drug treatment differs from prevention. Drug prevention involves preventing or reducing the extent of drug use. Drug treatment involves stopping drug use once it has begun.
10. The types of treatment settings are used for alleviating or eliminating addiction. *In-hospital* programs ensure intense treatment against drug abuse within an acute care hospital program. *Residential care programs* focus on 24-hour-per-day education and therapy, which

leads to rehabilitation. *Day hospitals* and *intensive outpatient service* provide care from three to four hours per day for patients who need additional structure while living independently.

11. The varieties of conscious states consist of *normal* (waking consciousness), *ergotropic* (arousal), and *trophotropic* (decreased arousal).
12. The six primary approaches to drug treatment are (a) medical, (b) psychological and psychotherapeutic, (c) social, (d) behavioral, and (e) innovative approaches. Medical treatments include detoxification and abstinence programs, maintenance programs, morphine, methadone and heroin maintenance, and opiate antagonists. Psychological and psychotherapeutic approaches focus on faulty or inadequate personality characteristics.
13. Two innovative treatment methods are hypnosis and acupuncture. Hypnosis is used to achieve relaxation, as in biofeedback. Acupuncture is accomplished by inserting electrically charged fine needles in certain nerve centers of the body, to redirect the body's natural electrical impulses.

References

Akers, R. L. *Drugs, Alcohol, and Society: Social Structure, Process, and Policy.* Belmont, CA: Wadsworth, 1992.

Alcoholics Anonymous World Services. *Alcoholics Anonymous: The Story of How Many Thousands of Men and Women Have Recovered from Alcoholism,* 3d ed. New York: Alcoholics Anonymous, 1976.

Archer, S. "Historical Perspective on the Chemistry and Development of Naltrexone." In *Narcotic Antagonists: Naltrexone Pharmaco-Chemistry and Sustained-Release Preparations,* edited by R. E. Willette and G. Barnett. NIDA Research Monograph 28. Washington, DC: National Institute on Drug Abuse, 1981.

Bailey, W. J. "Measuring the Impact of Drug Prevention Programs." *Prevention Newsline* 4, no. 4 (Summer 1991): 3–5.

Bangert-Downs, R. L. "The Effects of School-Based Substance Abuse Education—A Meta-Analysis." *Journal of Drug Education* 18, no. 3 (1988): 243–66.

Bassin, A. "Daytop Village." In *Readings in Social Psychology Today,* J. McConnell, contributing editor. Del Mar, CA: CRM Books, 1970, pp. 117–23.

Baumann, J., and A. Waterston. "Advertising Against Drugs: Themes from a Televised Anti-Drug Campaign." In *Drug Use in America: Social, Cultural, and Political Perspectives,* edited by P. J. Venturelli, 153–73. Boston: Jones and Bartlett, 1994.

Benson, H. "Systemic Hypertension and the Relaxation Response. *New England Journal of Medicine* 296, 1977: 1152–56.

Botvin, G. T. "Substance Abuse Prevention: Theory, Practice, and Effectiveness." In *Drugs and Crime,* edited by M. Tomy and J. Q. Wilson. Chicago: University of Chicago Press, 1990.

Carroll, E. "Notes on the Epidemiology of Inhalants." In *Review of Inhalants,* edited by C. W. Sharp and M. L. Brehm. NIDA Research Monograph no 15. Washington, DC: National Institute on Drug Abuse, 1977.

Clayton, R. R., A. Cattarello, L. E. Cay, and K. P. Walden. "Persuasive Communication and Drug Prevention: An Evaluation of the D.A.R.E. Program." In *Persuasive Communication and Drug Abuse Prevention,* edited by L. Donohew, H. Sypher, and W. Bukoski. Hillsdale, NJ: Erlbaum, 1991.

Clinard, M. B., and R. F. Meier. *Sociology of Deviant Behavior,* 8th ed. Fort Worth, TX: Harcourt, Brace, Jovanovich, 1992.

Cohen, A. Y. "The Journey Beyond Trips: Alternatives to Drugs." *Journal of Psychedelic Drugs* 3, no. 2 (Spring 1971): 7–14.

Cohen, A. Y. *Alternatives to Drug Abuse: Steps Toward Prevention.* NIDA Research Monograph no 14. Washington, DC: National Institute on Drug Abuse, 1973.

De Leon, G., and M. S. Rosenthal. "Therapeutic Communities." In *Handbook on Drug Abuse,* edited by R. L. DuPont, A. Goldstein, and J. O'Donnell. Washington, DC: National Institute on Drug Abuse, 1979.

DeLong, J. V. "Treatment and Rehabilitation." In *Dealing with Drug Abuse: A Report to the Ford Foundation,* 173–254. New York: Praeger, 1972.

Dowieko, H. E. *Concepts of Chemical Dependency.* Pacific Grove, CA: Brooks/Cole, 1990.

Eddy, N. B., H. Halbach, H. Isbell, and M. H. Seevers. "Drug Dependence: Its Significance and Characteristics." *Bulletin of the World Health Organization* 32 (May 1965): 721–33.

Eigen, L. D., and D. W. Rowden. *Prevention Works!* U.S. Department of Health and Human Services (USDHHS) and Substance Abuse and Mental Health Services Administration (SAMHSA). DHHS Publication no. (SMA) 93-246. Rockville, MD: National Clearinghouse for Alcohol and Drug Information, September 1993.

Findlay, S., D. Podolsky, and J. Silberner. "Wonder Cures from the Fringe." *U.S. News and World Report,* 111, no. 3, 23 September 1991, pp. 71–73.

Fischer, R. "A Cartography of the Ecstatic and Meditative States." *Science* 174 (1971): 897–904.

Forman, S. G., and J. A. Linney. "School-Based Prevention of Adolescent Substance Abuse: Programs, Implementation and Future Direction." *School Psychology Review* 17, no. 4 (1988): 550–58.

Ginzburg, H. M. *Naltrexone: Its Chemical Utility.* Rockville, MD: National Institute on Drug Abuse, 1986.

Gold, M. S., A. C. Pottash, D. R. Sweeney, and H. D. Kleber. "Opiate Withdrawal Using Clonidine." *JAMA* 243 (1980): 343–46.

Hopkins, Harold C. "Getting a Handle on Methadone." *FDA Consumer,* September 1973.

Huxley, A. *The Doors of Perception*. New York: Harper & Brothers, 1954.

Inciardi, J. A., R. Horowitz, and A. E. Pottieger. *Street Kids, Street Drugs, Street Crime*. Wadsworth, 1993.

Johnson, G. L. "Addiction and Withdrawal." *HAPS NEWS* (January 1992): 12.

Kennedy, B., M. Konstantareas, and S. Homatidis. "A Behavior Profile of Polydrug Abusers." *Journal of Youth and Adolescence* (1987): 115–27.

Klein, J. M., and S. I. Miller. "Three Approaches to the Treatment of Drug Addiction." *Hospital and Community Psychiatry* 37 (1986): 1083–85.

Levin, Jerome D. *Alcoholism: A Bio-Psycho-Social Approach*. New York: Hemisphere, 1990.

McGuire, W. J. "The Nature of Attitude and Attitude Change." In *Handbook of Social Psychology,* 2d ed., Vol. 3, edited by G. Lindzey and E. Aronson. Reading, MA: Addison-Wesley, pp. 136–314. 1969.

McGuire, W. J. "Attitudes and Attitude Change." In *The Handbook of Social Psychology,* 3d ed., Vol. II, edited by Gardner Lindzey and Elliot Aronson. New York: Random House, 1985, 233–346.

McNeece, C. A., and D. M. DiNitto. *Chemical Dependency: A Systems Approach*. Englewood Cliffs, NJ: Prentice Hall, 1994.

Nusbaumer, M. R. "Government Control of Deviant Drinking: The Manipulation of Morals and Medicine." In *Drugs in America: Social, Cultural, and Political Perspectives,* 13–22, edited by P. J. Venturelli. Jones and Bartlett, 1994.

O'Brien, C. P., and L. K. Y. Ng. "Innovative Treatments for Drug Addiction." In *Handbook on Drug Abuse,* edited by A. Goldstein, R. L. Dupont, and J. O'Donnell, 193–201. Washington, DC: National Institute on Drug Abuse, 1979.

Office of Applied Studies, Substance Abuse and Mental Health Services Administration (SAMHSA). *Preliminary Estimates from the 1992 National Household Survey on Drug Abuse: Selected Excerpts.* Washington, DC: Public Health Service, U.S. Department of Health and Human Services, June 1993.

Office of Justice Programs, Bureau of Justice Assistance. U.S. Department of Justice. *An Introduction to D.A.R.E.: Drug Abuse Resistance and Education,* 2d ed. Washington, DC: U.S. Government Printing Office, October 1991.

Palfai, Tibor, and Henry Jankiewicz. *Drugs and Human Behavior.* Dubuque, IA: Brown, 1991.

Pagano, R. R., R. M. Rose, R. M. Stivers, and S. Warrenburg. "Sleep During Transcendental Meditation." *Science* 191 (1976): 308–10.

Pickens, R. W., and T. Thompson. "Behavioral Treatment of Drug Dependence." In *Behavioral Intervention Techniques in Drug Dependence Treatment,* edited by Maxine L. Stitzer, J. Grabowski, Jack E. Henningfield, 53–67. Rockville, MD: National Institute on Drug Abuse, 1984.

Ray. W. J., J. M. Raczynski, R. Rogers, and W. H. Kimball. *Evaluation of Clinical Biofeedback*. New York: Plenum Press, 1979.

Renault, P. F. "Historical Perspective on the Chemistry and Development of Naltrexone." In *Narcotic Antagonists: Naltrexone Pharmaco-Chemistry and Sustained-Release Preparations,* edited by R. E. Willette and G. Barnett. NIDA Research Monograph 28. Washington, DC: National Institute on Drug Abuse, 1981.

Rudy, D. "Perspectives on Alcoholism: Lessons from Alcoholics and Alcohologists." In *Drug Use in America: Social, Cultural, and Political Perspectives,* edited by P. J. Venturelli, 23–29. Boston: Jones and Bartlett, 1994.

Schups, E., R. D. Bartolo, J. Moskowitz, C. S. Polley, and S. Cherigen. "A Review of 127 Drug Abuse Prevention Evaluations." *Journal of Drug Issues* 11 (1981): 17–43.

Sells, S. B. "Treatment Effectiveness." In *Handbook on Drug Abuse,* edited by A. Goldstein, R. L. DuPont, and J. O'Donnell, 105–118. Washington, DC: National Institute on Drug Abuse, U.S. Department of Health, Education, and Welfare, 1979.

Senate Task Force for a Drug Free America. "The War on Drugs Is Necessary." In *War on Drugs: Opposing Viewpoints,* edited by N. Bernards. San Diego, CA: Greenhaven Press, 1990.

Swan, N. "Experts Divided on Effectiveness of Acupuncture as a Drug Abuse Treatment." *NIDA Notes* 7, no. 5 (September–October 1992).

Swisher, J. D. "Prevention Issues." In *Handbook on Drug Abuse,* edited by R. L. DuPont, A. Goldstein, and J. O'Donnell. Washington, DC: National Institute on Drug Abuse, 1979.

Treaster, J. B. "Call it 'Harm Reduction' It's Not Legalization, but a User-Friendly Drug Strategy." *New York Times* 19 December 1993, p. E5.

Trebach, A. S. *The Heroin Solution.* New Haven, CT: Yale University Press, 1982.

U.S. Department of Education. *Learning to Live Drug Free: A Curriculum Model for Prevention.* Rockville, MD: National Clearinghouse for Alcohol and Drug Information, 1992.

U.S. Department of Health and Human Services (USDHHS). *The Future by Design: A Community Framework for Preventing Alcohol and Other Drug Problems Through a Systems Approach.* Department of Health and Human Services, Publication no. (ADM) 91-1760. Washington, DC: U.S. Government Printing Office, 1991.

U.S. Department of Justice. *Drugs and Crime Facts,* 1992. Washington, DC: Bureau of Justice Statistics, 1992.

Venturelli, P. J. *Drug Use in America: Social, Cultural, and Political Perspectives.* Boston: Jones and Bartlett, 1994.

Venturelli, P. J., editor. "Part IV–Drug Abuse Prevention." In *Drug Use in America: Social, Cultural, and Political Perspectives,* 143–47. Boston: Jones and Bartlett, 1994.

Waldorf, D. "Natural Recovery from Opiate Addiction: Some Social-Psychological Processes of Untreated Recovery." *Journal of Drug Issues* 13 (1983): 237–80.

Wallack, L., and K. Corbett. "Illicit Drug, Tobacco, and Alcohol Use Among Youth: Trends and Promising Approaches in Prevention." In *Youth and Drugs: Society's Mixed Messages,* edited by H. Resnik, S. E. Gardner, K. P. Lorian, and C. E. Marcas. OSAP Prevention Monograph no. 6, Office for Substance Abuse Prevention, Alcohol, Drug Abuse and Mental Health Administration. Rockville, MD: Public Health Service, U.S. Department of Health and Human Services, 1990.

Weil, A. *The Natural Mind.* Boston, MA: Houghton Mifflin, 1972.

White, J. M. *Drug Dependence.* Englewood Cliffs, NJ: Prentice Hall, 1991.

Wilson, M., and S. Wilson, eds. *Drugs in American Life,* Vol. 1. New York: Wilson, 1975.

World Health Organization. "Expert Committee on Addiction-Producing Drugs." *World Health Organization Technical Report* 273 (1964): 9–10.

GLOSSARY

abstinent cultures cultures in which alcohol is morally and socially prohibited
acute immediate or short-term effects after taking a single drug dose
addiction third phase in the addiction process, consisting of periodic or chronic dependence on a drug or several drugs; an insatiable desire to use drugs contrary to legal and/or social prohibitions
"addiction to pleasure" theory theory that assumes that it is biologically normal to continue a pleasure stimulus when once begun
adulterated contaminating substances are mixed in to dilute the drugs
agonistic a type of substance that activates a receptor
alcoholic a person who is addicted to alcohol
alcoholic cardiomyopathy congestive heart failure due to the replacement of heart muscle with fat and fiber
alcoholic hepatitis the second stage of alcohol-induced liver disease in which chronic inflammation occurs; reversible if alcoholic consumption ceases
alcohologists people who research alcohol addiction
altered perceptions changes in the interpretation of stimuli, resulting from marijuana use
alternatives approach one approach emphasizing the exploration of positive alternatives to drug abuse, based on replacing the pleasurable feelings gained from drug abuse with involvement in social and educational activities
ambivalent cultures cultures in which alcohol is prohibited *as well as* accepted in certain sectors
amnesiac causing the loss of memory
amotivational syndrome a lack of motivation and reduced productivity caused by regular marijuana use
anabolic substances that stimulate the conversion of nutrients into tissue
anabolic steroids compounds chemically like the steroids that stimulate production of tissue mass
analgesics drugs that relieve pain without affecting consciousness
analogs drugs with similar structures
anandamide a possible neurotransmitter acting at the marijuana (cannabinoid) receptor
androgens naturally occurring male hormones, such as testosterone
anesthesia a state characterized by loss of sensation or consciousness
anesthetic a drug that blocks sensitivity to pain
angina pectoris severe chest pain usually caused by a deficiency of blood to the heart muscle
anorexiants drugs that suppress the activity of the brain's appetite center, causing reduced food intake
antagonistic a type of substance that blocks a receptor
anticholinergic agents that antagonize the effects of acetylcholine
anti-inflammatory relieve symptoms of inflammation
antipyretics drugs that reduce fevers
antitussives drugs that block the coughing reflex
anxiolytics drugs that relieve anxiety
aphrodisiac a substance that stimulates or intensifies sexual desire
axon an extension of the neuronal cell body along which electrochemical signals travel

bactericidal kills bacteria
bacteriostatic stops replication and growth of bacteria
behavioral stereotypy meaningless repetition of a single activity
behavioral tolerance compensation of motor impairments by chronic alcohol users through behavioral pattern modification
biotransformation the process of changing the chemical properties of a drug, usually by metabolism
blood-brain barrier selective filtering between the cerebral blood vessels and the brain
broad spectrum effective against many species of bacteria
bronchodilators drugs that widen air passages

caffeinism symptoms caused by taking high chronic doses of caffeine
Cannabis sativa the hemp plant marijuana
carcinogenic able to cause cancer
catatonia a condition of physical rigidity, excitement, and stupor
catatonic pertaining to a state of arousal characterized by trancelike consciousness; sensory input is literally jammed, and the body is rigidly fixed
catecholamines a class of biochemical compounds, including the transmitters norepinephrine, epinephrine, and dopamine
chronic long-term effects, usually after taking multiple drug doses
cirrhosis scarring of the liver and destruction of fibrous tissues; results from alcohol abuse. Once cirrhosis begins, it is irreversible.
closed meetings meetings to which only alcoholics having a serious desire to completely stop drinking are invited
CNS (central nervous system) one of the major divisions of the nervous system, composed of the brain and the spinal cord
cocaine babies children exposed to cocaine while in the womb
codependency a relationship pattern in which nonaddicted family members identify with the alcohol addict; coalcoholism
compulsive users often addicted users
congeners nonalcoholic substances found in alcoholic beverages
congestive heart failure heart is unable to pump sufficient blood for the body's needs
control theories belief that if left to their own nature, individuals have a tendency to deviate from expected cultural values, norms, and attitudes

"crack" already processed and inexpensive "freebased" cocaine, ready for smoking
cumulative effect the buildup of a drug in the body after multiple doses taken at short intervals
cycling use of different types of steroids singly, but in sequence

DEA the Drug Enforcement Administration, the principal federal agency responsible for enforcing drug abuse regulations
delirium tremens (DTs) a condition that affects chronic abusers of alcohol during alcohol withdrawal; characterized by agitation, hallucinations, and involuntary body tremors
dendrites short branches of neurons that receive transmitter signals
dependence the physiological and psychological changes or adaptations that occur in response to the frequent administration of a drug
"designer" drugs illicit drugs that are chemically modified so they are not considered illegal but that retain abusive properties
detoxification elimination of a toxic substance, such as a drug, and its effects
diabetes mellitus disease caused by elevated blood sugar due to insufficient insulin
diabetes, type I associated with complete loss of insulin-producing cells in pancreas
diabetes, type II usually associated with obesity; there is not a loss of insulin-producing cells
"die-hards" slang term for drug users who strongly resist quitting
differential reinforcement the ratio between reinforcers favorable and disfavorable for sustaining drug use behavior
disinhibition the loss of conditioned reflexes due to depression of inhibitory centers of the brain
distillation heating fermented mixtures of cereal grains or fruits in a still to evaporate and be trapped as purified alcohol
distribution the movement of a drug in the bloodstream throughout the body
diuretic a drug or substance that increases the production of urine
dopamine the brain transmitter believed to mediate the rewarding aspects of most drugs of abuse
Drug Use Review a process conducted by pharmacists to improve the outcome of prescription drug therapy
drug any substance that modifies the nervous system and states of consciousness
drunken comportment cultural values and norms that cause an independent outcome of drinking behavior
dysphoric characterized by unpleasant mental effects; the opposite of euphoric

edema swollen tissue
elimination the final stage, in which the body exercises control over a drug by means of excretion (getting rid of the drug)
emphysema a common type of lung disease
enabling denial or making up of excuses for the excessive drinking of an alcohol addict to whom someone is close
endorphins neurotransmitters that have narcoticlike effects
enzyme induction an increase in the metabolic capacity of an enzyme system
epilepsy disease consisting of spontaneous repetitive seizures
equal-opportunity affliction drug use, in that it cuts across all members of society regardless of income, social class, and age category
ergogenic drugs drugs that enhance performance
ergotism poisoning by toxic substances from the ergot fungus *Claviceps purpurea*
ergotropic pertaining to the arousal state of consciousness
ethanol the consumable type of alcohol that is the psychoactive ingredient in alcoholic beverages; often called *grain alcohol*
ethylene glycol alcohol used as antifreeze
expectorants substances that stimulate mucus secretion and diminish mucus viscosity
experimenter a novel drug user

fermentation the biochemical process in which yeast converts sugar into alcohol
fetal alcohol syndrome (FAS) a condition affecting children born to alcohol-consuming mothers that is characterized by facial deformities, growth deficiency, and mental retardation
"flashback" the recurrence of an earlier drug-induced sensory experience in the absence of the drug
floaters drug users who vacillate from the need to seek pleasure to the need to relieve serious psychological problems
freebasing conversion of cocaine into its alkaline form for smoking

gastritis inflammation or irritation of the gut
gateway drugs drugs that often lead to the use of more serious drugs. Alcohol, tobacco, and marijuana are the most commonly used gateway drugs.
generic the official, nonpatented, nonproprietary name of a drug
genetic and biophysiological theories explanations of addiction in terms of genetic brain dysfunction and biochemical patterns
genitourinary having to do with the reproductive and urinary systems
glaucoma an eye disease manifested by increased intraocular pressure

habitual use second phase in the addiction process, in which a more patterned regular involvement with a particular drug(s) occurs
habituation repeating certain patterns of behavior until they become established or habitual
half-life the time required for the body to eliminate and/or metabolize half of a drug dose
hallucinogens substances that alter sensory processing in the brain, causing perceptual disturbances, changes in thought processing, and depersonalization
hepatotoxic effect when liver cells increase the production of fat, resulting in an enlarged liver
holistic health health perspective advocating knowledge about drug use to increase self-awareness and help others
homeostasis maintenance of internal stability; often biochemical in nature
hormones regulatory chemicals released by endocrine systems
human growth factor (HGF) a hormone that stimulates normal growth
hyperglycemia elevated blood sugar

hyperkinesis excessive movement
hyperpyrexia elevated body temperature
hypertension elevated blood pressure
hypnotics CNS depressants used to induce drowsiness and encourage sleep
hypothyroidism thyroid gland doesn't produce sufficient hormone
hypoxia a state of oxygen deficiency

"ice" a smokable form of methamphetamine
illicit drugs illegal drugs, such as marijuana, cocaine, and LSD.
initial use first phase in the addiction process, in which occasional use or experimentation with drugs without prior use occurs
interdiction the policy of cutting off or destroying supplies of illicit drugs
intergang happening between members of different gangs
intragang happening between members of the same gang
ischemia tissue deprived of sufficient blood and oxygen
isopropyl alcohol rubbing alcohol, sometimes used as an anesthetic
keratin layer the outermost protective layer of the skin
keratolytics caustic agents that cause the keratin skin layer to peel

labeling theory a theory stressing that other peoples' impressions have a direct influence over one's self-image
licit drugs legal drugs, such as coffee, alcohol, and tobacco

macroscopic explanations comprehensive, overall structural or general explanations for why people use drugs
"mainlining" intravenous injection of a drug of abuse
margin of safety the range in dose between the amount of drug necessary to cause a therapeutic effect and a toxic effect
Marinol FDA-approved THC in capsule form (dronabinol)
master status the overriding status position in the eyes of others that clearly identifies an individual; for example, doctor, lawyer, alcoholic, HIV positive
MDMA a type of illicit drug known as "Ecstasy" or "Adam" having stimulant and hallucinogenic properties
medical model the view that alcohol abuse is a disease that is innate and biologically determined in specific individuals
meditation a state of consciousness in which there is a constant level of awareness focusing on one object; for example, Yoga and Zen Buddhism
mental set the collection of psychological and environmental factors that influence an individual's response to drugs
metabolism chemical alteration of drugs by body processes
metabolites chemical products of metabolism
methyl alcohol wood alcohol or methanol
microscopic explanations closeup, detailed, mostly day-to-day explanations for why people use drugs
monoamine (MAO) inhibitors group of drugs used to treat severe depression
moral model the belief that people abuse alcohol because they choose to do so
the "munchies" hunger experienced while under the effects of marijuana
muscarinic a receptor type activated by ACh; usually inhibitory
mutagenic able to cause mutation (alter genes)
mydriasis pupil dilation
mystical rapture an ultimate state of consciousness similar to hallucination

narcolepsy a condition causing spontaneous and uncontrolled sleeping episodes
narrow spectrum effective against only a few species of bacteria
neurotransmitters chemical messengers released by neurons (nerve cells) for communication with other cells
Nicotiana tabacum the primary tobacco plant species cultivated in North America
nicotinic a receptor type activated by ACh; usually excitatory
NIDA the National Institute on Drug Abuse, the principal federal agency responsible for directing drug abuse–related research
noneuphoric opiate a drug or drugs used in maintenance programs that satisfies the craving but does not produce the euphoric effect, such as methadone
nonsteroidal anti-inflammatory drugs (NSAIDs) anti-inflammatory drugs that do not have steroid properties

open meetings meetings to which anyone having an interest in attending and witnessing is invited
opioid relating to the drugs that are derived from opium
oral hypoglycemics drugs taken by mouth to treat type II diabetes
overpermissive cultures cultures in which excessive use of alcohol is permitted

paradoxical an unexpected effect
patent medicines unregulated proprietary medicines often associated with fraudulent therapy
patterns of behavior consistent and related behaviors that occur together, such as marijuana use and euphoria, alcohol abuse and intoxication
peptic ulcers open sores that occur in the stomach or upper segment of the small intestine
permissive cultures cultures in which alcohol consumption is accepted
pharmacokinetics the study of factors that influence the distribution and concentration of drugs in the body
phocomelia a birth defect; impaired development of the arms or legs or both
placebo effects effects caused by suggestion and psychological factors, not the pharmacological activity of a drug
plateau effect the maximum drug effect, regardless of dose
plateauing developing tolerance to the effects of anabolic steroids
polydrug use using other types of drugs with alcohol
positive wellness an approach advocating the maintenance of health and wellness as a way of life
potency the amount of drug necessary to cause an effect
primary deviance inconsequential deviant behavior in which the perpetrator does not identify with the deviance
primary prevention prevention of any drug use

proprietary a brand or trademark name that is registered with the U.S. Patent Office
psychedelic substances that expand or heighten perception and consciousness
psychoactive drugs that affect mood or alter the state of consciousness
psychoactive drugs or psychoactive substances substances that affect the central nervous system and alter consciousness or perceptions
psychoactive effects how drug substances alter and affect the brain's mental functions
psychological dependence dependence that results because a drug produces pleasant mental effects
psychotogenic substances that initiate psychotic behavior
psychotomimetic substances that cause psychosis-like symptoms

rebound effect a form of withdrawal; paradoxical effects that occur when a drug has been eliminated from the body
receptor a special region in a membrane that is activated by natural substances or drugs to alter cell function
reinforcement any behavior that strengthens the likelihood that a behavior will be repeated
reinforcement theory a theory that asserts that alcohol use results from positive "stroking," which leads to satisfying feelings
relapse fourth phase in the addiction process, in which the user who stopped habitual use returns to regular use after having experienced some form of withdrawal symptoms
REM sleep the restive phase of sleep associated with dreaming
retrospective interpretation the social psychological process of redefining a person's reputation in a particular group
reverse tolerance an enhanced response to a given drug dose; opposite of tolerance
Reye's syndrome a potentially fatal complication of colds, flu, or chicken pox in children
"run" intense use of a stimulant, consisting of multiple administrations over a period of days

salicylates aspirin-like drugs
secondary deviance advanced type of deviant behavior that develops when the perpetrator identifies with the deviant behavior
secondary prevention prevention of casual drug use from progressing to dependence
secondhand smoke the smoke from burning tobacco that pollutes the air and is breathed by smokers and nonsmokers alike
sedatives CNS depressants used to relieve anxiety, fear, and apprehension
set an individual's expectation of what a drug will do to his or her personality
setting the physical and social environment where alcohol is consumed
"sidestream" smoke smoke released into the air directly from the lighted tip of a cigarette
sinsemilla one of the most potent types of marijuana available; means "without seeds"
smokeless tobacco two types exist: chewing and snuff tobacco. This type of tobacco consists of tobacco leaves that are shredded and twisted into strands.
snuff dipping placing a pinch of tobacco between the gums and the cheek
social influence the ability to inspire, motivate, or convince others to go along with or share in novel behavior
social learning theory a theory that asserts that the use of alcohol results from early socialization experiences
social lubricant the belief that drinking (misconceived as safe) that represses inhibitions and strengthens extraversion leads to increased sociability
social substance alcohol when it is not perceived as a drug
socialization the learning process responsible for becoming human
speakeasies places where alcoholic beverages were sold during the Prohibition Era
speed an injectable methamphetamine used by drug addicts
"speedball" a combination of amphetamine or cocaine with an opioid narcotic, often heroin
SPF (sun protection factor) number a designation to indicate ability to screen UV rays
ß-adrenergic stimulants drugs that stimulate a subtype of adrenaline and noradrenaline receptors
stacking use of several types of steroids together
steroids potent hormones released from the adrenal glands
structural analogs drugs that result from altered chemical structures of already illicit drugs. These drugs are produced for profit and mimic current effects of controlled substances.
structural influence theories theories that view the organization of a society, group, or subculture as responsible for drug use and abuse by its members
subculture theories explain drug use as caused by peer pressure
sudden infant death syndrome (SIDS) unexpected and unexplainable death that occurs while infants are sleeping
switching policy an FDA policy allowing the change of suitable prescription drugs to OTC status
sympathomimetic agents that mimic the effects of norepinephrine or epinephrine
synaptic cleft a minute gap between the neuron and target cell, across which neurotransmitters travel
synapse site of communication between a message-sending neuron and its message-receiving target cell
synergism the ability of one drug to enhance the effect of another; potentiation
synesthesia a subjective sensation or image of a sense other than the one being stimulated, such as an auditory sensation caused by a visual stimulus

teratogenic able to cause abnormal development of the fetus
thalidomide a sedative drug that, when used during pregnancy, can cause severe developmental damage to the fetus
therapeutic communities (TCs) programs that advocate a complete change in lifestyle, such as complete abstinence from drugs, elimination of deviant behavior, and development of employable skills

therapeutic index the toxic dose divided by the therapeutic dose; used to calculate margin of safety

threshold the minimum drug dose necessary to cause an effect

tobacco chewing the absorption of nicotine through the mucous lining of the mouth

tolerance a physical or biological attachment to a drug leading to a physical dependence

toxicity the capacity of a drug to do damage or cause adverse effects in the body

tricyclic antidepressants most commonly used group of drugs to treat severe depression

trophotropic pertaining to a state of consciousness in which there is decreased sensitivity to external stimuli and sedation

"uppers" a slang term for CNS stimulants

volatile readily evaporated at low temperatures

withdrawal unpleasant effects that occur when use of a drug is stopped

I N D E X